Sustainable Development Goals Series

The **Sustainable Development Goals Series** is Springer Nature's inaugural cross-imprint book series that addresses and supports the United Nations' seventeen Sustainable Development Goals. The series fosters comprehensive research focused on these global targets and endeavours to address some of society's greatest grand challenges. The SDGs are inherently multidisciplinary, and they bring people working across different fields together and working towards a common goal. In this spirit, the Sustainable Development Goals series is the first at Springer Nature to publish books under both the Springer and Palgrave Macmillan imprints, bringing the strengths of our imprints together.

The Sustainable Development Goals Series is organized into eighteen subseries: one subseries based around each of the seventeen respective Sustainable Development Goals, and an eighteenth subseries, "Connecting the Goals", which serves as a home for volumes addressing multiple goals or studying the SDGs as a whole. Each subseries is guided by an expert Subseries Advisor with years or decades of experience studying and addressing core components of their respective Goal.

The SDG Series has a remit as broad as the SDGs themselves, and contributions are welcome from scientists, academics, policymakers, and researchers working in fields related to any of the seventeen goals. If you are interested in contributing a monograph or curated volume to the series, please contact the Publishers: Zachary Romano [Springer; zachary.romano@springer.com] and Rachael Ballard [Palgrave Macmillan; rachael.ballard@palgrave.com].

Andrea Fiorillo • Serafino De Giorgi
Editors

Social Determinants of Mental Health

SIPS Società Italiana di Psichiatria Sociale
Affiliated to the World Association of Social Psychiatry

Springer

Editors
Andrea Fiorillo
Department of Psychiatry
University of Campania "Luigi Vanvitelli"
Napoli, Italy

Serafino De Giorgi
Mental Health Department
ASL Lecce
Lecce, Italy

ISSN 2523-3084 ISSN 2523-3092 (electronic)
Sustainable Development Goals Series
ISBN 978-3-031-70164-1 ISBN 978-3-031-70165-8 (eBook)
https://doi.org/10.1007/978-3-031-70165-8

This Springer imprint is published by the registered company Springer Nature Switzerland AG
The registered company address is: Gewerbestrasse 11, 6330 Cham, Switzerland

Preface

According to the World Health Organization (WHO), mental health is defined as a state of mental well-being, enabling people to cope with life stressors, to achieve their personal goals and to actively contribute to their community [1]. Mental health is a complex construct, which cannot just be explained as lack of mental disorders, lying on a continuum between physiological and pathological states.

Mental health conditions include different types of psychiatric disorders and behavioural disturbances, which are associated with significant levels of distress and impairment in social and personal functioning.

Thus, mental disorders have a complex etiopathogenesis, due to a complex interaction between the brain, human social relationships, and individual and social psychological domains. Although the etiopathogenesis of mental disorders is still not fully elucidated, paradigms that conceptualize mental disorders only as responses to genes or to adverse environmental situations or to problematic interpersonal relationships seem to be too simplistic. Establishing the superiority of a model over another is probably a useless exercise, which has led researchers and clinicians far from the identification of what really causes a given mental health problem. In this respect, mental disorders can be considered not different from other chronic diseases, such as diabetes, cardiovascular diseases, or cancer, for which the interaction between biological, physical, social, and psychological causal factors is well established [2].

In mental health, the social determinants are well-known and should represent the target for specific universal, preventive, and protective interventions aiming to prevent the onset of mental health problems, to promote positive attitudes towards mental health in the general populations [3]. The social determinants of mental health include early childhood adversities, physical and psychological violence, bullying, childhood neglect and maltreatment, lack of social and economic support, lack of social security, economic crisis, war-related traumas, belonging to minority groups, discrimination, and other forms of trauma. More recently, urbanization, pollution, and other environmental factors have also been identified as increasing the risk of developing mental health problems [4, 5].

Based on these premises, this book promoted by the Italian Society of Social Psychiatry (Società Italiana di Psichiatria Sociale, SIPS) includes contributions on the impact of social determinants on mental health, discussing the most up-to-date findings on social determinants of health and mental health. In particular, the first chapter addresses the relevance of the revised biopsychosocial model in explaining the etiopathogenesis of mental disorders (Fiorillo et al.), which seems to be more in line with recent findings from mental health research and practice and may serve as a foundation for a more granular understanding of the most severe mental disorders. Several chapters focus on specific social determinants, including employment and socioeconomic condition (Bellomo et al.), pollution and climate change (Tortorella et al.), urbanization (Percudani), and traumatic events (Carmassi). New social determinants of mental health are considered in other chapters; in particular, the risk of novel psychoactive substances (Martinotti et al.) and the impact of new technologies and digitalization (Volpe et al.) are addressed. Of course, for each chapter, not only are the risks discussed but also opportunities for mental health professionals to reduce such risk factors and increase protective factors for the general population and for those at risk of developing mental disorders.

This book is in line with the recent WHO report, "World Mental Health Report: Transforming Mental Health for All", which highlights the need for all countries to achieve meaningful progress towards better mental health for their populations by focusing on social determinants of mental health.

We really hope that psychiatrists and other mental health professionals will find this book useful for their clinical practice and will help them to pay more attention to the psychosocial determinants of mental health in order to develop more personalized treatment plans.

References

1. World Health Organization. Mental health definition. https://www.who.int/news-room/fact-sheets/detail/mental-health-strengthening-our-response
2. Fiorillo A, Giordano A. The biopsychosocial model of schizophrenia and cancer: unraveling the etiopathogenesis of complex diseases. Eur Psychiatry 2022;65(1):e86.
3. Kirkbride JB, Anglin DM, Colman I, Dykxhoorn J, Jones PB, Patalay P, Pitman A, Soneson E, Steare T, Wright T, Griffiths SL. The social determinants of mental health and disorder: evidence, prevention and recommendations. World Psychiatry 2024;23(1):58–90. https://doi.org/10.1002/wps.21160.
4. De Rosa C, Sampogna G, Luciano M, Del Vecchio V, Fabrazzo M, Fiorillo A. Social versus biological psychiatry: it's time for integration! Int J Soc Psychiatry 2018;64(7):617–21.
5. Deferio JJ, Breitinger S, Khullar D, Sheth A, Pathak J. Social determinants of health in mental health care and research: a case for greater inclusion. J Am Med Inform Assoc 2019;26(8–9):895–99.

Naples, Italy Andrea Fiorillo
Lecce, Italy Serafino De Giorgi

Contents

1 Organization of Community Mental Health Care in Italy

Serafino De Giorgi, Matteo Di Vincenzo, Riccardo De Giorgi, Gaia Sampogna, and Andrea Fiorillo

Abstract

In Italy, the approval of the 180 Law in 1978, also known as Basaglia Law, marked the transition from an asylum-based to a community-based mental health care system. According to the law, patients with mental disorders are treated in the community, are integrated into society, and their rights and preferences on treatments are recognized. Following the Italian model, similar acts were approved worldwide. By 2000, all psychiatric hospitals in Italy had been closed and all patients discharged.

Within the Italian National Health System, the Department of Mental Health is responsible for the provision of community-based mental health care. It includes several facilities, such as psychiatric wards located in general hospitals, residential units, mental health centres, and day-hospital and day-care facilities.

The main effects of the 180 Law include the shift from a custiodialistic to a therapeutic paradigm of mental health care and the respect for autonomy and dignity of patients with mental health problems. However, after more than 45 years from its approval, several unmet needs still persist, including low staffing levels, reduced use of community facilities as long-stay services, and economic disparities between regions.

Keywords

Mental health care · Community mental health system · Mental health centres Organization of healthcare · Social inclusion Rehabilitation

1.1 Historical Perspective on Italian Mental Health Care

In 1978, the Italian Parliament approved the 180 Law -commonly known as "Basaglia Law"- named after the psychiatrist Franco Basaglia (1924–1980). This reform marked the transition from an asylum-based to a community-based mental health care system, aimed at treating patients suffering from severe mental disorders outside of the psychiatric hospitals [1, 2]. Indeed, as an effect of the application of this law, psychiatric asylums were gradually closed down. This

S. De Giorgi
Department of Mental Health, Lecce, Italy
e-mail: serafinodegiorgi@gmail.com

M. Di Vincenzo · G. Sampogna · A. Fiorillo (✉)
Department of Psychiatry, University of Oxford, Oxford, UK
e-mail: dr.matteodivincenzo@gmail.com; andrea.fiorillo@unicampania.it; gaia.sampogna@unicampania.it

R. De Giorgi
Department of Psychiatry, University of Campania "L. Vanvitelli", Naples, Italy
e-mail: riccardo.degiorgi@psych.ox.ac.uk

A. Fiorillo, S. De Giorgi (eds.), *Social Determinants of Mental Health*, Sustainable Development Goals Series, https://doi.org/10.1007/978-3-031-70165-8_1

law imposed the closure of Italian psychiatric hospitals in favour of a community-based approach, and it returned civil rights to patients with mental disorders. When the 180 Law was approved, the infrastructures needed for the innovations were not yet established, so a significant burden was posed on relatives and family members of patients discharged from the hospital [3]. The law allowed regions to manage independently the allocated funds for psychiatric care, resulting in variations in the level of treatment provided [4]. With the Italian reform, it was defined the procedure for issuing involuntary treatments ("Voluntary and Obligatory Health Checks and Treatments for Mental Illness"), with the following conditions that must be present: there are psychic alterations such as to require urgent therapeutic interventions that are not accepted by the patient, and there are no conditions and circumstances that allow alternative measures to be taken. This limitation of freedom takes place with a view to safeguarding another constitutional relief—that of the right to health. Any doctor can propose a compulsory medical treatment if the conditions are met. The validation of this procedure must be done by a psychiatrist of the public service and provides for a forced 7-day, renewable, hospitalization. This document is sent to the mayor's office, which makes a validation ordinance within 48 h.

On December 23, 1978, the 180 Law was included into the 833 Law, which officially introduced the National Health System (NHS) in Italy, by redefining a comprehensive public health policy. The NHS was designed as tax-funded and based on universality, equality, and equity, in order to cover the health needs of the population. Nowadays, it absorbs 6.8% of the whole gross domestic product [5], while a further 2% is voluntarily and additionally spent on private health services by individual citizens. The NHS is articulated into 139 local health trusts across the country, each caring for catchment areas ranging from 60,000 to almost 3,500,000 residents. Since health care management is administered at a regional level, disparities exist in terms of economic indicators (per capita income, wealth distribution, unemployment rate, welfare level) which reflect the diverse allocation of resources for health among the different geographic areas.

In 1978, almost 80,000 individuals with mental disorders were living in psychiatric hospitals; they were 7704 twenty years later. By 2000, all psychiatric hospitals had been closed and all inpatients discharged [6]. In order to cover all geographic areas across the country, mental health services were disseminated, with the aim to reduce admissions to psychiatric wards located in the general hospitals [7]. From this moment on, people suffering from mental disorders had recognized the opportunity to choose treatments, to keep their rights, and to feel part of the society [8, 9]. This approach soon overcame Italian borders and many countries adopted similar models of care [10].

In the period 1994–1996 and 1998–2000, two programmes called *Progetto Obiettivo Tutela Salute Mentale* defined aims and organizational features of mental health departments, including staff characteristics. In 2020, the expenditure for mental health facilities in Italy amounted to approximately 3% of the total NHS resources, by excluding services for drug abuse and intellectual disabilities. In 2022, there were 9.9 beds per 100,000 population for ordinary inpatients and day-hospital cares in general hospitals, and 52 beds per 100,000 residents in community residential facilities at a national level [11].

Because the Italian community model was implemented earlier than in the rest of the world, and relevant efforts were made to move away from the institutional model, Italy can be viewed as a laboratory to assess the quality of mental health care delivered in a community-oriented system, especially for patients with severe mental disorders [6, 12].

1.2 The Organization of Mental Health Care

1.2.1 Mental Health Department

The Mental Health Department (MHD) is the health organization responsible for providing specialist mental health care in the community, as

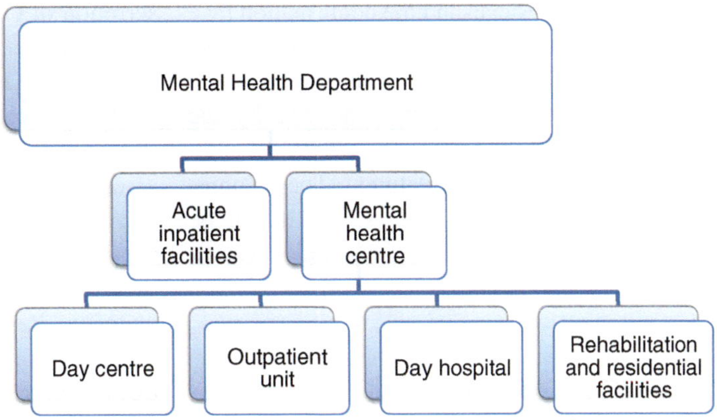

Fig. 1.1 Organization of mental health care in Italy

defined by the Progetto Obiettivo "Tutela Salute Mentale 1998–2000". MHDs include the following facilities: community mental health centres, day-care centres, general hospital psychiatric wards, and residential facilities. MHDs deal with prevention, treatment, and rehabilitation supporting mental health in a defined catchment area, by planning, organizing, and managing medical and social resources (Fig. 1.1). Moreover, MHDs promote informative campaigns and educational activities for the general population on mental health themes, in order to fight stigmatization and discrimination against mentally ill people. In addition, MHDs organize training courses for mental health professionals and research projects on the quality and effectiveness of pharmacological and nonpharmacological interventions.

1.2.2 Community Mental Health Centres

Community mental health centres (CMHCs) represent the cornerstone of the community-based system. They provide outpatient consultations and manage therapeutic and rehabilitative activities delivered by daily-care and residential facilities. Moreover, they are responsible for liaison consultations in hospital wards, patients' home assessment, and management of emergency. CMHCs are open every day for 12 or 24 h, based on regional organization. According to the PROG-CSM survey [13], the CMHC/resident ratio is about 1 CMHC per 80,460 inhabitants at national level. Each CMHC should include four psychiatrists, two psychologists, two social workers or rehabilitation therapists, and eight nurses, who provide integrated and personalized interventions for patients with severe mental disorders. The mean is about 24.8 full-time professionals per 100,000 residents, with some geographic differences (on average, 25.9 ± 11.5 professionals per 100,000 residents in Northern Italy, 28.3 ± 7.4 in Central Italy, and 23.7 ± 6.9 in Southern Italy). In 2022, almost 750,000 users accessed Italian CMHCs at least once, mainly for depression (33.2 per 10,000 residents) and psychotic disorders (30.6 per 10,000 residents) [11].

1.2.3 Acute Inpatient Units

Acute inpatient care is delivered in general hospital psychiatric wards (GHPWs), closely linked with CMHCs to guarantee a continuity of care. As established by the 180 Law, a maximum of 15 beds is allowed for each GHPW [14]. In 2022, more than 92,000 patients were discharged from psychiatric wards, after a mean length of stay of 12.7 days [11]. Admissions to GHPW can be either on a voluntary or a compulsory basis. Involuntary admission is regulated by a specific procedure, described in the 180 Law. According to the Italian regulation, the patient is suffering from a mental condition requiring urgent treatment, the person does not accept the treatments, and it is not possible to take appropriate extra hospital measures. The procedure includes the initial proposal by a physician and the confirmation by a psychiatrist working in a public hospital. These documents are sent to the mayor (the highest local health authority), which are authorized by the tutelary judge who is entrusted with the jurisdictional safeguard of such treatment. The involuntary treatment lasts for 7 days, but it can be revoked earlier or prolonged, if the clinical conditions still persist [15].

1.2.4 Day Centres

Day centres usually implement short- and medium-term rehabilitation programmes, that are semi-residential recovery-oriented facilities operated by the MHD or are accredited no-profit or for-profit structures. They are open 8 h per day from Monday to Saturday and can accommodate up to 20 patients per day. Multidisciplinary mental health professionals working in day centres include social workers, psychologists, rehabilitation technicians, and volunteers. Psychosocial rehabilitative interventions are delivered to small groups of subacute patients in order to increase their social skills, autonomy levels, and daily global functioning.

1.2.5 Community Residential Facilities

Community residential facilities are non-hospital services providing overnight assistance for patients with severe mental disorders, upon prescription of CMHCs. They are public or private (non-profit and for-profit). People living in these facilities have relatively stable mental health conditions, require rehabilitative interventions, and receive periodic clinical and functional assessment.

According to the Italian Ministry of Health, community residential facilities can be classified according to rehabilitation intensity and care intensity. Residential facilities aim to support residents to progress from more supported settings to more independent settings as they gain competences. The care pathway is organized so that people move on from residential facilities providing higher support to those providing intermediate support and then to those with minimal support [16] (Fig. 1.2). All patients receive tailored therapeutic plans, including rehabilitative, psychological, and pharmacological interventions, for relatively short periods. However, length of stay often exceeds 2 years [6].

1.2.6 Day-Hospital Facilities

Patients suffering from mental disorders can receive diagnostic assessments, administration of medications, and rehabilitative interventions in day-hospital facilities, which can be located within the hospital or in external settings. Day hospitals usually operate for 6 days a week, 8 h a day. The aim of day hospital is to provide personalized treatment plans limiting the need for hospital admissions. Availability of beds varies at regional level.

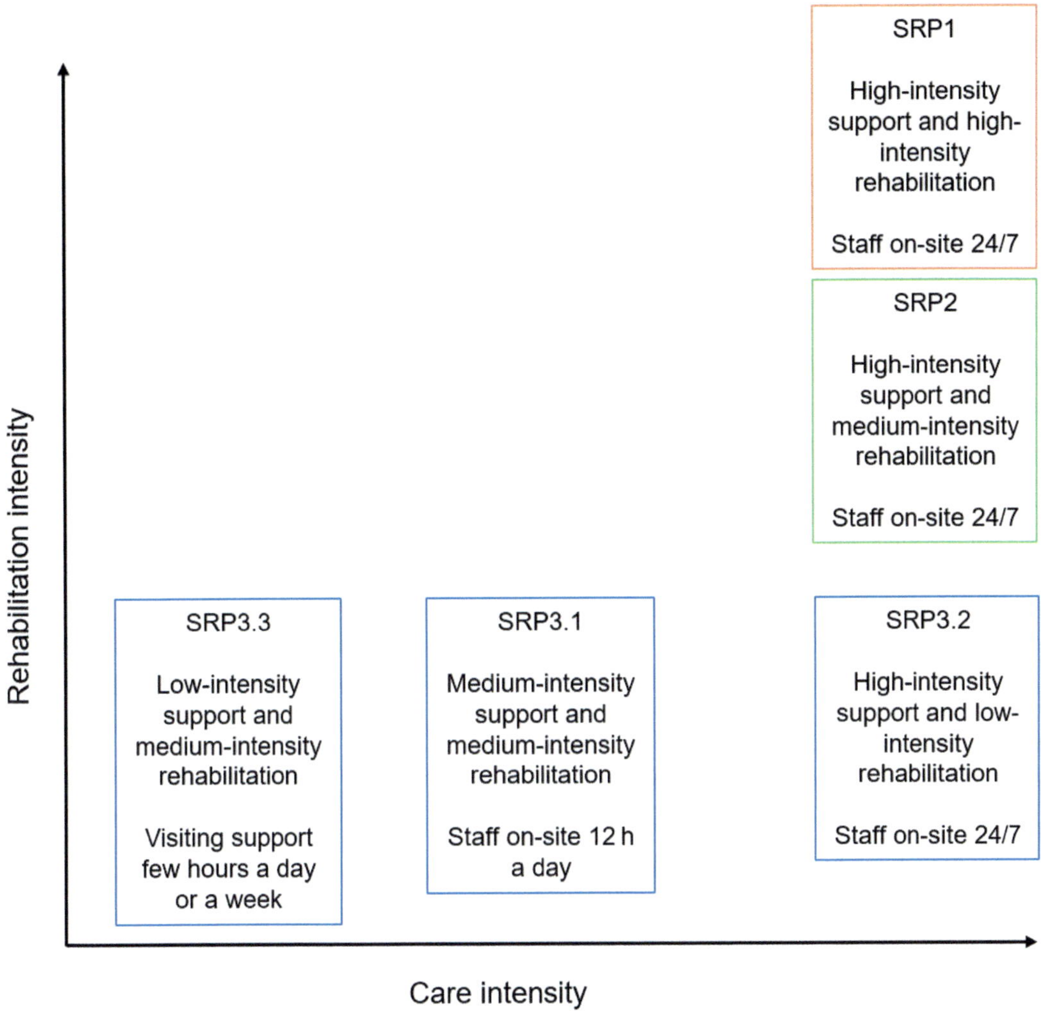

Fig. 1.2 Types of residential facilities

1.3 Service Use Data on Mental Health Care in Italian Regions

Provision of mental health care in Italy varies among the different regions. In particular, the prevalence of treated mental disorders, considered as a proxy indicator of the coverage capacity of community-based mental health care, ranges from 266.1 individuals per 10,000 population in the Autonomous Province of Bolzano-South Tyrol (Northern Italy) to 84.8 in Sardinia. Differences can also be detected in terms of incidence of treated mental disorders that is higher in Aosta Valley (Northern Italy) and lower in Friuli-Venezia Giulia (Northern Italy), Tuscany and Marche (Central Italy), and Molise and Basilicata (Southern Italy) [11].

The national rate of compulsory admissions is 1.0/10,000 residents, ranging from 2.3 in Umbria (Central Italy) to 0.1 in Basilicata (Southern Italy). Indeed, after the implementation of the 180 Law, the absolute number of compulsory admissions progressively declined, from more than 20,000 in 1978 to 5118 in 2022. Similarly, the proportion of compulsory psychiatric admissions progressively declined from 1978 to 2005, remaining stable thereafter, accounting for 6.2% of all psychiatric admissions in 2022 [11].

1.4 The Italian Mental Health Care System: What Else?

The approval of the 180 Law in 1978 marked significant and enduring changes in the provision of mental health care in Italy. First, the transition from a custodialistic to a therapeutic model, allowing mentally ill patients to be treated in their own environment and with the same rights as any other patient suffering from a chronic physical illness. It took around 20 years to complete the gradual closing down of all asylums, but at the end the whole process can be considered a happy-ending story [17]. Also, the dissemination of community-based mental health facilities opened the way for a community public health care system. The opening of psychiatric wards within general hospitals reduced the number of admissions and facilitated the integration of mental health care with other medical disciplines [6]. This new model of mental health care would have not been possible without multidisciplinary teams of professionals, which include psychiatrists, psychologists, psychiatric nurses, social workers, rehabilitation technicians, and other health workers providing tailored and integrated treatment for all patients, each professional with his/her level of expertise [18]. Finally, the 180 Law facilitated the collaboration between mental health professionals, patients, and family members, who are now considered effective members of the caring team.

However, some areas for concern still persist. The Italian NHS came into effect with the promulgation of the 833 Law on December 23, 1978. Since then, health care in Italy is provided on a regional basis, with significant variations across the different regions, especially between Northern vs. Central and Southern Italy, and the number of beds in psychiatric facilities cannot represent an indicator of public health quality, but harder indicators should be considered, such as suicide rates, involuntary admissions, and number of patients placed in forensic facilities [9].

Given this heterogeneity in mental health care provision, the "clinical pathways in patients with severe mental disorders in Italy" (QUADIM) study has been recently carried out to assess the quality indicators of healthcare pathways for patients with severe mental disorders in four regions, namely Lombardy, Emilia-Romagna, Lazio, and the Province of Palermo [19, 20]. Using the healthcare utilization databases, the authors found significant heterogeneity in terms of timing of starting medications, continuity of care, accessibility to psychotherapy and psychosocial interventions, monitoring of side effects and mortality among patients suffering from schizophrenia [21, 22], bipolar disorder [23], and personality disorders [24].

The QUADIM project confirmed that the quality of mental healthcare in Italy is extremely heterogenous. Although community care is accessible, continuous, and moderately intensive in almost all Italian regions, main gaps exist regarding delivery of psychosocial interventions. In particular, psychoeducation and psychological treatments are not frequently provided, and the intensity of treatments is moderate. Regional heterogeneity for the prevalent cases is high in almost all areas, while it is significantly lower for newly taken-in-care patients. Accessibility to home care and continuity of care between general practitioners and community mental health centres are relatively homogenous.

A relevant issue is the rate of employed mental health professionals, which significantly varies among different regions; thus, a reorganization of mental health services at a national level would be advisable, in order to reach adequate standards everywhere. Although more resources are urgently needed, an increase in resources alone is not sufficient.

Regional disparity also affects the provision of mental health to criminal offenders [25]. As consequence of a Government Decree on April 1, 2008, the national healthcare system became responsible for managing the health needs of patients under detention. Following the closing down of forensic psychiatric hospitals in 2015, MHDs provide mental health assistance to offenders both in prisons and in residential settings. In 2018, 37% of inmates in Emilia-Romagna were affected by psychiatric, behavioural, or substance use disorders; consequently, a multidisciplinary and case-management approach for mental healthcare in jails was proposed [26]. Forensic psychiatric units were created within the MHDs of Bologna, Parma, and Brescia in order to create continuity between forensic institutions and community facilities, to collaborate with penitentiary authorities and to support MHDs on legal matters [27]. Offenders who were judged not guilty "by the reason of insanity" but with "social dangerousness" can now be placed in residential institutions which replaced forensic psychiatric hospitals (the residences for the execution of measures of security, REMS).

The low levels of economic resources allocated to mental healthcare are associated with a significant burden on patients and their family members [28, 29]. Indeed, mental disorders are associated with high levels of family burden, making a priority the provision of supportive interventions to patients and their relatives [30–32]. Unfortunately, these interventions are only rarely available, mainly because mental health professionals are already overburdened, have difficulties in integrating these interventions in their routine work, and do not have adequate rooms or support to provide supportive family interventions within working hours [33].

Another area for concern is the separation between adult psychiatry and child and adolescent psychiatry (CAP), both in training of medical professionals and in the organization of clinical care. In some regions, CAP units are integrated in the MHDs, while in other contexts they are included in paediatric trusts and provide prevention, therapy, rehabilitation, social and school support to children and adolescents with mental problems independently from adult mental health services. The transition from child and adolescent psychiatry to adult mental health services is particularly important at this age, since treatment discontinuation can seriously damage mental health status of young patients [35]. Psychiatric services for early intervention in psychosis targeting people under the age of 18 are becoming more widespread in Italy, but significantly less than in other countries, and youth mental health services are completely missing [36].

Table 1.1 Staff and resources for mental health care in Italy (Source: WHO ATLAS [34])

Staff in mental health sector per 100,000	
Psychiatrists	6.39
Nurses	23.84
Social workers	2.41
Psychologists	3.94
Inpatient facilities per 100,000	
Beds for mental health in general hospitals	8.09
Beds in community residential facilities	42.83
Outpatient facilities	
Outpatient mental health facilities	1254
Day treatment facilities	843

Further reasons for concern include the low number of available mental health professionals, which is not adequate to satisfy the growing demands for care from the population (Table 1.1) and the potential use of residential facilities as long-stay residential services, with a subsequent lack of alternatives to acute inpatient admissions for many patients [14, 37, 38]. Patients should live in these facilities no more than 2 years, although with some regional variations. Finally, the use of involuntary admissions and of coercive measures remains a controversial issue in mental health practice in Italy and needs to be reconsidered [39, 40].

1.5 Conclusions

In conclusion, the organization of mental health care in Italy—albeit one of the oldest models in the whole Europe—is still modern and up to date. However, several concerns remain, including disparity of care provision at regional basis, low staffing levels, and improper use of residential facilities. Alongside with the achievement of patients' recovery, through a personalized approach of care including pharmacological, psychological, and psychosocial interventions, psychiatrists are called to deal with other challenges. At the level of the general population, dissemination of knowledge about mental health and fight against stigma remain priority areas of action. Prevention and treatment of new forms of mental health problems, as well as management of special patient populations, such as migrants; [41], adolescents [42, 43], and elderly people [44, 45], require new models of mental health care and a restructuring of mental health facilities.

References

1. Ferrannini L, Ghio L, Gibertoni D et al (2014) Thirty-five years of community psychiatry in Italy. J Nerv Ment Dis 202:432–439
2. Lora A (2009) An overview of the mental health system in Italy. Ann Ist Super Sanita 45(1):5–16
3. Badano V (2024) The Basaglia Law. Returning dignity to psychiatric patients: the historical, political and social factors that led to the closure of psychiatric hospitals in Italy in 1978. Hist Psychiatry 35(2):226–233
4. Ferrannini L, Peloso PF (2016) The closure of the psychiatric hospital as an original feature of rehabilitation in Italy. International Journal of Mental Health 45(1):1–6.
5. Organisation for Economic Co-operation and Development (2023) Country statistical profiles: key tables from OECD. https://www.oecd-ilibrary.org/docserver/f8002746-en.pdf?expires=1712781559&id=id&accname=guest&checksum=2062C1404A92D49A136B66B6EB16987A
6. Barbui C, Papola D, Saraceno B (2018) Forty years without mental hospitals in Italy. Int J Ment Health Syst 12:43
7. Amaddeo F, Barbui C, Tansella M (2012) State of psychiatry in Italy 35 years after psychiatric reform. A critical appraisal of national and local data. Int Rev Psychiatry 24:314–320
8. Castaldelli-Maia JM, Ventriglio A (2016) The impact of Basaglia on Brazilian psychiatry. Int J Soc Psychiatry 62(5):411–414
9. Mezzina C (2018) Forty years of the Law 180: the aspirations of a great reform, its successes and continuing need. Epidemiol Psychiatr Sci 27(4):336–345
10. Catanesi R, Manna A, Ventriglio A (2016) Community mental health services and responsibility of psychiatrists in Italy: lessons for the globe. Int J Soc Psychiatry 62(6):501–504
11. Ministero della Salute (2023) Rapporto sulla Salute mentale anno 2022. https://www.salute.gov.it/imgs/C_17_pubblicazioni_3369_allegato.pdf
12. Kilbourne AM, Beck K, Spaeth-Rublee B, Ramanuj P, O'Brien RW, Tomoyasu N, Pincus HA (2018) Measuring and improving the quality of mental health care: a global perspective. World Psychiatry 17(1):30–38. https://doi.org/10.1002/wps.20482. PMID: 29352529; PMCID: PMC5775149
13. Munizza C, Gonella R, Pinciaroli L, Rucci P, Picci RL, Tibaldi G (2011) CMHC adherence to National Mental Health Plan standards in Italy: a survey 30 years after national reform law. Psychiatr Serv 62(9):1090–1093
14. de Girolamo G, Barbato BA, Gaddini R, Miglio A, Morosini R, Norcio B, Picardi A, Rossi E, Rucci P, Santone G, Dell'Acqua G (2007) The characteristics and activities of acute psychiatric inpatient facilities: a national survey in Italy. Br J Psychiatry 191:170–177
15. Saya A, Brugnoli C, Piazzi G, Liberato D, Di Ciaccia G, Niolu C, Siracusano A (2019) Criteria, procedures, and future prospects of involuntary treatment in psychiatry around the world: a narrative review. Front Psych 10:271
16. Martinelli A, Killaspy H, Zarbo C et al (2022) DIAPASON consortium. Quality of residential facilities in Italy: satisfaction and quality of life of residents with schizophrenia spectrum disorders. BMC Psychiatry 22(1):717. https://doi.org/10.1186/s12888-022-04344-w. PMID: 36397009; PMCID: PMC9672559
17. Fiorillo A, Ventriglio A (2018) The legacy of Italian psychiatry. Int Rev Psychiatry 30(2):118–119
18. Pingani L, Fiorillo A, Luciano M, Catellani S, Vinci V, Ferrari S, Rigatelli M (2013) Who cares for it? How to provide psychosocial interventions in the community. Int J Soc Psychiatry 59(7):701–705
19. Corrao G, Monzio Compagnoni M, Barbato A, D'Avanzo B, Di Fiandra T, Ferrara L, Gaddini A, Saponaro A, Scondotto S, Tozzi VD, Carle F, Carbone S, Chisholm DH, Lora A (2022) From contact coverage to effective coverage of community care for patients with severe mental disorders: a real-world investigation from Italy. Front Psych 13:1014193
20. Monzio Compagnoni M, Caggiu G, Allevi L, Barbato A, Carle F, D'Avanzo B, Di Fiandra T, Ferrara L, Gaddini A, Giordani C, Sanza M, Saponaro A, Scondotto S, Tozzi VD, Corrao G, Lora A (2023) Assessment and monitoring of the quality of clinical pathways in patients with depressive disorders: results from a multiregional Italian investigation on mental health care quality (the QUADIM Project). J Clin Med 12(9):3297
21. Corrao G, Barbato A, D'Avanzo B, Di Fiandra T, Ferrara L, Gaddini A, Monzio Compagnoni M, Saponaro A, Scondotto S, Tozzi VD, Carle F, Lora A (2022) "QUADIM project", "Monitoring, assessing care pathways (M. A. P.)" working groups of the Italian Ministry of Health. Does the mental health system provide effective coverage to people with schizophrenic disorder? A self-controlled case series

study in Italy. Soc Psychiatry Psychiatr Epidemiol 57(3):519–529
22. Lora A, Monzio Compagnoni M, Allevi L, Barbato A, Carle F, D'avanzo B, Di Fiandra T, Ferrara L, Gaddini A, Leogrande M, Saponaro A, Scondotto S, Tozzi VD, Carbone S, Corrao G (2022) 'QUADIM project' and 'Monitoring and assessing diagnostic-therapeutic paths (MAP)' working groups of the Italian Ministry of Health. The quality of mental health care delivered to patients with schizophrenia and related disorders in the Italian mental health system. The QUADIM project: a multi-regional Italian investigation based on healthcare utilisation databases. Epidemiol Psychiatr Sci 31:e15
23. D'Avanzo B, Barbato A, Monzio Compagnoni M, Caggiu G, Allevi L, Carle F, Di Fiandra T, Ferrara L, Gaddini A, Sanza M, Saponaro A, Scondotto S, Tozzi VD, Giordani C, Corrao G, Lora A (2023) The quality of mental health care for people with bipolar disorders in the Italian mental health system: the QUADIM project. BMC Psychiatry 23(1):424
24. Sanza M, Monzio Compagnoni M, Caggiu G, Allevi L, Barbato A, Campa J, Carle F, D'avanzo B, Di Fiandra T, Ferrara L, Gaddini A, Saponaro A, Scondotto S, Tozzi VD, Lorusso S, Giordani C, Corrao G, Lora A (2023) Assessing the quality of the care offer for people with personality disorders in Italy: the QUADIM project. A multicentre research based on the database of use of Mental Health services. Int J Ment Health Syst 17(1):31
25. Peloso PF, D'Alema M, Fioritti A (2014) Mental health care in prisons and the issue of forensic hospitals in Italy. J Nerv Ment Dis 202(6):473–478
26. Pelizza L, Pupo S (2024) Mental health interventions in Italian prisons: are we ready for a new model? Suggestions from the Parma experience. Riv Psichiatr 59(1):35–42
27. Boaron F, Gerocarni B, Fontanesi MG, Zulli V, Fioritti A (2021) Across the walls. Treatment pathways of mentally ill offenders in Italy, from prisons to community care. J Psychopathol 27:34–39
28. Del Vecchio V, Luciano M, Sampogna G, De Rosa C, Giacco D, Tarricone I, Catapano F, Fiorillo A (2015) The role of relatives in pathways to care of patients with a first episode of psychosis. Int J Soc Psychiatry 61(7):631–637
29. Volpe U, Fiorillo A, Luciano M, Del Vecchio V, Palumbo C, Calò S, Piras S, Signorelli M, Filippo D, Piselli M, De Fazio P, Gotelli S, Bardicchia F, Cerveri G, Ferrari S, Mulè A, Ribolsi M, Sampogna G, De Rosa C, Sartorius N (2014) Pathways to mental health care in Italy: results from a multicenter study. Int J Soc Psychiatry 60(5):508–513
30. Fiorillo A, Del Vecchio V, Luciano M, Sampogna G, De Rosa C, Malangone C, Volpe U, Bardicchia F, Ciampini G, Crocamo C, Iapichino S, Lampis D, Moroni A, Orlandi E, Piselli M, Pompili E, Veltro F, Carrà G, Maj M (2015) Efficacy of psychoeducational family intervention for bipolar I disorder: a controlled, multicentric, real-world study. J Affect Disord 172:291–299
31. Luciano M, Sampogna G, del Vecchio V, Giacco D, Mulè A, de Rosa C, Fiorillo A, Maj M (2012) The family in Italy: cultural changes and implications for treatment. Int Rev Psychiatry 24(2):149–156
32. Sampogna G, Luciano M, Del Vecchio V, Malangone C, De Rosa C, Giallonardo V, Borriello G, Pocai B, Savorani M, Steardo L Jr, Lampis D, Veltro F, Bartoli F, Bardicchia F, Moroni AM, Ciampini G, Orlandi E, Ferrari S, Biondi S, Iapichino S, Pompili E, Piselli M, Tortorella A, Carrà G, Fiorillo A (2018) The effects of psychoeducational family intervention on coping strategies of relatives of patients with bipolar I disorder: results from a controlled, real-world, multicentric study. Neuropsychiatr Dis Treat 14:977–989
33. Fiorillo A, Del Vecchio V, Luciano M, Sampogna G, Sbordone D, Catapano F, De Rosa C, Malangone C, Tortorella A, Veltro F, Nicolò G, Piselli M, Bardicchia F, Ciampini G, Lampis D, Moroni A, Bassi M, Iapichino S, Biondi S, Graziani A, Orlandi E, Starace F, Baronessa C, Carrà G, Maj M (2016) Feasibility of a psychoeducational family intervention for people with bipolar I disorder and their relatives: results from an Italian real-world multicentre study. J Affect Disord 190:657–662
34. World Health Organization (2020) Mental health atlas. https://cdn.who.int/media/docs/default-source/mental-health/mental-health-atlas-2020-country-profiles/ita.pdf?sfvrsn=45d79fc8_4&download=true
35. Hendrickx G, De Roeck V, Maras A, Dieleman G, Gerritsen S, Purper-Ouakil D, Russet F, Schepker R, Signorini G, Singh SP, Street C, Tuomainen H, Tremmery S (2020) Challenges during the transition from child and adolescent mental health services to adult mental health services. BJPsych Bull 44(4):163–168
36. Meneghelli A, Ciancaglini P, Di Domenico M, Mazzola A, Ghio L, Preti A (2023) Implementation of early intervention clinical services within the National Health System in Italy: third wave survey with focus on structures, resources, and fidelity to the evidence-based model. Early Interv Psychiatry 17(9):884–892
37. de Girolamo G, Picardi A, Santone G et al (2005) The severely mentally ill in residential facilities: a national survey in Italy. Psychol Med 35:421–431
38. de Girolamo G, Bassi M, Neri G, Ruggeri M, Santone G, Picardi A (2007) The current state of mental health care in Italy: problems, perspectives, and lessons to learn. Eur Arch Psychiatry Clin Neurosci 257:83–91
39. Fiorillo A, De Rosa C, Del Vecchio V, Jurjanz L, Schnall K, Onchev G, Alexiev S, Raboch J, Kalisova L, Mastrogianni A, Georgiadou E, Solomon Z, Dembinskas A, Raskauskas V, Nawka P, Nawka A, Kiejna A, Hadrys T, Torres-Gonzales F, Mayoral F, Björkdahl A, Kjellin L, Priebe S, Maj M, Kallert T (2011) How to improve clinical practice on involuntary hospital admissions of psychiatric patients: sug-

gestions from the EUNOMIA study. Eur Psychiatry 26(4):201–207
40. Luciano M, De Rosa C, Sampogna G, Del Vecchio V, Giallonardo V, Fabrazzo M, Catapano F, Onchev G, Raboch J, Mastrogianni A, Solomon Z, Dembinskas A, Nawka P, Kiejna A, Torres-Gonzales F, Kjellin L, Kallert T, Fiorillo A (2018) How to improve clinical practice on forced medication in psychiatric practice: suggestions from the EUNOMIA European multicentre study. Eur Psychiatry 54:35–40
41. Forte A, Trobia F, Gualtieri F, Lamis DA, Cardamone G, Giallonardo V, Fiorillo A, Girardi P, Pompili M (2018) Suicide risk among immigrants and ethnic minorities: a literature overview. Int J Environ Res Public Health 15(7):1438
42. Bloomfield MAP, Chang T, Woodl MJ, Lyons LM, Cheng Z, Bauer-Staeb C, Hobbs C, Bracke S, Kennerley H, Isham L, Brewin C, Billings J, Greene T, Lewis G (2021) Psychological processes mediating the association between developmental trauma and specific psychotic symptoms in adults: a systematic review and meta-analysis. World Psychiatry 20(1):107–123
43. Guloksuz S, Pries LK, Ten Have M, de Graaf R, van Dorsselaer S, Klingenberg B, Bak M, Lin BD, van Eijk KR, Delespaul P, van Amelsvoort T, Luykx JJ, Rutten BPF, van Os J (2020) Association of preceding psychosis risk states and non-psychotic mental disorders with incidence of clinical psychosis in the general population: a prospective study in the NEMESIS-2 cohort. World Psychiatry 19:199–205
44. Fiorillo A, Malik A, Luciano M, Del Vecchio V, Sampogna G, Del Gaudio L, Rojnic Kuzman M, Jovanovic N, Nawka A, Volpe U (2013) Challenges for trainees in psychiatry and early career psychiatrists. Int Rev Psychiatry 25(4):431–437
45. Fiorillo A, Maj M (2018) The role of psychiatry in modern medicine. Int Rev Psychiatry 30(2): 169–175

2 The Biopsychosocial Model Revised for Mental Health

Gaia Sampogna, Roberto Brugnoli, and Andrea Fiorillo

Abstract

Mental health and mental disorders are complex phenomena involving specific brain functions, the area of human relationships, and several individual and social psychological domains. Although the etiopathogenesis of mental disorders is still not fully understood, paradigms that conceptualize mental disorders only as responses to genes or to adverse environmental situations or to problematic interpersonal relationships seem to be too simplistic. Establishing the superiority of a model over another is probably a useless exercise, considering that mental disorders are complex disorders that reflect the complex interplay between a complex organ (i.e., the brain) and an even more complex function, that is that of human relationships. The biopsychosocial model, which encompasses social, biological, and personal factors, seems the best model for explaining the etiopathogenesis of mental disorders. This model, which is well recognized in other branches of medicine—such as cancer—is currently living a renaissance in mental health research and practice.

Keywords

Biopsychosocial model · Social determinants · Mental health · Mental disorders

2.1 Background

Mental health is a complex phenomenon that can be approached from many angles, with a recent renewed interest for interdisciplinary approaches.

The World Health Organization (WHO) defines mental health as "a state of mental well-being that enables people to cope with life stressors, realize their abilities, learn well and work well, and contribute to their community." Mental health is an integral component of health and well-being that underpins individual and collective abilities to make decisions, build relationships, and shape the world we live in. Thus, mental health is much more than the mere absence of mental disturbances. It exists on a complex continuum, which is experienced differently from one person to another, with varying degrees of difficulty and distress and potentially different clinical and social outcomes. Mental health conditions include not only proper mental disorders and psychosocial disabilities but also

G. Sampogna · A. Fiorillo (✉)
Department of Psychiatry, University of Campania "L. Vanvitelli", Naples, Italy
e-mail: gaia.sampogna@unicampania.it; andrea.fiorillo@unicampania.it

R. Brugnoli
Department of Psychiatry, Fondazione Policlinico Universitario Agostino Gemelli IRCCS, Rome, Italy
e-mail: roberto.brugnoli@uniroma1.it

A. Fiorillo, S. De Giorgi (eds.), *Social Determinants of Mental Health*, Sustainable Development Goals Series, https://doi.org/10.1007/978-3-031-70165-8_2

other less severe mental health problems which cause significant distress, impairment in functioning, or risk of self-harm.

Several social determinants—such as poverty, unemployment, war, migration, environmental pollution, climate change—and personal factors, including specific cognitive traits or temperaments or genetic liabilities, such as polygenic variants, may act both as risk and protective factors for mental disorders.

In the last century, the etiopathogenesis of mental disorders has been explained through different models; however, it has been recently highlighted that paradigms conceptualizing mental disorders only as responses to genes or to adverse environmental situations or to problematic interpersonal relationships seem to be too simplistic [1]. Furthermore, establishing the superiority of a model over another is probably a useless exercise, considering that mental disorders are complex disorders that reflect the complex interplay between a complex organ (i.e., the brain) and an even more complex function, that is that of human relationships. The biopsychosocial model, which encompasses social, biological, and personal factors, seems the best model for explaining the etiopathogenesis of mental disorders. This approach, which is well recognized in other branches of medicine—such as cancer—is currently living a renaissance in mental health research and practice.

2.2 The Original Biopsychosocial Model

The "biopsychosocial model" of mental disorders was originally proposed by George Engel back in 1960s. An internist with a training in psychoanalysis, Engel started from the biomedical model of medical illnesses but considered the isolated biological, psychological, social, and environmental components of the various illnesses. Since his publication of "A Unified Concept of Health and Disease" in 1960 and his work "The Need for a New Medical Model: A Challenge for Biomedicine" in 1977, clinicians and researchers worldwide started to consider the integrative model more appropriate to explain the causes of most physical and mental disorders.

Engel contended that medical illnesses—and particularly mental disorders—result from a complex and dynamic interplay between physiological, psychological, and social variables.

As a consequence of this conceptualization, he proposed the first biopsychosocial approach, which became widely accepted for a comprehensive case formulation model and adapted to several illnesses, including schizophrenia [2]. Since 1980s, the biopsychosocial formulation became the organizing principle for psychiatric education and training, gaining wide acceptability across the globe.

The biopsychosocial formulation is a tentative working hypothesis which attempts to explain the biological, psychological, and sociocultural factors which have been combined to create and maintain the presenting clinical problem (American Psychiatric Association Commission on Psychotherapy). It is a guide to treatment planning and selection. It will be changed, modified, or amplified as the clinician learns more and more about the patient's history.

Recently, the sociocultural dimension of case formulation has received increased attention with the recognition that culture and ethnicity are often ignored or mishandled through ignorance or personal bias on the part of the therapist. In fact, the DSM-5 has included a Cultural Formulation Interview (CFI) in order to help clinicians to address important cultural factors [3].

However, in the past 20 years, the biopsychosocial model has been increasingly criticized for being vague, useless, and even incoherent clinically, scientifically, and philosophically. The combination of these two points defines a crisis in the conceptual foundations of medicine and healthcare [4]. Thomas R. Insel (2012) stated that "mental illnesses are not different from heart disease, diabetes or any other chronic illness. All chronic diseases have behavioral components as well as biological components, the only difference here is that the organ of interest is the brain instead of the heart or pancreas. But the same basic principles apply." Furthermore, Jerome Wakefield (2007) highlighted that by placing too much attention on the biological causes of mental disorders, we may overlook important environmental, behavioral, and social factors that contribute to mental disorders. But also considering mental disorders as due only to psychological or social factors seems to be too reductionist. Establishing the superiority of a model over another is not an easy task, considering that mental disorders are complex disorders reflecting the complex interplay between a complex organ, which is the brain, and an even more complex function that is that of human relationships [5]. Thus, a balanced view—considering biological, psychological, and social factors—is again needed in order to correctly understand mental health and manage mental disorders.

2.3 The Biopsychosocial Model: Revised

Since then, several models have been proposed for integrating biological and social aspects. These models have considered social factors as antecedents to biological processes (i.e., the biological consequences of social disadvantage accumulate over time), as modifiers of genetic effects (i.e., the gene-environment effect [6]), or as an integral part of biological systems (i.e., biological and social aspects are intrinsically related as demonstrated in animal studies in which the social context changes the neuronal response to serotonin). However, how social factors are integrated with biological ones is still a matter of debate and no clear answers can be provided at the current level of knowledge.

The emotional tone of a person, his/her personality, the surrounding environment, and other social parameters do influence the manifestation of illness. This principle applies to basically all complex conditions, including cancer, neurological illnesses, and mental disorders.

Schizophrenia and cancer are complex disorders causing severe impairment and premature mortality. They both include a wide range of different illnesses, with different symptoms, course, and outcome. While the causes of severe mental disorders, such as schizophrenia, depression, and bipolar disorder, remain largely unknown, research into the etiopathogenesis of cancer has led to clarify its main genetic and environmental factors. Hopefully, a similar pathway will be applied to mental disorders if the approach used for understanding the etiopathological mechanism of cancer is going to be translated to severe mental disorders. In fact, nowadays, schizophrenia is conceptualized as a neurodevelopmental disorder, lying on a continuum, from mild psychotic experiences observed in the general population to frank psychotic episodes. This conceptualization is very similar to that of neoplasia. Several genetic loci are responsible for the liability to the illness, and several biological (e.g., hormones), environmental (e.g., pollution), or behavioral (e.g., healthy lifestyles) factors either protect against or prompt the illness. Such conceptualization of cancer has paved the way to a personalized approach to the disorder. This model has been recently proposed also for mental disorders, since cancer and mental disorders share the same environmental and behavioral risk factors, while responsible genes are still far to be identified [7].

The interplay between biological and psychosocial phenomena does not allow to draw certain linear causal links. What is causal, that is, responsible for a cause–effect between two observable events, may appear casual, that is, the result of chance and randomness, as we are often unable to determine a direct relationship. In mechanisms as complex as cancer and schizophrenia, scientists often fail to discriminate between what is causal from what is random or chaotic.

Mental disorders, exactly as cancer is, are heterogeneous, multifactorial "genetic diseases of environmental origin," in which genetic and environmental (chemical, physical, and biological) factors contribute. In fact, evidence is accumulating which confirm the role of social determinants of health as risk or protective factors for the development of severe mental disorders. The hope is that sooner or later we will be able to find a genomic alteration caused by stressful environmental factors in patients with schizophrenia [7].

2.4 Genetic Determinants of Mental Disorders

A study carried out by the Brainstorm Consortium [8] published on *Science* for quantifing the genetic sharing of 25 brain disorders from genome-wide association studies. The authors found that mental disorders share common variant risks, whereas neurological disorders appear more distinct from one another and from psychiatric disorders. These results highlight the importance of a common genetic variation as a risk factor for brain disorders and the value of heritability-based methods in understanding their etiology.

Molecular genetic methods allow estimation of genetic correlations between psychiatric disorders and subclinical traits of these disorders based on additive, common genome-wide variants. Such studies report strong genetic correlations across disorders and traits for ADHD and major depressive disorder, with a moderate estimate for autism spectrum disorder. An alternative approach is to calculate the polygenic risk scores (PRSs) based on discovery genome-wide association studies (GWASs) of psychiatric disorders; PRSs capture an individual's common variant risk for a phenotype. Although some preliminary evidence supports shared genetic risks across disorders and traits for some psychiatric phenotypes, the evidence is still controversial. In a large population study, Taylor et al. [9] found that genetic factors associated with psychiatric disorders are also associated with milder variation in characteristic traits in the general population for many psychiatric phenotypes.

2.5 The Gene–Environment Model

Intriguing findings on genetic and environmental causation suggest a need to reframe the etiology of mental disorders. Molecular genetics show that mental illnesses are due to the contribution of thousands of common and rare genetic variants. Epidemiological studies have identified dozens of environmental exposures associated with psychopathology. The effect of environment is likely conditional on genetic factors, resulting in gene–environment interactions. The impact of environmental factors also depends on previous exposures, resulting in environment–environment interactions. Most known genetic and environmental factors are shared across multiple mental disorders. Schizophrenia, bipolar disorder, and major depressive disorder, in particular, are closely causally linked. Synthesis of findings from twin studies, molecular genetics, and epidemiological research suggests that joint consideration of multiple genetic and environmental factors has much greater explanatory power than separate studies of genetic or environmental causation. Multifactorial gene–environment interactions are likely to be a generic mechanism involved in the majority of cases of mental illness, which is only partially tapped by existing gene–environment studies. Future research may cut across psychiatric disorders and address poly-causation by considering multiple genetic and environmental measures across the life course with a specific focus on the first two decades of life. Integrative analyses of poly-causation including gene–environment and environment–environment interactions can realize the potential for discovering causal types and mechanisms that are likely to generate new preventive and therapeutic tools.

2.6 Social Determinants of (Mental) Health

We cannot exactly predict when and to which extent a certain environmental insult can cause a specific mental (or physical) disorder, but it is well established that the combination of genetic alterations and environmental factors under certain conditions can lead to the onset of various illnesses.

Therefore, the social determinants of mental health play an essential role in the etiopathogenesis of mental disorders. The social determinants of mental health can be grouped in five main domains: demographic, economic, life context, cultural, and environmental, which can influence the mental health of the population. The impact of structural and economic conditions on mental health has been highlighted by studies focused on poverty and income inequality [10], and on the different exposure to adverse life events—including humanitarian emergencies, war, or interpersonal violence [11, 12].

As recently highlighted by the WHO [13], a significant role is played by the environmental domain. In fact, climate change is associated with a heightened risk of environmental disasters, such as floods, fires, hurricanes, thus affecting the mental health and general well-being of the population. In particular, the Intergovernmental Panel on Climate Change (IPCC) has documented an association between recent climate changes and increased levels of anxiety, depression, insomnia, and suicidal behavior [14]. The impact of climate change on the mental health of the general population is mediated by several factors such as age, gender, educational level, and socioeconomic status. Furthermore, the association between some climate changes and some mental disorders, such as seasonal affective disorders, is well established since decades.

Recent studies carried out in different countries have documented that environmental pollutants and global warming are predictive factors of increased access to emergency room for mental health problems [15–19].

All nongenetic factors, including infections, childhood maltreatment and neglect, cannabis use, alcohol, smoking, bullying, and air, water, and soil pollution, can make the genome more "instable," modifying its structure [20]. Thus, the environment would "trigger" complex and specific cellular pathways that, through epigenetic modification, can become transmissible from one generation to another [20–27].

The concept that environmental factors, to which each of us is involuntarily exposed, represent a negligible risk today is outdated, particularly in light of growing incidence of cancer and schizophrenia in children and adolescents. Thus, there is the need for an integrated and multilevel approach, which integrates politics, health education, and an efficient health system.

2.7 The Biopsychosocial Model and Its Implications for Ordinary Clinical Practice

The predisposing, precipitating, perpetuating and protective factors (defined as "4Ps") of the revised biopsychosocial model include different factors reported in (Table 2.1). Predisposing factors are areas of vulnerability that increase the risk for the presenting problem. Examples include genetic (i.e., family history) predisposition for mental disorders or prenatal exposure to alcohol. Precipitating factors are considered as stressful events (that could be either positive or negative) that may be precipitants of the symptoms. Examples include conflicts about identity, relationship conflicts, or transitions. Perpetuating factors are any conditions in the patient, family, community, or larger systems that exacerbate rather than solve the problem. Examples include relationship conflicts, lack of education, financial and occupation stress (or lack of employment). Protective factors include the patient's own areas of competency, skill, talents, interest, and supportive elements. Protective factors counterbalance the predisposing, precipitating, and perpetuating factors.

It can be useful to develop a formulation table, in order to identify all factors occurring in the specific case of the individual patient. It is important to consider that not all boxes must be filled in, since many factors can act both as precipitating and perpetuating factors.

Table 2.1 Biopsychosocial model of mental disorders and 4Ps model

	Biological	Psychological	Social
Predisposing	• Temperament • Personality characteristics • Family history • Perinatal problems • Neurodevelopmental history	• Attachment style • Cognitive style • Self-esteem	• Poverty • Low socioeconomic status • Early traumatic events • Migration • Discrimination • Racism
Precipitating	• Serious medical illness or injury • Use of alcohol or drugs • Medication non-adherence	• Attachment style • Cognitive style • Self-esteem	• Loss/separation from family member • Interpersonal trauma • Work/academic/financial stressors • Recent immigration, loss of home
Perpetuating	• Serious medical illness or injury • Use of alcohol or drugs • Medication non-adherence	• Attachment style • Cognitive style • Self-esteem	• Loss/separation from family member • Interpersonal trauma • Work/academic/financial stressors • Recent immigration, loss of home
Protective	• Good overall health • Absence of family history • No substance use	• Positive sense of self • Adaptive coping mechanisms • Good coping skills	• Positive relationships • Supportive community • Religious/spiritual beliefs • Good interpersonal supports • Financial/disability support

Based on [28]

2.8 Conclusions

The WHO report "World Mental Health Report: Transforming Mental Health for All" highlights the need for all countries to achieve meaningful progress toward better mental health for their populations by focusing on deepening the value given to mental health, improve the physical, social, and economic characteristics of environments, and strengthen mental health care so that the full spectrum of mental health needs is met through a community-based network of accessible, affordable, and quality services and supports. The revised biopsychosocial model seems more aligned with the recent findings coming from mental health research and practice and may represent the basis for a full and granular understanding of the most severe mental disorders [29–31].

References

1. Cicchetti D, Doyle C (2016) Child maltreatment, attachment and psychopathology: mediating relations. World Psychiatry 15(2):89–90
2. Zubin J, Spring B (1977). Vulnerability: A new view of schizophrenia. J Abnor Psychol. 86(2):103–126.
3. Weir K (2012) The roots of mental illness. How much of mental illness can the biology of the brain explain? APA's Monitor Psychol 43(6):30
4. Bolton D, Gillett G (2019) The biopsychosocial model of health and disease: new philosophical and scientific developments [Internet]. Palgrave Pivot, Cham. PMID: 31886965
5. Maj M (2016) The need for a conceptual framework in psychiatry acknowledging complexity while avoiding defeatism. World Psychiatry 15:1–2
6. Uher R, Zwicker A (2017) Etiology in psychiatry: embracing the reality of poly-gene-environmental causation of mental illness. World Psychiatry

16(2):121–129. https://doi.org/10.1002/wps.20436. PMID: 28498595; PMCID: PMC5428165
7. Fiorillo A, Giordano A (2022) The biopsychosocial model of schizophrenia and cancer: unraveling the etiopathogenesis of complex diseases. Eur Psychiatry 65(1):e86
8. Brainstorm Consortium (2018) Analysis of shared heritability in common disorders of the brain. Science 360(6395):eaap8757
9. Taylor MJ, Martin J, Lu Y, Brikell I, Lundström S, Larsson H, Lichtenstein P (2019) Association of genetic risk factors for psychiatric disorders and traits of these disorders in a Swedish population twin sample. JAMA Psychiatry 76(3):280–289
10. Reuben A, Manczak EM, Cabrera LY, Alegria M, Bucher ML, Freeman EC, Miller GW, Solomon GM, Perry MJ (2022) The interplay of environmental exposures and mental health: setting an agenda. Environ Health Perspect 130(2):25001
11. Howard LM, Wilson CA, Chandra PS (2022) Intimate partner violence and mental health: lessons from the COVID-19 pandemic. World Psychiatry 21(2):311–313
12. Micklitz HM, Glass CM, Bengel J, Sander LB (2023) Efficacy of psychosocial interventions for survivors of intimate partner violence: a systematic review and meta-analysis. Trauma Violence Abuse 6:15248380231169481
13. WHO (2022) Mental health and climate change: policy brief. June 2022.
14. Intergovernmental Panel on Climate Change, report March 2023. https://www.ipcc.ch/report/ar6/syr/
15. Bernardini F, Attademo L, Trezzi R, Gobbicchi C, Balducci PM, Del Bello V, Menculini G, Pauselli L, Piselli M, Sciarma T, Moretti P, Tamantini A, Quartesan R, Compton MT, Tortorella A (2019) Air pollutants and daily number of admissions to psychiatric emergency services: evidence for detrimental mental health effects of ozone. Epidemiol Psychiatr Sci 29:e66
16. Cherry KE, Miller LR, Bordes PJ, Calamia MR, Elliott EM, Sampson L, Galea S (2023) Longitudinal assessment of mental health after a flood: roles of social support, hope, recovery stressors, and prior lifetime trauma. Aging Ment Health 30:1–11
17. Rothschild J, Haase E (2023) Women's mental health and climate change Part II: socioeconomic stresses of climate change and eco-anxiety for women and their children. Int J Gynaecol Obstet 160(2):414–420
18. Tortorella A, Menculini G, Moretti P, Attademo L, Balducci PM, Bernardini F, Cirimbilli F, Chieppa AG, Ghiandai N, Erfurth A (2022) New determinants of mental health: the role of noise pollution. A narrative review. Int Rev Psychiatry 34(7–8):783–796
19. Vergunst F, Berry HL, Minor K, Chadi N (2022) Climate change and substance-use behaviors: a risk-pathways framework. Perspect Psychol Sci 28:17456916221132739
20. Silove D, Ventevogel P (2022) Living through interminable adversity: the mental health of the Afghan people. World Psychiatry 21(1):55–56
21. Cianconi P, Betrò S, Janiri L (2020) The impact of climate change on mental health: a systematic descriptive review. Front Psychiatry 11:74
22. De Rosa C, Sampogna G, Luciano M, Del Vecchio V, Fabrazzo M, Fiorillo A (2018) Social versus biological psychiatry: it's time for integration! Int J Soc Psychiatry 64(7):617–621
23. Engel GL (1960) A unified concept of health and disease. Perspect Biol Med 3:459–485
24. Engel GL (1978) The biopsychosocial model and the education of health professionals. Ann NY Acad Sci 310:169–187
25. Engel GL (1977) The need for a new medical model: a challenge for biomedicine. Science 196:129–136
26. Fiorillo A, Maj M (2018) The role of psychiatry in modern medicine. Int Rev Psychiatry 30(2):169–175
27. Fiorillo A (2019) The complexity of vulnerability to psychosis. Epidemiol Psychiatr Sci 28(2):138–139
28. Sampogna G, Luciano M, Fiorillo A (2023) The psychiatric formulation. In: Tasman A et al (eds) Tasman's psychiatry. Springer, Cham. https://doi.org/10.1007/978-3-030-42825-9_120-1
29. Fried EI, Robinaugh DJ (2020) Systems all the way down: embracing complexity in mental health research. BMC Med 18(1):205
30. Heinz A, Liu S (2022) Challenges and chances for mental health care in the 21st century. World Psychiatry 21(3):423–424. https://doi.org/10.1002/wps.21006. PMID: 36073712; PMCID: PMC9453898
31. Sampogna G, Luciano M, Del Vecchio V, Giallonardo V, Pocai B, Fiorillo A (2020) Unmet needs in modern psychiatric practice. In: Pompili M, Fiorillo A, McIntyre R, Sartorius N (eds) New directions in psychiatry. Springer, pp 1–13

3 How Social Determinants of Mental Health Influence Clinical Dimensions of Mental Disorders

Chiara Alessandra Capogrosso,
Riccardo Matteo Cioni, Cristina Crocamo,
Francesco Bartoli, and Giuseppe Carrà

Abstract

Social determinants of health have been examined for several years in many fields of medicine. The importance of considering these factors when discussing mental health is indisputable, as the role of environmental interference cannot and must not be minimised. This chapter aims to provide an overview of the social determinants of mental health, making a distinction between *individual-level* and *area-level* determinants. From a public health standpoint, it seems increasingly important to distinguish between factors acting on a personal level and those acting on areas. Indeed, this makes it possible to better understand how the pressures exerted by certain factors are distributed, in a more or less targeted manner, throughout society, influencing different clinical domains. In order to provide a comprehensive approach, we will address transversal dimensions of psychiatric disorders, such as *aggressivity*, *suicide*, *psychosocial functioning* and *loneliness*. These dimensions are represented to varying degrees in the large spectrum of mental disorders, reflecting the multifaceted nature of this field and aiming to provide an alternative point of view to standard nosology.

Keywords

Area-level social determinants of mental health · Individual-level social determinants of mental health · Aggressivity · Suicide
Social functioning · Loneliness

3.1 Introduction

When assessing mental health issues, the experienced clinicians collect information on the individual's personal history, family history and social conditions that may have had an impact on his health. Assuming what impact catastrophic events—such as the coronavirus disease-2019 (COVID-19) pandemic, or the migration journey from war-torn countries, or the natural calamities driven by climate change—might have on mental health is rather obvious, whereas more proximate factors tend to be less valued, although they are

C. A. Capogrosso · R. M. Cioni · C. Crocamo
F. Bartoli
Department of Medicine and Surgery, University of Milano-Bicocca, Monza, Italy
e-mail: c.capogrosso@campus.unimib.it; r.cioni1@campus.unimib.it; cristina.crocamo@unimib.it; francesco.bartoli@unimib.it

G. Carrà (✉)
Department of Medicine and Surgery, University of Milano-Bicocca, Monza, Italy

Division of Psychiatry, University College London, London, UK
e-mail: giuseppe.carra@unimib.it

A. Fiorillo, S. De Giorgi (eds.), *Social Determinants of Mental Health*, Sustainable Development Goals Series, https://doi.org/10.1007/978-3-031-70165-8_3

more common and relatable. Since medical research is adopting a preventative approach, the social determinants-i.e. the conditions in which people are born, grow, work, live and age, and the wider set of forces and systems shaping the conditions of daily life-have acquired a pivotal role in their association with mental health. These forces include social, economic, cultural, environmental, political factors and phenomena that shape health-related behaviours as well as physical and mental health outcomes [1].

Structural determinants may be defined as those that drive the distribution of power, money, and resources in society. This policy-makers level includes economic policies such as welfare state, employment facilities, income support, social security, and education. A review of these determinants has shown a reduction of mental health inequalities in more comprehensive and gender inclusive welfare states [2]. Stakeholders should try to minimise these inequalities: differences in gender, ethnicity, income, and education confer advantage to some and disadvantage to others, even in the distribution of mental disorders.

It is inherent in the definition of social determinants that the influence that environmental factors can have over time is highly variable. A number of social determinants present in childhood and adolescence can heighten the risk of mental disorders throughout the life of the individual. These social determinants include area-level ones, such as growing up in certain neighbourhoods, housing conditions, and education, and individual ones, such as being a victim of neglect, abuse, or having a parent with a mental illness, or who misuses substances, or who has criminal behaviours [3]. Social determinants, such as housing and urbanisation, being related to the social functioning clinical dimension, become relevant for the older population group [4].

Priority needs, fundamental necessities of individuals, such as food, water, and healthcare, are usually given for granted, but inequalities around the world make them a relevant subject for research during catastrophic events or in both low-income and high-income countries (e.g., where privatised healthcare systems are present). These basic and essential factors have long been studied as drivers of mental well-being, since their unstable provision is correlated to depression and anxiety [5].

Data on the way social determinants specifically alter clinical dimensions of disease are hard to synthesise and analyse due to the great number of correlated variables and factors. However, the two main mental disorder classification systems have embraced the role of social determinants in their current versions in the attempt of integrating them into daily clinical psychiatric practice.

The latest version of the *Diagnostic and Statistical Manual* (DSM-5-TR) includes paragraphs on sex, gender, and cultural factors associated with each disorder [6]. However, structural and social determinants of health are not clearly explained and still have no place in the DSM. Furthermore, the DSM addresses social determinants in a heterogeneous way, letting one believe that they may be relevant only for some disorders [7].

The International Classification of Diseases (ICD) instead has included a number of non-diagnostic codes to describe a large number of circumstances or problems that influence health, including employment, homelessness, and other psychosocial conditions, in the attempt of including social determinants of the disease in the coding system of diagnoses in a concise yet clear way [8]. However, such codes are rarely used in everyday practice making them an important if only formal addition to the ICD [9].

Although established, the causal relationship between mental disorders and social determinants is far from being clear. Nonetheless, increasing evidence sheds light on the significant interaction between genetics and environment in pushing psychopathological symptoms over the threshold of psychiatric diagnoses, while the stress response of the hypothalamic-pituitary-adrenal (HPA) axis and the immune system have been shown to play a role in mediating social factors and the development of psychiatric disorders [10]. The relationship between social adversity and mental health problems appears bidirectional: social adversity increases the risk of poor mental health and having mental health issues increases the risk of poor social circumstances and limited social connections [11]. Severe mental illness is a significant social and economic burden for patients, their families and the whole society, thus confronting and treating it can induce a virtuous cycle that will both reduce the mental disorder's strain on individuals and have a positive impact on communities as a whole [12].

3.2 Social Determinants: Individual Level and Area Level

Social determinants can be divided into individual-level and area-level ones. While area-level social determinants include all those factors related to the social, cultural and economic context in which an individual is raised and lives, individual ones refer to the specific history of the person's life [13].

3.2.1 Individual-Level Social Determinants of Mental Health

3.2.1.1 Gender

Gender refers to socially constructed characteristics of women and men. As a social construct in each culture, society and era, genders can acquire different meanings and different characteristics transforming norms, behaviours, roles associated with each one as well as relationships with each other. Gender differences in mental disorders are apparent, although everyone, regardless of gender, can be affected by mental disorders. Such differences are shaped by biological factors and social influences. For example, common mental disorders, such as anxiety and depressive disorders, are more present among women than men [14]. Men, instead, show higher rates of substance misuse or suicide compared to women [15, 16], and are more susceptible to neurodevelopmental disorders [17]. In addition, gender inequality, the social processes whereby people are treated differently under similar circumstances on the basis of gender, may be at the root of gender differences also in mental health [18].

3.2.1.2 Ethnicity

Ethnicity is a complex social construct that influences identity and group social relationships. Ethnic identity and how ethnicities are classified are place-, time-, and context-specific [19]. Ethnicity is an individual social determinant that defines inequalities in mental healthcare since it is itself a differentiation and individualisation factor accompanied by group-specific cultural and social aspects. For example, black people often find it difficult to make their concerns heard: mistrust of mental health services generates reluctance to seek help among people of black ethnicity, but also exacerbates individuals' sense of vulnerability when services are accessed [20]. This may reflect unconscious biases both in staff and in individuals accessing services, especially considering that evidence has shown that people who grew up in a racist environment are more likely to develop a greater racial consciousness [21].

The stronger association between racism and mental health, compared with physical health, raises questions about the mechanisms by which racism affects health. Racism impacts health by reducing access to employment, housing and education, but it is also implicated in neuroendocrinological mechanisms, such as the hypothalamic-pituitary-adrenal (HPA) axis dysregulation that can negatively affect physical and mental health and that is implicated in the etiopathogenesis of psychotic disorders [22, 23]. From a neurobiological point of view, racism impacts on the imbalance of cognitive-affective brain regions, such as the prefrontal cortex, anterior cingulate cortex, amygdala and thalamus, replicating pathways that lead to anxiety, depression and psychosis [24].

3.2.1.3 Migration

Migration is a complex phenomenon that is becoming increasingly important due to the displacement of entire communities because of wars, genocides or natural catastrophes. In 2020, around 3–4% of the world population lived outside of their country of birth [25].

The terms migrants and refugees cannot be used interchangeably, since migrant is an umbrella term referring to anyone who moves away from their usual place of residence, whereas refugees are migrants who have left their countries due to a threat to their lives or freedom [26]. Any form of migration however can act as a social determinant of mental disorders in all its stages. Immigrants from certain regions may have been exposed to political instability, poverty, natural disaster, or other adverse social conditions that may have an impact on their health. The migration journey can be long and encompass various traumatic experiences, including torture. In the post-migratory stage, immigrants (especially non-white ones) frequently face racial discrimination, difficulties in finding and keeping employment and housing [27]. The relationship between migration and risk of schizophrenia is well established, and extends to children of migrants. In fact, a recent national cohort study performed by Dykxhoorn et al. [28] found that the risk of psychosis appears higher among visible minorities regardless of sex, age or socioeconomic status. Bipolar disorder instead has not been found to be higher in migrants but, with some instances, it has lower rates compared to the native population. Although there is not a large body of literature on the frequency of bipolar disorder among migrants, the findings concerning psychosis are largely replicated and it is therefore now assumed that migration-related exposures substantially increase the risk of schizophrenia spectrum disorders [28, 29]. With regard to the prevalence of common mental disorders among migrants, current evidence is conflicting and unclear, also due to the numerous factors that can negatively affect the psychic sphere (e.g. status of refugee or asylum seeker, lack of social support) [30–32].

3.2.1.4 Religious Affiliation

Ninety per cent of the world's population declares to be religious or spiritual [33]. Religion refers to an established tradition characterised by common beliefs and rituals concerning the sacred, whereas spirituality is a personal, less regulated or ritualised form of belief [33]. Although its role is still controversial and difficult to determine with an acceptable grade of certainty, recent studies suggest that spirituality and religious involvement may promote mental health due to the identification in a community, the use of supportive faith-based community networks, and by providing individuals with some form of goal or meaning in life. Thus, religious involvement has been associated with a better capacity in coping with stress, and an overall decrease in rates of depression, suicide, anxiety and substance abuse [34, 35].

3.2.1.5 Early Childhood Adverse Experiences and Trauma

Early childhood and adolescence are fundamental building blocks of a person's future well-being. Warm, responsive, nurturing environments, with protection from adverse experiences, ensure the best outcomes for children. Although parental love and attention greatly matter, family's income, education, housing and the neighbourhoods in which children live [36] are equally important in reducing the risk of mental disorders in later life.

Adverse conditions during childhood affect biological mechanisms that regulate stress responses and have lifelong impacts [37, 38]. A cross-sectional retrospective study comparing surveys from 21 countries found that adversities, such as childhood experiences of family dysfunction–parental mental illness, substance misuse, criminal behaviour, domestic violence, physical and sexual abuse, or neglect, tend to be interrelated and that they are associated with mental disorders at all stages of life [39]. Psychological traumas are likely to represent transdiagnostic factors across different diagnostic criteria and spectra, with highly suggestive evidence showing with any mental disorder [40].

As with other social determinants, the relationship with mental disorders and attempts at understanding causal pathways is extremely complex and would be better described as a vicious cycle instead of a linear relationship. Moreover, childhood adversity is associated with a number of other social determinants as mentioned above, including social isolation and poverty [41].

3.2.1.6 Housing

Poor housing conditions and unaffordable housing are associated with the risk of mental health problems. For example, improving housing conditions for those living in cold and damp homes reduces the likelihood of experiencing depression and anxiety [42]. A recent systematic review reported evidence from longitudinal studies further supporting the hypothesis that prior exposure to housing disadvantage is consistently associated with worse mental health, in particular depression. Housing is a key social determinant of mental health, and policy interventions directed at reducing housing disadvantage may achieve substantial mental health benefit [43]. A cross-sectional study looking at the interaction between housing quality, neighbourhood quality and psychological well-being in eight European cities found that both low-quality housing and low-quality neighbourhoods are associated with lower psychological well-being but living in a better-quality neighbourhood buffers the impact of living in low-quality housing on well-being [44]. A good-quality neighbourhood environment that encourages supportive neighbourly relationships and opportunities for psychological restoration benefits mental well-being.

Looking at fear of crime, in a longitudinal study in Great Britain, participants who were more fearful regarding crime were nearly twice as likely to have depression as those with lower fear of crime. They also were less likely to socialise and exercise [45], suggesting an association between fear of crime and depression, as both social and physical activities support mental health.

3.2.1.7 Income

Socio-economic status has also been proposed as an important correlate of both illicit drug use [46] and severe mental illnesses [47]. Poverty, even using basic measures like family income, increases the odds of both mental illnesses and substance use disorders [48]. In particular, income inequality seems a powerful driver of poor mental health, although the mechanisms underlying its impact, possibly involving stress due to social comparisons and loss of social capital, have led to heterogeneous findings [49]. Data from the National Survey on Drug Use and Health (NSDUH) in 2015 showed that women and people living in poverty were more likely to suffer from severe mental illnesses. In the US, poverty—family income under 100% of the federal threshold—was associated with concurrent severe mental illnesses and cannabis use, regardless of multiple clinical and socio-demographic characteristics [50].

The stress of having insufficient income to have a socially acceptable living standard creates adverse conditions for mental health also in the younger population. A recent umbrella review synthesised data on mental health of children and adolescents during COVID-19 pandemic, concluding that family financial constraints played an important role in determining poor mental health [51]. Indeed, children from low-income families are more at risk of mental health problems than their peers in better-off families [52].

3.2.1.8 Digital Environment

The technological advances of recent decades have led individuals to a paradigmatic shift in the way they interact with the world: the increase in the speed and breadth of knowledge turnover within the economy and society has made digital approaches essential to stay connected and engaged in mainstream culture.

Digitalisation may affect the traditional concept of social determinants of health. From a tech-influenced perspective, these can be translated as numbers of online friends, or as complex social biomarkers, such as timing, frequency, content, and patterns of posts and degree of interaction with online communities [53]. Focusing on mental health, Phan et al. [54] have recently showed that social cohesion is a major protective factor against moderate to severe depressive symptoms. The increase in Internet usage can socially distance peers and it can lead to more numerous exposures to cyberbullying, thus negatively affecting mental well-being [54]. On the other hand, technology has made everything traceable: in contrast with traditional bullying, cyberbullying may leave digital footprints that can be reported to family members, teachers, or other community members [54].

Although the importance of digital approaches—such as digital phenotyping and apps—is widely recognised in mental health [55], further studies on how the digital environment can alter social determinants are needed.

3.2.2 Area-Level Social Determinants of Mental Health

3.2.2.1 Deprivation

Deprivation refers to a general lack of resources and opportunities in the area in which an individual is raised, grows and lives. Different domains may concur in defining area-level deprivation: income deprivation; employment deprivation; health deprivation and disability; education, skills and training deprivation; barriers to housing and services; crime; and living environment deprivation. Area socio-economic deprivation increases the prevalence of common mental disorders in neighbourhood and regional levels [56]. Recently, Lee et al. [57] revisited aspects of the social drift and causation hypotheses by examining associations between increased risks of severe mental illnesses: acknowledging the higher prevalence and incidence of affective and non-affective psychoses among people living in more deprived areas was not any epidemiological evidence of downward social drift. With regard to addictions, the role of deprivation is still unclear: in fact, substance use disorder and gambling rates do not seem to be influenced by area-level disadvantage [58, 59].

3.2.2.2 Urbanisation

Urbanisation affects mental health through a combination of social, economic and environmental factors [60]. Currently, 55% of the world population resides in urban areas. By 2050, that percentage will be at least 68%, mostly in developing and emerging economies [61]. Green spaces may, according to some evidence, reduce stress and increase subjective well-being [62]. Sex, socio-economic position and types of exposures mediate the association between green space and mental health [63]. A number of explanations for the benign influence of urban green spaces on mental health have been proposed: increased physical activity, which is related to improvements in mood; increased sense of belonging, and opportunities for social interaction; and psychological restoration [64]. Furthermore, natural surroundings reduce stress markers, such as cortisol and blood pressure, compared to more unnatural urban environments possibly for evolutionary and physiological reasons, even if the exposure is limited to the individual's childhood [65, 66].

3.2.2.3 COVID-19 Pandemic

Coronavirus Disease-2019 (COVID-19) has been a global public health crisis in 2020. To prevent the severe acute respiratory syndrome coronavirus-2 (SARS-Cov-2) spread, many countries have required citizens who may have been exposed to the virus to self-isolate either at home or in professional quarantine facilities [67]. Restrictions and fear of contagion may have impacted the daily routine of people all over the world, generating uncertainty and negatively impacting psychological well-being. Great concern exists about the consequences of the pandemic, in terms of the short- and long-term impact on the mental health of both the general population and, particularly, of individuals already suffering from a psychiatric disease [68].

Several studies contributed to the effort of disentangling the relationship between COVID-19 pandemic and mental health. The meta-analysis by Dragioti et al. [69] estimated the increase in the prevalence rates of anxiety, depression, stress and sleep problems between 9% and 31%. Different subpopulations were found to be more vulnerable to psychiatric symptoms, such as pregnant women, healthcare workers, COVID-infected patients and their caregivers, and people with mental disorders, who were the most impacted groups in terms of anxious/depressive symptoms, stress, sleep problems and post-traumatic stress disorder (PTSD) [69, 70]. Data on severe mental illness are less clear. Indeed, the long-term effects of COVID-19 cannot be assessed through the analysis of surveys developed and distributed early in the pandemic. It is worth noting that even in the case of the COVID-19 pandemic, although it may be assessed as a single social determinant, the repercussions on the economy, the job market and the altered access to healthcare services have determined a variety of consequences that demonstrate the difficulty in assessing and understanding the entangled way in which social determinants influence mental disorders.

3.2.2.4 Air Pollution

The association between air pollution and mental disorders has been studied more and more extensively since 2021. Air pollution has been associated with a small but consistent increase in the rate of affective disorders, suicide and cognitive decline [71]. However, psychotic and anxiety disorders do not have significant evidence linking them to air pollutants. Its role in mental health may be mediated by a number of biological pathways, including oxidative stress reaction and neuroinflammation [72]. It has been reported that there are different knowledge gaps about bioaerosols exposure, indoor and outdoor pollution and urban design and their impact on mental health over the life course [73].

3.3 Clinical Dimensions

Social determinants' theoretical concept permeates health in all its declinations. There is a large body of evidence supporting the role of these factors both in severe and in common mental disorders. Nonetheless, disentangling the association between social determinants and widespread psychiatric dimensions may be of primary concern for everyday clinical practice. Transdiagnostic clinical dimensions are aspects of mental disorders that are assessed in a number of different severe mental illnesses. The association of some of these clinical dimensions with social determinants of mental health has been studied in a number of studies, warranting a broader assessment of the socio-ecological context in which the disorder was developed instead of focusing only on the affected individual. There are sufficient amounts of data on a few clinical dimensions associated with important behavioural consequences, such as aggressivity, suicide, psychosocial functioning and loneliness.

3.3.1 Aggressivity

From an epidemiological point of view, violence is a leading cause of mortality and morbidity [74]. Aggressivity is the quality of a person who commits verbal or physical acts that target other people, animals, or objects with the aim of causing harm. While sometimes the aggressors are not aware of the implications of their actions or the harm is coincidental, an instrumental or proactive aggression involves intentionally harming an individual to achieve a desired goal. In contrast, impulsive aggression is often referred to as hostile or reactive aggression that has no identifiable goal. In impulsive aggression, the perpetrator is driven by anger, and the act is an inconsiderate and unplanned response to perceived provocation [75].

Understanding the controversial relationship between psychiatric disorders and aggressive behaviour has proven particularly difficult, without mentioning the stigmatisation issues that such research quest entails [76].

As regards the correlation of social determinants of mental health and aggressivity, available data suggest that persons living with serious mental illness are at a modestly increased risk of committing violence [77] and several determinants, such as sex, age and socio-economic status, heighten the risk of aggressive behaviours [76]. Although a common clinical response to aggressivity is the use of pharmacological options, it would be unwise to not assess nonclinical variables, such as female sex, household composition, social interaction and lack of vocational or leisure activity. Thus, violence risk management must consider the individual in the context of his/her community and life context [78–80]. Being a perpetrator or a victim of aggressive behaviour has been shown in some populations to define a subgroup of people with a higher risk of psychiatric disorders and a higher association with economic disparities and other social determinants [81]. Overall, the association of social determinants as factors in aggressive behaviour in people with mental disorders is clear. This would let one presume that morbidity and mortality of aggressive behaviours enacted by people suffering from mental disorders could be reduced by a broader public health approach on social determinants, instead of an individualised pharmacotherapy.

3.3.2 Suicide

People with severe mental illness are at higher risk of suicide-related behaviours [82]. According to the World Health Organization, as reported elsewhere in this book, suicide is defined as the act of deliberately ending one's life, and it is considered a preventable form of premature death [83]. Suicide is associated with clearly established clinical risk factors, with a history of suicide attempts and suffering from a mood disorder being the most consistent ones [83, 84]. However, social determinants are also associated with suicide. Social isolation, for example, is a complex phenomenon that has been associated with an increased risk of suicide, while social support has been hypothesised as a possible protective factor [85]. Obviously, a bidirectional relationship between mental disorders and social isolation makes interventions on this problem complex. In a study performed by Hu et al. [86], a social support intervention proved effective in preventing suicidal behaviours, especially in females and adults, confirming Moutillon-Toudic's findings.

Additional evidence has shown that people suffering from major depressive disorder who had suicidal behaviours compared to ones without suicidal behaviours had a higher correlation with work loss [87]. This may highlight the association with work instability and suicidal behaviours in people with severe mental illness. A clear association between suicide and financial stressors, including loss of income, bankruptcy and loss of job or retirement, was not found in a large prospective cohort study by Yu et al. [82]. Rural residence and male sex were instead correlated with a higher risk of suicide.

In a cohort of veterans, comparing participants who committed suicide and matched controls, a number of social determinants extracted through natural language processing showed an association between suicide and social isolation, job or financial insecurity, housing instability, legal problems, violence, barriers to care, transition of care and food insecurity [88].

3.3.3 Psychosocial Functioning

Functioning can be defined as the psychological capacity to cope and carry on with the day-to-day activities that a person finds meaningful and necessary, such as work, studies, leisure time and hobbies, self-care and care for others. This capacity is commonly assessed in psychiatric practice since its disruption is considered fundamental in the diagnosis of many mental disorders. Understanding the correlation between mental health, social determinants and functioning is a complex task due to their interconnectedness. Furthermore, functioning can have a significant degree of variation in chronic disorders such as schizophrenia and bipolar disorder.

Some studies have shown that a degree of pervasive and persistent deficit in functioning is present even in individuals whose symptoms went into remission [89], and that social and occupational adjustment problems persist in individuals suffering from bipolar disorder even if they do not manifest inter-episode symptoms [90].

Fenn et al. [91], when assessing functioning in bipolar disorder, concluded that the presence of depressive symptoms was the only consistently reported clinical predictor of social adjustment, so surprisingly socio-demographic factors were more important than clinical ones in determining deficits in functioning. Unsurprisingly, living with a significant other raises opportunity to engage in a spectrum of social activities and to have a richer social life [92].

With respect to schizophrenia spectrum disorder, a socio-developmental model has been hypothesised to integrate biological findings with the evidence on the social factors that heighten the risk of psychosis development [93]. This model describes how social adversity has a bidirectional effect on dopamine production in certain brain areas leading to the development of psychotic symptoms. As regards employment, a number of interventions have been developed and used to help people with severe mental illnesses to get and keep a job [94]. This has been shown to be particularly significant due to the overall improvement of quality of life in people with severe mental illnesses who were employed in a stable way [95]. Employment, other than being satisfactory in and of itself, is an assured way for people with severe mental illness to maintain social connectedness and reduce isolation and social retreat, especially in a culture where social disconnectedness has reached high levels and in the United States has been compared to heart disease and cancer [96].

3.3.4 Loneliness

Loneliness can be defined as a complex set of feelings derived from the absence of satisfaction of intimate and social needs [97]. It refers to the subjective aspects of social isolation. In fact, socially isolated individuals may not feel lonely, and vice versa, being social isolation as the objective portrayal of a social situation characterised by poor social ties [85]. In terms of mental health, loneliness and social isolation are not just strongly correlated with depression [98], but can increase vulnerability to developing future depressive episodes [99, 100]. It is important to distinguish social disconnection from loneliness. Social disconnection is based on the objective quantity of the interactions. Thus, people may feel lonely even when surrounded by friends and family. Social disconnection refers to an objective, long-standing lack of social/family relationships and minimal participation in social/family activities [101]. Taken together, loneliness has been a significant and growing concern for a number of years [102]; however, it is now being more widely recognised as a critical public health issue with the arrival and continued impact of the COVID-19 pandemic [103]. The role of social determinants on loneliness has been widely investigated. A study conducted during the COVID-19 pandemic in Canada showed that individuals from lower-income households, those living alone or with their parents, and young females experienced higher anxiety and depression scores, and greater loneliness [104]. In fact, loneliness was significantly higher for those with an annual income <$50,000/year compared with an income category of >$50,000/year. As expected, and in line with other studies during the pandemic [105], respondents living alone had higher levels of loneliness than those living with other family members and/or with a spouse. Unexpectedly, individuals living with their parents displayed similarly high levels of loneliness as those living alone. During COVID-19, younger age was associated with higher loneliness, depression and anxiety symptoms. While extensive literature exists regarding loneliness among older adults [106], loneliness might actually be a larger problem in younger adults, as feelings of loneliness can stabilise or decline with increased age [107].

3.4 Conclusions

As discussed, there is abundant evidence on the correlation between social determinants and mental disorders. Unfortunately, social determinants have a peripheral meaning in daily psychiatric practice, while they take centre-stage in social psychiatry research settings. Nonetheless, numerous community-mental health strategies have been shown to effectively act in helping individuals with mental disorders in non-pharmacological ways addressing social aspects of disease [108]. This should not be seen only in a preventative way, since social determinants do not only 'determine' risk of developing mental disorders, but also continually determine a worse prognosis, heighten risk of relapse and act, as long as they are present, in worsening outcomes of mental disorders [109].

The recognition and evaluation of social determinants cannot be disregarded: research should focus on more balanced use of different types of assessments, i.e. self-report-based, informant report-based, objective and community-based [110]. Keeping in mind the division between area-level and individual-level social determinants, individual-level ones may be easier to assess and alter in psychiatric practice.

Interventions implemented by governments consist of various policies that promote well-being and address key social determinants, such as poverty, racism, discrimination, food insecurity, lack of housing and unemployment. The use of these interventions, of course, is deeply connected to political leanings and historical aspects of the country in which they are developed or implemented. Supported employment interventions for individuals with severe mental illness or housing interventions are a way of tackling mental disease by considering social determinants and their effects in a more individualised way. Furthermore, better access to healthcare, programmes for early psychosis intervention and services addressing homelessness, criminal justice, global mental health and mental health promotion and prevention have all demonstrated efficacy in reducing the burden of social determinants on mental health [10].

Social determinants should not be viewed as individual patient's vulnerabilities but as structural inequalities of the social and economic context in which we live. Thus, research and awareness on social determinants of health should not lead the physician towards giving for granted a worse prognosis in patients with a problematic economic and social background, but rather provide a broader scope in which to view the mental health of each of us.

The evidence on social determinants reminds us of the multifaceted nature of mental disorders, and that only through the integration of social, psychological and biological perspectives of mental health we can lessen the burden of severe mental illness in the future. The importance of education, employment and racial discrimination, to name just a few, on the development of severe mental illness proves once more the importance of developing ways to build networks with teachers, police officers, employers, and other non-medical professionals who may provide support to the individual and improve the prognosis of mental disorders [34].

Acknowledgements None.

Competing Interests The authors have no conflicts of interest to declare that are relevant to the content of this chapter.

References

1. Marmot M (2005) Social determinants of health inequalities. Lancet 365(9464):1099–1104. https://doi.org/10.1016/S0140-6736(05)71146-6
2. McAllister A, Fritzell S, Almroth M, Harber-Aschan L, Larsson S, Burström B (2018) How do macro-level structural determinants affect inequalities in mental health?—a systematic review of the literature. Int J Equity Health 17(1):180. https://doi.org/10.1186/s12939-018-0879-9
3. Cotton NK, Shim RS (2022) Social determinants of health, structural racism, and the impact on child and adolescent mental health. J Am Acad Child Adolesc Psychiatry 61(11):1385–1389. https://doi.org/10.1016/j.jaac.2022.04.020
4. Zheng Z, Chen H (2020) Age sequences of the elderly' social network and its efficacies on well-being: an urban-rural comparison in China. BMC Geriatr 20(1):372. https://doi.org/10.1186/s12877-020-01773-8
5. Alegría M, Zhen-Duan J, O'Malley IS, DiMarzio K (2022) A new agenda for optimizing investments in community mental health and reducing disparities. Am J Psychiatry 179(6):402–416. https://doi.org/10.1176/appi.ajp.21100970
6. American Psychiatric Association (2022) Diagnostic and statistical manual of mental disorders: DSM-5-TR (fifth edition, text revision). American Psychiatric Association Publishing, Arlington, WA
7. Aggarwal NK (2023) Improving the integration of social determinants of mental health in the DSMs. JAMA Psychiatry 80(9):865–866. https://doi.org/10.1001/jamapsychiatry.2023.1301
8. World Health Organization (2019) International classification of diseases. Eleventh Revision (ICD-

11). https://icd.who.int/browse11. Accessed 31 Oct 2023
9. Kinderman P, Allsopp K, Zero R, Handerer F, Tai S (2023) Minimal use of ICD social determinant or phenomenological codes in mental health care records. J Ment Health 32(1):216–225. https://doi.org/10.1080/09638237.2021.1952944
10. Alegría M, Alvarez K, Cheng M, Falgas-Bague I (2023) Recent advances on social determinants of mental health: looking fast forward. Am J Psychiatry 180(7):473–482. https://doi.org/10.1176/appi.ajp.20230371
11. Johnson S (2017) Social interventions in mental health: a call to action. Soc Psychiatry Psychiatr Epidemiol 52(3):245–247. https://doi.org/10.1007/s00127-017-1360-6
12. Thornicroft G (2011) European mental health policy: the key issue is social inclusion. Eur J Public Health 21:548–549. https://doi.org/10.1093/eurpub/ckr123
13. Jeste DV, Pender VB (2022) Social determinants of mental health: recommendations for research, training, practice, and policy. JAMA Psychiatry 79(4):283–284. https://doi.org/10.1001/jamapsychiatry.2021.4385
14. Yeretzian ST, Sahakyan Y, Kozloff N, Abrahamyan L (2023) Sex differences in the prevalence and factors associated with anxiety disorders in Canada: a population-based study. J Psychiatr Res 164:125–132. https://doi.org/10.1016/j.jpsychires.2023.06.018
15. Hedegaard H, Curtin SC, Warner M (2018) Suicide rates in the United States continue to increase. NCHS Data Brief 309:1–8
16. Office of Disease Prevention and Health Promotion (2019) Drug and alcohol use. In: Healthy people 2030. US Department of Health and Human Services, Washington, DC. https://health.gov/healthypeople/objectives-and-data/browse-objectives/drug-and-alcohol-use/reduce-proportion-adults-who-used-drugs-past-month-su-07/data?group=Sex&from=2018&to=2019&state=United%20States&populations=#edit-submit. Accessed 31 Oct 2023
17. Affleck W, Carmichael V, Whitley R (2018) Men's mental health: social determinants and implications for services. Can J Psychiatry 63(9):581–589. https://doi.org/10.1177/0706743718762388
18. Otten D, Tibubos AN, Schomerus G, Brähler E, Binder H, Kruse J et al (2021) Similarities and differences of mental health in women and men: a systematic review of findings in three large German cohorts. Front Public Health 9:553071. https://doi.org/10.3389/fpubh.2021.553071
19. Ford ME, Kelly PA (2005) Conceptualizing and categorizing race and ethnicity in health services research. Health Serv Res 40(5 Pt 2):1658–1675. https://doi.org/10.1111/j.1475-6773.2005.00449.x
20. Lawrence V, McCombie C, Nikolakopoulos G, Morgan C (2021) Ethnicity and power in the mental health system: experiences of white British and black Caribbean people with psychosis. Epidemiol Psychiatr Sci 30:e12. https://doi.org/10.1017/S2045796020001043
21. Cénat JM, Farahi SMMM, Dalexis RD (2023) Prevalence and determinants of depression, anxiety, and stress symptoms among black individuals in Canada in the context of the COVID-19 pandemic. Psychiatry Res 326:115341. https://doi.org/10.1016/j.psychres.2023.115341
22. Cavaleri D, Capogrosso CA, Guzzi P, Bernasconi G, Re M, Misiak B et al (2023) Blood concentrations of anterior pituitary hormones in drug-naïve people with first-episode psychosis: a systematic review and meta-analysis. Psychoneuroendocrinology 158:106392. https://doi.org/10.1016/j.psyneuen.2023.106392
23. Paradies Y, Ben J, Denson N, Elias A, Priest N, Pieterse A, Gupta A, Kelaher M, Gee G (2015) Racism as a determinant of health: a systematic review and meta-analysis. PLoS One 10(9):e0138511. https://doi.org/10.1371/journal.pone.0138511
24. Berger M, Sarnyai Z (2015) More than skin deep: stress neurobiology and mental health consequences of racial discrimination. Stress 18(1):1–10. https://doi.org/10.3109/10253890.2014.989204
25. McAuliffe M, Triandafyllidou A (2021) World migration report 2022. International Organization for Migration. https://worldmigrationreport.iom.int/wmr-2022-interactive/. Accessed 31 Oct 2023
26. United Nations High Commissioner for Refugees (2019) Migrant definition. In: Emergency handbook. https://emergency.unhcr.org/protection/legal-framework/migrant-definition. Accessed 31 Oct 2023
27. Whitley R, Wang J, Fleury MJ, Liu A, Caron J (2017) Mental health status, health care utilisation, and service satisfaction among immigrants in Montreal: an epidemiological comparison. Can J Psychiatry 62(8):570–579. https://doi.org/10.1177/0706743716677724
28. Dykxhoorn J, Hollander AC, Lewis G, Magnusson C, Dalman C, Kirkbride JB (2019) Risk of schizophrenia, schizoaffective, and bipolar disorders by migrant status, region of origin, and age-at-migration: a national cohort study of 1.8 million people. Psychol Med 49(14):2354–2363. https://doi.org/10.1017/S0033291718003227
29. Cantor-Graae E, Pedersen CB (2013) Full spectrum of psychiatric disorders related to foreign migration: a Danish population-based cohort study. JAMA Psychiatry 70(4):427–435. https://doi.org/10.1001/jamapsychiatry.2013.441
30. Hasan SI, Yee A, Rinaldi A, Azham AA, Mohd Hairi F, Amer Nordin AS (2021) Prevalence of com-

mon mental health issues among migrant workers: a systematic review and meta-analysis. PLoS One 16(12):e0260221. https://doi.org/10.1371/journal.pone.0260221
31. Patanè M, Ghane S, Karyotaki E, Cuijpers P, Schoonmade L, Tarsitani L et al (2022) Prevalence of mental disorders in refugees and asylum seekers: a systematic review and meta-analysis. Glob Ment Health (Camb) 9:250–263. https://doi.org/10.1017/gmh.2022.29
32. Swinnen SG, Selten JP (2007) Mood disorders and migration: meta-analysis. Br J Psychiatry 190:6–10. https://doi.org/10.1192/bjp.bp.105.020800
33. Koenig HG (2009) Research on religion, spirituality, and mental health: a review. Can J Psychiatry 54(5):283–291. https://doi.org/10.1177/070674370905400502
34. Carrà G, Bartoli F, Canestro A, Capogrosso CA, Bebbington PE, Crocamo C (2023) Influence of intrinsic and extrinsic religiosity on youth cannabis use: a structural equation modelling analysis on national survey on drug use and health (NSDUH) 2015–2019. J Psychiatr Res 166:178–185. https://doi.org/10.1016/j.jpsychires.2023.09.016
35. Hodapp B, Zwingmann C (2019) Religiosity/spirituality and mental health: a meta-analysis of studies from the German-speaking area. J Relig Health 58(6):1970–1998. https://doi.org/10.1007/s10943-019-00759-0
36. Pillas D, Marmot M, Naicker K, Goldblatt P, Morrison J, Pikhart H (2014) Social inequalities in early childhood health and development: a European-wide systematic review. Pediatr Res 76(5):418–424. https://doi.org/10.1038/pr.2014.122
37. Shonkoff JP, Garner AS (2012) Committee on psychosocial aspects of child and family health; committee on early childhood, adoption, and dependent care; section on developmental and behavioral pediatrics. The lifelong effects of early childhood adversity and toxic stress. Pediatrics 129(1):e232–e246. https://doi.org/10.1542/peds.2011-2663
38. Taylor SE (2010) Mechanisms linking early life stress to adult health outcomes. Proc Natl Acad Sci U S A 107(19):8507–8512. https://doi.org/10.1073/pnas.1003890107
39. Kessler RC, McLaughlin KA, Green JG, Gruber MJ, Sampson NA, Zaslavsky AM et al (2010) Childhood adversities and adult psychopathology in the WHO world mental health surveys. Br J Psychiatry 197(5):378–385. https://doi.org/10.1192/bjp.bp.110.080499
40. Hogg B, Gardoki-Souto I, Valiente-Gómez A, Rosa AR, Fortea L, Radua J et al (2023) Psychological trauma as a transdiagnostic risk factor for mental disorder: an umbrella meta-analysis. Eur Arch Psychiatry Clin Neurosci 273(2):397–410. https://doi.org/10.1007/s00406-022-01495-5
41. Allen SF, Gilbody S, Atkin K, van der Feltz-Cornelis CM (2023) The associations among childhood trauma, loneliness, mental health symptoms, and indicators of social exclusion in adulthood: a UK Biobank Study. Brain Behav 13(4):e2959. https://doi.org/10.1002/brb3.2959
42. Public Health England, Institute of Health Equity (2014) Local action on health inequalities: fuel poverty and cold home-related health problems. https://www.instituteofhealthequity.org/resources-reports/local-action-on-health-inequalities-fuel-poverty-and-cold-home-related-health-problems. Accessed 31 Oct 2023
43. Singh A, Daniel L, Baker E, Bentley R (2019) Housing disadvantage and poor mental health: a systematic review. Am J Prev Med 57(2):262–272. https://doi.org/10.1016/j.amepre.2019.03.018
44. Jones-Rounds ML, Evans GW, Braubach M (2014) The interactive effects of housing and neighbourhood quality on psychological well-being. J Epidemiol Community Health 68(2):171–175. https://doi.org/10.1136/jech-2013-202431
45. Stafford M, Chandola T, Marmot M (2007) Association between fear of crime and mental health and physical functioning. Am J Public Health 97(11):2076–2081. https://doi.org/10.2105/AJPH.2006.097154
46. Williams CT, Latkin CA (2007) Neighborhood socioeconomic status, personal network attributes, and use of heroin and cocaine. Am J Prev Med 32:S203–S210. https://doi.org/10.1016/j.amepre.2007.02.006
47. Walker ER, Druss BG (2017) Cumulative burden of comorbid mental disorders, substance use disorders, chronic medical conditions, and poverty on health among adults in the U.S.A. Psychol Health Med 22(6):727–735. https://doi.org/10.1080/13548506.2016.1227855
48. Lund C (2014) Poverty and mental health: towards a research agenda for low and middle-income countries. Commentary on Tampubolon and Hanandita (2014). Soc Sci Med 111:134–136. https://doi.org/10.1016/j.socscimed.2014.04.010
49. Burns J (2015) Poverty, inequality and a political economy of mental health. Epidemiol Psychiatr Sci 24(2):107–113. https://doi.org/10.1017/S2045796015000086
50. Carrà G, Bartoli F, Riboldi I, Trotta G, Crocamo C (2018) Poverty matters: cannabis use among people with serious mental illness: findings from the United States survey on drug use and health, 2015. Int J Soc Psychiatry 64(7):656–659. https://doi.org/10.1177/0020764018795213
51. Hossain MM, Nesa F, Das J, Aggad R, Tasnim S, Bairwa M et al (2022) Global burden of mental health problems among children and adolescents during COVID-19 pandemic: an umbrella review. Psychiatry Res 317:114814. https://doi.org/10.1016/j.psychres.2022.114814
52. Pickett KE, Wilkinson RG (2007) Child wellbeing and income inequality in rich societies: ecological cross sectional study. BMJ 335(7629):1080. https://doi.org/10.1136/bmj.39377.580162.55
53. Abnousi F, Rumsfeld JS, Krumholz HM (2019) Social determinants of health in the digital

age: determining the source code for nurture. JAMA 321(3):247–248. https://doi.org/10.1001/jama.2018.19763
54. Phan TC, Chau B, Do HN, Vu TBT, Vu KL, Nguyen HD et al (2022) Determinants of mental health among youths and adolescents in the digital era: roles of cyber and traditional bullying, violence, loneliness, and environment factors. Front Public Health 10:971487. https://doi.org/10.3389/fpubh.2022.971487
55. Smith KA, Blease C, Faurholt-Jepsen M, Firth J, Van Daele T, Moreno C et al (2023) Digital mental health: challenges and next steps. BMJ Ment Health 26(1):e300670. https://doi.org/10.1136/bmjment-2023-300670
56. Fone D, White J, Farewell D, Kelly M, John G, Lloyd K et al (2014) Effect of neighbourhood deprivation and social cohesion on mental health inequality: a multilevel population-based longitudinal study. Psychol Med 44(11):2449–2460. https://doi.org/10.1017/S0033291713003255
57. Lee SC, DelPozo-Banos M, Lloyd K, Jones I, Walters JTR, Owen MJ et al (2020) Area deprivation, urbanicity, severe mental illness and social drift—a population-based linkage study using routinely collected primary and secondary care data. Schizophr Res 220:130–140. https://doi.org/10.1016/j.schres.2020.03.044
58. Carrà G, Crocamo C, Bebbington PE (2017) Gambling, geographical variations and deprivation: findings from the adult psychiatric morbidity survey. Int Gambl Stud 17(3):459–470. https://doi.org/10.1080/14459795.2017.1355405
59. Karriker-Jaffe KJ (2011) Areas of disadvantage: a systematic review of effects of area-level socioeconomic status on substance use outcomes. Drug Alcohol Rev 30(1):84–95. https://doi.org/10.1111/j.1465-3362.2010.00191.x
60. Gong P, Liang S, Carlton EJ, Jiang Q, Wu J, Wang L et al (2012) Urbanisation and health in China. Lancet 379(9818):843–852. https://doi.org/10.1016/S0140-6736(11)61878-3
61. Halbreich U (2023) Impact of urbanization on mental health and well being. Curr Opin Psychiatry 36(3):200–205. https://doi.org/10.1097/YCO.0000000000000864
62. Kruize H, van der Vliet N, Staatsen B, Bell R, Chiabai A, Muiños G et al (2019) Urban Green space: creating a triple win for environmental sustainability, health, and health equity through behavior change. Int J Environ Res Public Health 16(22):4403. https://doi.org/10.3390/ijerph16224403
63. Bratman GN, Anderson CB, Berman MG, Cochran B, de Vries S, Flanders J et al (2019) Nature and mental health: an ecosystem service perspective. Sci Adv 5(7):eaax0903. https://doi.org/10.1126/sciadv.aax0903
64. Roe JJ, Thompson CW, Aspinall PA, Brewer MJ, Duff EI, Miller D et al (2013) Green space and stress: evidence from cortisol measures in deprived urban communities. Int J Environ Res Public Health 10(9):4086–4103. https://doi.org/10.3390/ijerph10094086
65. Engemann K, Pedersen CB, Arge L, Tsirogiannis C, Mortensen PB, Svenning JC (2019) Residential green space in childhood is associated with lower risk of psychiatric disorders from adolescence into adulthood. Proc Natl Acad Sci U S A 116(11):5188–5193. https://doi.org/10.1073/pnas.1807504116
66. Mantler A, Logan AC (2015) Natural environments and mental health. Adv Integr Med 2(1):5–12. https://doi.org/10.1016/j.aimed.2015.03.002
67. Gloster AT, Lamnisos D, Lubenko J, Presti G, Squatrito V, Constantinou M et al (2020) Impact of COVID-19 pandemic on mental health: an international study. PLoS One 15(12):e0244809. https://doi.org/10.1371/journal.pone.0244809
68. Verdolini N, Amoretti S, Montejo L, García-Rizo C, Hogg B, Mezquida G et al (2021) Resilience and mental health during the COVID-19 pandemic. J Affect Disord 283:156–164. https://doi.org/10.1016/j.jad.2021.01.055
69. Dragioti E, Li H, Tsitsas G, Lee KH, Choi J, Kim J et al (2022) A large-scale meta-analytic atlas of mental health problems prevalence during the COVID-19 early pandemic. J Med Virol 94(5):1935–1949. https://doi.org/10.1002/jmv.27549
70. Crocamo C, Bachi B, Calabrese A, Callovini T, Cavaleri D, Cioni RM et al (2021) Some of us are most at risk: systematic review and meta-analysis of correlates of depressive symptoms among healthcare workers during the SARS-CoV-2 outbreak. Neurosci Biobehav Rev 131:912–922. https://doi.org/10.1016/j.neubiorev.2021.10.010
71. King JD, Zhang S, Cohen A (2022) Air pollution and mental health: associations, mechanisms and methods. Curr Opin Psychiatry 35(3):192–199. https://doi.org/10.1097/YCO.0000000000000771
72. Zundel CG, Ryan P, Brokamp C, Heeter A, Huang Y, Strawn JR et al (2022) Air pollution, depressive and anxiety disorders, and brain effects: a systematic review. Neurotoxicology 93:272–300. https://doi.org/10.1016/j.neuro.2022.10.011
73. Bhui K, Newbury JB, Latham RM, Ucci M, Nasir ZA, Turner B et al (2023) Air quality and mental health: evidence, challenges and future directions. B J Psych Open 9(4):e120. https://doi.org/10.1192/bjo.2023.507
74. Whiting D, Gulati G, Geddes JR, Fazel S (2022) Association of schizophrenia spectrum disorders and violence perpetration in adults and adolescents from 15 countries: a systematic review and meta-analysis. JAMA Psychiatry 79(2):120–132. https://doi.org/10.1001/jamapsychiatry.2021.3721
75. Anderson CA, Bushman BJ (2002) Human aggression. Annu Rev Psychol 53:27–51. https://doi.org/10.1146/annurev.psych.53.100901.135231
76. Girasek H, Nagy VA, Fekete S, Ungvari GS, Gazdag G (2022) Prevalence and correlates of aggressive behavior in psychiatric inpatient populations. World J Psychiatry 12(1):1–23. https://doi.org/10.5498/wjp.v12.i1.1

77. Labrum T, Zingman MA, Nossel I, Dixon L (2021) Violence by persons with serious mental illness toward family caregivers and other relatives: a review. Harv Rev Psychiatry 29(1):10–19. https://doi.org/10.1097/HRP.0000000000000263
78. Monahan J, Steadman H (eds) (1994) Violence & mental disorder: developments in risk assessment. University of Chicago Press, Chicago, IL
79. Susser M (1973) Causal thinking in the health sciences: concepts and strategies of epidemiology. Oxford University Press, New York, NY
80. Swanson JW, Swartz MS, Van Dorn RA, Elbogen EB, Wagner HR, Rosenheck RA et al (2006) A national study of violent behavior in persons with schizophrenia. Arch Gen Psychiatry 63(5):490–499. https://doi.org/10.1001/archpsyc.63.5.490
81. Scott-Storey K, O'Donnell S, Busolo D, DiTommaso E, Malcolm J, Taylor P et al (2022) Cumulative lifetime violence severity, social determinants and anxiety in a national sample of Canadian men. BMC Psychiatry 22(1):265. https://doi.org/10.1186/s12888-022-03865-8
82. Yu R, Chen Y, Li L, Chen J, Guo Y, Bian Z et al (2021) Factors associated with suicide risk among Chinese adults: a prospective cohort study of 0.5 million individuals. PLoS Med 18(3):e1003545. https://doi.org/10.1371/journal.pmed.1003545
83. World Health Organization (2014) Preventing suicide: a global imperative. https://www.who.int/publications/i/item/9789241564779. Accessed 31 Oct 2023
84. Yoshimasu K, Kiyohara C, Miyashita K (2008) Stress Research Group of the Japanese Society for hygiene. Suicidal risk factors and completed suicide: meta-analyses based on psychological autopsy studies. Environ Health Prev Med 13(5):243–256. https://doi.org/10.1007/s12199-008-0037-x
85. Motillon-Toudic C, Walter M, Séguin M, Carrier JD, Berrouiguet S, Lemey C (2022) Social isolation and suicide risk: literature review and perspectives. Eur Psychiatry 65(1):e65. https://doi.org/10.1192/j.eurpsy.2022.2320
86. Hu FH, Zhao DY, Fu XL, Zhang WQ, Tang W, Hu SQ et al (2023) Effects of social support on suicide-related behaviors in patients with severe mental illness: a systematic review and meta-analysis. J Affect Disord 328:324–333. https://doi.org/10.1016/j.jad.2023.02.070
87. Lundberg J, Cars T, Lampa E, Ekholm Selling K, Leval A, Gannedahl A et al (2023) Determinants and outcomes of suicidal behavior among patients with major depressive disorder. JAMA Psychiatry 80:e232833. https://doi.org/10.1001/jamapsychiatry.2023.2833
88. Mitra A, Pradhan R, Melamed RD, Chen K, Hoaglin DC, Tucker KL et al (2023) Associations between natural language processing-enriched social determinants of health and suicide death among US veterans. JAMA Netw Open 6(3):e233079. https://doi.org/10.1001/jamanetworkopen.2023.3079
89. Coryell W, Scheftner W, Keller M, Endicott J, Maser J, Klerman GL (1993) The enduring psychosocial consequences of mania and depression. Am J Psychiatry 150:720–727. https://doi.org/10.1176/ajp.150.5.720
90. MacQueen GM, Young LT, Joffe RT (2001) A review of psychosocial outcome in patients with bipolar disorder. Acta Psychiatr Scand 103:163–170. https://doi.org/10.1034/j.1600-0447.2001.00059.x
91. Fenn HH, Bauer MS, Altshuler L, Evans DR, Williford WO, Kilbourne AM et al (2005) Medical comorbidity and health-related quality of life in bipolar disorder across the adult age span. J Affect Disord 86(1):47–60. https://doi.org/10.1016/j.jad.2004.12.006
92. Monk TH, Kupfer DJ, Frank E, Ritenour AM (1991) The social rhythm metric (SRM): measuring daily social rhythms over 12 weeks. Psychiatry Res 36(2):195–207. https://doi.org/10.1016/0165-1781(91)90131-8
93. Howes OD, Murray RM (2014) Schizophrenia: an integrated sociodevelopmental-cognitive model. Lancet 383(9929):1677–1687. https://doi.org/10.1016/S0140-6736(13)62036-X
94. Suijkerbuijk YB, Schaafsma FG, van Mechelen JC, Ojajärvi A, Corbière M, Anema JR (2017) Interventions for obtaining and maintaining employment in adults with severe mental illness, a network meta-analysis. Cochrane Database Syst Rev 9(9):CD011867. https://doi.org/10.1002/14651858.CD011867.pub2
95. Gold PB, Macias C, Rodican CF (2016) Does competitive work improve quality of life for adults with severe mental illness? Evidence from a randomized trial of supported employment. J Behav Health Serv Res 43(2):155–171. https://doi.org/10.1007/s11414-014-9392-0
96. Green MF, Lee J, Wynn JK (2020) Experimental approaches to social disconnection in the general community: can we learn from schizophrenia research? World Psychiatry 19(2):177–178. https://doi.org/10.1002/wps.20734
97. Ernst JM, Cacioppo JT (1999) Lonely hearts: psychological perspectives on loneliness. Appl Prev Psychol 8(1):1–22. https://doi.org/10.1016/S0962-1849(99)80008-0
98. Pitman A, Suleman S, Hyde N, Hodgkiss A (2018) Depression and anxiety in patients with cancer. BMJ 361:k1415. https://doi.org/10.1136/bmj.k1415
99. Cacioppo JT, Hawkley LC, Thisted RA (2010) Perceived social isolation makes me sad: 5-year cross-lagged analyses of loneliness and depressive symptomatology in the Chicago health, aging, and social relations study. Psychol Aging 25(2):453–463. https://doi.org/10.1037/a0017216

100. Cruwys T, Dingle GA, Haslam C, Haslam SA, Jetten J, Morton TA (2013) Social group memberships protect against future depression, alleviate depression symptoms and prevent depression relapse. Soc Sci Med 98:179–186. https://doi.org/10.1016/j.socscimed.2013.09.013
101. Cornwell EY, Waite LJ (2009) Social disconnectedness, perceived isolation, and health among older adults. J Health Soc Behav 50(1):31–48. https://doi.org/10.1177/002214650905000103
102. Cacioppo JT, Cacioppo S (2018) The growing problem of loneliness. Lancet 391(10119):426. https://doi.org/10.1016/S0140-6736(18)30142-9
103. Killgore WDS, Cloonan SA, Taylor EC, Miller MA, Dailey NS (2020) Three months of loneliness during the COVID-19 lockdown. Psychiatry Res 293:113392. https://doi.org/10.1016/j.psychres.2020.113392
104. McQuaid RJ, Cox SML, Ogunlana A, Jaworska N (2021) The burden of loneliness: implications of the social determinants of health during COVID-19. Psychiatry Res 296:113648. https://doi.org/10.1016/j.psychres.2020.113648
105. Li LZ, Wang S (2020) Prevalence and predictors of general psychiatric disorders and loneliness during COVID-19 in the United Kingdom. Psychiatry Res 291:113267. https://doi.org/10.1016/j.psychres.2020.113267
106. Courtin E, Knapp M (2017) Social isolation, loneliness and health in old age: a scoping review. Health Soc Care Community 25(3):799–812. https://doi.org/10.1111/hsc.12311
107. Beam CR, Kim AJ (2020) Psychological sequelae of social isolation and loneliness might be a larger problem in young adults than older adults. Psychol Trauma 12(S1):S58–S60. https://doi.org/10.1037/tra0000774
108. Carrà G, Bartoli F, Capogrosso CA, Cioni RM, Moretti F, Piacenti S et al (2022) Innovations in community-based mental health care: an overview of meta-analyses. Int Rev Psychiatry 34(7–8):770–782. https://doi.org/10.1080/09540261.2022.2113043
109. Jester DJ, Thomas ML, Sturm ET, Harvey PD, Keshavan M, Davis BJ et al (2023) Review of major social determinants of health in schizophrenia-spectrum psychotic disorders: I. Clinical outcomes. Schizophr Bull 49(4):837–850. https://doi.org/10.1093/schbul/sbad023
110. Sturm ET, Thomas ML, Sares AG, Dave S, Baron D, Compton MT et al (2023) Review of major social determinants of health in schizophrenia-spectrum disorders: II. Assessments. Schizophr Bull 49(4):851–866. https://doi.org/10.1093/schbul/sbad024

4 Initiatives for Ending Stigma and Discrimination in Mental Health

Matteo Di Vincenzo, Salvatore Cipolla, Eleonora Arsenio, and Gaia Sampogna

Abstract

Stigma attached to mental disorders represents a major obstacle for affected people and their relatives. Stigma is a complex phenomenon, which has been conceptualized as a problem of knowledge, behaviors, and attitudes. Several types of stigma have been described, including public stigma, structural stigma, experienced stigma, felt/perceived stigma, self-stigma or internalized stigma, and associative/courtesy stigma. To counteract stigma, different approaches have been developed, which can be classified into education-based, protest-based, and contact-based strategies. Although many international anti-stigma initiatives and campaigns have been implemented, there is still much work to be done.

Keywords

Stigma · Discrimination · Anti-stigma strategies · Anti-stigma initiatives · Anti-stigma campaigns · Mental health · Mental disorders

M. Di Vincenzo · S. Cipolla · E. Arsenio
G. Sampogna (✉)
Department of Psychiatry, University of Campania "L. Vanvitelli", Naples, Italy
e-mail: gaia.sampogna@unicampania.it

4.1 Background

Since the Greeks learned the art of drawing the skin from the Persians, the application of a mark (*stigma*, in ancient Greek) was a distinctive and punitive sign used to indicate thieves, slaves, and war prisoners. Marked people suffered from lifelong ostracism by the other members of the Greco-Roman society. Since then, stigma has been a synonymous of humiliation, shame, and loss of honor.

Nowadays, the term "stigma" is used to indicate a permanent discredit that limits a person's social status, preventing them from being accepted into ordinary social relationships [1]. Stigma is frequently associated with people suffering from mental disorders, indicating the set of negative connotations that are prejudicially attributed to them determining discrimination and social exclusion [2].

Mental disorders began to be viewed with disdain since a link with sin was created in the seventeenth century in Western Europe: in the *Malleus Maleficarum* ("The Witches' Hammer") the description of some witches seemed to represent mental disorders, such as depression and schizophrenia, which at that time were considered deals with the devil who needed to be punished [3]. Similarly, with the advent of Confucianism, in Eastern culture, mental disorders began to be associated with a sense of guilt

A. Fiorillo, S. De Giorgi (eds.), *Social Determinants of Mental Health*, Sustainable Development Goals Series, https://doi.org/10.1007/978-3-031-70165-8_4

and shame because it prevented one from operating in a harmonious and positive way [4].

One of the main purposes of mental asylums was to physically separate unwanted people (insane people) from the rest of the society.

4.2 Conceptualization of Stigma

The sociologist Ervin Goffman proposed the first conceptualization of the phenomenon of stigma. He defined stigma as “an attribute considered undesirable and unpleasant by society, which differentiates a person from other members of the community that he/she should be part of.” Thus, a specific attribute can be stigmatizing when it produces discredit on a social level and a person holding this attribute is regarded as someone marked and discredited [1].

The concept of stigma has evolved over time to become a complex construct, derived from a specific social process. The Labeling Theory [5] describes a process that begins with the attribution of the label “mentally ill,” which evokes negative stereotypes (for example “dangerousness”) learned during childhood. In turn, these stereotypes evoke negative emotional responses (prejudice) and the expression of discriminatory behavior (rejection or distancing) [6]. Consequently, those who prejudicially label mentally ill people as dangerous, useless, unpredictable will be more predisposed to respond in an angry or punitive way and will be in favor of more coercive laws and treatments, further implementing stigmatizing behaviors.

The conceptualization made by Goffman and Sheff describes stigma as a social phenomenon, rooted in interpersonal relationships and shaped by the culture and structure of a society. In the “Modified Labeling Theory,” Link and Phelan [7] describe the phases of the broad process that links stigmatization to interactions between individuals and groups, as synthetized in Fig. 4.1.

Although the focus of the present chapter is on stigma attached to mental disorders, the process of stigmatization can be applied to many different conditions and can involve a large number of minorities [7]: people suffering from obesity, cancer, or other chronic diseases, people with human immunodeficiency virus (HIV) infection or other contagious diseases, or people from ethnic or sexual minorities [8–11].

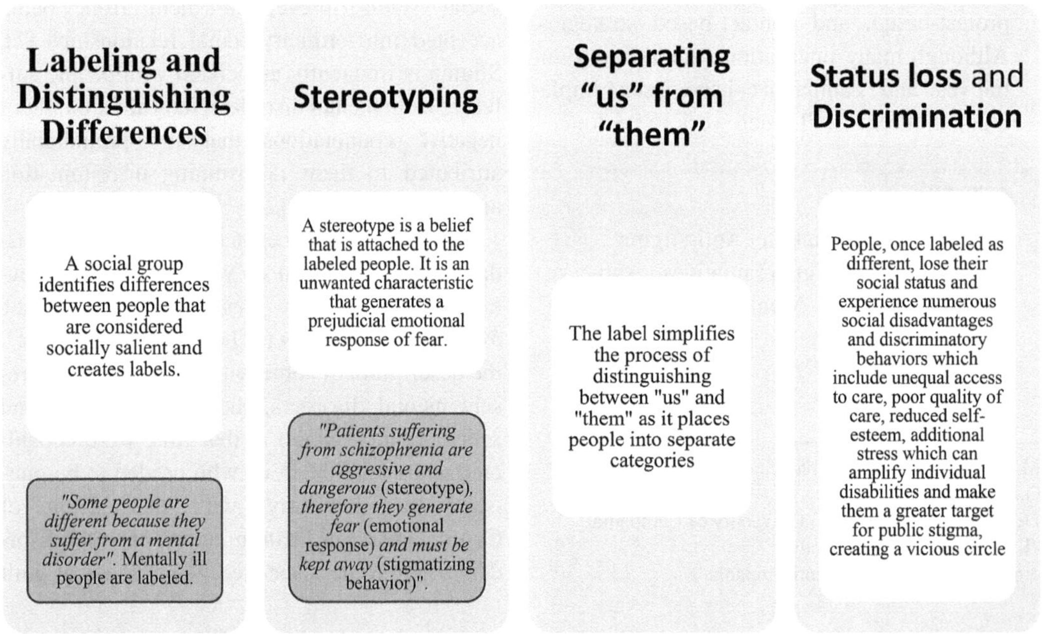

Fig. 4.1 Modified Labeling Theory

4.3 Types of Stigma

In Table 4.1 we report different types of stigma, which have been identified [12].

Public stigma is the discriminatory reaction of the general population toward people suffering from mental disorders. *Structural stigma*, defined as the "societal-level conditions, cultural norms, and institutional practices that constrain the opportunities, resources, and well-being for stigmatized populations" [13], refers to the inequities and injustices inherent in social structures that arbitrarily restrict the means and freedoms of a specific population [7, 14, 15]. Structural stigma related to mental illness is increasingly recognized as one of the most significant barriers to the well-being of people with mental disorders. Examples of this so-called *structural stigma* are the sensationalist headlines in newspapers or the laws in the USA that restrict parental rights to people who have a history of mental disorder [16].

Experienced stigma refers to a person's experience of real discrimination and/or restriction. It contrasts with *felt/perceived stigma (or anticipated stigma)*, which refers to the stigma that people with a (potentially) stigmatizing condition may fear or perceive in the community. Perceived stigma can influence the expectations of people with mental disorders, who expect that others will adopt devaluing attitudes or discriminatory behaviors toward them. Anticipated stigma is widespread in people with mental disorders, regardless of whether or not they have experienced a direct episode of discrimination [17]. *Self-stigma* or *internalized stigma* refers to the negative attitudes, including internalized shame, that people with mental disorders have about their own condition [18]. When a negative public perception is internalized by people with mental disorders, it has a negative impact on self-esteem and self-identification. According to the "why try" effect, people reporting high levels of self-stigma avoid undertaking actions or activities because they feel incapable or are certain of failure. Therefore, low self-esteem and low self-efficacy prevent individuals from achieving important goals, such as looking for a job, living independently, or having social interactions and affective relationships [16, 19].

Table 4.1 Types of stigma

Public stigma	The stigma perpetuated by the general population
Structural stigma	Institutions, laws, and regulations that systematically disadvantage discriminated people
Experienced stigma	Experience of real discrimination and/or restriction reported by people suffering from mental disorder
Felt/perceived stigma	Stigma perceived as present in the community by people with a (potentially) stigmatized condition
Self-stigma or internalized stigma	Negative perception internalized by people suffering from mental disorders
Associative or courtesy stigma	The effect of stigma on those who have a close relationship with labeled people

In the framework of a more pragmatic approach, Thornicroft [20] conceptualized stigma and stigmatization as due to the interaction among three different components: knowledge (ignorance), attitude (prejudice), and behavior (discrimination), respectively reflecting cognitive, emotional, and behavioral aspects. The effects of stigma not only affect the people directly labeled, but also all those who live or work or have a close social relationship with individuals suffering from mental disorders [21], defined as *associative* or *courtesy stigma* [1, 22]. Associative stigma involves family members of people with mental disorders [23] and mental health professionals [24], who are often avoided or discriminated due to the presence of stereotypes and prejudices about their work.

4.4 Consequences of Stigma

Stigma and discrimination represent a significant obstacle for the full recovery of patients with mental disorders, having an impact on help-seeking, the care process as a whole, and the participation in rehabilitation activities. People with severe mental disorders are subjected to a double challenge: on the one hand, they deal with the direct consequences of their disorder and, on the other hand, they challenge stereotypes, prejudices, discrimination, and social exclusion [2]. A precise estimation of stigma prevalence is complex. There is a tendency to provide "socially desirable responses," which reduces the possibility that people from the general population do not declare their prejudices against people with mental disorders or do not report their discriminating behaviors.

Stigma toward people suffering from mental disorders is strongly influenced by culture, tradition, access to education, health services, and personal experience [25]. A survey carried out in 27 countries found that the most frequent forms of discrimination concern social, family, and intimate and work relationships [26]. Less than 10% of the sample described "positive discrimination," i.e., the existence of advantages deriving from having a diagnosis of a mental disorder. Patients frequently reported avoidant behaviors due to the "why try" effect. Moreover, anticipated stigma was more frequent than experienced stigma: 69% of participants experienced anticipatory discrimination when looking for a job, but less than 50% had actually experienced this discrimination; 60% declared they felt stigmatized when starting an intimate relationship, but 50% had never been discriminated. These findings have been confirmed in a similar study on patients suffering from major depression, showing that people feeling higher levels of anticipatory stigma decide to give up pursuing their goals [27].

Anticipatory and internalized stigma and the "why try" effect can be considered as interrelated dimensions, contributing to the self-exclusion of people with mental disorders from the community. They are associated with a series of negative clinical and social outcomes, such as poor quality of life, lack of empowerment, shame, guilt, and increased symptom severity [28, 29]. Stigma represents a social barrier to recovery [30], since the vicious circle triggered by stigma leads to social isolation, inability to work, alcohol or drug abuse, and to the onset of other psychiatric disorders. For many people, the consequences of stigma are even worse than the experience of the mental disorder itself [27, 28, 31].

Help-seeking is significantly influenced by stigma. For example, people may decide to ignore their mental health to avoid the effects of a stigmatizing label on themselves. This phenomenon, known as "label avoidance," also includes the fear/shame of a diagnosis of mental disorder and the poor compliance with pharmacological treatments.

4.5 Strategies to Fight Stigma

To combat stigma toward people with mental disorders, three different strategies have been described: protest, education, and contact [32]. *Protest*-based interventions aim to eliminate negative stereotypes through public declarations, media reports or advertisements, and celebrity testimonials. *Education*-based interventions provide correct and evidence-based information on mental disorders and/or provide scientific explanation of stereotypes ("myth vs. facts"). *Contact* involves the direct contact of the general population with people suffering from mental disorders.

Educational programs raise awareness on mental health among the general population [7], and are particularly effective with specific target populations, such as students, adolescents, family members, or patients themselves. Contact-based strategies are the most effective way to combat stigma since one's own prejudices are undermined [31].

A meta-analysis analyzed the effectiveness of anti-stigma interventions based on protest, education, and contact and highlighted that personal contact has a greater effect-size for adults, educational interventions maintain their effectiveness on adolescents, while protest-based interventions were smaller in number and less effective [33]. The comparison between the effects of education-based and contact-based anti-stigma programs revealed that the former increases knowledge on mental disorders modifying discriminatory attitudes and behaviors, while the latter produces a double effect compared to educational programs. In fact, direct contact facilitates discussion between the general population and stigmatized people who have the opportunity to talk about their illness experience firsthand [34].

4.6 Examples of Anti-Stigma Initiatives Worldwide

Several initiatives and campaigns have been promoted worldwide in order to increase awareness on mental health and mental disorders and to fight stigma attached to people with severe mental disorders. Scientific associations, governmental institutions, as well as charities and private

Table 4.2 Anti-stigma initiatives implemented by scientific societies

Scientific society	Initiative	Aims and features
World Psychiatric Association (WPA)	*Fighting Stigma and Discrimination because of Schizophrenia—Open the Doors*	Rehabilitation of the image of psychiatry; educational interventions' adoption of patients' point of view
	WPA Stigma Section	Research promotion and dissemination of information, knowledge, and public awareness about stigma
European Psychiatric Association (EPA)	*EPA guidance*	Focus on the image of psychiatry and psychiatrists
American Psychiatric Association (APA)	*National poll on stigma at workplace*	
	Do's and don'ts during conversations with patients	
Association for Improvement of Mental Health Programmes (AIMHP)	*Together against stigma*	

Table 4.3 Anti-stigma initiatives implemented by governmental and public institutions

Country	Institution	Initiative	Aims and features
Australia	Government	*Beyond Blue*	Information
Canada	Mental Health Commission of Canada	*Opening Minds*	Information and accessible training programs
Denmark	Government and Regions	*En Af Os (One of Us)*	Information and shared experiences
Ireland	Partnership of Associations	*See Change*	Information and shared experiences
Italy	Ministry of Health	*Da vicino nessuno è normale (Up close no one is normal)*	Information
New Zealand	Government	*Like Minds, Like Mine*	Information
Scotland	Government	*See Me*	Information and shared experiences
Spain	Department of Health	*Idecada4 (1 in 4)*	Information
Spain	Catalan Government and Municipality of Barcelona	*Obertament (Open Mind)*	Information
International	World Health Organization (WHO)	*Myth* vs. *fact*	Educational
International	World Federation of Mental Health (WFMH)	*World Mental Health Day*	Information—disease awareness

foundations have been very active in promoting anti-stigma campaigns worldwide.

A variety of initiatives has been developed and promoted worldwide, but it is out of the scope of the present chapter to systematically review and summarize all past, on-going, and future anti-stigma initiatives (Tables 4.2 and 4.3).

4.6.1 Scientific Associations

World Psychiatric Association (WPA) Since 1996, the most important society of psychiatrists and mental health professionals worldwide promotes initiatives aimed at fighting stigma of people suffering from mental disorders. The promotion of a positive image of psychiatry, educational interventions on mental disorders, as well as the adoption of patients' views were central in the "*Fighting Stigma and Discrimination because of Schizophrenia - Open the Doors*" campaign, which was implemented in 18 countries. Furthermore, the WPA supports the *Global Anti-Stigma Alliance (GASA)*, an informal network gathering 25 organizations across 14 countries, aimed at developing knowledge and best practices in mental health care.

European Psychiatric Association (EPA) An EPA guidance paper [35] examined the image of psychiatry and psychiatrists, prone to prejudges and discriminatory attitudes as well. Strategies and recommendations were proposed by an international panel of experts, by calling out the efforts of mental health professionals, patients, families, stakeholders, and mass-media.

American Psychiatric Association (APA) In 2019, APA promoted a nation wide poll on stigma at workplace, finding workers' concerns about discussing mental health problems at work and retaliation or being fired in the case of mental health treatment being sought. Moreover, most workers reported they would support and guide troubled co-workers in seeking help. Currently, on its website (https://www.psychiatry.org/), APA explains how to address stigma, indicates do's and don'ts during conversations with patients, and collects links of American associations and foundations that actively operate in combating stigma.

Association for the Improvement of Mental Health Programmes (AIMHP) The Association for the Improvement of Mental Health Programmes (AIMHP) was founded in 2004. Its objective is to make a contribution to the improvement and promotion of mental health programs worldwide. AIMHP aims to achieve its goals by means of consultation, organizing talks and seminars, initiating and coordinating studies, other theoretical and practical work, and by any other appropriate means that can improve the care of people with mental illness and their families and raise the value given to mental health by individuals and societies. The association has been involved in the global anti-stigma program WPA "Open the doors." Moreover, the Association has promoted several international meetings entitled "Together against stigma," held in Germany, England, Canada, Turkey, and Japan.

4.6.2 Governmental and Public Institutions

Beyond Blue: Australia In 2000, eight Australian governments started a project aimed at providing public information about depression, anxiety, and suicide prevention, and delivering online support. It promoted anti-stigma campaigns and encouraged help-seeking and dissemination of knowledge through its website (www.beyondblue.org.au).

Opening Minds: Canada As an initiative of Mental Health Commission of Canada, since 2009 Opening Minds aims at changing Canadian people's mindset toward patients suffering from mental disorders, removing any type of stigma and reaffirming the role of affected people in the society. Youth, workplace well-being, mental health professions, and media represent the pillars on whom Opening Minds focuses its efforts. Accessible training programs, supporting mental health in communities and workplaces, are delivered about the themes of suicide prevention, adequate mental health care access, workplace well-being, substance use, along with stigma and discrimination (https://mentalhealthcommission.ca/opening-minds/).

En Af Os (One of Us): Denmark The network, including governmental and regional institutions, as well as philanthropic foundations in Denmark, aims at promoting social inclusion and reducing stigma of people suffering from psychiatric disorders. Social contacts with people with lived experience of mental health problems as well as production of information material addressed to media operators are among the activities of this partnership (https://www.sst.dk/da/en-af-os).

See Change: Ireland Established in 2010 as a partnership of Irish associations, this program aims at challenging discrimination and empowering equality, respect, and rights of patients with mental health problems. See Change works by implementing national, regional, and community anti-stigma campaigns, giving voice to "ambassadors" with lived experiences, and building partnerships with other organizations (https://seechange.ie).

Da vicino nessuno è normale: Italy The Italian Ministry of Health celebrated the 40th anniversary of the "Legge Basaglia" (1978) by supporting the campaign "Da vicino nessuno è normale" (Up close no one is normal). Italian mayors were asked to promote in their own municipalities and cities initiatives for breaking down prejudices around mental health, by sharing information through handouts and social media.

Like Minds, Like Mine: New Zealand This campaign, funded by the New Zealand Government in 1997, promotes public awareness of mental disorders and social inclusion of people who experience them, by creating guidelines for media reporting, disseminating information through its website (https://www.likeminds.org.nz), and organizing public initiatives in the community and at workplaces. Specific focus on populations living with social disadvantage and ethnic minority, being more prone to develop mental health problems, is performed as well.

See Me: Scotland Funded by Scottish government in 2002, See Me works by delivering awareness initiatives, promoting social contacts with patients sharing their lived experiences of mental disorder, and developing policies and practices within the target settings (young population groups, workplaces, schools, health and social workers). On its webpage (https://www.seemescotland.org), it is reported that 20 years after See Me foundation, 96% of Scots declare that "they would be willing to help someone who is struggling with their mental health."

Idecada4: Spain Idecada4 (1 in 4) aims at fighting stigma and encourages the recovery of people with mental disorders. It was founded in 2007 as a cross-sectional plan of three agencies of Department of Health. Healthcare professionals, patients with their families, schools, universities, workplaces, and media represent the agents toward whom actions are addressed. Social media campaigns, videos, workshops, and reports are the activities *Idecada4* usually perform in order to disseminate new awareness and knowledge in the field of mental health.

Obertament: Catalonia, Spain Since its foundation in 2010, Obertament (Open Mind) combats stigma among the general population of Catalonia, reaching 9–11% of it. Youth education, primary health care, and workplaces represent the main concerns of this project, whose commitment has also produced guidelines for media in the framework of the *Media Observatory* and initiatives for schools (Table 4.3).

World Health Organization (WHO) The WHO is committed to fight misconceptions, stigma, and discrimination surrounding mental health. In particular, the WHO's Comprehensive Mental Health Action Plan 2013–2030 calls on Member States to adopt strategic interventions to reduce stigmatization, discrimination, and human rights violations against people with mental health conditions. In particular, the WHO has promoted an educational program, with the production of informative materials focused on "myth and fact" related to mental disorders.

World Federation of Mental Health (WFMH) The WFMH is a non-profit association that is committed to promote the advancement of mental health awareness, prevention of mental disorders, advocacy, and best practice recovery-focused interventions worldwide. Every year on October 10, it is celebrated the World Mental Health Day, in order to increase awareness of mental health issues around the world and to mobilize efforts in support of mental health. The WFMH is actively involved in the promotion of activities for improving awareness around mental health issues.

4.6.3 Charities and Private Foundations

SANE Australia: Australia Within this charity, which was founded in 1986 to focus on schizophrenia-related issues, the Stigma Watch promotes public awareness, and deals with the stigmatizing language used by mass-media. Indeed, information and training materials are specifically delivered for journalists.

Meeting for Minds (M4M): Australia A non-profit organization founded in 2014 in Australia and currently operating in five countries, which supports the direct collaboration of people experiencing psychiatric disorders in scientific research, and organizes workshops, conferences, and other events about mental health with patients.

Bell Let's Talk: Canada Founded in 2010 for fundraising and disseminating information about mental health. During the *Bell Let's Talk day*, once a year, 5 cents were donated for each call/text people of Canada made/sent to talk about psychiatric issues. Thus, nation-wide conversations took place alongside the accumulation of donations. After 5 years, more than 1000 randomly surveyed Canadians mostly reported higher awareness about mental health.

Time to Change (TTC): England, Wales This campaign was established in October 2007 by the charities MIND and Rethink Mental Illness, with the specific aim to reduce mental disorder-related stigma and discrimination level by 5% throughout the first year. Supported by several English financial and industrial companies, until 2021 it has promoted a series of initiatives such as sharing lived experiences, development of information material addressed to students and teachers, and initiatives for improving communication by media around the topic of mental health problems (http://www.time-to-change.org.uk). Over the years, TTC has crossed England borders developing anti-stigma programs in low-income countries belonging to Commonwealth and launching *Time to Change Wales* in 2012 with the efforts of the charities MIND Cymru, Gofal, and Hafal.

An innovative approach introduced by the TTC campaign has been the inclusion of a social marketing campaign, using mass-media channels, social media, and social contact events. The novel aspect of TTC program is the explicit target to change behavior. The key active ingredients are forms of contact between people with and without experience of mental illness. Mass-media/communication campaigns are often considered part of a social marketing intervention (e.g., a mass-media campaign is used as a promotional tool for a social marketing product) and they can be effective in increasing awareness on the targeted topic and motivating people to change their behavior [36–40].

SANE: England SANE is committed to promote the rights of people with mental health problems and to provide support and information to patients and caregivers. The improvement of attitude and understanding toward mental disorder at public level is one of its main goals. Moreover, it disposes of a helpline that delivers support to people with mental disorders.

Samen Sterk Zonder Stigma: The Netherlands Samen Sterk Zonder Stigma (Together Strong Against Stigma) was a project using population-based approach that promoted increasing awareness in the field of mental disorder, by addressing initiatives among psychiatry professionals, in the general population, among young people, and in the workplaces, where employers were invited to talk about these topics. Moreover, a focus on media aimed at encouraging a responsible and non-stigmatizing narration of stories involving people with mental disorder. Although this project is over, its website (https://samensterkzonderstigma.nl) continues to disseminate knowledge.

Unidos Para Ajuadar: Portugal Unidos Para Ajuadar (United to Help) was established in 2007 by the Portuguese non-governmental organization (NGO) ENCONTRAR+SE. The project aims to increase public awareness and to reduce discrimination due to mental disorders, with a specific focus on youth people and discrimination in the workplace. They included school-based interventions, rehabilitation programs for the community, and the production of songs against prejudices and stigma.

Hjärnkoll: Sweden Almost 300 "ambassadors," directly experiencing mental issues or living with a relative suffering from a psychiatric disorder, share their stories "to show that mental illness is nothing to be afraid of. We just have different ways of functioning, and we all benefit from the differences being taken care of, humanly and financially," as is reported on the website (https://hjarnkoll.se/vad-vi-gor/). Differences among psychiatric diagnoses, best practices in assistance, and the relation between mental health and youth or migrations are some of the topics addressed by *Hjärnkoll* ambassadors during their speeches.

Bring Change to Mind (BC2M): United States of America In 2010, the actress and activist Glenn Close founded the charity in order to promote a dialogue about mental disorder and reduce stigma, by organizing campaigns, involving middle- and high-school students, and providing tools for sharing experiences and learning more (https://www.bringchange2mind.org).

The Carter Center: United States of America Mental health is one of the areas of focus of the Jimmy and Rosalynn Carter's foundation. In particular, The Rosalynn Carter Fellowship for Mental Health Journalism promotes responsible description of news involving people suffering from psychiatric disorders, with the use of balanced and non-stigmatizing language. Moreover, the Carter Center supports patients' rights, informs public policy, and works for achieving "equity for mental health comparable to other health care" (https://www.cartercenter.org/health/mental_health/index.html).

Stamp Out Stigma: United States of America Founded in the framework of the Association for Behavioral Health and Wellness, this campaign aims to promote open talking about mental and substance use disorders. Recognizing the prevalence of mental health problems, Reeducating ourselves, families, and friends, and Reducing stigma represent the Three R's on which this initiative is based (https://stampoutstigma.com/).

This Is My Brave: United States of America It is a theatre show where individuals experiencing mental disorder tell their own successful story, despite a diagnosis of depression, bipolar disorder, anxiety disorder, post-traumatic stress disorder (PTSD), or other (https://thisismybrave.org).

The Mental Health Coalition: United States of America This is a network of leading mental health organizations, brands, and individuals, which focus their efforts to end mental health-related stigma and improve the way for talking about mental disorders. Equity, diversity, anti-racism, and accessibility are the pillars of its actions, while evidence-based information is provided through its website (https://www.thementalhealthcoalition.org/). Its fight against stigma also comes through the sharing of stories with the tag line "How are you really?"

Table 4.4 Anti-stigma initiatives implemented by governmental and public Institutions

Country	Initiative	Aims and features
Australia	*SANE Australia*	Information and training for mass-media workers
Australia	*Meeting for Minds (M4M)*	Information and collaboration of people experiencing psychiatric disorders in scientific research
Canada	*Bell Let's Talk*	Information and fundraising
England and Wales	*Time to Change*	Information, shared experiences, and training for mass-media workers
England	*SANE*	Research, information, and support to patients and families
Netherlands	*Samen Sterk Zonder Stigma (Together Strong Against Stigma)*	Information
Portugal	*Unidos Para Ajuadar (United to help)*	Information and rehabilitation
Sweden	*Hjärnkoll (Mind control)*	Information and shared experiences
USA	*Bring Change to Mind (BC2M)*	Information and shared experiences
USA	*The Carter Center*	Information, guidelines for mass-media, and support to patients
USA	*Stamp Out Stigma*	Information
USA	*This Is My Brave*	Shared experiences
USA	*The Mental Health Coalition*	Information
USA	*Safe Space Radio*	Information and shared experiences
USA	*NAMI's Stigma Free*	Information at workplace
USA	*Healthy Minds with Dr. Jeffrey Borenstein*	Information and shared experiences

Safe Space Radio: United States of America Since 2008, it has put on the air more than 300 episodes about living with depression, anxiety, schizophrenia, and borderline personality disorder, combining guidance by experts to the testimonies by people with lived experiences. Such stories can be listened by linking to its website (https://safespaceradio.com).

NAMI's Stigma Free: United States of America National Alliance on Mental Illness promotes a campaign specifically aimed at reducing stigma "through powerful words and actions." Among the Stigma Free pledges, there is the transformation of companies/workplaces into "Stigma Free zones" by increasing safety and support (https://www.nami.org/Get-Involved/Pledge-to-Be-StigmaFree).

Healthy Minds with Dr. Jeffrey Borenstein: United States of America It is a series produced by Brain & Behavior Research Foundation, consisting of inspiring storytelling performed by people with the experience of mental disorder. As well, experts provide updated information about diagnosis and treatments (https://www.pbs.org/show/healthy-minds-with-dr-jeffrey-borenstein/) (Table 4.4).

4.7 Conclusions

Stigma and discrimination trigger a vicious cycle that feeds on itself and involves in various ways people suffering from mental disorders and their loved ones, mental health professionals, and the whole society. Moreover, stigma represents a significant obstacle in accessing physical and mental healthcare services, and in achieving recovery [41]. Many initiatives and campaigns aimed at eliminating prejudices toward people with mental health problems have been established and carried out, mostly involving specific stakeholders and target groups, such as patients, families, mental health professionals, school-aged students, and workers. Despite an increasing evidence-based knowledge, stigma and discrimination due to mental health problems continue to be an issue, especially in those geographic areas where initiatives cannot yet be implemented at the public level [42, 43]. Interventions based on social contact, actively involving people with an experience of mental disorder, and providing guidance to mass-media on how to spread out a non-stigmatizing language, are good strategies for overcoming social marginalization for patients with mental disorders [41].

Authors' Contribution All authors actively contributed to the present chapter and approved it.

References

1. Goffman E (1963) Stigma: notes on the management of spoiled identity. Touchstone. https://books.google.it/books?id=7CNUUMKTbIoC
2. Lasalvia A, Tansella M (2008) Fighting discrimination and stigma against people with mental disorders. Epidemiol Psichiatr Soc 17(1):1–9
3. Anderson RD (1970) The history of witchcraft: a review with some psychiatric comments. Am J Psychiatry 126(12):1727–1735. https://doi.org/10.1176/ajp.126.12.1727
4. Tsang HWH, Angell B, Corrigan PW, Lee Y-T, Shi K, Lam CS, Jin S, Fung KMT (2007) A cross-cultural study of employers' concerns about hiring people with psychotic disorder: implications for recovery. Soc Psychiatry Psychiatr Epidemiol 42(9):723–733. https://doi.org/10.1007/s00127-007-0208-x
5. Scheff TJ (1966) Being mentally ill: a sociological theory. Aldine Publishing Company, London. https://books.google.it/books?id=6iXy3_TBYW8C
6. Corrigan P, Markowitz FE, Watson A, Rowan D, Kubiak MA (2003) An attribution model of public discrimination towards persons with mental illness. J Health Soc Behav 44(2):162–179
7. Link BG, Phelan JC (2001) Conceptualizing stigma. Annu Rev Sociol 27:363–385
8. Eylem O, de Wit L, van Straten A, Steubl L, Melissourgaki Z, Danışman GT, de Vries R, Kerkhof AJFM, Bhui K, Cuijpers P (2020) Stigma for common mental disorders in racial minorities and majorities a systematic review and meta-analysis. BMC Public Health 20(1):879. https://doi.org/10.1186/s12889-020-08964-3
9. Misra S, Ke C, Srinivasan S, Goyal A, Nyriyenda MJ, Florez JC, Khunti K, Magliano DJ, Luk A (2023) Current insights and emerging trends in early-onset type 2 diabetes. Lancet Diabetes Endocrinol 11(10):768–782. https://doi.org/10.1016/S2213-8587(23)00225-5
10. Yip CCH, Chan KKS (2022) Stigma resistance among sexual minorities. Sex Res Soc Policy 19(2):647–655. https://doi.org/10.1007/s13178-021-00580-z
11. Zollweg SS, Belloir JA, Drabble LA, Everett B, Taylor JY, Hughes TL (2023) Structural stigma and alcohol use among sexual and gender minority adults: a systematic review. Drug Alcohol Depend Rep 8:100185. https://doi.org/10.1016/j.dadr.2023.100185
12. Van Brakel WH (2006) Measuring health-related stigma—a literature review. Psychol Health Med 11(3):307–334. https://doi.org/10.1080/13548500600595160
13. Hatzenbuehler ML, Link BG (2014). Introduction to the special issue on structural stigma and health. Social Science & Medicine 103:1–6.
14. Corrigan PW, Watson AC (2004). At issue: Stop the stigma: call mental illness a brain disease. Schizophr Bull 30(3):477–9.
15. Kelly BD (2006). The power gap: freedom, power and mental illness. Soc Sci Med. 63(8):2118–28.
16. Corrigan PW (2005) On the stigma of mental illness: practical strategies for research and social change. American Psychological Association, Washington, DC. https://books.google.it/books?id=XNtxQgAACAAJ
17. Uçok A, Brohan E, Rose D, Sartorius N, Leese M, Yoon CK, Plooy A, Ertekin BA, Milev R, Thornicroft G, INDIGO Study Group (2012) Anticipated discrimination among people with schizophrenia. Acta Psychiatr Scand 125(1):77–83. https://doi.org/10.1111/j.1600-0447.2011.01772.x
18. Watson AC, Corrigan P, Larson JE, Sells M (2007) Self-stigma in people with mental illness. Schizophr Bull 33(6):1312–1318. https://doi.org/10.1093/schbul/sbl076
19. Corrigan PW, Larson JE, Rüsch N (2009) Self-stigma and the "why try" effect: impact on life goals and evidence-based practices. World Psychiatry 8(2):75–81. https://doi.org/10.1002/j.2051-5545.2009.tb00218.x

20. Thornicroft G (2006) Shunned: discrimination against people with mental illness. Oxford University Press, Oxford. https://books.google.it/books?id=R1NQEAAAQBAJ
21. Sartorius N (2007) Stigma and mental health. Lancet 370(9590):810–811. https://doi.org/10.1016/S0140-6736(07)61245-8
22. Mehta SI, Farina A (1988) Associative stigma: perceptions of the difficulties of college-aged children of stigmatized fathers. J Soc Clin Psychol 7(2–3):192–202. https://doi.org/10.1521/jscp.1988.7.2-3.192
23. Phelan JC, Bromet EJ, Link BG (1998) Psychiatric illness and family stigma. Schizophr Bull 24(1):115–126. https://doi.org/10.1093/oxfordjournals.schbul.a033304
24. Stuart H, Sartorius N, Liinamaa T, Images Study Group (2015) Images of psychiatry and psychiatrists. Acta Psychiatr Scand 131(1):21–28. https://doi.org/10.1111/acps.12368
25. Corrigan PW, Bink AB, Fokuo JK, Schmidt A (2015) The public stigma of mental illness means a difference between you and me. Psychiatry Res 226(1):186–191. https://doi.org/10.1016/j.psychres.2014.12.047
26. Thornicroft G, Brohan E, Rose D, Sartorius N, Leese M, INDIGO Study Group (2009) Global pattern of experienced and anticipated discrimination against people with schizophrenia: a cross-sectional survey. Lancet 373(9661):408–415. https://doi.org/10.1016/S0140-6736(08)61817-6
27. Lasalvia A, Zoppei S, Van Bortel T, Bonetto C, Cristofalo D, Wahlbeck K, Bacle SV, Van Audenhove C, Van Weeghel J, Reneses B, Germanavicius A, Economou M, Lanfredi M, Ando S, Sartorius N, Lopez-Ibor JJ, Thornicroft G (2013) Global pattern of experienced and anticipated discrimination reported by people with major depressive disorder: a cross-sectional survey. Lancet 381(9860):55–62. https://doi.org/10.1016/S0140-6736(12)61379-8
28. Brohan E, Elgie R, Sartorius N, Thornicroft G, GAMIAN-Europe Study Group (2010) Self-stigma, empowerment and perceived discrimination among people with schizophrenia in 14 European countries: the GAMIAN-Europe study. Schizophr Res 122(1–3):232–238. https://doi.org/10.1016/j.schres.2010.02.1065
29. Ritsher JB, Phelan JC (2004) Internalized stigma predicts erosion of morale among psychiatric outpatients. Psychiatry Res 129(3):257–265. https://doi.org/10.1016/j.psychres.2004.08.003
30. Stuart H, Arboleda-Florez J, Sartorius N (2012) Paradigms lost: fighting stigma and the lessons learned. Oxford University Press, Oxford. https://doi.org/10.1093/med/9780199797639.001.0001
31. Evans-Lacko S, London J, Japhet S, Rüsch N, Flach C, Corker E, Henderson C, Thornicroft G (2012) Mass social contact interventions and their effect on mental health related stigma and intended discrimination. BMC Public Health 12(1):489. https://doi.org/10.1186/1471-2458-12-489
32. Corrigan PW, River LP, Lundin RK, Penn DL, Uphoff-Wasowski K, Campion J, Mathisen J, Gagnon C, Bergman M, Goldstein H, Kubiak MA (2001) Three strategies for changing attributions about severe mental illness. Schizophr Bull 27(2):187–195. https://doi.org/10.1093/oxfordjournals.schbul.a006865
33. Corrigan PW, Morris SB, Michaels PJ, Rafacz JD, Rüsch N (2012) Challenging the public stigma of mental illness: a meta-analysis of outcome studies. Psychiatr Serv 63(10):963–973. https://doi.org/10.1176/appi.ps.201100529
34. Corrigan PW, Fong MWM (2014) Competing perspectives on erasing the stigma of illness: what says the dodo bird? Soc Sci Med 1982(103):110–117. https://doi.org/10.1016/j.socscimed.2013.05.027
35. Bhugra D, Sartorius N, Fiorillo A, Evans-Lacko S, Ventriglio A, Hermans MH, Vallon P, Dales J, Racetovic G, Samochowiec J, Roca Bennemar M, Becker T, Kurimay T, Gaebel W (2015) EPA guidance on how to improve the image of psychiatry and of the psychiatrist. Eur Psychiatry 30(3):423–430. Epub 2015 Feb 27. https://doi.org/10.1016/j.eurpsy.2015.02.003
36. Evans-Lacko S, Henderson C, Thornicroft G (2013) Public knowledge, attitudes and behaviour regarding people with mental illness in England 2009-2012. Br J Psychiatry Suppl 55:s51–s57. https://doi.org/10.1192/bjp.bp.112.112979
37. Henderson C, Thornicroft G (2013) Evaluation of the time to change programme in England 2008-2011. Br J Psychiatry Suppl 55:s45–s48. https://doi.org/10.1192/bjp.bp.112.112896
38. Sampogna G, Bakolis I, Evans-Lacko S, Robinson E, Thornicroft G, Henderson C (2017a) The impact of social marketing campaigns on reducing mental health stigma: results from the 2009-2014 time to change programme. Eur Psychiatry 40:116–122. https://doi.org/10.1016/j.eurpsy.2016.08.008
39. Sampogna G, Bakolis I, Robinson E, Corker E, Pinfold V, Thornicroft G, Henderson C (2017b) Experience of the time to change programme in England as predictor of mental health service users' stigma coping strategies. Epidemiol Psychiatr Sci 26(5):517–525. Epub 2016 Jul 28. PMID: 27466083; PMCID: PMC6998878. https://doi.org/10.1017/S204579601600041X
40. Sampogna G, Gehlen L, Giallonardo V, Robinson EJ, Thornicroft G, Henderson C (2020) Mental health service users' responses to anticipated discrimination and the time to change program in England. Eur Psychiatry 64(1):e5. PMID: 33342457; PMCID: PMC8057446. https://doi.org/10.1192/j.eurpsy.2020.114

41. Thornicroft G, Sunkel C, Alikhon Aliev A, Baker S, Brohan E, El Chammay R, Davies K, Demissie M, Duncan J, Fekadu W, Gronholm PC, Guerrero Z, Gurung D, Habtamu K, Hanlon C, Heim E, Henderson C, Hijazi Z, Hoffman C, Hosny N, Huang FX, Kline S, Kohrt BA, Lempp H, Li J, London E, Ma N, Mak WWS, Makhmud A, Maulik PK, Milenova M, Morales Cano G, Ouali U, Parry S, Rangaswamy T, Rüsch N, Sabri T, Sartorius N, Schulze M, Stuart H, Taylor Salisbury T, Vera San Juan N, Votruba N, Winkler P (2022) The lancet commission on ending stigma and discrimination in mental health. Lancet 400(10361):1438–1480. Epub 2022 Oct 9. https://doi.org/10.1016/S0140-6736(22)01470-2
42. Evans-Lacko S, Courtin E, Fiorillo A et al (2014) The state of the art in European research on reducing social exclusion and stigma related to mental health: a systematic mapping of the literature. Eur Psychiatry 29:381–389
43. Gaebel W, Rössler W, Sartorius N (2016) The stigma of mental illness - end of the story? Springer International, Cham, pp 1–656

Mental Health and the Role of New Communication Technologies

5

Laura Orsolini, Giulio Longo, and Umberto Volpe

Abstract

The development of digital communication technologies recently led to a progressive change in the way we perform daily activities, rapidly transforming society into a global digital eco-system. Although digitalization determined an improvement in some aspects of life, it also led to the emergence of new technology-based psychopathologies, including problematic use of digital tools and new technological addictions (i.e., Internet addiction, smartphone addiction, social media addiction, internet gaming disorder). Furthermore, new digital technologies and tools determined significant modifications of the characteristics of several existing mental disorders. For example, several social media, forums/blogs, and dedicated websites may reinforce psychological dynamics underpinning eating disorders or provide means to enact them and facilitate their expression. Some social media 'game challenges' recently contributed to the spread of non-suicidal self-harm behaviours, particularly among teens. The rise of Internet clearly promoted the onset and perpetration of techno-assisted sexual violence and cyberbullying. Despite the pathoplastic potential associated to new communication technologies, digital tools should not be demonised at all, given the abundant evidence concerning their efficacy in the management and treatment of several mental disorders. Nowadays, digital psychiatry has a great potential to integrate and implement several diagnostic and therapeutic interventions, to support and make more effective psychiatric clinical practice. Therefore, a more balanced approach to digital communication technologies should be taken by mental health professionals, in order to increase awareness of their risks but also to gain knowledge about the benefits of such new communication tools.

Keywords

Digitalisation · Internet · Internet addiction
Gaming disorder · Mental sisorders
Smartphone addiction · Social media
Technology · Technopaties
Telecommunications

5.1 Introduction and Historical Background

Communication modalities have profoundly evolved over time [1]. The first communication mode was nonverbal communication, character-

L. Orsolini · G. Longo · U. Volpe (✉)
Unit of Clinical Psychiatry, Department of Clinical Neurosciences/DIMSC, Polytechnic University of Marche, Ancona, Italy
e-mail: u.volpe@staff.univpm.it

A. Fiorillo, S. De Giorgi (eds.), *Social Determinants of Mental Health*, Sustainable Development Goals Series, https://doi.org/10.1007/978-3-031-70165-8_5

ised by unstructured gestures and sounds; a shift to verbal communication was due to the development of languages through the organisation of sounds emitted through the human phonatory apparatus [2]. For facilitating communication between people at a distance, initial technologies involved the use of smoke and fire signals to convey messages, such as those historically widespread among the Greeks, Romans, or Persians [3]. A further evolution occurred with the development of writing. In particular, the history of human communication can be divided into two blocks. The first phase began with writing, while the second phase started with the invention of the telegraph [4]. The first phase can be furtherly divided into a first part involving script writing and a later part based on printing. From the telegraph onward, the development of the computers and their related technologies has profoundly changed communication [4]. Nowadays, society is witnessing a fast technological revolution, due to the advent of new digital devices, technologies, and communication forms [1, 3], such as use of smartphones, computers, tablets, and consoles. Despite technological tools are perceived like something very recent and modern, it is well documented that their historical roots go back to early decades of the twentieth century [1]. Hereby, we provided a comprehensive summary of the historical background and more recent developments of the main communication technologies.

5.1.1 The First Milestone: The Advent of Telephony

The 'era of telecommunications' actually started in 1794, when a message was transmitted on the Paris–Lille optical telegraph line [3]. However, the first real steps towards the development of technology allowing to communicate at distance in real time (i.e., telephony) occurred in 1809, when Samuel Thomas von Soemmering, a versatile inventor, developed an electrochemical telegraph. Later, in 1837, William Fothergill Cooke and Charles Wheatstone, two British inventors, constructed an electrical five-needle telegraph [3]. The invention of the telephone began to take shape in 1849, when the Italian inventor Antonio Meucci discovered the electronic transmission of voice, leading to the creation of a rudimentary prototype of the telephone between 1862 and 1870 [5]. The first electric phone was indeed patented in 1876 by Alexander Graham Bell [1]. A further revolution in the context of telephony occurred in 1895, thanks to another Italian inventor Guglielmo Marconi who firstly sent out a 'wireless' message using radio waves, opening up new communication scenarios and winning the Nobel Prize in Physics in 1909 [3]. The first transcontinental call occurred between the United States and France in 1915 to test the potential of radio communication [3]. While wired telephones dominated daily communication for most of the twentieth century, the development of a handheld wireless telephone became a reality only in 1973, when it was firstly designed by Martin Cooper, an engineer at Motorola, who was fascinated by Captain Kirk's 'communicator' from the TV show Star Trek [1]. Subsequently, the convergence of computer and mobile phone technology led to a further evolution of mobile phones with the advent of 'smartphones', i.e., phones with multipurpose features that go beyond simple voice telecommunication [6]. The first prototype of a smartphone, able to deliver wireless email and mobile faxing, was officially marketed in 2002 by Blackberry; the first iPhone was released by Apple in 2007 and the first Android smartphone 1 year later [1].

5.1.2 The Second Milestone: The Invention of the Computer

Blissmer [7] traced the historical premises for the development of the computer during the seventeenth century, with the invention of logarithms and the development of the first calculators. Later, Blaise Pascal and Gottfried von Leibniz, two philosophers and mathematicians, developed the first mechanical calculators to perform the four classical arithmetic operations [1]. The evolution of calculators continued until 1886, when Herman Hollerith, an engineer, founded the Tabulating Machine Company (TMC), which later became the International Business Machine (IBM), the first company to produce 'computers', in 1924 [8]. The first computers were realised to fulfil specific tasks (i.e., numbering people and objects, calculating coordinates, making forecasts, or breaking codes) [1]. The first computer commercialised was the UNIVersal Automatic Computer (UNIVAC) in 1951, which became famous for accurately predicting the results of the 1952 US presidential election [1]. Until the 1970s, the computers were designed as large hardware computer systems. In 1971, Intel produced the first microprocessor which greatly favoured the development of the first desktop computer (the 'Altair 8800'), in 1975 [1]. The Altair 8800 was announced by 'Popular Electronics' magazine as the 'world's first mini-computer kit to rival commercial models' [1]. In the same year, Bill Gates and Paul Allen left the Altair company to found Microsoft. In 1976, Steve Wozniak and Steve Jobs founded Apple, which released its first microcomputer in 1977, named the 'Apple II', which led to the official birth of home-based or 'personal' computers [1]. In the 1980s, computers became small enough to be placed in most offices. Computers have also become extremely popular worldwide, thanks to the advent of the more compact home-based models (e.g., Apple Macintosh or Commodore Amiga) and the development of more user-friendly operating systems (e.g., Microsoft Windows) [1]. In the 1990s, with the growth and capillary spread of networks and the Internet, both companies and single individuals began to buy computers, spreading everywhere in the homes of the general population. However, another revolutionary change was about to happen when turning into the new century, which would have allowed individual/personal computers to connect to a worldwide digital web.

5.1.3 The Third Milestone: Internet and the Web

The origin of the Internet dates back to 1969, when the US Department of Defence set up ARPANET (Advanced Research Projects Agency network), a computer network created to face Russian technological development during the cold war years [1]. The United States feared a Russian attack that could have damaged classic communication systems, so ARPANET allowed data to be exchanged via a different method [1]. In the 1970s, Vint Cerf, an American engineer, developed the 'Transmission Control Protocol' and the Internet Protocol (TCP/IP), making it possible to improve communication between two computers [1], leading to a progressive growth of the network, to the so-called modern Internet. In 1971, the email was first introduced as a communication tool to exchange written messages by Internet [9]. In 1979, the first discussion forums (Usenet) were born [10]. In 1982, there was the first contact with countries outside the United States, Norway, and Great Britain [9]. In 1981, the Minitel network was born in France, which soon became the largest network after the American one [9]. In 1984, CERM in Geneva was commissioned to upgrade its network to the TCP/IP protocol [11]. In 1991, Tim Berners-Lee, an English computer scientist, developed the World Wide Web (WWW) at CERN, a graphical interface for accessing the Internet via a common communication language and hyperlinks [1]. Over the last few years, Google search algorithm has revolutionised the access to the WWW: Google was developed in 1996 by three computer scientists, Larry Page, Sergey Brin, and Scott Hassan. The name 'Google' was inspired by the mathematical term *googol* (i.e., a number equivalent to ten raised to the power of a hundred or, more in general, an amount to designate to a very large integer), just wrongly transcripted during domain registration. According to the founders, it was meant to represent the amount of information to be qualitatively indexed for the purpose of optimising the navigation of web users. The evolution of the Internet continued, reaching the present day, where the Internet has spread in almost every field of daily life activities [12].

5.1.4 The Fourth Milestone: New Communication Modalities—The Advent of Social Media

Social media are defined as 'Internet-based channels that allow users to opportunistically interact and selectively self-present, either in real-time or asynchronously, with both broad and narrow audiences who derive value from user-generated content and the perception of interaction with others' [13]. The earliest forms of social networks can be found in listservs such as CompuServe, Bulletin Board Systems (BBS), and America Online (AOL), which were meeting points for people to share files and ideas. These listservs allowed communication by 'time sharing' computers. Specifically, one computer was used as a central hub through which other computers accessed it remotely, allowing messages and/or files exchange [14]. CompuServe was developed in 1969 by Jeff Wilkins, for business scopes [1], but, around the 1980s and 1990s, numerous BBSs and websites, such as AOL, became major points of social aggregation and conversation on the Internet, allowing remote and distant users to meet up with each other and interact through the Internet [1]. The first prototype of social network was 'SixDegrees', released in 1997, in which people are asked to create a profile by entering personal information and ten email addresses of friends and/or family members [1]. SixDegrees was shut down in 2001, during the rise and birth of more modern social networks [1]. In 2002, Jonathan Abrams, a Netscape engineer, created Friendster [15]. Originally, the website was conceived as a platform for creating personal profiles, including birth date or favourite foods with the aim to be only connected with distant friends and/or family members [15]. Friendster allowed users to become 'friends' only by inserting the friend's last name or his/her email address [15]. In 2003, MySpace and LinkedIn were born [1]. LinkedIn is a social network whose purpose is to create a network for professional connections, allowing people to create collaborations, find new job opportunities, and increase productivity. Myspace was similar to Friendster but differed by allowing users to customise their profiles through the use of multimedia, like photos, music, and videos. In 2004, Mark Zuckerberg, a Harvard student, created Facebook [16]. Initially, it was supposed to be accessible for Harvard students only, even though the success and growing interest of the social media allowed the rapid dissemination and spread beyond Harvard University towards other universities [16]. In fact, Mark Zuckerberg clearly differentiated Facebook from other already developed social media by including a 'news feed' section on the users' home page [1]. In 2008, YouTube was first launched, with the aim to be a simple video hosting platform; however, it rapidly became a social media platform, thanks to the comments' sections and the creation of communities [1]. Nowadays, YouTube is one of the most widely used social platforms [17] and it maintains a substantial user base with 2 billion monthly users and 81% of individuals in the 15–25 age group in the United States using the platform [18]. On an average day, users spend around 11.5 min watching YouTube contents, with a significant 70% of these views originating from mobile devices [18]. Around 95% of teenagers in the United States use YouTube and 60% of them use it constantly or several times/day [17]. Twitter was firstly introduced only in 2006, based on the idea of creating a tool able to keep in touch with friends in an easier way than other social networks [19]. The name was supposed to recall the twittering of a bird, this is because the messages were meant to be short (140 characters) and quick [20]. Twitter was and still is characterised by a maximum character limit, currently at 280 characters [1]. In 2023, after its acquisition by Elon Musk, Twitter changed its name to 'X' [21]. In 2021, 23% of the US adult population reported using Twitter [22]. In 2022, Twitter had 368.4 million users, although that number of active users is falling following Elon Musk's acquisition [23, 24]. In 2010, Instagram, a social network entirely based on the publication of photo content, was rapidly introduced in the social media scenario. In 2011, Instagram also introduced the 'hashtags', which would allow photos to be aggregated under specific keywords [1]. Hashtags are in fact words or phrases (composed of several joined written words), preceded by the hash symbol (#), that serve to tag and track topics of interest. In 2012, one of the most popular dating apps, 'Tinder', was developed and launched in the market, followed by many other dating apps, with the aim to allow people to link up with each other and find occasional relationships and/or partners. In 2014, it was initially introduced musically, which then became, in 2018, TikTok, one of the most popular social networks among youngsters [25]. TikTok allows people to share short videos by adding sounds, filters, and songs [25]. Other social media platforms are currently downloaded and used worldwide; many more will be probably developed and released by the time of the publication of this chapter.

5.1.5 Online Video Games

New communication modalities were recently developed and spread also through online video games and their associated communication tools, such as the voice channel and the verbal statements (i.e., 'callouts') delivered by using chats associated with video games which were adopted as communication means between team members in multiplayer online video games to coordinate working team and team situation awareness as well as to provide up-to-date information about the locations of opposing players. Indeed, since 1952, when Sandy Douglas, a computer scientist, developed an electronic version of the game Tic-tac-toe, to play against the first programmable computer of Cambridge University [26, 27], the era of video games and lately online video games drastically evolved. In 1958, William Higinbotham, an American physicist, developed the first truly interactive electronic game, 'Tennis for Two', where two players played a tennis match with a single knob programmed on an oscilloscope [26, 27]. In 1961, Massachusetts Institute of Technology (MIT) student Steve Russell created Spacewars, officially starting the era of video games [26]. In 1966, Ralph Baer invented 'Brown Box', a prototype of the first multiplayer multi-game system [1]. In 1972, the first console was developed, the Magnavox Odyssey, which led other companies to produce their own consoles (Atari, Coleco, URL, GHP) [26]. Indeed, the 1980s and 1990s facilitated the beginning of the so-called Golden Age for video games, during which several video gaming companies that revolutionised the world of video games, such as Commodore, Atari, SEGA, Nintendo, Sony, Microsoft, flourished [27]. During the same years, the first online multiplayer video game also was introduced and furtherly developed, by allowing the growth of the Massive Multiplayer Online (MMO) games [26, 27]. The console war continued for years until the 2000s where Nintendo, Microsoft, and Sony emerged as winners [27]. A further revolution in the video game medium occurred in 2006 when Nintendo launched the Nintendo Wii [27]. This console allowed the player to reproduce through an opposite joypad the body movements in the game world [27]. Indeed, this innovation in video games also determined the further developments of virtual reality (VR) and augmented reality (AR) as potential new communication tools [27]. Within this context, the Xbox Kinect, PlayStation Move, and Nintendo Wii were developed to allow users' body movements to be transferred directly into the virtual world through cameras placed on the television [27]. These devices represent the first recent applications of VR and AR.

5.1.6 Virtual Reality (VR) and Augmented Reality (AR)

VR is a simulation of a digital environment, through a human–machine interface, in which the individual can interact with the surrounding virtual environment in real time, by means of specific technologies such as visors, helmets, cyber suits and gloves equipped with sensors, and so forth [28]. AR is an enhanced and augmented version of reality, obtained by adding digital information through the use of devices such as smartphones, tablets, or more complex technological systems [29]. History of VR and AR is strictly connected. The birth of VR has its historical roots with the invention of the stereoscope, in 1833, by the businessman Sir Charles Wheaton. The stereoscope consists of a system of mirrors that reflect two images placed to the right and left side of the eyes, giving the effect of a single image with solidity and dimensionality [1]. In 1930, the first Sensorama machine was invented, which allowed an immersive movie experience [30]. The Sensorama consisted of a cabin in which to place the head, while inside it recreated all the sensations that one would experience if one were inside the observed video (e.g., wind, vibrations from a motorcycle, etc.) [30]. Between the 1900s and 1960s, a few mechanical VR devices were developed [31]. The most interesting was Edwin Link's 1928 flight simulator [31]. In 1968, Ivan Sutherland and Bob Sproull, two computer scientists, produced the first head-mounted VR display, called the 'Sword of Damocles' [32]. This device was indeed an AR device because it allowed digital images to be overlaid on the room all around [32]. In the 1980s, a stereoscopic Head-Mounted Display (HMD) called Virtual Visual Environment Display (VIVED) was patented by National Aeronautics and Space Administration (NASA). This device was used to train astronauts for space missions [1]. During those years, Visual Programming Language (VPL) laboratories produced further HMD devices, as well as rudimentary VR gloves [33]. Lately, in the 1990s, several companies developed their own augmented reality displays (e.g. SEGA, Nintendo), but due to limited technical skills and too unadvanced technology, they were not very successful [33]. In 1995, artist Char Davies of the Softimage group developed Osmose, an art installation characterised by computer-generated environments accessible via HMDs and cybervest [34]. However, the main important applications of VR and VA have occurred since the 2010s. In 2012, Oculus produced the Oculus Rift SDK I, a breakthrough tethered stereoscopic HMD (software and hardware) with a head-tracking sensor built into the lightweight headset [35]. In 2012, Google announced Google Glass, a device for AR, which, however, never reached the consumer market [36]. In 2014, Google Cardboard was announced, which allowed users to use VR through their smartphones [37]. In 2015, Microsoft announced HoloLens, an AR device characterised by 'a high-definition stereoscopic 3D optical see-through head-mounted display which uses holographic waveguide elements in front of each eye to present the user with high-definition holograms spatially correlated and stabilised within your physical surroundings' [38]. At the same time, Valve, HTC, and Samsung produced their respective VR systems [33]. In 2016, the PlayStation VR was created, and in the same year, one of the most important augmented reality applications, Pokemon GO, was released [1]. Magic Leap also announced the first generation of all-in-one consumer AR glasses [33]. In 2019, Facebook launched Facebook Horizon, a VR-based social network world [39], then renamed Meta Platforms, announcing that they were developing a greater and immersive virtual world, the metaverse [40]. In 2023, Apple announced its VR-based device, named Apple Vision Pro, featuring a mix of VR and AR [41]. Mixed reality can be obtained by switching from VR to AR and vice versa, the user is able to see what is around it and at the same time use their hands and voice to navigate between apps [41].

5.1.7 The Future Milestones: Artificial Intelligence and Chatbots

The term artificial intelligence (AI) refers to an intelligent computer system capable of reproducing the functioning and behaviour of the human mind [42]. The history of AI is not only rooted in computer science, but it refers to many disciplines including mathematics, philosophy, linguistics, psychology, economics, neuroscience, and engineering [43]. AI has developed considerably since the early 1950s. Alan Turing, a prominent British mathematician, discussed it within his 1950 article 'Computing Machinery and Intelligence', by developing the Turing test which identifies an 'intelligent' machine [43]. However, the term AI was only created in 1956, during the summer workshop '*Dartmouth Summer Research Project on Artificial Intelligence*' (DSRPAI) organised in New Hampshire by John McCarthy, a computer scientist [44]. After this initial boom, there was a gradual slowdown of AI (named 'Winter AI') mainly due to technical difficulties and poor technological advancements [44]. While in the 1980s, the spread of computers facilitated a research resurgence with further, even though small, advances in the early 2000s due to the spread of the Internet [44]. In 2010, the development of machine learning (ML) and deep learning (DL) techniques established the era of the 'Spring AI fever' [45].

ML is a specific application of AI involving the construction of mathematical algorithms capable of self-learning, i.e., learning from analysed data without prior instruction on how to handle the data and able to identify specific/mathematical patterns, based on the analysis of received inputs [46]. These patterns are virtually verified and used to create prediction models of variables' trends, correct errors, and improve the performance of the same algorithms [46]. Another AI-based application is represented by the chatbots, i.e., software able to simulate human conversations by allowing users to interact with digital devices as if they were communicating with a real person [47]. The first-ever chatbot ('ELIZA') was developed in 1966 by Joseph Weizenbaum, a German computer scientist at the Massachusetts Institute of Technology (MIT). *ELIZA* sought to simulate the conversational skills of a psychotherapist [47]. The term was coined by Michael Mauldin in 1996, who created the chatbot *TinyMUD*, an artificial video gamer [48]. One of the evolutions of chatbots, occurred from 2010s, concerns the development of voice assistants (e.g., Apple's Siri, Google's Assistant, Amazon's Alex, and Microsoft's Cortana), with whom people can communicate through voice or text messages asking for information [48]. Nowadays, AI is under development to create predictive models of mental disease(s) through self-learning from specific inputs provided [46, 47].

Overall, despite the promising and beneficial technological advancements in the digitalization and new communication modalities, the process indeed determined a set of changes in an individual's daily life activities as well as a differential impact on mental health which will be discussed in the below paragraph.

5.2 Digitalization and the Impact on Mental Health

The digital devices and new communication tools are now fully integrated in everyone's daily lives [49]. New technologies have been developed not only as a communication mean but also to deliver education, social relationships, jobs, business, travel, online shopping, entertainment as well as medical consultation [50]. The sociologist Manuel Castells [51] anticipated this new digitally delivered societal era (aka 'Information Age') and our post-modern digitally delivered society as the 'Network Society'. Within the 'Network Society', social dynamics, particularly among younger generations (aka 'digital natives'), are indeed regulated by the direction of Internet information flows, governed by technologies [51, 52]. Consequently, the consolidation of a 'Network Society' significantly impacted and led to many individual and interpersonal changes, such as establishing new 'virtual' friends and favouring peer-to-peer social communication, finding love, shopping, accessing inexhaustible sources of information and studying, reducing perceived feelings of loneliness, sharing own experiences, and creating support networking [52–59].

However, despite the many potential applications and positive impacts on daily life activities of the new communication technologies, a series of potential technologically driven and web-mediated mental health issues have been occurred with digital devices and the Internet. A quick overview of the most frequently reported mental health issues related to new communication technologies is provided in the next paragraphs.

5.2.1 Problematic Internet Use and Internet-based psychopathologies

Problematic Internet Use (PIU) is one of the most commonly investigated mental health issues related to Internet use [60]. Indeed, PIU has been historically variably named as 'Internet addiction', 'excessive Internet use', 'pathological Internet use', 'compulsive Internet use', and 'Internet use disorder' [61]. However, PIU seems the most accurate term as the condition is not unanimously considered a pathological addiction and it is still unclear the pathological threshold level of Internet use to discriminate between a non-pathological use and a behavioural addiction [61]. PIU was firstly defined in 1996 as 'an uncontrolled and excessive Internet use' [60]. The diagnostic threshold for diagnosing a PIU is 'spending more than 6 hours daily online (not for work and/or educational activities), with an associated global functioning impairment of daily activities due to a loss of control over behaviours secondary to the need to use Internet and online devices' [62]. Indeed, PIU currently represents an 'umbrella' term composed of different types of technological activities facilitated through the Internet, including online gaming, video streaming, social media engagement, and so forth [63–65]. Despite methodological disparities across studies in terms of assessment tools and diagnostic criteria, a recent meta-analysis indicated a global prevalence of around 7% for PIU, with significant geographical differences across countries [66]; European rates range from 2% in Norway to 22% in Italy [67]. Factors such as low parental involvement, negative peer relationships, parental unemployment, and male sex are significant contributors to the onset of PIU [68].

Although the aetiopathogenesis of PIU is still unclear, the two proposed theoretical frameworks are: (a) the cognitive-behavioural model and (b) the interaction of Person-Affect-Cognition-Execution (I-PACE) model. The former includes distal (i.e., factors that predispose and promote the maintenance of the disorder, such as depression, social anxiety, positive reinforcement) and proximal factors (i.e., maladaptive cognitions about oneself and the world, such as low self-efficacy, self-doubt, negative self-appraisal) as possible causal determinants in the onset and/or maintenance of PIU [61], while the I-PACE model considers PIU as a multifactorial disease [67], involving personality (e.g., low self-esteem, impulsivity, etc.), psychosocial (e.g. loneliness, isolation, poor social support, low parental involvement, etc.), biopsychological (e.g., genetics, childhood experiences), and psychopathological variables (e.g., ADHD, depression, social anxiety, autism spectrum disorder, etc.). The second factor (A and C component) consists of motivation for use (e.g., escapism from reality), coping strategies (e.g., avoidance), internet-related cognitive biases (e.g., expectancies, illusions), and affective and cognitive responses (i.e., cue reactivity, craving, urge for mood regulation, attentional bias). The third factor (E component) includes patients' executive functions, conditioning factors, and inhibitory control [61, 67, 69].

Furthermore, PIU has been associated with several psychiatric disorders, such as anxiety, depression, autism spectrum disorder, personality traits, ADHD, Hikikomori, and psychosomatic illnesses [70–80]. From a clinical and psychopathological perspective, PIU has been associated with the emergence of risky behaviours and occurrence of potentially detrimental mental health consequences (Table 5.1). An accurate differential diagnosis is needed to discriminate between primary and secondary PIU (i.e., due to an underpinned psychiatric disorder), as the treatment plan should be addressed to firstly

Table 5.1 Mental health issues related to Internet use

Mental health issues related to Internet use
• Problematic use of Internet
• Anxiety disorders
• Depression
• Loneliness
• Isolation

manage causal psychiatric disorder [81]. Current evidence suggest interventions such as cognitive-behavioural therapy (CBT), including brief manualized CBT programmes and mobile app-based coaching programmes, online-based motivational interventions, school-based psychoeducational media literacy interventions on Internet use, psychosocial interventions, solution-focused approaches, and, in some cases, combined CBT and psychopharmacotherapy (e.g., bupropion, atomoxetine, methylphenidate, etc.); the effectiveness of these interventions is moderate-to-large effect size [67].

5.2.2 Smartphone-Based Psychopathologies

Overall, despite the spread of smartphones increased the opportunities to obtain and share any type of information in the real-time, to be entertained, to be relaxed, to apparently improve individual performance and efficiency, to meet new people, to earn and increase own social status [82], the widespread dissemination of smartphones also facilitated the development of problematic smartphone use (PSU) as well as the emergence of specific smartphone-based psychopathologies [83]. PSU refers to the difficulty of staying separated from one's smartphone, with the consequent development of anxious symptoms associated with withdrawal symptoms upon detachment [82]. The prevalence of PSU widely varies according to socioeconomic and cultural differences (Table 5.2), with a supposed increasing trend in the next years [90]. Due to the lack of a clear theoretical and clinical conceptualisation as well as universally recognised definition, PSU is currently not included as a diagnosis either in the ICD-11 [91] or DSM-5-TR [92].

Table 5.2 Problematic smartphone use (PSU) prevalence among European countries

Country	PIU prevalence
Korea	30.9%
United Kingdom	10%
India	31%
Italy	33%
Switzerland	16.9%
Taiwan	16.7%

Sources: [84–89].

Etiopathogenesis of PSU is multifactorial, including socio-demographic and psychopathological domains, such as female sex, number of daily and weekly hours spent on a smartphone, presence of the 'reassurance seeking' smartphone use modality, high levels of neuroticism, pre-existing anxiety, stress, depressive symptoms, insomnia, perceived higher loneliness, low self-esteem, exposition to excessive rigid and/or permissive parenting styles, dysfunctional family dynamics, a history of emotional abuse, poor school performance, and low motivation to study [82, 93–96]. The onset of PSU may be facilitated by the presence of impulsive features, characterised by antisocial personality traits, disinhibition and attention deficits, sensation-seeking, and reward sensitivity [82, 93, 96]. A higher risk to develop PSU is also associated with low conscientiousness levels, due to low levels of self-control and premeditation for risky behaviours [82, 93, 96], while protective factors include good sociability, good network of 'real' friends, and good self-control [94].

Overall, excessive smartphone use has been associated with risky behaviours and potentially detrimental physical and mental health consequences (Table 5.3). For example, risky behaviours due to improper and/or excessive smartphone use may comprise those occurring

Table 5.3 Health issues related to pathological smartphone use

Mental issues	Organic issues
• Problematic smartphone use • Anxiety disorders • Depression • Loneliness • Isolation • Stress • Insomnia • *Phubbing* • Attention impairment • FOMO • Nomophobia	• Chronic headaches • Dizziness • Dry eyes • Blurred vision • Fatigue • Burning • Itching • Gliomas • Blood–brain barrier alterations • Musculoskeletal damage (neck, shoulders, hands)

while driving, walking, sleeping, and so forth. Numerous car accidents and deaths have been reported each year caused by individuals engaged in phone calls or texting while driving [97]. In 2021, the National Highway Traffic Safety Administration (NHTSA) stated that 8% of all reported crashes are caused by smartphone-related distractions, while in fatal crashes the rate rises to 12% [98]. Texting while driving is estimated to increase the risk of traffic accidents by 23 times, dialling a phone increases it by 2.8 times, while talking on or listening to the phone increases it by 1.3 times [97]. Moreover, numerous episodes of collisions, accidents, and falls are caused by pedestrians who were distracted by their smartphone [82, 99].

Regarding physical health issues, some studies reported that excessive smartphone use could cause chronic headaches, dizziness, dry eyes, blurred vision, eyes fatigue, eyes burning, eyes itching, gliomas, and blood–brain barrier alterations [97, 100]. Moreover, damages to the neck and shoulders, accompanied by chronic pain, as well as hand dysfunctions resulting from musculoskeletal damage, have also been reported due to the position assumed while using the smartphone [82].

Moreover, PSU can also cause sleep problems due to the late-night use of mobile phones, but also to the effects of the blue light emitted by mobile phone display which may simulate solar radiation, by consequently prompting melatonin production and altering circadian rhythm [97, 101, 102]. PSU has been also associated with poor school performance, lower physical activity, higher obesity rates, poor well-being, risky sexual or aggressive behaviours, anxiety and depression symptomatology [52, 82, 95, 96]. Excessive smartphones use may also lead individuals to detach from reality, to reduce/eliminate social interactions, peer-to-peer communications, by triggering feelings of rejection and neglect by their peers and friends [96]. This phenomenon is referred to so-called *phubbing* which results in a reduced satisfaction with emotional and loving relationships [95, 96]. Excessive smartphones use may also lead to attention impairment, with a selective attention addressed only to smartphone-related activities [52]. The driven motivation can be certainly due to the quality of accessible digital content, as well as to different attractive smartphone-based dynamics. The smartphone user is usually in a state of constant anticipation of information, by, hence, addressing the selective attention towards any smartphone notifications/adverts. This phenomenon, known as '*checking behaviours*', refers to the frequent and quick inspection of the smartphone in search of the incoming information [52]. This activity represents a positive reinforcement upon receiving such information, by determining an information reward which, in turns, results in preferring multi-tasking media that allow individuals to interact simultaneously with multiple media but contextually to remain on the surface level of information. This behaviour may significantly lead to cognitive deterioration, as documented by imaging studies that identified an increased activity in the right prefrontal region—a region devoted to suppressing distractor stimuli—which results in a loss of grey matter [52].

Overall, the ability to access an immense amount of information has also changed the way individuals can learn. Indeed, having the smartphone always available simply pushes people towards 'transactive memory', which refers to the ability to store information in a sort of external memory determining a 'cognitive offloading', which means reducing the information learned [52]. In fact, even though 'cognitive offloading' could allow the memory not to be overloaded, it may result in a different learning modality, in which the individual may easily learn where to find the information without really learning the notions. This determines a reduced activation of the ventral brain areas involved in the ability to recall information [52]; conversely, it has been observed an increase in the frontal, occipital, parietal, and temporal connecting fibres integrity, which would improve the ability to detect elements that are not immediately visible [52].

Furthermore, PSU could lead to stress-related symptomatology (the so-called *technostress*). In the past, this term was used to describe a reduction in workplace performance resulting from employees' sustained efforts to stay competent in evolving fields of information and communication technology [95, 96].

PSU determined the emergence of two new smartphone-related psychopathologies: nomophobia and FOMO. The term nomophobia is a neologism originated from the expression '*no mobile phone phobia*', firstly described in 2010 [103, 104]. The term refers to the discomfort, anxiety, nervousness, and distress generated by the individual's loss of connection from his/her cell phone or any other technological mean that allows connection to the Internet. Some authors define it as a syndrome characterised by the pathological fear of staying '*out of touch with technology*' [105]. Indeed, it is essential to perform an accurate differential diagnosis with the following disorders, before confirming the diagnosis: panic attack disorder, body dysmorphic disorder, avoidant personality disorder, atypical depression, dysthymia, obsessive-compulsive disorder [104]. In a recent meta-analysis, the prevalence of moderate-to-severe nomophobia in the population was around 70.8%, while severe nomophobia was reached by 21% of the general population [106]. Recent studies demonstrated that nomophobia is linked to personality traits such as extraversion, dysfunctional obsessive beliefs, neuroticism, disinhibition, and maladaptive coping strategies and it is more frequently observed among females and younger people [106–109].

The concept of 'fear of missing out' (FOMO) was initially used in the marketing world and only later adopted by mental health professionals [110, 111]. FOMO is characterised by '*a pervasive apprehension that others might be having rewarding experiences from which one is absent*' [111]. FOMO is more represented among youngsters, with no gender differences [111–113]. The development of FOMO is related to the 'self-determination theory pathway'. This framework is characterised by the composition of three psychopathological needs: (a) need for relatedness (the need to be accepted by others), (b) competence (the need to be competent and effective in anything); (c) autonomy (the need to decide for oneself) [111–113]. FOMO has been more likely described among individuals with lower levels of satisfaction in the above-mentioned dimensions [111–113]. FOMO is a major driver for the development of PSU and problematic internet use, and it is associated with the presence of impulsivity, poor self-control, lower life satisfaction, and neuroticism [53, 111–113]. In contrast, it is negatively associated with consciousness traits [112]. FOMO often may be both a consequence of pre-existing depressive-anxiety symptomatology and a causal factor, by also determining PSU and PIU onset [111–113].

Current evidence suggests cognitive-behavioural therapy (CBT), mindfulness-based cognitive therapy (MBCT), psychoeducation-based sleep hygiene interventions, app-based combined CBT, MBCT, and psychoeducational interventions, and psychosocial and lifestyle interventions including physical activity-based programmes.

5.2.3 Social Media-Based Psychopathologies

Overall, it has been estimated that about 4.59 billion people used social media worldwide in 2022, with a supposed increasing trend over the next few years [114]. *Approximately 68% and 73% of the American adult population declared to be attracted and regularly engaged, respectively, in Facebook- and YouTube-related activities* [115]. *Problematic Social Networks Use (PSNU) is emerging as a potential detrimental mental health condition secondary to an excessive and inappropriate/maladaptive use of social media. It is usually preferred the term PSNU* (versus *'social media addiction'), as there are still ongoing studies aimed to investigate whether PSNU could be classified within the behavioural addictions* [64, 65, 116–118]. *Indeed, social media addiction refers to the problematic and compulsive use of social media platforms, leading to substantial functioning impairment that persists over a prolonged period* [64, 65]. *The prevalence of PSNU has been reported to be around 5% worldwide, with a country-based variability ranging from 4.5% in Hungary to 12% in China* [119]. *Females, middle-aged, and older people are the most vulnerable to the development of PSNU* [120].

Furthermore, PSNU has been associated to other mental health issues in comorbidity such as depression, anxiety (especially, social anxiety), stress-related disorders and stress levels, attention deficit hyperactivity disorder (ADHD), obsessive-compulsive disorder (OCD), psychosomatic disorders, eating disorders (ED), substance use disorder (SUDs), Internet Gaming Disorder (IGD), and sleep disorders, even though some studies supported the hypothesis that PSNU could be secondary to pre-existing psychopathological conditions or a concausal condition rather than a merely comorbidity [119–121]. For instance, the relationship between social media use and depressive symptomatology has been supposed to be indeed bidirectional. PSNU has been described to lead to reduced self-esteem, which may worsen depressive symptoms, which in turn may prompt an increase in PSNU as a maladaptive coping mechanism. This distortion is driven by the Hyperpersonal Model, whereby social users are constantly exposed to idealised and unreal contents, leading individuals to consider others on social media exaggeratedly more successful, brilliant, and happy than themselves [122]. This effect appears to be more impactful depending on the number of hours spent on social media, and it has been observed to be particularly significant among males, especially if they need psychological and/or psychiatric help [121]. Conversely, social media could represent an escape valve and coping strategy for managing depressive-anxiety symptomatology [122]. Overall, a set of potential identified risk factors of PSNU have been reported and listed in Table 5.4. Furthermore, a set of personality traits have been significantly associated as potential predictors of PSNU, such as the 'Dark Triad' personality (aka, Narcissism, Machiavellianism, and emotional dysregulation), due to emotional regulation and impulsivity issues [79, 80, 119, 123]. Both types of narcissism have been identified as personality traits more likely associated with the onset of PSNU. The grandiose narcissism is characterised by the presence of grandiosity, dominance, and aggression, while the vulnerable narcissism is characterised by hypersensitivity, defensiveness, and need for approval. Indeed, social networks may represent an excellent tool for such individuals to express control over their presentation, receive attention, spread their thoughts to a larger audience, and obtain feedback.

Table 5.4 Risk factor for problematic social network use (PSNU)

Risk factor for PSNU
• Pre-existing mental health impairment • Low self-esteem • Impulsivity • Positive outcome expectation • Stress • Lower emotional intelligence • External motivation of social reward • Faulty metacognition (such as punishment, worry, beliefs about responsibility, superstition, and cognitive monitoring) • Anxious attachment (as opposed to secure attachment which is a protective factor) • Personality trait (emotional stability, extraversion, conscientiousness, neuroticism) • History of childhood maltreatment • Lower family support • Low family functioning • Poor support from friends

Sources: [119, 120].

Overall, one of the most detrimental consequences of PSNU is the negative impact that it can have on the subjects' work and school and overall functioning in daily life activities, due to the impaired sustained and selective attention to other routine daily activities different from those 'virtually' experienced on social media [122]. It has been also reported an increased perception of loneliness, following the development of PSNU [120]. Moreover, PSNU could also promote the occurrence of PSNU [124]. For example, TikTok offers such immersive functionality that it engages users to the fullest. More time is spent by the user on the platform, higher is the probability that the social network will be able to collect punctual psychological features of the individual, which allows the system to offer more individual-tailored content and, hence, attract him/her to stay connected through the social and using the smartphone. Similarly, the user's 'likes' are used by AI to endlessly refine and personalise the content shown to users. This satisfies the patient's needs, according to the 'gratification theory', thus driving them to spend more time on the social network and, hence, on the smartphone. At the same time, creating content and posting videos also helps satisfy the subject's need for fame and attention-seeking, according to the 'social impact' and 'self-affirmation' theories [124]. Obviously, all these functionalities could lead to potentially serious mental health issues, particularly among teenagers and young adults who currently represent the most vulnerable population to techno-mediated mental health issues but also the most frequently reported users of all social media [124].

Among the most frequently described social media-driven psychopathologies, there are the social media-mediated EDs, cyberbullying, and the death challenges. Overall, it has been overly demonstrated that the advent of new media (i.e., fashion journals, satellite TV, etc.) indeed encouraged the spread of unachievable beauty standards and determined an increase in the emergence of altered eating styles and eating disorders [125, 126]. Similarly, with the spread of the Internet and social media, a further diffusion of EDs has been also reported [127–129]. In fact, most social networks (particularly Instagram and Snapchat) could lead to an individual's body dissatisfaction, which could facilitate the development and/or maintenance and/or worsening of EDs [127, 128, 130]. In fact, social networks facilitate the process of internalisation of excessive and unrealistic beauty standards which are usually hyper-idealised on social networks, such as photos of lean and toned bodies or retouched images posted on social media, with subsequent unrealistic and unreachable comparisons and consequent own body dissatisfaction [127, 128]. Moreover, social media incentivise the process of the so-called self-objectification, particularly among females, through which the individual strongly believes that own value is only based on his/her physical appearance, thus, incentivising body surveillance, body comparisons, and body/food self-control [127, 128]. Conversely, '*body positivity movements*' are currently emerging to promote more realistic and 'imperfect' body standards, through different social media channels [127, 128].

Cyberbullying represents another social media-driven psychopathology. The first case of cyberbullying was described in 1998 when a 14-year-old boy was expelled from school for spreading threatening content against other students on the Internet [131]. Cyberbullying is described as 'the wilful and repeated harm inflicted through the use of computers, cell phones, and other electronic devices'. The prevalence of cyberbullying has been estimated to be around 33.1%, while perpetration of violent modality is reported in approximately 25% of cases [132]. Females are more likely to be at-risk to be cyberbullying victims, compared to the male counterpart as well as LGBTQ+ individuals [131, 132]. The main modalities through which cyberbullying is perpetuated involve using social media, texting, and chatting. Among the most 'targeted topics' of cyberbullying activities are listed: (a) individual's general appearance (55%), (b) individual's body shape (37%), and (c) racial and ethnic discrimination (16%). Cyberbullying is mainly acted and perpetrated anonymously (i.e., without direct contact with the abused victim) [131]. Predictors of cyberbullying behaviours are represented by online exposure, earlier involvement in online activities, younger age, living in urban areas, more impulsive, antisocial, and less empathetic personality traits, previous victimisation experiences (i.e., the subject expresses his or her superiority and strength, externalising feelings of anger and relieving the sadness of having been victimised in the past), and specific parenting styles (authoritarian parenting style associated with low parental control) [131, 132]. Cyberbullied individuals may develop a variety of mental disorders including depression and anxiety disorders, PTSD, sleep disorders, isolation, somatic symptoms (i.e., headaches, abdominal pain, etc.), alcohol use disorder (AUD) and/or SUD, and paranoia, suicidality, interpersonal, and conduct disorders [131].

Furthermore, another social media-driven phenomenon has been described, particularly among adolescents and young people, named 'Death Challenges' [133–135]. One of the most famous death challenges is represented by the 'Blue Whale Challenge', spread in 2013 in Russia [134]. This challenge pushed teenagers and young adults to complete a series of 50 tasks within a span of 50 days, all assigned by a 'curator'. The level of challenge in these tasks escalates progressively, starting with actions that pose a severe risk to one's life, such as etching a whale onto their skin with a sharp object, scaling buildings, or enduring prolonged sleep deprivation. Ultimately, the culmination of this dangerous game leads to the player's tragic act of suicide, wherein they are compelled to leap from the roof of the city's tallest building [134, 136]. Another 'death challenge' is represented by the 'Blackout Challenge' (aka the 'Choking Game') during which participants are engaged in forced asphyxiation. This is accomplished by applying pressure to the neck using their hands or ligatures, all to experience a sensation akin to being 'high' without using drugs. Those involved in the challenge often report a brief feeling of euphoria before losing consciousness, a result of the reduced blood flow to the brain [137]. Individuals engaged in these activities are usually recorded in videos which are then uploaded on the most commonly used social media platforms, such as TikTok, YouTube, and Instagram. The potential dangers associated with this practice encompass a range of adverse consequences, including bruising, short-term memory loss, seizures, concussions, retinal haemorrhage, stroke, brain damage, and even death. Furthermore, several documented cases have been published, underscoring the occurrence of unintentional deaths resulting from this perilous challenge [138, 139].

Current evidence suggests interventions such as cognitive-behavioural therapy (CBT), mindfulness-based cognitive therapy (MBCT), app-based interventions (combining CBT, MBCT, and psychoeducational interventions), and psychosocial and lifestyle interventions including physical activity-based programmes may be useful in treating the above conditions.

5.2.4 Forum and Online Communities

With the rise of the Internet and the web 2.0, online communities and other networking online platforms such as fora and blogs emerged and were rapidly populated. Online communities are composed of a group of people with common interests who meet 'virtually' to discuss a particular Internet service and/or belong to a particular Internet platform [140]. Over time, 'extreme communities' have also emerged, which are characterised by use/spread/comment of/on material that may be considered 'extreme' by the general population and may face censorship [141]. Such communities, originally developed on online forums and websites, currently spread also through different social media platforms [142]. 'Extreme communities' include those specifically addressed to individuals with EDs, those promoting non-suicidal self-injury (NSSIs) behaviours or SUDs and the 'incel communities'.

Communities specifically addressed to EDs are mainly represented by 'pro-ana' forums (promoting anorexia) and 'pro-mia' forums (promoting bulimia) [142]. In such sites, patients suffering from EDs virtually meet up to share and discuss their conditions, exchanging information and advice on eating behaviours/disorders. In particular, such forums lead to reinforcement and maintenance of EDs, by promoting the development of an ED identity [142]. Users share tips on how to lose weight (e.g., alternative methods of consuming calories, medications, and how to get them, etc.), how to hide the disorder from family and friends, and how to reduce their calorie intake, thus reinforcing the disorder [143]. In addition, this kind of interaction also results in increased negative affect and reduced self-esteem, as well as increased number of hospitalisations [142]. It has been demonstrated that those who have visited such websites daily for at least 12 months are characterised by the highest level of ED pathology and functional impairment, engaging in the most dangerous activities [142]. Some patients have also established mechanisms of competition with others, pushing them to very severe thinness [142]. In addition, '*thinspiration*' threads (threads that promote thinness and are intended to inspire those who view them) are posted, allowing readers to compare their bodies to the already validated body to be used as a model [142, 144]. Indeed, these behaviours reinforce the disorder, by pushing patients to identify themselves with their disorder. The two underlying themes of self-identification with the disorder are keeping the disorder a secret and help in maintaining a sense of the pro-anorexic self as abnormality [142, 145]. This is corroborated by disclosures of loyalty to anorexia and associated behaviours, self-loathing and self-deprecation, advice giving (e.g., tips and techniques to lose weight, managing offline social situations), and group encouragement and cohesion [142, 145]. It has been shown that the reason for enrolling in such platforms is a poor social support perceived from offline relationships [142, 146]. A study conducted on a sample of healthy subjects found that exposure to such sites may lead individuals to perceive their bodies heavier, to increase exercise, to reduce self-esteem, to increase negative affect, to increase comparison of their bodies with others, and to think about how they will vary in the near future [147].

Another type of 'extreme community' promotes NSSI. Indeed, the risks associated with online NSSI are related to the fact that such forums normalise and reinforce risky behaviours among users [142]. On such sites, participants share NSSI-related feelings and experiences (specifying the emotional pain and distress), videos and photos of the self-injurious conduct. Often these individuals do not seek help to manage the mental pain they experience and prefer to use the online platform to share their feelings and psychological distress. Similarly to pro-ana and pro-mia forums, users share information about self-injury strategies (e.g., ways to cut, burn skin, what medications to take to facilitate self-injury, etc.), how to hide NSSI from family and friends (e.g., suggesting hidden cutting locations), first aid tips (e.g., disinfect wounds, promote healing, etc.). At the same time, exposure to self-injurious content may trigger such behaviours in more vulnerable people [142].

Similarly to pro-NSSI forums, there are also communities promoting suicide. The first one was described in Japan, where the phenomenon of 'Net Suicides' was firstly identified [148]. Mass suicides occurred because of pacts made between people who never met each other, except online [148]. On such forums and websites, information on how to commit suicide was exchanged and such pacts were agreed upon. The phenomenon is now worldwide spread [141, 149]. It has been also confirmed that (social) media may influence, particularly young people, in pushing suicide through emulation [149]. This is referred to as 'Werther Effect' to recall the wave of suicides among young readers that occurred after the publication of the book *The Sorrows of Young Werther* written by Johann Wolfgang Goethe in 1774. One study has been demonstrated that exposure to forums and sites that incentivize suicide may lead to an increased suicidal ideation, by normalising and prompting the suicide act [150, 151].

Other communities promoting pro-drug behaviours and activities are those represented by the e-psychonauts' communities [152]. The term 'psychonaut' comes from the German psychonaut, a neologism for those individuals who are seeking new psychoactive substances to attempt exploring their inner selves, so much that they also define themselves as 'mind navigators' and/or 'chemicals' experimenters' [153]. These are usually male subjects with high novelty seeking and reduced harm avoidance, which drive themselves to consume any new substance placed on the market, independently by the safety and tolerability profile [153]. Nowadays, these subjects use online forums and websites to share information about newly produced substances, their experiences, and histories and about places where they can safely purchase such substances [152, 153]. Such sites are also rich in technical, pharmacological, and phytological information, all facilitated by the anonymity given by the Internet [152–155].

Finally, one of the most represented communities on the web is the recent 'incel community'. The term *'incel'* is derived from 'involuntary celibacy', which refers to those individuals who do not have loving and sexual relationships, although the desire to have them [156, 157]. This term was born in 1997, when a college student, Alana, created a website to document her struggles in dating. This site was intended to create a support and discussion group for similar experiences. After a few years, Alana gave up the site to other users after entering into a stable relationship. She rediscovered the group in 2014, following an incel attack in California in which six people died. In particular, she discovered that the site was turned into a meeting place for men who were not in loving or sexual relationships and whose anger was often directed towards women [156, 157]. Such individuals believe that society is organised on a hierarchical system based on physical appearance [156]. According to this ideology, incels do not have emotional or sexual relationships because women are only interested in good-looking subjects, regardless of other characteristics of the person [156]. According to recent estimates, more than half of the world's incels are located in Europe or North America [156]. From a psychopathological perspective, such individuals are characterised by higher levels of depressive and anxiety symptoms, a higher rate of ASD diagnosis, higher levels of social isolation, loneliness levels, intolerance of interpersonal rejection, lower self-esteem, anxious/avoidant attachment styles, dating anxiety, high ruminations of self-criticism, feelings of guilt, tendency to manipulation, a greater tendency to victimisation, and higher levels of suicidal ideation, compared to the general population [156, 157].

Continuously new communities and forums on the web are being founded. Recent topics include discussion forums on paraphilias and unusual sexual practices as well as on rare diseases such as Body Integrity Identity Disorder, where users discuss about their desire to amputate themselves limbs or cause themselves very serious damage (e.g., becoming blind or causing themselves severe spinal damage to become paralysed) [158].

5.2.5 Chat-Related Psychopathology

Nowadays, it is possible to meet new people online, not only with social media but also through the so-called *dating apps*. Online dating is defined as the use of internet-enabled information and communication technology aimed at connecting individuals with potential partners for different types of intimate relationships, like dating, long-term relationship, sexual encounters, and so forth [159]. Online dating was initially promoted through advertising websites, then through websites which ask you to register and that use individual details to run algorithms to pair individuals, and, finally, through the use of dating apps [159]. The first-ever produced app in 2008 was Grindr, a dating app for homosexual people, while the most famous one is Tinder. In 2021, the Tinder app had 430 million downloads since its launch with 1.5 million dates per week [159]. Before 1990, the number of couples who met online was 0, while in 2009 it rose up to 22% [159]. At the same time, in 2013, 11% of US people had used a dating app at least once in their lives, compared to the current 30% [159]. However, dating apps have been reported to potentially determine negative mental health issues due to the risky behaviours derived by using these dating apps. For example, technology-facilitated sexual violence is characterised by 'a range of criminal, civil, or otherwise harmful sexually aggressive and harassing behaviors that are perpetrated with the aid or use of communication technologies' [159]. Technology-facilitated violence could be perpetrated in different ways, in particular *sextortion* (i.e., coercion via threats to publish sexual content like photos or videos or information), *image-based abuse* (i.e., spread intimate photos without consent), *doxxing* (i.e., publishing private personal information), cyberbullying, online sexual harassment (i.e., a form of sexual harassment that initially starts on the Internet, generally through email, Internet forums, or online messaging programs), *cyberstalking* (i.e., using technology to stalk virtually someone), online grooming for sexual assault (i.e., building trust and making connections with someone to procure sexual cooperation), *hate speech*, online impersonation (i.e., using an identity different from one's for malicious purposes), *hacking* (i.e., stealing personal information or banking accounts), sending unsolicited nude or genital images [159–161]. Prevalence rates of these behaviours are limited and often discordant. In studies focusing on adult populations in Australia, instances of technology-facilitated sexual violence were documented in 62.3% of cases, a trend that increased up to 71.8% within the 18–24 age bracket [162]. In contrast, a study involving Canadian college students projected a higher prevalence, reaching up to 84.3% [163]. Risk factors for sexual violence victimisation are: female gender, sexual and gender minorities, persons of colour, and lack of social support [159, 163]. Four reasons for which platforms would drive violence are [159]: (a) disinhibition, whereby the use of social media leads to altered behaviour by driving violence (mainly due to anonymity); (b) technoculture approach, whereby such activities would be norm-governed; (c) risky lifestyle, whereby social media would not necessarily lead to violence but would be supported by the victim's conduct; and (d) social embedding, whereby violence would be supported by cultural aspects of the subject that are also perpetrated offline. Identified risk factors for the violence perpetuation include male sex, antisocial traits, and sexist beliefs [159]. The consequences of such violence on the victims may determine the onset of depressive symptoms, anxiety disorders, post-traumatic stress disorder, loneliness, emotional regulation disorders, low perceived self-control, and low self-esteem [164, 165].

Another communication-related issue includes the phenomenon of the '*revenge porn*', which firstly emerged in 2005 and belongs to the category of '*non-consensual pornography*' [166]. It refers to the dissemination of sexually explicit images or videos without the consent of the persons portrayed and may have potentially devastating mental health consequences for the subjected person. Typically, '*revenge porn*' is more prevalent among women and is performed following a breakup of an emotional relationship with the intention to attack the ex-partner, being a kind of revenge against the ex-partner [166]. It may cause lowered self-esteem, a sense of inadequacy, relationship and emotional difficulties, embarrassment in public, depressive symptoms, suicidal attempt, anxiety disorders, loneliness and stigmatisation, self-harm, and post-traumatic stress disorder in the victim [167, 168]. It can also have work and social consequences, for example, becoming more prone to experience bullying, isolation, and other sexual abuse (like rape) [166, 168]. Those who disseminate such content have high levels of impulsivity and a low empathic and emotional intelligence [166–168]. Revenge porn is often a consequence of what is called *'sexting'* [166, 168, 169], which was introduced in 2005 by the Daily Telegraph, from the union of the terms '*sex*' and '*texting*', indicating '*sending and receiving sexual content (e.g., photos, videos) via the Internet and mobile phones*' [167]. However, there is not still agreement on the definition, and it often varies among investigators [167, 168]. Women are at higher risk of feeling pressured and coerced into sending pornographic material [169]. Similarly to revenge porn, sexting exposes the subject to the risk of receiving unsolicited pornographic material, of experiencing sexual abuse, stalking, and to take risky behaviours, substance abuse, and risky sexual activities. Those with anxious or avoidant attachment and in the presence of risky behaviours, psychological difficulties, sensation-seeking, substance use, unprotected sex, chatting with strangers, pornography use, and neuroticism are more prone to this activity [169]. Depression and anxiety symptoms could be both the mental health consequences and the cause of these activities [167].

Other chats are those associated with online video games which indeed become a tool for virtual socialisation [170]. However, within online video game-related chats, elements of hostility and harassment have been documented among online games, with the development of behaviours such as '*trash talking*' (e.g., a form of verbal aggression aimed at asserting one's superiority over the rival) and '*trolling*' (e.g., the disruptive and provocative action exercised against other users) [132, 170]). Such behaviours are often directed at opponents or towards unskilled teammates [170]. Men experience such attacks most often, while women experience more violent forms [170]. Another at-risk category is represented by LGBTQIA+ community and persons of colour [170].

Consequences include low self-esteem, hopelessness, reduced educational attainment, loneliness, school absenteeism, and even the development of suicidal ideation and suicide attempts [170]. Women report higher levels of emotional distress than men [170]. A protective factor towards cyber-aggression includes playing together with long-time friends [171]. This type of behaviour is called *'griefing'*, and those who take pleasure in ruining the gaming experience of others are called *'griefers'*, often prompting other gamers to quit gaming [172]. Four categories of griefing behaviours have been identified: (a) harassment (i.e., to cause emotional distress); (b) power imposition (manifested by the imposition of one's own power superiority towards those at a lower level); (c) scamming (e.g., in which the subject tries to cheat other players); and (d) greed play (i.e., a game scheme that involves grabbing all the benefits at the expense of other players) [173]. Nowadays, video game companies are moving to the direction of punishing subjects who have unpleasant behaviours. For example, the company Blizzard introduced bonuses in case of prosocial behaviours, while Ubisoft imparts a temporary ban for subjects with nasty behaviours [170]. Many subjects consider such behaviours as normal and part of the experience, labelling those who suffer from such activities as over-sensitive and overreacting. Indeed, this type of violence is mediated by normative beliefs, prompting individuals to disregard such activity as harmful and is facilitated by the anonymity granted by the medium [170].

5.2.6 Online Video Gaming and Internet Gaming Disorder (IGD)

There are two main types of uses of video games (i.e., offline and online), even though some video games also allow individuals to play both online and offline [174]. The offline video gaming is usually solitary and with a predetermined endpoint [174]; the online video gaming is instead often endless and played interactively and simultaneously with other players, including competition, responsibilities, cooperation, and obligations [174]. Online video gaming is much more likely represented in Internet Gaming Disorder (IGD) individuals.

Among all new technology-related disorders, IGD represents the only one officially recognised by the scientific community and included in the DSM-5-TR [92] and in the ICD-11 [175] (Table 5.5).

IGD was anecdotally reported about 40 years ago, by Keepers [176], who described a case of a young man who experienced a pathological preoccupation with video gaming, while a more detailed list of symptoms was identified in 1995 along with some predictive signs of video gaming addiction [177, 178]. Today, IGD is characterised as a disorder in which video gaming activity is all-consuming, resulting in an impaired social and work functioning [179]. The IGD prevalence is variable across different studies due to lack of homogeneity of the samples (i.e., gender, social, cultural differences, screening tools). The overall percentage of individuals with IGD is around 1–2%, and up to 4.6% when samples include adolescents only [179, 180].

IGD is associated with physical and psychological problems (Table 5.6), including impaired vision, eye strain, muscle tension, back pain, joint problems, sleep deprivation, poor nutrition, and metabolic issues (such as obesity) [181]. From a psychological viewpoint, a decreased self-esteem, social withdrawal, ruminations on the possible next video gaming opportunity, poor social relationships, low self-interest, tolerance of video gaming activity, school/work failures, loneliness, increased hostility and aggression, inability to control video gaming activity, loss of interest, and low interest in scolding [179, 181]. Moreover, IGD individuals could have ADHD, depression, anxiety disorders (particularly, social anxiety), suicidal ideation, SUDs, sleep disorders, other technopathies, PTSD, autistic traits, conduct disorders, and self-harm in comorbidity [179, 180, 182]. IGD could act both as a causal factor of the above-mentioned disorders (particularly anxiety and depression) or represent a coping mechanism [179, 180, 182]. The chronicity

Table 5.5 Diagnostic criteria for Internet Gaming Disorder (IGD) in DSM-V-TR and ICD-11

DSM-V-TR	ICD-11
Persistent and recurrent use of the Internet to engage in games, often with other players, leading to clinically significant impairment or distress as indicated by five (or more) of the following in a 12-month period:	Essential (required) features:
1. Preoccupation with Internet games. (The individual thinks about previous gaming activity or anticipates playing the next game; Internet gaming becomes the dominant activity in daily life.) Note: This disorder is distinct from Internet gambling, which is included under gambling disorder.	• A persistent pattern of gaming behaviour ('digital gaming' or 'video gaming'), which may be predominantly online (i.e., over the internet or similar electronic networks) or offline, manifested by all of the following:
2. Withdrawal symptoms when Internet gaming is taken away. (These symptoms are typically described as irritability, anxiety, or sadness, but there are no physical signs of pharmacological withdrawal).	– Impaired control over gaming behaviour (e.g., onset, frequency, intensity, duration, termination, context).
3. Tolerance—the need to spend increasing amounts of time engaged in Internet games.	– Increasing priority given to gaming behaviour to the extent that gaming takes precedence over other life interests and daily activities.
4. Unsuccessful attempts to control the participation in Internet games.	– Continuation or escalation of gaming behaviour despite negative consequences (e.g., family conflict due to gaming behaviour, poor scholastic performance, negative impact on health).
5. Loss of interests in previous hobbies and entertainment as a result of, and with the exception of, Internet games.	• The pattern of gaming behaviour may be continuous or episodic and recurrent but is manifested over an extended period of time (e.g., 12 months).
6. Continued excessive use of Internet games despite knowledge of psychosocial problems.	• The gaming behaviour is not better accounted for by another mental disorder (e.g., Manic Episode) and is not due to the effects of a substance or medication.
7. Has deceived family members, therapists, or others regarding the amount of Internet gaming.	• The pattern of gaming behaviour results in significant distress or impairment in personal, family, social, educational, occupational, or other important areas of functioning.
8. Use of Internet games to escape or relieve a negative mood (e.g., feelings of helplessness, guilt, anxiety).	Specifiers for online or offline behaviour:
9. Has jeopardised or lost a significant relationship, job, or educational or career opportunity because of participation in Internet games. Note: Only nongambling Internet games are included in this disorder. Use of the Internet for required activities in a business or profession is not included; nor is the disorder intended to include other recreational or social Internet use. Similarly, sexual Internet sites are excluded.	• Gaming disorder, predominantly online: This refers to gaming disorder that predominantly involves gaming behaviour that is conducted over the internet or similar electronic networks (i.e., online).
Specify current severity: Internet gaming disorder can be mild, moderate, or severe depending on the degree of disruption of normal activities. Individuals with less severe Internet gaming disorder may exhibit fewer symptoms and less disruption of their lives. Those with severe Internet gaming disorder will have more hours spent on the computer and more severe loss of relationships or career or school opportunities.	• Gaming disorder, predominantly offline: This refers to gaming disorder that predominantly involves gaming behaviour that is not conducted over the internet or similar electronic networks (i.e., offline).

Table 5.6 Health issues related to Internet gaming disorder

Mental issues	Organic issues
• Decreased self-esteem	• Impaired vision
• Social withdrawal	• Eye strain
• Hostility and aggression	• Muscle tension and postural problems leading to back pain and joint problems
• Loss of interest	• Poor nutrition and sedentary lifestyle with metabolic issues
• Anxiety disorders	
• Depression	
• Suicidal ideation	
• Loneliness	
• Insomnia	
• Self-harm	

of IGD depends on the presence of comorbidity, impulsive traits, poor school performance, and poor social resources. Contrarily, factors that promote recovery include older age, early intervention, low levels of depressive symptoms and of attention deficits [179].

IGD induces a number of changes in brain functioning observed in neuroimaging studies [178], including increased activation of the anterior cingulate cortex, orbitofrontal cortex (OFC), nucleus accumbens, dorsal striatum, insula, and parahippocampus [178]. In addition, the severity of disease correlates with the connectivity of the posterior cingulate cortex with the right precuneus, thalamus, caudate, nucleus accumbens, supplementary motor area, and lingual gyrus correlates [178]. Reduced cortical thickness in the OFC, inferior temporal gyrus, right middle occipital and right inferior occipital, atrophy in the right OFC, bilateral insula, and right supplementary motor area, and an increase in the right thalamus were also observed [178]. These findings suggest a dysfunction of the corticolimbic system, with an alteration of the dopaminergic reward system and the development of cognitive dysfunction [178].

Men are at higher risk of developing IGD than women, with a 2:1 ratio [179, 180, 182], which is due not only to a greater involvement in video gaming but also because males are more involved in riskier games (e.g., competitive games or Massively Multiplayer Online Role-Playing Game, MMORPG) [179]. Younger individuals are at higher risk due to cultural, neurological (a less developed prefrontal cortex), and social (e.g., clashing with parental authority, need of belonging and identity aspects) reasons [180, 182]. Other risk factors include maladaptive personality traits, such as disinhibition, neuroticism, novelty seeking, introversion, great inhibition, borderline traits, poor histrionic traits, narcissistic traits, avoidant traits, schizoid traits, impulsivity, poor capacity for emotional regulation, low self-esteem, loneliness, shyness, poor self-control, risky behaviour, hostility, aggression, inclination to boredom, poor conscientiousness, resourcefulness, agreeableness, irritability, poor extraversion, high tendency to take risks, deficit in decision-making, poor ability to delay gratification, disorganised attachment, and low self-efficacy [179, 180]. SUD represents another facilitating factor for the development of IGD [182]. Social risk factors include poor social network, isolation, poor functioning, poor educational attainment, limited alternatives, unemployment, poor school and work skills, absenteeism, poverty, playing with friends, being invited to play, being part of a group, relational trauma, and conflict with peers [179, 182]. Family factors, such as single-parent, blended families, poor paternal devotion, poor parental control, less warm families, poor family functioning, poor relationships with parents, oppressive/hostile parents, negative parental role models, anxious parents, family conflict, overprotection, and parental rejection may also increase the risk of IGD [180, 182].

Finally, factors related to game-play, such as games without an ending (replayability and limitless rewards), MMO games, competitive games, online games, video game reward systems, particularly immersive games, games with forbidden content, having achieved high skills or rare rewards, glory, regular membership fees, narrative elements, graphical realism, monetisation, curiosity, role-playing, may also contribute to the development of this addiction [179, 182].

5.2.7 Online Pornography and Related Psychopathologies

The advent of the Internet changed the way users nowadays watch pornography. In fact, there has been a first shift from 'print media' to 'videotapes' and more recently to the Internet. The spread of online pornography was facilitated by the '*Triple-A-Engine*' (i.e., accessibility, affordability, and anonymity of the Internet) [183]. Adolescents are easily exposed to online pornography, amounting to 93.2% for boys and 62.1% for girls. Thus, the Internet is often the first source of information regarding sexual activity.

Cybersex is defined as '*a type of online sexual activity, which can be solitary or shared with others, can involve technologies like webcams and microphones, and is not necessarily indicative of a disorder*' [64, 65]. Those who use online pornography are usually classified in three ways: (a) recreational (i.e., intermittent and controlled use); (b) compulsive (i.e., compulsive use associated with sexual dysfunction and/or preoccupation for sexual activity); and (c) at-risk (i.e., who are preoccupied with their use of online porn, with high time consumption and potential mental health serious consequences) [64, 65]. Generally, the use of online pornography is associated with internalising unrealistic expectations about one's body and their sexual performance, leading to a decline in self-esteem and confidence. There is also an increase in aggression when exposed to violent pornographic content. Watching porn excessively also may cause depressive and anxiety symptoms, difficulty in forming connections, low levels of social integration, unreal and distorted expectations of couple dynamics, objectification of women, risky sexual behaviour, sexual promiscuity, and alcohol and drug use [97]. Moreover, early exposure to pornography is associated with antisocial behaviour [97]. The Internet has also facilitated the onset, maintenance, and exacerbation of what is referred to as sexual addiction or Problematic Online Pornography Use (POPU) [183]. The latter is characterised by the presence of feelings of loss of control and persistent use, despite the negative consequences [183]. The Internet allows not only access to pornography but also to search for possible sexual partners through dating apps, which is promoted by high levels of impulsivity [183]. It is very difficult to define the prevalence of individuals with online sexual disorders since anonymity does not allow for a true estimate [183]. The most frequent consequences of POPU include erectile dysfunction, psychosexual dissatisfaction, and the development of comorbidities (anxiety disorders, depressed mood, substance use, sexual dysfunction, smoking, alcohol or coffee use, drug use, and IGD) [183]. Further studies should be conducted to better characterise and define this disorder.

5.2.8 Online Shopping and Related Psychopathologies

Although the term 'online shopping addiction' (OSA) is commonly used in recent literature, there are no definitive and consistent definitions and clinical characterisation of the condition so far. Overall, OSA is conceptualised as a clustering of predisposing factors that may be associated with specific at-risk behaviours which may determine the development of OSA, rather than being defined by a strict set of diagnostic criteria [64, 65]. Potential predisposing factors include low self-esteem, cognitive overload, low self-regulation, psychological enjoyment, anonymity, and negative cognitions [64, 65]. Such addiction leads to the development of economic problems and emotional distress that often result in depressive-anxiety symptoms. E-commerce platforms are also contributing to the development of OSA by proposing targeted products based on users' searches on the various platforms [64, 65].

5.2.9 Psychopathologies Related to Work-From-Home and Distance Learning

Finally, it is important to describe the mental health consequences following the introduction and maintenance of work-from-home (WFH) and distance learning (DL), introduced or implemented mainly during the SARS-CoV-2 pandemic [184–186]. Indeed, both WFH and DL were alternative modalities that allowed the enforcement of social isolation, which was crucial for the prevention and spread of COVID-19 disease [187].

The term WFH is a working arrangement allowing individuals to shift work from their office to their homes [188]; DL refers to conducting and participating in didactic activities via telematics. Despite many advantages offered by both modalities, particularly during the pandemic, specific mental issues related to both communication technology modalities were described (Table 5.7).

Although WFH has been associated with a plethora of potential mental health issues experienced by the general population, the effects were higher particularly in parents. In fact, they substantially needed to adapt their daily routine, with subsequent higher stress levels, due to increased visibility and heightened childcare responsibilities compelled parents working remotely, compared to those who work at their offices [189, 190]. WFH has been associated with higher distress, mainly due to role transition, particularly the difficulty to separate 'work' from 'private' life [189–191]. Indeed, mental health consequences include lack of social interactions and support, domestic abuse, disrupted routines, lack of structure, technical issues related to new technologies, overload of work, mood and anxiety disorders, cognitive impairment, loneliness, sleep disorders, and isolation [189–191]. The sedentary nature of such people also would promote the aggravation of both physical and mental health issues [192].

Table 5.7 Health issues related to work-from-home and distance learning

Mental issues	Organic issues
• Stress	• Sedentary lifestyle
• Mood disorder	
• Anxiety disorders	
• Cognitive impairment	
• Loneliness	
• Sleep disorders	
• Isolation	
• Suicidal thoughts	
• Emotional dysregulation	
• Substance use	
• NSSIs	
• Poor well-being	

Overall, the in-person social interaction between children and adolescents within a school environment plays an important role in their cognitive and emotional development, influencing social, academic, and familiar functioning [130, 193, 194]. Recent studies found that children and adolescents who experienced school closures were more prone to develop psychological repercussions, primarily marked by feelings of loneliness and confusion [130, 194]. During the COVID-19 pandemic, the prevailing emotion reported was a fear regarding personal and familial safety [194]. Within the familial context, adolescents not only had to manage their individual anxieties but also navigate the burden of their parents' distress and apprehensions [194]. Although the data could be influenced by the effects of the pandemic, the possible consequences of DL are suicidal thoughts, anxiety and depressive disorders, emotional dysregulation, psychological stress, substance use, NSSIs, and poor well-being [130, 193–196]. Females are more prone to develop mental health consequences due to DL compared to males [194, 195]. The onset of such mental health issues would be attributed to the lack of social interactions with one's peers, which would lead to the development of feelings of loneliness with high levels of inadequacy [130, 194, 196]. The causes include the possibility of poorer quality of lessons, as well as technical issues related to new technologies, domestic abuse, disrupted routines and lack of structure, poverty, and inability to purchase the necessary supplies to attend classes [130, 195, 196].

Further studies should be carried out to confirm the causal relationship between work/school online activities and mental health issues, independently by the COVID-19 pandemic. Indeed, evidence suggests caution in using and implementing such alternative modalities, particularly among more vulnerable individuals such as children, adolescents, and subjects with pre-existing mental health conditions.

5.3 Conclusions

Technology and digitalisation have indeed revolutionised our daily life and clearly impacted on the behaviour of humans as well as on their physical and mental health. Despite the integration of new communication technologies significantly improved some aspects of human quality of life, mental health issues were described following the introduction and excessive use of digital technologies. However, only IGD is defined through specific diagnostic criteria in both ICD-11 and DSM-5-TR. There are still ongoing studies aimed to more precisely define the psychopathology of problematic behaviours (such as PIU, PSNU, PSU, online pornography, etc.) related to digital technologies and to provide clinicians with unanimously recognised diagnostic criteria and effective treatment tools for these mental health issues. The current exclusion of such nosographic entities from diagnostic manuals is indeed problematic from diagnostic, preventive, and treatment perspectives. To date, it is not possible to officially recognise 'at-risk' individuals nor to provide early preventive strategies, thus increasing the risk of chronicity. Even more cogently, the lack of official assessment tools and diagnostic criteria may imply suboptimal treatment of disabling mental health conditions and slowing down the search for more specific diagnostic and treatment algorithms.

Conversely, digital technologies may reveal themselves not only a source of psychiatric burden but also a potential asset for mental health care, as professionals may greatly benefit from the implementation of new communication technologies within their psychiatric clinical practice. Currently, there are various mental health interventions effectively and safely administered through new communication technologies, including telepsychiatry (both synchronously or asynchronously; [197, 198]), digital phenotyping (by using smartphones and/or wearable sensors for momentary assessment and real-time interventions; [28]) and digital therapeutics (at least, those with a larger evidence-base and already approved by regulatory entities; [28, 199]). Moreover, VR/AR systems may enable the delivery of new customisable mental health interventions, with an increased user engagement and in a safe environment [200]. Furthermore, the development of video games specifically programmed with educational or/and therapeutic goals (i.e., 'serious games') further increased the therapeutic and rehabilitation opportunities in the field of youth mental health [201]. Finally, AI-based applications allow mental health professionals to analyse a larger amount of data, to detect early onset or worsening of psychiatric symptoms, to assess response to treatment, to build new theoretical explanatory models of psychopathology, and to identify novel therapeutic strategies [202, 203]. Machine learning, a specific application of AI, allowed the construction of mathematical algorithms that can self-learn from analysed data without prior instruction on how to handle data, by allowing predictive models: such approaches may be particularly useful in psychiatry for differential diagnosis, early identification of prodromal signs and/or symptoms, and clinical risk mental health conditions or treatment response [46, 203]. In addition, other AI applications (such as chatbots, software simulating human conversations) may be very useful in mental health care easing users' interaction with digital devices [47, 204].

A balanced approach could allow clinicians to adequately evaluate which patients could be the most promising candidates to achieve benefit by digital psychiatry and which patients instead should be accurately monitored due to their high risk to potentially develop detrimental mental health issues following an excessive and/or inappropriate/maladaptive modality of digital communication technologies. Further studies should deepen mental health issues related to digital communication technologies, particularly focusing on their treatment as well as integrated and sequential approaches in case of comorbidity with other psychiatric conditions.

References

1. Grant AE, Meadows JH (2020) Communication technology update and fundamentals, 17th edn. Routledge, p 535
2. Miyagawa S, Ojima S, Berwick RC, Okanoya K (2014) The integration hypothesis of human language evolution and the nature of contemporary languages. Front Psychol 5:564. https://doi.org/10.3389/fpsyg.2014.00564. PMID: 24936195; PMCID: PMC4048833
3. Huurdeman A (2003) The worldwide history of telecommunications. Wiley-Interscience, Hoboken
4. Kittler F (1996) The history of communication media. ctheory, 7-30
5. Catania B (2001) Antonio Meucci: telephone pioneer. Bull Sci Technol Soc 21(1):55–76
6. Economist (2009) Brain scan—father of the cell phone. The Economist website. http://www.economist.com/node/13725793?story_id=13725793
7. Blissmer RH (1991) Introducing computers: concepts, systems, and applications, 1991–92 edn. Wiley, Austin
8. Campbell-Kelly M, Aspray W, Wilkes MV (1996) Computer a history of the information machine. Nature 383(6599):405–405
9. Zakon RF (1997) Hobbes' Internet timeline [online], http://www.zakon.org/robert/internet/timeline
10. Singhal M, Hura GS (2001) Data and computer communications: networking and internetworking. Taylor & Francis, London, p 758
11. Fluckiger F (2000) The European researchers' network. La Recherche 328 (translation); https://cern.ch/Fluckiger/Articles/F.Fluckiger-The_European_Researchers_Network.pdf
12. Google Company (2012) Our history in depth. Archived from the original on April 1, 2012 https://web.archive.org/web/20120401005940/http://www.google.com/about/company/history/
13. Carr CT, Hayes RA (2015) Social media: defining, developing, and divining. Atlantic J Commun 23:46–65. https://doi.org/10.1080/15456870.2015.972282
14. Banks MA (2007) The Internet, ARPANet, and consumer online. All Business. (2007, January). https://www.questia.com/magazine/1G1-158091728/the-internetarpanet-and-consumer-online
15. Milian M (2009, July) Friendster founder on social networking: I invented this stuff (updated). The Los Angeles Times. http://latimesblogs.latimes.com/technology/2009/07/friendsterjonathan-abrams.html
16. Brügger N (2015) A brief history of Facebook as a media text: the development of an empty structure. First Monday
17. Vogels EA, Gelles-Watnick R, Massarat N (2022) Teens, social media and technology 2022
18. Cooper P (2020, January 13) 23 YouTube statistics that matter to marketers in 2020. https://blog.hootsuite.com/youtubestatsmarketers/
19. Beaumont C (2008, November) The team behind Twitter: Jack Dorsey, Biz Stone and Evan Williams. Telegraph. http://www.telegraph.co.uk/technology/3520024/The-teambehind-Twitter-Jack-Dorsey-Biz-Stone-and-Evan-Williams.html
20. Sarno D (2009). Twitter creator Jack Dorsey illuminates the site's founding document. Part I. Los Angeles Times. https://www.latimes.com/archives/blogs/technology-blog/story/2009-02-18/twitter-creator-jack-dorsey-illuminates-the-sites-founding-document-part-i
21. Davis W (2023). Twitter is being rebranded as X, su The Verge. https://www.theverge.com/2023/7/23/23804629/twitters-rebrand-to-x-may-actually-be-happening-soon
22. Auxier B, Anderson M (2021) Social media use in 2021. Pew Research Center 1:1–4
23. Dinesh S, Odabaş M (2023) 8 facts about Americans and Twitter as it rebrands to X
24. Statista (2022) Number of Twitter users worldwide from 2019 to 2024. https://www.statista.com/statistics/303681/twitter-users-worldwide/
25. Tidy J, Smith GS TikTok: the story of a social media giant, BBC news, 5 August 2020. https://www.bbc.com/news/technology-53640724
26. Ivory JD (2015) A brief history of video games. The video game debate: unravelling the physical, social, and psychological effects of digital games, 1–21
27. Kent SL (2010) The ultimate history of video games, volume 1: from Pong to Pokemon and Beyond... the story behind the craze that touched our lives and changed the world, vol 1. Crown
28. Torous J, Bucci S, Bell IH, Kessing LV, Faurholt-Jepsen M, Whelan P, Carvalho AF, Keshavan M, Linardon J, Firth J (2021) The growing field of digital psychiatry: current evidence and the future of apps, social media, chatbots, and virtual reality. World Psychiatry 20(3):318–335. https://doi.org/10.1002/wps.20883. PMID: 34505369; PMCID: PMC8429349
29. Hugues O, Fuchs P, Nannipieri O (2011) New augmented reality taxonomy: technologies and features of augmented environment. In: Furht B (ed) Handbook of augmented reality. Springer, New York. https://doi.org/10.1007/978-1-4614-0064-6_2
30. Luna R (2021) Il Sensorama, la macchina per realtà virtuale che non venne capita. La repubblica. https://www.repubblica.it/tecnologia/2021/08/28/news/il_sensorama_la_macchina_per_realta_virtuale_che_non_venne_capita-315540396/
31. Jerald J (2015) The VR book: human-centered design for virtual reality. Morgan & Claypool
32. Tricart C (2017) Virtual reality filmmaking: techniques & best practices for VR filmmakers. Taylor & Francis
33. Steinicke F (2016) Being really virtual. In: Immersive natives and the future of virtual reality. Springer, pp 19–32
34. Davies C (1998) OSMOSE: Notes on being in Immersive virtual space

35. Parisi T (2016) Learning virtual reality: developing immersive experiences and applications for desktop, web and mobile. O'Reilly Media, Inc
36. Bilton N (2015) Why Google glass broke. New York Times. https://www.nytimes.com/2015/02/05/style/why-google-glassbroke.html
37. Newman J (2014) The weirdest thing at Google I/O was this cardboard virtual reality box. http://time.com/2925768/theweirdest-thing-at-google-io-was-this-cardboard-virtual-realitybox/
38. Aukstakalnis S (2017) Practical augmented reality: a guide to the technologies, applications, and human factors for AR and VR. Pearson Education, Inc
39. Constine J (2019, September 25) Facebook announces horizon, a VR massive-multiplayer world. TechCrunch. Archived from the original on December 7, 2021 https://web.archive.org/web/20211207063211/https://techcrunch.com/2019/09/25/facebook-horizon/
40. Milmo D (2021, October 28) Enter the metaverse: the digital future Mark Zuckerberg is steering us toward. The Guardian. theguardian.com/technology/2021/oct/28/facebook-mark-zuckerberg-meta-metaverse
41. Apple (2023) Apple Vision Pro. https://www.apple.com/apple-vision-pro/
42. Fiske A, Henningsen P, Buyx A (2019) Your robot therapist will see you now: ethical implications of embodied artificial intelligence in psychiatry, psychology, and psychotherapy. J Med Internet Res 21(5):e13216. https://doi.org/10.2196/13216. PMID: 31094356; PMCID: PMC6532335
43. Russell S, Norvig P (2009) Artificial intelligence: a modern approach. Pearson
44. Haenlein M, Kaplan A (2019) A brief history of artificial intelligence: on the past, present, and future of artificial intelligence. Calif Manag Rev 61(4):5–14. https://doi.org/10.1177/0008125619864925
45. Mitchell M (2019) Artificial intelligence: a guide for thinking humans. Farrar, Straus and Giroux
46. Graham S, Depp C, Lee EE et al (2019) Artificial Intelligence for mental health and mental illnesses: an overview. Curr Psychiatry Rep 21:116
47. Pham KT, Nabizadeh A, Selek S (2022) Artificial intelligence and chatbots in psychiatry. Psychiatry Q 93:249–253
48. Adamopoulou E, Moussiades L (2020) Chatbots: history, technology, and applications. Mach Learn Appl 2:100006
49. Schallmo DRA, Williams CA (2018) History of digital transformation. In: Digital transformation now!. Springer briefs in business. Springer, Cham. https://doi.org/10.1007/978-3-319-72844-5_2
50. European Commission (2020) Digital economy and society index (DESI) 2020—use of internet services. https://digital-strategy.ec.europa.eu/en/policies/desi-use-internet
51. Castells M (1996) The rise of the network society, the information age: economy, society and culture, vol I. Blackwell, Cambridge, MA/Oxford. ISBN 978-0-631-22140-1
52. Firth J, Torous J, Stubbs B, Firth JA, Steiner GZ, Smith L, Alvarez-Jimenez M, Gleeson J, Vancampfort D, Armitage CJ, Sarris J (2019) The "online brain": how the Internet may be changing our cognition. World Psychiatry 18(2):119–129. https://doi.org/10.1002/wps.20617. PMID: 31059635; PMCID: PMC6502424
53. Oberst U, Wegmann E, Stodt B, Brand M, Chamarro A (2017) Negative consequences from heavy social networking in adolescents: the mediating role of fear of missing out. J Adolesc 55:51–60. https://doi.org/10.1016/j.adolescence.2016.12.008. Epub 2016 Dec 27. PMID: 28033503
54. Lattie EG, Lipson SK, Eisenberg D (2019) Technology and college student mental health: challenges and opportunities. Front Psych 10:246. https://doi.org/10.3389/fpsyt.2019.00246. PMID: 31037061; PMCID: PMC6476258
55. Torous J, Jän Myrick K, Rauseo-Ricupero N, Firth J (2020) Digital mental health and COVID-19: using technology today to accelerate the curve on access and quality tomorrow. JMIR Ment Health 7(3):e18848. https://doi.org/10.2196/18848. PMID: 32213476; PMCID: PMC7101061
56. Figueroa CA, Aguilera A (2020) The need for a mental health technology revolution in the COVID-19 pandemic. Front Psych 11:523. https://doi.org/10.3389/fpsyt.2020.00523. PMID: 32581891; PMCID: PMC7283500
57. Torous J, Wykes T (2020) Opportunities from the coronavirus disease 2019 pandemic for transforming psychiatric care with telehealth. JAMA Psychiatry 77(12):1205–1206. https://doi.org/10.1001/jamapsychiatry.2020.1640. PMID: 32391857
58. Zahn C, Leisner D, Niederhauser M, Roos AL, Iseli T, Soldati M (2022) Effects of game mode in multiplayer video games on intergenerational social interaction: randomized field study. JMIR Form Res 6(2):e29179. https://doi.org/10.2196/29179. PMID: 35171097; PMCID: PMC8892273
59. Orben A (2020) Teenagers, screens and social media: a narrative review of reviews and key studies. Soc Psychiatry Psychiatr Epidemiol 55(4):407–414. https://doi.org/10.1007/s00127-019-01825-4. Epub 2020 Jan 10. PMID: 31925481
60. Young KS (1996) Psychology of computer use: XL. Addictive use of the Internet: a case that breaks the stereotype. Psychol Rep 79:899–902
61. El-Guebaly N, Carrà G, Galanter M, Baldacchino AM (eds) (2015) Textbook of addiction treatment: international perspectives, vol 4. Springer Milan
62. Young KS (1998) Internet addiction: the emergence of a new clinical disorder. Cyber Psychol Behav 1:237–244
63. World Health Organization (2014) Public health implications of excessive use of the internet, computers, smartphones and similar electronic devices: Meeting report. In Proceedings of the Main Meeting Hall, Foundation for Promotion of Cancer Research, National Cancer Research Centre, Tokyo, Japan, 27–29 August 2014

64. Sherer J, Levounis P (2022a) Technological addictions. Curr Psychiatry Rep 24:399–406. https://doi.org/10.1007/s11920-022-01351-2
65. Sherer J, Levounis P (2022b) Technological addictions. Psychiatr Clin N Am 45:577–591
66. Pan Y-C, Chiu Y-C, Lin Y-H (2020) Systematic review and meta-analysis of epidemiology of internet addiction. Neurosci Biobehav Rev 118:612–622
67. Pontes HM (ed) (2022) Behavioral addictions: conceptual, clinical, assessment, and treatment approaches. Springer Nature
68. Durkee T, Kaess M, Carli V, Parzer P, Wasserman C, Floderus B, Apter A, Balazs J, Barzilay S, Bobes J et al (2012) Prevalence of pathological internet use among adolescents in Europe: demographic and social factors. Addiction 107:2210–2222
69. Orsolini L, Longo G, Volpe U (2023) The mediatory role of the boredom and loneliness dimensions in the development of problematic internet use. Int J Environ Res Public Health 20:4446. https://doi.org/10.3390/ijerph20054446
70. Chundawat DS, Yadav KC, Mudgal SK, Yadav Y, Gaur R, Malhotra V (2022) A study on psychosomatic problems related to the problematic internet use among adolescents at selected schools of Aspur Block, Dungarpur, Rajasthan. Mymensingh Med J 31:539–546
71. El Archi S, Barrault S, Brunault P, Ribadier A, Varescon I (2022) Co-occurrence of adult ADHD symptoms and problematic Internet use and its links with impulsivity, emotion regulation, anxiety, and depression. Front Psych 13:792206
72. Fineberg NA, Menchón JM, Hall N, Dell'Osso B, Brand M, Potenza MN, Chamberlain SR, Cirnigliaro G, Lochner C, Billieux J et al (2022) Advances in problematic usage of the internet research—a narrative review by experts from the European network for problematic usage of the internet. Compr Psychiatry 118:152346
73. Kato TA, Shinfuku N, Tateno M (2020) Internet society, internet addiction, and pathological social withdrawal: the chicken and egg dilemma for internet addiction and hikikomori. Curr Opin Psychiatry 33(3):264–270. https://doi.org/10.1097/YCO.0000000000000601
74. Ko C-H, Hsiao S, Liu G-C, Yen J-Y, Yang M-J, Yen C-F (2010) The characteristics of decision making, potential to take risks, and personality of college students with Internet addiction. Psychiatry Res 175:121–125
75. Lakkunarajah S, Adams K, Pan AY, Liegl M, Sadhir M (2022) A trying time: Problematic Internet Use (PIU) and its association with depression and anxiety during the COVID-19 Pandemic. Child Adolesc Psychiatry Ment Health 16:49
76. Orosz G, Benyó M, Berkes B, Nikoletti E, Gál É, Tóth-Király I, Bőthe B (2018) The personality, motivational, and need-based background of problematic Tinder use. J Behav Addict 7:301–316
77. Pettorruso M, Valle S, Cavic E, Martinotti G, di Giannantonio M, Grant JE (2020) Problematic Internet use (PIU), personality profiles and emotion dysregulation in a cohort of young adults: trajectories from risky behaviors to addiction. Psychiatry Res 289:113036
78. Tao R, Huang X, Wang J, Zhang H, Zhang Y, Li M (2010) Proposed diagnostic criteria for internet addiction. Addiction 105:556–564
79. Orsolini L, Cicolini A, Salvi V, Volpe U (2022) The "Well-Dressed Snake Personality": an insight into narcissistic/psychopathic personalities. J Psychol Psychother Res 9:104–115. https://doi.org/10.12974/2313-1047.2022.09.5
80. Orsolini L, Yılmaz-Karaman IG, Longo G, Bellagamba S, Kato TA, Volpe U (2022) Sex-differences in hikikomori traits as predictors of problematic internet use in Italian university students. J Psychiatr Res 155:211–218
81. Akerele E (ed) (2022) Substance and non-substance related addictions: a global approach. Springer Nature
82. Elhai JD, Dvorak RD, Levine JC, Hall BJ (2017) Problematic smartphone use: a conceptual overview and systematic review of relations with anxiety and depression psychopathology. J Affect Disord 207:251–259. https://doi.org/10.1016/j.jad.2016.08.030. Epub 2016 Oct 2. PMID: 27736736
83. Panova T, Carbonell X (2018) Is smartphone addiction really an addiction? J Behav Addict 7(2):252–259. https://doi.org/10.1556/2006.7.2018.49. Epub 2018 Jun 13. PMID: 29895183; PMCID: PMC6174603
84. Yen C-F, Tang T-C, Yen J-Y, Lin H-C, Huang C-F, Liu S-C, Ko C-H (2009) Symptoms of problematic cellular phone use, functional impairment and its association with depression among adolescents in Southern Taiwan. J Adolesc 32(4):863–873. https://doi.org/10.1016/j.adolescence.2008.10.006
85. De Pasquale C, Sciacca F, Conti DD, Dinaro C, Nuovo SD (2013) Personality and dissociative experiences in smartphone users. Life Span Disabil 1:129–146
86. Lopez-Fernandez O, Honrubia-Serrano L, Freixa-Blanxart M, Gibson W (2014) Prevalence of problematic mobile phone use in British adolescents. Cyberpsychol Behav Soc Netw 17(2):91–98. https://doi.org/10.1089/cyber.2012.0260
87. Nikhita CS, Jadhav PR, Ajinkya SA (2015) Prevalence of mobile phone dependence in secondary school adolescents. J Clin Diagn Res 9(11):VC06–VC09. https://doi.org/10.7860/JCDR/2015/14396.6803
88. Haug S, Castro RP, Kwon M, Filler A, Kowatsch T, Schaub MP (2015) Smartphone use and smartphone addiction among young people in Switzerland. J Behav Addict 4(4):299–307. https://doi.org/10.1556/2006.4.2015.037
89. Cha S-S, Seo B-K (2018) Smartphone use and smartphone addiction in middle school students in Korea: prevalence, social networking service, and

game use. Health Psychol Open 5(1):1–15. https://doi.org/10.1177/2055102918755046
90. Olson JA, Sandra DA, Colucci ÉS, Bikaii AA, Chmoulevitch D, Nahas J, Raz A, Veissière SPL (2022) Smartphone addiction is increasing across the world: a meta-analysis of 24 countries. Comput Hum Behav 129:107138. https://doi.org/10.1016/j.chb.2021.107138
91. World Health Organization [WHO] (2015) Public health implications of excessive use of the internet, computers, smartphones and similar electronic devices: Meeting report, Main meeting Hall, Foundation for promotion of Cancer research, national Cancer research Centre, Tokyo, Japan. August 2014, Geneva, Switzerland: WHO27–29
92. American Psychiatric Association (2022) Diagnostic and statistical manual of mental disorders, fifth edition, text revision. American Psychiatric Association, Washington, DC
93. Billieux J, Maurage P, Lopez-Fernandez O, Kuss DJ, Griffiths MD (2015) Can disordered mobile phone use be considered a behavioral addiction? An update on current evidence and a comprehensive model for future research. Curr Addict Rep 2:156–162
94. Fischer-Grote L, Kothgassner OD, Felnhofer A (2019) Risk factors for problematic smartphone use in children and adolescents: a review of existing literature. Neuropsychiatrie 33(4):179–190. https://doi.org/10.1007/s40211-019-00319-8. Epub 2019 Sep 6. PMID: 31493233; PMCID: PMC6901427
95. Horwood S, Anglim J (2019) Problematic smartphone usage and subjective and psychological well-being. Comput Hum Behav 97:44–50. https://doi.org/10.1016/j.chb.2019.02.028
96. Pivetta E, Harkin L, Billieux J, Kanjo E, Kuss DJ (2019) Problematic smartphone use: an empirically validated model. Comput Hum Behav 100:105–117., ISSN 0747-5632,. https://doi.org/10.1016/j.chb.2019.06.013
97. Jacobson C, Bailin A, Milanaik R, Adesman A (2016) Adolescent health implications of new age technology. Pediatr Clin N Am 63(1):183–194. https://doi.org/10.1016/j.pcl.2015.09.001
98. National Center for Statistics and Analysis (2023, May) Distracted driving in 2021. Research Note. Report No. DOT HS 813 443. National Highway Traffic Safety Administration
99. Kong X, Xiong S, Zhu Z, Zheng S, Long G (2015) Development of a conceptual framework for improving safety for pedestrians using smartphones while walking: challenges and research needs. Procedia Manuf 3:3636–3643. https://doi.org/10.1016/j.promfg.2015.07.749
100. Park JS, Choi MJ, Ma JE, Moon JH, Moon HJ (2014) Influence of cellular phone videos and games on dry eye syndrome in university students. J Korean Acad Community Health Nurs 25(1):12–23. https://doi.org/10.12799/jkachn.2014.25.1.12
101. Demirci K, Akgönül M, Akpinar A (2015) Relationship of smartphone use severity with sleep quality, depression, and anxiety in university students. J Behav Addict 4(2):85–92. https://doi.org/10.1556/2006.4.2015.010.km
102. Randler C, Wolfgang L, Matt K, Demirhan E, Horzum MB, Beşoluk Ş (2016) Smartphone addiction proneness in relation to sleep and morningness–eveningness in German adolescents. J Behav Addict 5(3):465–473. https://doi.org/10.1556/2006.5.2016.056
103. King AL, Valença AM, Nardi AE (2010) Nomophobia: the mobile phone in panic disorder with agoraphobia: reducing phobias or worsening of dependence? Cogn Behav Neurol 23(1):52–54. https://doi.org/10.1097/WNN.0b013e3181b7eabc
104. King AL, Valença AM, Silva AC, Sancassiani F, Machado S, Nardi AE (2014) "Nomophobia": impact of cell phone use interfering with symptoms and emotions of individuals with panic disorder compared with a control group. Clin Pract Epidemiol Ment Health 10:28–35. https://doi.org/10.2174/1745017901410010028. PMID: 24669231; PMCID: PMC3962983
105. Bragazzi NL, Del Puente G (2014) A proposal for including nomophobia in the new DSM-V. Psychol Res Behav Manag 7:155–160. https://doi.org/10.2147/PRBM.S41386. PMID: 24876797; PMCID: PMC4036142
106. Humood A, Altooq N, Altamimi A, Almoosawi H, Alzafiri M, Bragazzi NL, Husni M, Jahrami H (2021) The prevalence of nomophobia by population and by research tool: a systematic review, meta-analysis, and meta-regression. Psych 3(2):249–258. https://doi.org/10.3390/psych3020019
107. Bragazzi NL, Re TS, Zerbetto R (2019) The relationship between nomophobia and maladaptive coping styles in a sample of Italian young adults: insights and implications from a cross-sectional study. JMIR Ment Health 6(4):e13154. https://doi.org/10.2196/13154. PMID: 30763254; PMCID: PMC6505371
108. Dib JE, Hallit R, Akel M, Chalhoub C, Hachem M, Hallit S, Obeid S (2022) Association between personality traits/dimensions and fear of no mobile phone connectivity (nomophobia): results of a Lebanese national study. Prim Care Companion CNS Disord 24(5):21m03036. https://doi.org/10.4088/PCC.21m03036. PMID: 36126917
109. García-Masip V, Sora B, Serrano-Fernandez MJ, Boada-Grau J, Lampert B (2023) Personality and nomophobia: the role of dysfunctional obsessive beliefs. Int J Environ Res Public Health 20(5):4128. https://doi.org/10.3390/ijerph20054128. PMID: 36901141; PMCID: PMC10002437
110. Herman D (2000) Introducing short-term brands: a new branding tool for a new consumer reality. J Brand Manage 7(5):330–340. https://doi.org/10.1057/bm.2000.23
111. Przybylski AK, Murayama K, DeHaan CR, Gladwell V (2013) Motivational, emotional, and behavioral correlates of fear of missing out. Comput Human

Behav 29(4):1841–1848. https://doi.org/10.1016/j.chb.2013.02.014
112. Fioravanti G, Casale S, Benucci SB, Prostamo A, Falone A, Ricca V, Rotella F (2021) Fear of missing out and social networking sites use and abuse: a meta-analysis. Comput Hum Behav 122:106839. https://doi.org/10.1016/j.chb.2021.106839
113. Elhai JD, Levine JC, Alghraibeh AM, Alafnan AA, Aldraiweesh AA, Hall BJ (2018) Fear of missing out: testing relationships with negative affectivity, online social engagement, and problematic smartphone use. Comput Hum Behav 89:289–298. https://doi.org/10.1016/j.chb.2018.08.020
114. Statista (2022) Number of social media users worldwide from 2018 to 2027 (in billions). https://www.statista.com/statistics/278414/number-of-worldwide-social-network-users/
115. Smith A, Anderson M (2018) Social media use 2018: demographics and statistics. Pew Research Center Internet & Technology. Retrieved from http://www.pewinternet.org/2018/03/01/social-media-use-in-2018/
116. Billieux J, van Rooij AJ, Heeren A, Schimmenti A, Maurage P, Edman J, Kardefelt-Winther D (2017) Behavioural Addiction Open Definition 2.0—using the open science framework for collaborative and transparent theoretical development. Addiction 112(10):1723–1724. https://doi.org/10.1111/add.13938
117. Kardefelt-Winther D (2017) Conceptualizing Internet use disorders: addiction or coping process? Psychiatry Clin Neurosci 71(7):459–466. https://doi.org/10.1111/pcn.12413
118. Pontes HM, Kuss DJ, Griffiths MD (2015) Clinical psychology of Internet addiction: a review of its conceptualization, prevalence, neuronal processes, and implications for treatment. Neurosci Neuroecon 4:11–23. https://doi.org/10.2147/NAN.S60982
119. Weinstein AM (2023) Problematic social networking site use-effects on mental health and the brain. Front Psych 13:1106004. https://doi.org/10.3389/fpsyt.2022.1106004. PMID: 36741578; PMCID: PMC9893026
120. Paakkari L, Tynjälä J, Lahti H, Ojala K, Lyyra N (2021) Problematic social media use and health among adolescents. Int J Environ Res Public Health 18(4):1885. https://doi.org/10.3390/ijerph18041885. PMID: 33672074; PMCID: PMC7919645
121. Huang C (2022) A meta-analysis of the problematic social media use and mental health. Int J Soc Psychiatry 68(1):12–33. https://doi.org/10.1177/0020764020978434. Epub 2020 Dec 9. PMID: 33295241
122. Hou Y, Xiong D, Jiang T, Song L, Wang Q (2019) Social media addiction: Its impact, mediation, and intervention. Cyberpsychology: J Psychosocial Res Cyberspace 13(1):article 4. https://doi.org/10.5817/CP2019-1-4
123. Hussain Z, Wegmann E, Griffiths MD (2021) The association between problematic social networking site use, dark triad traits, and emotion dysregulation. BMC Psychol 9(1):160. https://doi.org/10.1186/s40359-021-00668-6. PMID: 34663456; PMCID: PMC8525015
124. Montag C, Yang H, Elhai JD (2021) On the psychology of TikTok use: a first glimpse from empirical findings. Front Public Health 9:641673. https://doi.org/10.3389/fpubh.2021.641673
125. Becker AE, Burwell RA, Gilman SE, Herzog DB, Hamburg P (2002) Eating behaviours and attitudes following prolonged exposure to television among ethnic Fijian adolescent girls. Br J Psychiatry 180:509–514. https://doi.org/10.1192/bjp.180.6.509
126. Crisp AH (2002) A tale of corruption. Br J Psychiatry 180:480–482. https://doi.org/10.1192/bjp.180.6.480
127. Fioravanti G, Bocci Benucci S, Ceragioli G et al (2022) How the exposure to beauty ideals on social networking sites influences body image: a systematic review of experimental studies. Adolescent Res Rev 7:419–458. https://doi.org/10.1007/s40894-022-00179-4
128. Vandenbosch L, Fardouly J, Tiggemann M (2022) Social media and body image: recent trends and future directions. Curr Opin Psychol 45:101289. https://doi.org/10.1016/j.copsyc.2021.12.002. Epub 2021 Dec 14. PMID: 35030460
129. Saiphoo A, Vahedi Z (2019) A meta-analytic review of the relationship between social media use and body image disturbance. Comput Hum Behav 101:259–275. https://doi.org/10.1016/j.chb.2019.07.028
130. Kwaning K, Ullah A, Biely C, Jackson N, Dosanjh KK, Galvez A, Arellano G, Dudovitz R (2023) Adolescent feelings on COVID-19 distance learning support: associations with mental health, social-emotional health, substance use, and delinquency. J Adolesc Health 72(5):682–687. https://doi.org/10.1016/j.jadohealth.2022.12.005. Epub 2023 Jan 16. PMID: 36653259; PMCID: PMC9870620
131. Aboujaoude E, Savage MW, Starcevic V, Salame WO (2015) Cyberbullying: review of an old problem gone viral. J Adolesc Health 57(1):10–18. https://doi.org/10.1016/j.jadohealth.2015.04.011
132. Zhu C, Huang S, Evans R, Zhang W (2021) Cyberbullying among adolescents and children: a comprehensive review of the global situation, risk factors, and preventive measures. Front Public Health 9:634909. https://doi.org/10.3389/fpubh.2021.634909. PMID: 33791270; PMCID: PMC8006937
133. Bernacki JM, Davies WH (2012) Prevention of the choking game: parent perspectives. J Inj Violence Res 4(2):73–78. https://doi.org/10.5249/jivr.v4i2.119. Epub 2011 Apr 16. PMID: 21502782; PMCID: PMC3426904
134. Lupariello F, Curti SM, Coppo E, Racalbuto SS, Di Vella G (2019) Self-harm risk among adolescents and the phenomenon of the "blue whale challenge": case series and review of the literature. J Forensic

Sci 64(2):638–642. https://doi.org/10.1111/1556-4029.13880. Epub 2018 Jul 23. PMID: 30036450

135. Khasawneh A, Chalil Madathil K, Dixon E, Wiśniewski P, Zinzow H, Roth R (2020) Examining the self-harm and suicide contagion effects of the blue whale challenge on YouTube and Twitter: qualitative study. JMIR Ment Health 7(6):e15973. https://doi.org/10.2196/15973. PMID: 32515741; PMCID: PMC7312265
136. Macnab AJ, Deevska M, Gagnon F, Cannon WG, Andrew T (2009) Asphyxial games or "the choking game": a potentially fatal risk behaviour. Inj Prev 15(1):45–49. https://doi.org/10.1136/ip.2008.018523. PMID: 19190276
137. Andrew TA, Fallon KK (2007) Asphyxial games in children and adolescents. Am J Forensic Med Pathol 28(4):303–307. https://doi.org/10.1097/PAF.0b013e318148bdb2. PMID: 18043016
138. Egge MK, Berkowitz CD, Toms C, Sathyavagiswaran L (2010) The choking game: a cause of unintentional strangulation. Pediatr Emerg Care 26(3):206–208. https://doi.org/10.1097/PEC.0b013e3181d1e3e3. PMID: 20216282
139. Soengkoeng R, Moustafa AA (2022) Digital self-harm: an examination of the current literature with recommendations for future research. Discov Psychol 2:19. https://doi.org/10.1007/s44202-022-00032-8
140. Eysenbach G, Powell J, Englesakis M, Rizo C, Stern A (2004) Health related virtual communities and electronic support groups: systematic review of the effects of online peer to peer interactions. BMJ 328:1166. https://doi.org/10.1136/bmj.328.7449.1166
141. Bell V (2007) Online information, extreme communities and internet therapy: is the internet good for our mental health? J Ment Health 16(4):445–457
142. Lewis SP, Arbuthnott AE (2014) Non-suicidal self-injury, eating disorders, and the Internet. In: Claes L, Muehlenkamp J (eds) Non-suicidal self-injury in eating disorders. Springer, Berlin/Heidelberg. https://doi.org/10.1007/978-3-642-40107-7_16
143. Harshbarger JL, Ahlers-Schmidt CR, Mayans L, Mayans D, Hawkins JH (2009) Pro-anorexia websites: what a clinician should know. Int J Eat Disord 42(4):367–370. https://doi.org/10.1002/eat.20608
144. Norris ML, Boydell KM, Pinhas L, Katzman DK (2006 Sep) Ana and the Internet: a review of pro-anorexia websites. Int J Eat Disord 39(6):443–447. https://doi.org/10.1002/eat.20305
145. Gavin J, Rodham K, Poyer H (2008) The presentation of "pro-anorexia" in online group interactions. Qual Health Res 18(3):325–333. https://doi.org/10.1177/1049732307311640
146. Ransom DC, La Guardia JG, Woody EZ, Boyd JL (2010) Interpersonal interactions on online forums addressing eating concerns. Int J Eat Disord 43(2):161–170. https://doi.org/10.1002/eat.20629. PMID: 19308991
147. Bardone-Cone AM, Cass KM (2007) What does viewing a pro-anorexia website do? An experimental examination of website exposure and moderating effects. Int J Eat Disord 40(6):537–548. https://doi.org/10.1002/eat.20396. PMID: 17525952
148. Reid D, Weigle P (2014) Social media use among adolescents: benefits and risks. Adolesc Psychiatry 4(2). https://doi.org/10.2174/221067660402140709115810
149. Becker K, Mayer M, Nagenborg M, El-Faddagh M, Schmidt MH (2004) Parasuicide online: Can suicide websites trigger suicidal behaviour in predisposed adolescents? Nord J Psychiatry 58(2):111–114. https://doi.org/10.1080/08039480410005602. PMID: 15204216
150. Dunlop SM, More E, Romer D (2011) Where do youth learn about suicides on the Internet, and what influence does this have on suicidal ideation? J Child Psychol Psychiatry 52(10):1073–1080. https://doi.org/10.1111/j.1469-7610.2011.02416.x. Epub 2011 Jun 10. PMID: 21658185
151. Marchant A, Hawton K, Stewart A, Montgomery P, Singaravelu V, Lloyd K et al (2017) A systematic review of the relationship between internet use, self-harm and suicidal behaviour in young people: The good, the bad and the unknown. PLoS One 12(8):e0181722. https://doi.org/10.1371/journal.pone.0181722
152. Davey Z, Schifano F, Corazza O, Deluca P (2012) Psychonaut web mapping group. e-Psychonauts: conducting research in online drug forum communities. J Ment Health 21(4):386–394. https://doi.org/10.3109/09638237.2012.682265
153. Orsolini L, Papanti GD, Francesconi G, Schifano F (2015) Mind navigators of chemicals' experimenters? A web-based description of e-psychonauts. Cyberpsychol Behav Soc Netw 18(5):296–300. https://doi.org/10.1089/cyber.2014.0486. PMID: 25965863
154. Orsolini L, Papanti D, Corkery J, Schifano F (2017) An insight into the deep web; why it matters for addiction psychiatry? Hum Psychopharmacol 32(3). https://doi.org/10.1002/hup.2573. PMID: 28657187
155. Orsolini L, St John-Smith P, McQueen D, Papanti D, Corkery J, Schifano F (2017) Evolutionary considerations on the emerging subculture of the E-psychonauts and the novel psychoactive substances: a comeback to the shamanism? Curr Neuropharmacol 15(5):731–737. https://doi.org/10.2174/1570159X15666161111114838
156. Sparks B, Zidenberg AM, Olver ME (2022) Involuntary Celibacy: a review of Incel ideology and experiences with dating, rejection, and associated mental health and emotional sequelae. Curr Psychiatry Rep 24(12):731–740. https://doi.org/10.1007/s11920-022-01382-9. Epub 2022 Nov 17. PMID: 36394688; PMCID: PMC9780135

157. Sparks B, Zidenberg AM, Olver ME (2023) One is the loneliest number: Involuntary celibacy (Incel), mental health, and loneliness. Curr Psychol:1–15. https://doi.org/10.1007/s12144-023-04275-z. Epub ahead of print. PMID: 36747916; PMCID: PMC9892684
158. Blom RM, Hennekam RC, Denys D (2012) Body integrity identity disorder. PLoS One 7(4):e34702. https://doi.org/10.1371/journal.pone.0034702
159. Filice E, Abeywickrama K, Parry D, Johnson C (2022) Sexual violence and abuse in online dating: a scoping review. Aggress Violent Behav 67:101781. https://doi.org/10.1016/j.avb.2022.101781
160. Brown C, Hegarty K (2018) Digital dating abuse measures: a critical review. Aggress Violent Behav 40:44–59. https://doi.org/10.1016/j.avb.2018.03.003
161. Douglas H, Harris BA, Dragiewicz M (2019) Technology-facilitated domestic and family violence: women's experiences. Br J Criminol 59(3):551–570. https://doi.org/10.1093/BJC/AZY068
162. Powell A, Henry N (2016) Technology-facilitated sexual violence victimization: results from an online survey of Australian adults. J Interpers Violence 34(17):3637–3665. https://doi.org/10.1177/0886260516672055
163. Snaychuk LA, O'Neill ML (2020) Technology-facilitated sexual violence: prevalence, risk, and resiliency in undergraduate students. J Aggress Maltreat Trauma 29(8):984–999. https://doi.org/10.1080/10926771.2019.1710636
164. Gewirtz-Meydan A, Volman-Pampanel D, Opuda E, Tarshish N (2023) Dating apps: a new emerging platform for sexual harassment? A scoping review. Trauma Violence Abuse 25(1):752–763. https://doi.org/10.1177/15248380231162969
165. Holladay KR, Hagedorn WB, Boote D (2020) The influence of cyber-sexual assault on the mental health outcomes of survivors. J Counsel Sexol Sexual Wellness Res Pract Educ 2(2):93–103
166. Veronica V, Di Giacomo D (2022) Implicazioni psicologiche del fenomeno del revenge porn: prospettive cliniche [Psychological aspects of Revenge Porn phenomena: clinical perspective]. Riv Psichiatr 57(1):10–17. https://doi.org/10.1708/3749.37322. PMID: 35166725
167. Gassó AM, Klettke B, Agustina JR, Montiel I (2019) Sexting, mental health, and victimization among adolescents: a literature review. Int J Environ Res Public Health 16(13):2364. https://doi.org/10.3390/ijerph16132364. PMID: 31277335; PMCID: PMC6650829
168. Doyle C, Douglas E, O'Reilly G (2021) The outcomes of sexting for children and adolescents: a systematic review of the literature. J Adolesc 92:86–113. https://doi.org/10.1016/j.adolescence.2021.08.009. Epub 2021 Aug 25. PMID: 34454257
169. Smith PK, Thompson F, Davidson J (2014) Cyber safety for adolescent girls: bullying, harassment, sexting, pornography, and solicitation. Curr Opin Obstet Gynecol 26(5):360–365. https://doi.org/10.1097/GCO.0000000000000106
170. Hilvert-Bruce Z, Neill JT (2020) I'm just trolling: the role of normative beliefs in aggressive behaviour in online gaming. Comput Hum Behav 102:303–311
171. Grandprey-Shores K, He Y, Swanenburg KL, Kraut R, Riedl J (2014, February) The identification of deviance and its impact on retention in a multiplayer game. In: Proceedings of the 17th ACM conference on Computer supported cooperative work & social computing, pp 1356–1365
172. Blackburn J, Kwak H (2014, April) STFU NOOB! predicting crowdsourced decisions on toxic behavior in online games. In: Proceedings of the 23rd international conference on World wide web, pp 877–888
173. Foo CY, Koivisto EM (2004, September) Defining grief play in MMORPGs: player and developer perceptions. In: Proceedings of the 2004 ACM SIGCHI international conference on advances in computer entertainment technology, pp 245–250
174. Smohai M, Urbán R, Griffiths MD, Király O, Mirnics Z, Vargha A, Demetrovics Z (2017) Online and offline video game use in adolescents: measurement invariance and problem severity. Am J Drug Alcohol Abuse 43(1):111–116. https://doi.org/10.1080/00952990.2016.1240798. Epub 2016 Nov 3. PMID: 27808562.
175. WHO (2018) ICD-11 clinical descriptions and diagnostic guidelines for mental and behavioural disorders
176. Keepers GA (1990) Pathological preoccupation with video games. J Am Acad Child Adolesc Psychiatry 29:49–50
177. Király O, Griffiths MD, Demetrovics Z (2015) Internet gaming disorder and the DSM-5: conceptualization, debates, and controversies. Curr Addict Rep 2:254–262. https://doi.org/10.1007/s40429-015-0066-7
178. Han DH, Hyun GJ, Park JH, Renshaw PF (2016) Internet gaming disorder. In: Neuropathology of drug addictions and substance misuse, pp 955–961. https://doi.org/10.1016/B978-0-12-800634-4.00094-9
179. King DL, Delfabbro PH (2020) Video game addiction. In: Adolescent addiction. Academic Press, pp 185–213
180. Mestre-Bach G, Fernandez-Aranda F, Jiménez-Murcia S (2022) Exploring Internet gaming disorder: an updated perspective of empirical evidence (from 2016 to 2021). Compr Psychiatry 116:152319. https://doi.org/10.1016/j.comppsych.2022.152319. Epub 2022 Apr 28. PMID: 35526417
181. Chen KH, Oliffe JL, Kelly MT (2018) Internet gaming disorder: an emergent health issue for men. Am J Mens Health 12(4):1151–1159. https://doi.org/10.1177/1557988318766950. Epub 2018 Apr 1. PMID: 29606034; PMCID: PMC6131461
182. Paulus FW, Ohmann S, von Gontard A, Popow C (2018) Internet gaming disorder in children and adolescents: a systematic review. Dev Med Child Neurol 60(7):645–659. https://doi.org/10.1111/dmcn.13754. Epub 2018 Apr 6. PMID: 29633243

183. Sussman S, Tsai JY (2020) Sexual addiction. In: Adolescent addiction. Academic Press, pp 241–263
184. Addimando L (2022) Distance learning in pandemic age: lessons from a (no longer) emergency. Int J Environ Res Public Health 19(23):16302. https://doi.org/10.3390/ijerph192316302. PMID: 36498375; PMCID: PMC9737831
185. Chu AMY, Chan TWC, So MKP (2022) Learning from work-from-home issues during the COVID-19 pandemic: Balance speaks louder than words. PLoS One 17(1):e0261969. https://doi.org/10.1371/journal.pone.0261969. PMID: 35025893; PMCID: PMC8758108
186. Galanti T, Guidetti G, Mazzei E, Zappalà S, Toscano F (2021) Work from home during the COVID-19 outbreak: the impact on employees' remote work productivity, engagement, and stress. J Occup Environ Med 63(7):e426–e432. https://doi.org/10.1097/JOM.0000000000002236. PMID: 33883531; PMCID: PMC8247534
187. Hsiang S, Allen D, Annan-Phan S et al (2020) The effect of large-scale anti-contagion policies on the COVID-19 pandemic. Nature 584:262–267. https://doi.org/10.1038/s41586-020-2404-8
188. Haines VY III, St-Onge S, Archambault M (2002) Environmental and person antecedents of telecommuting outcomes. J Organ End User Comput 14:32–50
189. Xiao Y, Becerik-Gerber B, Lucas G, Roll SC (2021) Impacts of working from home during COVID-19 pandemic on physical and mental wellbeing of office workstation users. J Occup Environ Med 63(3):181–190. https://doi.org/10.1097/JOM.0000000000002097. PMID: 33234875; PMCID: PMC7934324
190. Memon MA, Shaikh S, Mirza MZ, Obaid A, Muenjohn N, Ting H (2023) Work-from-home in the new normal: a phenomenological inquiry into employees' mental health. Int J Environ Res Public Health 20:48. https://doi.org/10.3390/ijerph20010048
191. Shankar N (2021) Work from home during COVID-19-disequilibrium of mental health and wellbeing among employees. EXCLI J 20:1287–1289. https://doi.org/10.17179/excli2021-4029. PMID: 34602926; PMCID: PMC8481794
192. Falk GE, Mailey EL, Okut H, Rosenkranz SK, Rosenkranz RR, Montney JL, Ablah E (2022) Effects of sedentary behavior interventions on mental well-being and work performance while working from home during the COVID-19 pandemic: a pilot randomized controlled trial. Int J Environ Res Public Health 19(11):6401. https://doi.org/10.3390/ijerph19116401. PMID: 35681986; PMCID: PMC9180109
193. Hertz MF, Kilmer G, Verlenden J, Liddon N, Rasberry CN, Barrios LC, Ethier KA (2022) Adolescent mental health, connectedness, and mode of school instruction during COVID-19. J Adolesc Health 70(1):57–63. https://doi.org/10.1016/j.jadohealth.2021.10.021. Epub 2021 Oct 22. PMID: 34930571; PMCID: PMC8531003
194. Saulle R, De Sario M, Bena A, Capra P, Culasso M, Davoli M, De Lorenzo A, Lattke LS, Marra M, Mitrova Z, Paduano S, Rabaglietti E, Sartini M, Minozzi S (2022) School closures and mental health, wellbeing and health behaviours among children and adolescents during the second COVID-19 wave: a systematic review of the literature. Epidemiol Prev 46(5–6):333–352. https://doi.org/10.19191/EP22.5-6.A542.089. PMID: 36384255
195. Hawrilenko M, Kroshus E, Tandon P, Christakis D (2021) The association between school closures and child mental health during COVID-19. JAMA Netw Open 4(9):e2124092. https://doi.org/10.1001/jamanetworkopen.2021.24092. Erratum in: JAMA Netw Open. 2021 Sep 1;4(9):e2132935. PMID: 34477850; PMCID: PMC8417763
196. Wang Y (2023) The research on the impact of distance learning on students' mental health. Educ Inf Technol (Dordr):1–13. https://doi.org/10.1007/s10639-023-11693-w. Epub ahead of print. PMID: 37361750; PMCID: PMC10007642
197. Caroppo E, Lanzotti P, Janiri L (2020) Interventi a distanza in salute mentale: usi e prospettive dei Digital Health Interventions al tempo di COVID-19. Interventi a distanza in salute mentale:1–122
198. Hilty DM, Luo JS, Morache C et al (2002) Telepsychiatry. Mol Diag Ther 16:527–548. https://doi.org/10.2165/00023210-200216080-00003
199. US Food and Drug Administration (2020) What is digital health? Sept 22, 2020. https://www.fda.gov/medical-devices/digital-healthcenter-excellence/what-digital-health
200. Kim S, Kim E (2020) The use of virtual reality in psychiatry: a review. Soa Chongsonyon Chongsin Uihak 31:26–32
201. Dewhirst A, Laugharne R, Shankar R (2022) Therapeutic use of serious games in mental health: scoping review. BJPsych Open 8:e37
202. Torous J, Keshavan M, Gutheil T (2014) Promise and perils of digital psychiatry. Asian J Psychiatry 10:120–122
203. Lee EE, Torous J, De Choudhury M, Depp CA, Graham SA, Kim HC et al (2021) Artificial intelligence for mental health care: clinical applications, barriers, facilitators, and artificial wisdom. Biol Psych Cogn Neurosci Neuroimag 6(9):856–864
204. Lovejoy CA, Buch V, Maruthappu M (2019) Technology and mental health: the role of artificial intelligence. Eur Psychiatry 55:1–3. https://doi.org/10.1016/j.eurpsy.2018.08.004. Epub 2018 Oct 28. PMID: 30384105

Transforming Mental Health Systems for Youth: An Unavoidable Priority

6

Paola Calò

Abstract

The transition from adolescence to adulthood is the peak period for the onset of mental and substance use disorders that have a serious impact on the productive years of adult life. About 30 years ago, the "WHO Burden of Disease Study," developed to estimate prevalence, severity, and treatment of mental disorders in 14 countries, suggested that "mental illnesses are the chronic diseases of the young," and pointed out the needs to move to the value of treating mild cases, especially in young at risk for progressing to more serious disorders.

In recent years, the mental health of young people has been steadily undermined by several socioeconomic forces, and concerns have increased during the coronavirus disease-2019 (COVID-19) pandemic, with data documenting the wave of distress, mental illness, and suicidal behavior flowing into emergency departments.

Thinking about the reallocation of treatment resources, these early stages of illness need to be targeted for preventive interventions to be most effective. A clearer definition of these early stages is essential to guide clinicians in selecting the most appropriate treatments to the phase of the illness, with the assumption that interventions delivered during this period will be both more effective and less harmful than treatments delivered later.

We must acknowledge the magnitude of the problem and reallocate treatment resources to substantially decrease the unmet needs of mental disorders, overcoming structural barriers to this reallocation.

In an under-resourced mental health system, considering that young people are often reluctant to seek help from mainstream health services, digital technologies can be useful to detect emerging mental disorders outside established clinical pathways, and constitute an important prerequisite for population-based preventive approaches.

Keywords

Youth mental health · Prevention · Transition
Adolescent vulnerability · Mental health services

6.1 Background

Childhood, adolescence, and early youth are crucial phases for the onset of mental disorders; thus, recognition and treatment strategies, from a preventive perspective to scientifically based

P. Calò (✉)
Department of Mental Health Lecce, Community Mental Health Centre, Campi Salentina, Italy
e-mail: paola.calo.6a@asl.lecce.it

A. Fiorillo, S. De Giorgi (eds.), *Social Determinants of Mental Health*, Sustainable Development Goals Series, https://doi.org/10.1007/978-3-031-70165-8_6

clinical and organizational changes, must be a priority for public health services.

It is estimated that more than 13% of adolescents aged 10–19 years live with a diagnosed mental disorder; moreover, in the last years, the problems of adolescence are rapidly changing, and the emergencies in the transition phase to adulthood no longer consist of alcohol abuse, eating disorders, unwanted pregnancies, and smoking, thanks to greater education and public health campaigns that have increased awareness of the risk among parents and children. The current alarm, raised by psychiatrists, pedagogists, sociologists, psychologists, and child neuropsychiatrists on the escalation of malaise and clinical emergencies in very young people, concerns anxiety, mood, and somatization disorders, but also complex psychiatric and behavioral syndromes, such as domestic withdrawal "hikikomori" type, self-harm, accentuation of obsessive symptoms, aggravation of eating disorders, and psychoses.

The coronavirus disease-2019 (COVID-19) pandemic has had a sharp impact on the mental health of young people; compared to the pre-pandemic period, the number of adolescents taken into care for mental health problems increased by over 30%, for panic attacks, anxiety, depression, and eating disorders.

The fear of contagion and economic worries, the interruption of routine, and the rarefaction of supportive relationships have affected the entire population without distinction, but psychologically the most fragile groups.

The report released by UNICEF highlighted that at least 1 in 5 children and adolescents aged between 5 and 24 years experienced depression, fear, and uncertainty about the future in the first months of the year. Anxiety and depression account for about 40% of these mental disorders, followed by attention-deficit/hyperactivity disorder, conduct disorder, intellectual disability, bipolar disorder, eating disorders, autism, schizophrenia, and a group of personality disorders [1].

Suicide is the fifth most prevalent cause of death for adolescents aged 10–19 years; for adolescents aged 15–19 years, it is the fourth most common cause of death, after road injury, tuberculosis, and interpersonal violence. For girls aged 15–19 years, it is the third most common cause of death, and the fourth for boys in the same age group.

During the pandemic, the fear of getting sick and isolated acted as a detonator: the rules on distancing were too strict, and the suspension of school attendance was too prolonged. The absence of sport, social, and recreational activities, forced coexistence in the family, and the increase in hours spent in front of the computer or smartphone did the rest.

Despite these findings, young people are often reluctant to seek help from mainstream health services, because mental health is widely stigmatized and misunderstood.

6.2 The Impact of Mental Illness on Young People

Consistent epidemiological evidence highlights that about 75% of all major syndromes start before the age of 25 years [2–4] (Fig. 6.1).

Not only children with a mental disorder may present with mental health problems later in life [5], but also children and adolescents with symptoms that do not fully meet the criteria for the diagnosis of a mental disorder are at increased risk for impaired mental health in adulthood [6].

Mental health problems affect the developmental opportunities of children and adolescents and may have effects into adulthood, in terms of impaired mental health, lower life satisfaction, poorer quality of life, and indicators of sexual and reproductive health in young adulthood [7]. The availability of protective (personal, familial, and social) factors in childhood or adolescence may also have an impact on mental health, life satisfaction, and health-related quality of life in young adulthood.

Due to an often complicated and difficult-to-access care system, help-seeking for young people with mental health concerns can be impeded by several barriers, including stigma and a preference for self-reliance. Online help-seeking may offer an additional domain where young people can seek help for mental health difficulties [8].

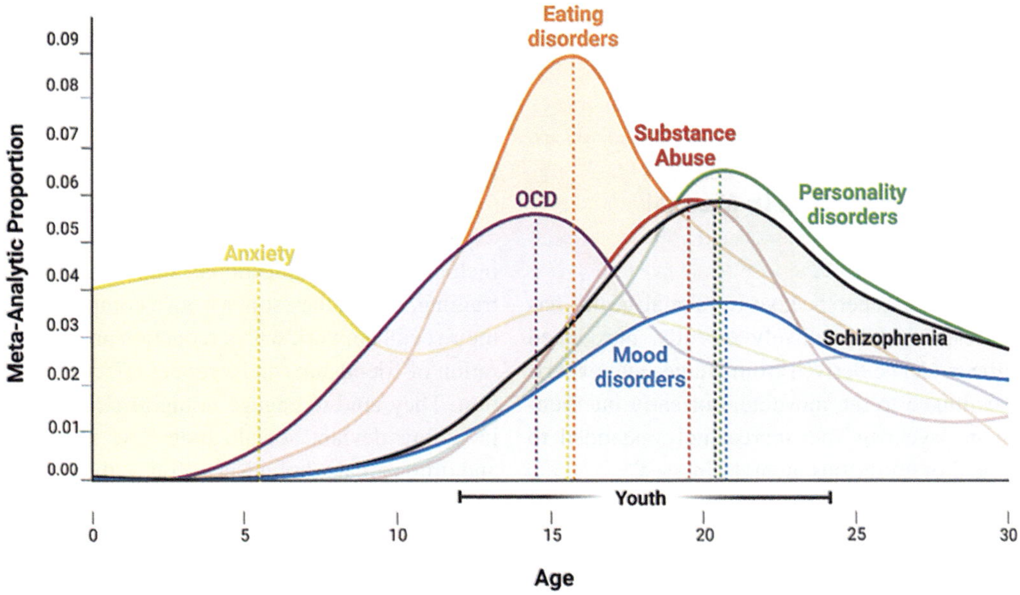

Fig. 6.1 Age of onset of mental disorders. Distribution of age of onset of mental disorders in the general population based on *t*-analysis by Solmi et al. [2]: Meta-analytic epidemiologic proportion (*y*-axis) for anxiety disorders (5.5/15.5 years), substance use disorder (19.5 years), schizophrenia/psychotic disorders (20.5 years), eating disorders (15.5 years), personality disorders (20.5 years), and obsessive-compulsive (14.5 years) and mood disorders (20.5 years) (International Statistical Classification of Diseases and Related Health Problems 10th Revision (ICD-10) blocks). The dotted horizontal lines represent the peak age of onset for each disorder category. (Reproduced from Uhlhaas et al. [4])

6.3 Adolescent Neurodevelopment and Vulnerability

Along the years of transition from adolescence to adulthood important changes take place in the structure and functioning of the brain, which will support the transition to the varied demands of adult life.

This phase is also characterized by special opportunities for growth, particularly in the domain of social functioning [9, 10]. However, adolescence is also associated with a vulnerability to psychopathology, particularly depression, anxiety, or psychosis [3, 11].

Adolescence is a time of dynamic structural and functional brain changes, driven by a series of maturational processes that result in the refinement of the neuronal circuitry, particularly in the frontal cortex [12].

Across different regions of the brain, early maturation of those responsive to reward (e.g., subcortical brain regions) and later maturation of brain regions involved in thoughtful, effortful control of behavior (e.g., prefrontal cortex) underlie enhanced reward-seeking, exploration, and risk-taking [13, 14]. These mechanisms may also result in adolescence being a period of enhanced flexibility in learning and adapting to new environments [15].

Hormonal changes and consequent physical maturation linked to pubertal development in adolescence impact multiple aspects of brain development, social cognition, and peer relationships, which are associated with mood and anxiety disorders [16].

One future direction with strong implications for both mental health and social processes is to understand the role that digital devices and social media play in these processes [17]. Mental health can be significantly shaped by one's social, economic, and local environment, particularly during childhood and adolescence [18].

6.4 Prevention and Early Intervention in Mental Health

The preventive perspective in mental health has been established relatively recently, introduced by the evidence derived from studies and experiences linked to the movement of early intervention in psychosis, but increasingly extended to the field of all serious mental illnesses.

Although more than a quarter of the world's population is between 10 and 24 years of age, the well-being of this period of life has not gained adequate attention and use of resources. Yet adolescence and early adulthood are phases of life in which health opportunities are decisive and in which the pattern of future health of adults and of a community is established. However, adolescents and young adults meet complex difficulties, particularly in asking for and finding the necessary help [19]. The level of psychophysical well-being derives from the interaction between prenatal and early childhood development, and from specific biological and social role changes that accompany puberty.

The opportunity to put adolescents at the center of global health policies has the potential not only to benefit young people directly, but also to have wide-ranging effects on the health of adults and national economic development.

Effective preventive interventions that target mental ill-health in young people need to be applied and scaled up. And finally, the impact of these preventive interventions on health in young people, but also in adults, needs to be monitored and reviewed.

Many public health agendas are now adopting a preventive approach—universal measures, selective measures, or indicated prevention—to particular group of populations depending on an assessment of risks, costs, and benefits of each case [20].

Researchers have proposed that subthreshold syndromes can be considered as risk factors for full-threshold disorders and that these subthreshold syndromes could be targeted by preventive interventions as a step toward indicated prevention for serious mental illness [21, 22].

Youth with mental health disorders often experience difficulties in a variety of settings, including their educational and professional training. Often, they suffer from a compromise in their social network with a reduction and deterioration of friendships and frequent affective isolation. They tend to engage in high-risk behaviors including deviant socialization, law violations, and drug and alcohol misuse. Today, the problem of mental health is by far one of the most critical, since it can impact many areas, including that of adaptation, functioning, social, and future productivity [23–26].

Preventive interventions that target mental health in young people have an excellent chance of reducing the incidence of subsequent mental disorders, and their associated morbidity and costs to the individual and society. Early detection interventions may allow for more effective healthcare pathways, by taking action long before health problems worsen or by preventing their onset [27]. They also allow for more personalized care in terms of tailoring health interventions to the specific sociodemographic and health-related risk factors as well as activating interventions specific to the illness stage [28]. In this regard, the application of the clinical staging model has been suggested to improve health benefits, by addressing the needs of people at different stages along the continuum between health and disease [29].

Despite being challenging, reformulating health services from this perspective may increase prevention and early intervention effectiveness, disease control, and overall care, positively impacting the health and well-being outcomes of a broader population [30]. Not to be overlooked, it may potentially reduce disease burden and healthcare system costs [31].

Clinical and epidemiological research are increasingly focusing their attention on the states or conditions that precede psychiatric illnesses, and on early identification and treatment strategies. It is established that the quality of life and social functioning worsen even before illness onset [32]. From this derives the need to recompose the life of each person into a continuum that does not include caesuras that delay times and methods of intervention. Trained professionals in collaboration with informed family members can identify the risk factors and signs of a nascent disorder, both of which are often present, as early as the age of 12–14 years, and begin protective courses or effective and safe treatments. It becomes of crucial importance to recognize with sufficient certainty from a diagnostic and clinical point of view the early stages of the disease and high-risk conditions using the currently available biological, behavioral, and cognitive tools.

An organization of Mental Health Services placed in the natural context of life and divided into facilities should facilitate working methods and approaches that are permeable to changes in the structure of society, and the evolution of knowledge. It would be necessary to encourage change in professionals and overcome the limitation of fragmentation of skills and responsibilities in favor of the early intervention approach, which represents the real innovation in the mental health panorama and which has powerful elements of innovation, evolution, and development of services. Adolescents and young people need services, approaches, and interventions suited to them. Some authors propose a transformative early intervention paradigm for research and clinical care, rethinking mental health as "youth mental health" [4]. Strategies include pre-psychotic and prodromal interventions to prevent the emergence of mental illnesses, with the appropriate methods of intervention and service models based on:

- Time: act promptly with a preventive perspective, with a smooth and effective transition from a child and adolescent mental health service (CAMHS) to an adult mental health service (AMHS).
- The place: with very low-access thresholds (not stigmatizing, with specific hospital access facilities for adolescent psychiatric patients).
- The way: evidence-based practices, including a period of shared management, and building of territorial multidisciplinary teams.

The expression Early Intervention can therefore indicate two different forms of preventive intervention:

- Intervention before the development of the disorder with subjects at risk, in the prodromal phase.
- Intervention immediately after the onset, in the early period.

6.5 At-Risk Mental State and Early Psychosis

Schizophrenia is a severe, chronic, and debilitating neuropsychiatric disorder with an estimated prevalence between 0.3 and 0.8%, affecting approximately 24 million people worldwide [33, 34].

Psychosis is currently considered a complex syndrome, characterized by positive symptoms, especially delusions and hallucinations, and typically associated with negative symptoms, mood or personality disorders, substance abuse, traumatic stress, and organic diseases.

Schizophrenic psychoses and related syndromes are characterized by a progression of symptoms and multiple disabilities of a social nature that further worsen during the illness, fueling the vicious symptom/disability cycle. Psychotic disorders, with mood disorders, represent the leading cause of disability in young people [35].

6.5.1 Psychotic Risk (or Mental State at Risk)

Even if the importance of paying attention to the period preceding psychotic onset was already present in the reflections in the past, certainly the most propulsive orientation came from the results of the retrospective ABC study [36], from which it emerged that approximately two-thirds of those who subsequently developed psychosis presented non-specific signs, warnings, and symptoms in the 2–3 years preceding the onset—in some cases up to 5 years earlier—which could be grouped in the cognitive (difficulty with attention and concentration) and affective (depressed mood, insecurity, anxiety) spectrum. They are generally followed by behavioral anomalies, physiological disorders, and finally by what we could call positive symptoms, even in attenuated form (perceptual alterations, anomalous beliefs, eccentric behaviors that differ in their intensity and content from those typical of adolescence or youth subcultures operating in a given historical moment). From the first recognizable appearance of these signals, the *duration of untreated illness* is decisive in producing the first effects in a progressive shattering of the individual's personal and social path.

There is now a vast literature, clinical experience, and research supporting the need to prevent the suffering and reduce the personal and social costs of the disease as promptly and effectively as possible, with the most appropriate use of resources. Although the Diagnostic and Statistical Manual of Mental Disorders (DSM-5), after a long debate [37], has not yet attributed an autonomous nosological status to the psychotic risk situations, placing them among unspecified psychotic disorders with the definition of Attenuated Psychosis Syndrome, randomized controlled studies, reviews, meta-analyses, and guidelines are providing valuable and safe indications in this field. Two fundamental objectives have been proposed:

- The identification of people at risk.
- The appropriate intervention for them.

6.5.2 Risk Factors and Signals

Since psychoses are increasingly considered to be a neurodevelopmental disorder with a polygenic inheritance [38], research is focused on polygenic factors and their phenotypic expressions. Although evidence is still lacking on involved genes, it has been hypothesized that these expressions are greatly influenced both by variants of rare genes with large effects, and by the interactions of various genes with reduced effects, and finally by the interaction of genes with the environment. This last possibility, now supported by an extremely robust body of research, is particularly useful in helping to determine people who could develop psychosis.

The factors mostly associated with the risk of developing psychosis are:

- A family history of mental disorders.
- Birth and life in urban areas.
- Second-generation immigration.
- Pre/perinatal factors, including maternal stress, distress during management (pre-eclampsia, viral infections), and obstetric complications (hypoxia, central nervous system (CNS) damage, low birth weight).
- Delay in reaching the fundamental stages of childhood development.
- Schizoid or schizotypal personality.
- Stressful life events, including trauma.
- Substance abuse.
- Premorbid poor functioning.

As recognized in the scientific literature, we currently refer to two complementary approaches in the definition of psychotic risk: the ultra-high-risk (UHR) criterion and the basic symptoms criterion. Different definitions and different corresponding tools are used for these two different criteria [39].

UHR is a construct aiming to operationally identify people who are at imminent risk of developing psychosis [40–42], which includes at least one of the following criteria:

- Attenuated psychotic symptoms (APS): presence of at least one attenuated psychotic symptom: ideas of reference, paranoid ideation, unusual content of thought or magical thinking, ideas of grandiosity, or unusual perceptual experiences.
- Brief intermittent psychotic episode (BLIPS): presence of at least one episode with hallucinations, delusions, or formal thought disorder.

- Genetic risk: psychiatric familiarity and schizotypal personality especially if accompanied by functional decline.

The most frequently used tools to identify these situations are:

- Comprehensive Assessment of At-Risk Mental State (CAARMS) [41].
- Structured Interview for Prodromal Symptoms (SIPS) and Scale of Prodromal Symptoms (SOPS) [43].
- Early Recognition Inventory (ERIraos) [44–46].
- Basel Screening Instrument for Psychosis (BSIP) [47].

The basic symptoms criterion aims to recognize more nuanced signals and to initiate intervention even earlier, before full symptoms and/or functional decline appear. These are very subtle subjective experiences, which concern the affective, cognitive, verbal, somatic–perceptive, motor, and vegetative dimensions, felt as different from one's "normal" self and rarely recognizable by an external observer. They include:

- The basic cognitive–perceptual symptoms (COPER) criterion for risk recognition.
- The cognitive impairment criterion (COGDIS) for recognizing high risk [48, 49].

These criteria are evaluated through the following tools:

- Bonn Scale for the Assessment of Basic Symptoms (BSABS) [50].
- Schizophrenia Proneness Instrument, adult and children version (SPI-A, SPI-CY) [51, 52].
- Examination of anomalous self-experiences (EASE) [53].

In this field, the primary outcome is the assessment of transition to psychosis, which is associated with several clinically meaningful real-world outcomes [54]. Thus, identifying the transition to psychosis in individuals at clinical high risk for psychosis (CHR-P) is of paramount importance for clinical care [55].

The risk of transition to psychosis in individuals at CHR-P as estimated by a meta-analysis [56] was 18% at 6 months, 22% at 1 year, 29% at 2 years, and 36% at 3 years.

In an updated meta-analysis of 130 longitudinal studies including 9222 individuals at clinical high risk for psychosis from 74 cohorts, the risk of developing psychosis continued increasing after 2 years, cumulating to 25% at 3 years and reaching 35% at 10 years [57]. The probability of transitioning to psychosis in individuals at clinical high risk is substantial and continues increasing in the long term, suggesting that an extended duration of clinical monitoring and preventive care may be beneficial.

However, some authors have underlined the need for new identification and diagnosis strategies, by adopting a transdiagnostic approach, which on the one hand considers the psychotic experiences not necessarily predictive of psychotic onset, in the complex and varied psychopathology of seeking help; on the other hand, it highlights the importance of having as aim of the intervention not only the prevention of transition, but also other possible unfavorable pathological and functional trajectories [58–60].

6.5.3 Treatment of at-Risk Mental States

Some research programs investigating the prepsychotic period have integrated research into clinical services. The first research clinic was the Personal Assessment and Crisis Evaluation (PACE) clinic in Melbourne, Australia. Like PACE, there are many in the USA, Canada, Australia, and several European countries specialized in integrated research and service clinics. These "prodromal" or high-risk clinics may offer combinations of treatment packages including engagement, supportive therapy, case management, stress management, cognitive behavioral therapy (CBT), family-based treatment and pharmacotherapy.

Early interventions for groups at high risk of psychosis are promising for alleviating symptoms such as subthreshold psychotic symptoms, reducing the progression of deterioration in the quality of life, and increasing the quality of life of individuals. However, a meta-analysis investigating whether specific interventions are useful for the prevention of transition to psychosis did not show any evidence regarding the efficacy of any specific intervention [61].

Cognitive behavioral therapy (CBT) should be considered as an early preventive approach for individuals at high risk of psychosis, considering its high tolerability and absence of side effects.

A meta-analysis including 5 studies with 24- and 48-month follow-up periods and 10 studies with 12-month follow-up periods on the effect of CBT on decreasing the risk of transition to psychosis found that CBT reduced the risk of transition to psychosis by 54% at 12-month and by 37% at 24–48 months [62]. If CBT is not sufficiently effective and the symptoms progress (less insight and more frequent symptoms), pharmacological interventions—such as short-term use of antipsychotics—can be appropriate [63].

While mood stabilizers and antidepressants can be used in cases of predominant symptoms associated with mood fluctuations or anxiety, pharmacological interventions also include new and experimental pharmacotherapies and food supplements, such as omega-3 long-chain polyunsaturated fatty acids (PUFA), whose efficacy was not recently confirmed [64].

6.6 Early Psychosis: Assessment and Treatment

Mental health is an important health concern for young people; yet, most young people are reluctant to seek help from standard mental health services [65, 66]. Paradoxically, the life stage between 12 and 25 years of age is characterized by both the highest level of need for effective mental health care and the lowest level of service use.

The help-seeking process is difficult and complicated by personal and contextual factors, such as access and stigma; several approaches to improve help-seeking by young people consider the role of Internet and online resources [8], as discussed elsewhere in this book.

Despite that in the last 15–20 years there has been a worldwide movement to detect and intervene as early as possible for those with a psychotic illness, individuals usually come into contact with mental health services for the first time during their psychotic onset.

The phase of psychotic onset, or the acute phase of illness, usually happens between 15 and 25 years, which is in common with the onset of higher prevalence mental illnesses, such as depression and anxiety, and is characterized by the full-blown phase of psychotic illness, or fully fledged psychosis [67], in which psychotic symptoms become manifest.

Inpatient hospitalization can be very disruptive to the goals (e.g., schooling) of young people with first-episode psychosis (FEP) and is often experienced as traumatic [68].

The onset of psychosis, or "first-episode psychosis" (FEP), often coincides with the moment in which patients come into contact with services for the first time [69]. Despite treatment advances, inpatient psychiatric hospitalization rates for individuals with first-episode psychosis remain high. Even with early intervention services (EIS), a third or more of individuals are hospitalized over the first 2 years of treatment. In this period, psychotic positive and negative symptoms, alone or together with other symptoms (mood alterations, personality disorders, post traumatic stress disorder (PTSD), organic comorbidities), become manifest [67]. The type of symptoms, and their prevalence, influence the treatment approach. Unfortunately, both the phase in which psychosis has not been recognized yet and the one in which, even if recognized, it is not adequately treated, have a variable duration, with consequent treatment delays for patients. In people with a newly diagnosis of psychotic disorders, hospitalization may impact subsequent service engagement.

The acute phase or crisis (*stage 1*), which is characterized by florid psychotic symptoms (sustained symptoms lasting 4 weeks or more; 102),

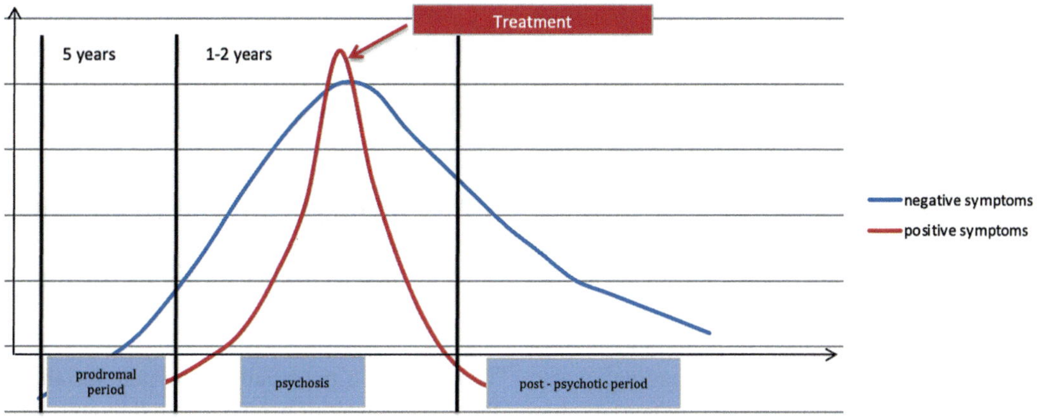

Fig. 6.2 Course of illness over time [70]

is followed by an early recovery phase or post-acute phase in the first 6–12 months following the acute episode (*stage 2*) (Fig. 6.2).

Interventions in this phase are associated with improvements in psychotic symptoms, but also with higher patients' satisfaction with treatment, improved personal well-being, better quality of life, and greater involvement in school and work, with an overall reduced family burden [71–73].

The benefits of early interventions are crucial for the secondary prevention of illness progression to clinical *stage 3*, in particular to prevent relapse into a second episode of psychosis. This is significant, because relapses interfere with the social and vocational development of individuals suffering from a first episode of psychosis [74].

The early phase of psychosis (including the period of untreated psychosis) is a *critical period* of illness progression, in which long-term outcome is predictable, and biological, psychological, and psychosocial influences are developing and show maximum plasticity [75].

An early intervention strategy, in the first 5 years from the onset of psychosis, can limit the chronicity and disability associated with the disorder [76], thus justifying the need for patients with FEP to remain within early intervention programs for at least 2–5 years [77] and receive effective treatment. The critical period is the one in which patients are at the highest risk of disengagement, relapses, and suicidal risk. During this period interventions have their greatest impact [78].

The purpose of using the word psychosis rather than a diagnostic label such as schizophrenia is firstly to avoid premature judgment about the course of illness as there is a very high diagnostic instability after presentation for treatment. In addition to clinical symptoms, people with schizophrenia spectrum disorders are often targets of negative attitudes and social labels that lead to stigma, which can precipitate initial episodes of psychosis, trigger relapses, and promote a more severe course[79]). Some authors have highlighted that, in patients with FEP, symptomatic remission for at least 3 months of both positive and negative symptoms in the first 2 years from the onset of the full-blown clinical picture, is predictive of the achievement of good personal and social functioning [80].

6.6.1 Prognosis and Related Factors

Given the global burden of psychotic disorders, the identification of patients at higher risk of adverse outcomes should be a priority. Risk factors associated with a poor outcome have been identified, including male sex, early age at onset, belonging to an ethnic minority, and family history of mental disorders. In addition to these non-modifiable factors, other replicated predictors of worse clinical, functional, and cognitive outcomes are:

(a) An insidious onset, with negative symptoms and functional deterioration preceding positive symptoms by a substantial period.
(b) A long duration of untreated psychosis (DUP), which correlates with a worse symptomatic outcome and quality of life. Many studies have replicated the finding that longer DUP is regularly associated with a more chronic long-term course of the disorder and a poorer outcome [81].
(c) Negative symptoms, which are more closely related to poor patient functioning, worse quality of life, and lowered productivity than positive symptoms, which can be better addressed by available treatment options [70].
(d) Substance use disorders: in patients with psychotic disorders, the lifetime prevalence of substance use disorders is higher than in the general population [82], including those in their first psychotic episode, ranging from 30 to 70% [83]. Co-occurring substance use disorder has been associated with clinical exacerbations, non-compliance with treatment, poor global functioning, violence, suicide, and increased rates of relapse and re-hospitalization [84].
(e) Premorbid difficulties (poorer premorbid adjustment, history of developmental disorder) and greater symptom severity (especially negative symptoms) at baseline, which are consistently found to be significant predictors of worse clinical, functional, and cognitive outcomes [85].
(f) Disengagement: The proportion of individuals disengaging from Early Intervention Services before 2 years varies from 21 to 40% across studies [86]. Predictors of disengagement are related to sociodemographic factors, clinical features, and psychological issues. Patients with a lower level of family support, reduced adherence to medication, and higher substance use are at higher risk of disengagement in FEP [87]. FEP patients who disengage or are only superficially engaged are at greater risk of relapse [88] and worse long-term outcomes. A possible solution to decrease disengagement and to favor re-engagement of these young individuals might be to provide the option of low-intensity monitoring and support, also via remote technology [89].

6.7 Management and Treatment of Psychosis and Schizophrenia in Young People

The DUP is a potentially important variable in the management of people with a first episode of psychosis—that becoming the focus of intervention strategies. For psychotic illnesses, early intervention is seen as an intuitive and sensible way to limit the damage. Delays in accessing appropriate care may be influenced by the time between help-seeking and the start of appropriate treatment. Ease of access to care is important because it provides relief from the distress that psychotic and non-psychotic symptoms can cause.

Mental health services should be accessible and provide a timely assessment for people experiencing their first episode of psychosis.

Guidelines recommend that an expert assessment should be set for any person suspected of developing a psychotic disorder for the first time, including symptom evaluation and an assessment of cognitive functions; potential targets for intervention; personal, social, and work functioning; quality of life; and adherence and satisfaction with treatment.

Although there may be a natural reluctance to widen access and enhance the quality of assessment because of a lack of resources in community psychiatry settings, this should make the work of the service easier and result in a reduced need for inpatient care and involuntary treatment.

An optimal early-phase detection should extend the investigation to environmental risk factors, the presence of obstetric complications and developmental abnormalities, family history, and psychosocial disabilities. It is also essential to collect data on alcohol and substance abuse, both in the past and currently. Some centers also include a genetic and neurobiological assessment.

The treatment path for patients at the first psychotic episode or at high risk of psychosis has the aim not only of preventing chronicity but also of shortening illness duration with a positive medium-term effect on the course of the disorder.

However, the treatment should be phase-specific. In the earlier phases of illness, the approach should be more benign and potentially more effective than in later phases.

The acute phase is usually the time for the first contact with a mental health service. The presentation will determine the initial setting for treatment (i.e., inpatient or outpatient care). This first presentation of suspected psychosis is considered a psychiatric emergency requiring immediate treatment, in order to reduce both DUP and distress caused to the individual and caregivers. In a first psychotic episode, pharmacotherapy is usually the first choice [69, 90]. Clinicians must pay particular attention to the therapeutic strategy, as the response and the side effects are potentially able to influence future engagement and adherence to treatment. Concomitant drug abuse should be taken into account.

People with FEP generally show a more rapid symptom remission and usually respond to lower antipsychotic doses than those with a full-blown illness [91].

Despite high response rates to antipsychotic medications, FEP is followed by frequent antipsychotic discontinuation and elevated relapse rates soon after maintenance treatment [92]. With subsequent episodes, the time to respond progressively increases and the likelihood of response decreases [93, 94].

In this cohort of patients the clinical use of medication differs, because they are more sensitive to the effects of antipsychotic medication and more vulnerable to their adverse effects, such as extrapyramidal side effects (EPS), especially akathisia and withdrawal dyskinesia, prolactin abnormalities, and weight gain, than those in later phases of the illness [95].

Overall rates of non-adherence to antipsychotic medications for FEP patients are higher than 50% within the first year of treatment, suggesting that malleable factors linked to non-adherence need to be targeted in interventions provided. Factors influencing adherence can be categorized into four groups: (1) environment-related, (2) patient-related, (3) medication-related, and (4) illness-related.

Treatment guidelines for FEP recommend oral antipsychotic dosages in the lower half of the treatment range and lower than those that are required for multi-episode schizophrenia, with individualized dosages for their patients based on symptom improvement and tolerability, according to the "start low, go slow" principle [96]. However, higher dosages may be needed than those used in FEP clinical trials, recommended by guidelines for FEP or multi-episode patients, or approved by the food and drug administration (FDA). Higher dosages also may be reasonable to overcome drug–drug interactions (e.g., cigarette smoking-mediated cytochrome P450 1A2 induction, resulting in increased olanzapine metabolism; [97]), or to establish antipsychotic failure if adequate trials at lower dosages have resulted in a suboptimal response and the patient is not experiencing tolerability or safety concerns.

An analysis from the Recovery After an Initial Schizophrenia Episode Project's Early Treatment Program (RAISE-ETP), a nationwide multisite effectiveness study for patients with first-episode schizophrenia spectrum disorders, found that, of participants identified who may benefit from therapy modification, 8.8% were prescribed an antipsychotic (often, olanzapine, risperidone, and haloperidol) at a higher-than-recommended dosage [98].

Most guidelines suggest antipsychotic monotherapy, because combining antipsychotics has been shown to independently predict both shorter treatment duration and discontinuation before 1 year [99]. The benefits of antipsychotic polypharmacy outweigh the risks in some situations and may be reasonable for FEP patients (managing coexisting symptom domains, e.g., mood changes, negative symptoms, disorganization, and mitigating antipsychotic-induced side effects; [100]).

Guidelines do not explicitly recommend long-acting injectable (LAI) antipsychotics in FEP, because of limited evidence.

To improve prescription of antipsychotics for first-episode schizophrenia patients, in the light of the serious neurobiological adverse effects of psychotic relapses, including neuroinflammation and oxidative stress, some studies have considered using LAI treatment for FEP, and showed significant differences in outcomes. Thus, long-acting injectable antipsychotics are recommended in FEP to proactively combat the high relapse rate and more easily identify antipsychotic failure. The guidelines issued by the World Federation of Societies of Biological Psychiatry contain LAI dosage recommendations for FEP [101].

According to the *International Clinical Practice Guidelines in Early Psychosis* [102], there are no differences in efficacy between first-generation antipsychotics (FGAs) and second-generation antipsychotics (SGAs), but tolerability and compliance are better with SGAs. Second-generation antipsychotic long-acting injectables (SGA-LAIs) have increased the number of options available to personalize the pharmacological treatment of schizophrenia [103]. A treatment plan with SGA-LAIs may be of significant advantage in terms of neuroprotective effect, especially compared to first-generation antipsychotics (FGAs), which have a well-known neurotoxicity [104, 105].

Young people experiencing psychosis are more likely to have significant weight gain and metabolic changes within weeks of starting antipsychotic treatment, especially with SGA. The most common causes of premature death before suicide in these patients are cardiovascular diseases, which are due to a combination of high rates of smoking, weight gain, and metabolic changes.

Healthcare professionals have to work cohesively to protect and maintain the physical health of young people experiencing psychosis, through education and promotion of healthy lifestyle, focusing on healthy nutrition and diet, physical activity, and reduced tobacco use (Healthy Active Lives—HeAL—Declaration, International Early Psychosis Association conference in Amsterdam, 2010).

Interrupting the use of antipsychotics in patients with a first episode of schizophrenia or schizoaffective disorder increases the risk of recurrence by about fivefold [106]. Even when patients with FEP have responded to antipsychotic treatment and achieved remission, maintenance therapy is recommended for at least 1–2 years; in case of early suspension, clinical monitoring for relapses must be implemented for at least 2 years.

More evidence on early intervention approaches demonstrates that pharmacotherapy alone is not sufficient to promote adequate recovery. Several randomized controlled trials have shown that the cognitive behavioral approach is superior to both routine care and treatment as usual (TAU) to reduce the distress experienced by people with psychosis and to improve their quality of life [107].

The primary aim of CBT for psychosis is not necessarily to reduce the frequency of psychotic symptoms but, rather, to help patients to achieve their own specific goals about the problems they have identified.

Moreover, family intervention may contribute to reducing relapse and hospital admission rates in patients with a first episode of psychosis [108].

In the OPUS 20-year follow-up trial, the longest follow-up of a randomized clinical trial testing early intervention services (EIS) among individuals with first-episode schizophrenia spectrum disorder, no differences in 2 years of EIS vs. TAU among individuals with diagnosed schizophrenia spectrum disorders at 20 years were found [109]. To maintain positive long-term outcomes, further initiatives are recommended in the period following the first episode of psychosis, including psychosocial interventions and, in particular, family psychoeducational intervention and social skill training [110].

Findings also suggest the need to involve family members as early as possible in the treatment of their loved ones, not only with psychoeducational interventions, but also through other structured focused interventions, such as the management of Expressed Emotions and the improvement of problem-solving techniques [108, 111].

Cognitive rehabilitation is effective in improving cognition in patients with schizophrenia. Although no studies have examined the long-term neurobiological effects of cognitive rehabilitation in early schizophrenia, cognitive enhancement therapy can protect against gray matter loss and may even support gray matter growth in medial–temporal areas of the brain. Thus, there is some evidence that cognitive rehabilitative approaches can positively affect the brain in early-course schizophrenia [112].

Over the last 100 years, different methods of vocational intervention have been developed, but there is a paucity of evidence about their outcome. However, it is well recognized that people with schizophrenia face several barriers to access employment. One of the key problems that contribute to high unemployment rate is the level of education of people with mental illness, which usually has its onset in a period of life that is mostly associated with secondary education and the commencement of higher training or employment.

Supported education involves a series of supports that help to addressing the barriers that prevent people with psychiatric disabilities from pursuing educational goals with individualized, practical assistance ([113]).

Societal attitudes, stigma, and work-related legislation are other barriers that act against employment of young person with psychosis [114].

The supported employment approach combined with interventions targeting the significant deficits associated with schizophrenia, such as neurocognitive therapy and job-related social skill training, appears to hold the key to successfully addressing the work disability.

There are now hundreds of early intervention programs worldwide, of varying intensity and duration, which focus on the special needs of young people and their families. Early intervention in psychosis is an evidence-based practice that shows great benefits for those who are treated according to this paradigm.

Early intervention services are based on a low threshold for access and an optimistic view of outcomes. The course of mental disorders is seen as fluid and malleable, and the examination of risk factors that can influence outcomes has revealed that many of these are reversible [67].

Children of people with severe mental illness are a largely neglected, yet identifiable, population, which represent an enormous potential for developmentally tailored primary and secondary preventive strategies and approaches, such as flexible support for families and routine systematic screening and early intervention [115].

The significant impact of the COVID-19 pandemic underlines the importance of identifying markers of risk and resilience in young adults, an age group at particularly high risk for the development of psychopathologies, and the importance of maintaining access to inclusive mental healthcare services during any new COVID-19 waves, or potential future pandemics [116].

Integrating digital technologies into more traditional therapeutic models appears to support better clinical outcomes for youth. As the COVID-19 pandemic has largely increased the utilization of telehealth, mobile mental health technologies—such as smartphone apps, virtual reality, chatbots, and social media—have also gained attention.

The use of smartphone devices in mental health care provides ubiquitous connectivity/Internet access for a sizeable proportion of the global population, and social media represent a source of social support for many who have been socially isolated and lonely [117], with low purchasing and running costs. There is a need to build new service delivery models that incorporate technology, ensuring the involvement of young people in the process of continuous improvement.

Youth mental health research requires coordination, planning, and adequate funding. By addressing mental health issues in young people, we can enhance their overall productivity and ability to contribute to society, both socially and economically.

Young people Not in Education, Employment, or Training (NEETs) are at increased risk for mental disorders and suicidal ideation. By investing in youth mental health, we can improve educational outcomes, leading to a more skilled and productive workforce. This, in turn, can have a positive impact on a country's economy and overall development.

Supporting the mental health of youth will require a whole-of-society effort to address longstanding challenges, strengthen the resilience of young people, support their families and communities, empower youth workers, and train youth mental health workforce.

This includes raising awareness on correct terminology, methodology, and new developments in the field of youth mental health (emerging disorders, new digital solutions, etc.); guaranteeing continuity of care; better planning of the transition between child and adolescent services and those for adult; and promoting an anti-stigma cultural change.

6.8 Youth Suicide

Youth suicide is a significant global public health concern and one of the leading causes of death among 5- to 24-year-olds.

Comorbidity of psychiatric disorders, particularly mood, disruptive, and substance abuse disorders, significantly increases the risk for youth suicide and suicidal behavior [118]. One of the key factors mediating the relationship between depression and suicidal ideation is hopelessness, which increases the risk among already suicidal patients [119].

Depression, anxiety, isolation, and decreased social support have likely contributed to increased suicide risk in youth associated with the coronavirus disease-2019 (COVID-19) pandemic and related lockdown measures [120]. A warning of a mental health crisis among youth, particularly in youth with intellectual and developmental disabilities, those belonging to racial/ethnic and sexual/gender minority groups, or those living in low-income, rural, or immigrant households, has been recently issued (*Protecting Youth Mental Health: The US Surgeon General's Advisory*, [121]).

Mental health and suicide researchers and providers suggest that suicide prevention should be implemented in multiple settings, especially in schools, through school-based mental health and suicide prevention training, connecting at-risk students with needed services [122]. Selective interventions can be useful for subgroups of the population who are not necessarily showing signs of suicide-related behavior but have specific risk factors (e.g., symptoms of mental illness).

6.9 Management of Substance Use and Associated Mental Health in Youth

The prevalence of alcohol, tobacco, and other drug misuse varies greatly among young people, particularly when we compare substance use during the early teens to that in the mid-twenties. It increases rapidly from early to late adolescence, peaks during the transition to young adulthood, and declines through adulthood. Furthermore, there is accumulating evidence showing that the initiation of substance use early in life contributes to higher levels of use and abuse later in life. Early onset is also associated with later negative health, social, and behavioral outcomes including physical and mental health problems, violent and aggressive behavior, and adjustment problems within the family and at workplace [123].

Young people with mental health problems are a particularly high-risk population, given the high rates of co-occurring substance misuse [124] as well as the impact of substance use on clinical and functional outcomes [125]. It is therefore critical to provide young people with information regarding the link between mental illness and substance use, as well as brief interventions that discourage their regular use. A flexible treatment approach is needed to address individual cognitive, emotional, social, and environmental differences that are typical in young people [126].

References

1. Keeley B, de Oliveira JD, Dooley T et al (2021) The state of the World's children. ON MY MIND promoting, protecting and caring for children's mental health, United Nations Children's fund (UNICEF). ISBN: 978-92-806-5285-7
2. Solmi M, Radua J, Olivola M et al (2022) Age at onset of mental disorders worldwide: large-scale meta-analysis of 192 epidemiological studies. Mol Psychiatry 27:281–295
3. Kessler RC, Berglund P, Demler O et al (2005) Lifetime prevalence and age-of-onset distributions of DSM-IV disorders in the National Comorbidity Survey Replication. Arch Gen Psychiatry 62:593–602
4. Uhlhaas PJ, Davey CG, Mehta UM et al (2023) Towards a youth mental health paradigm: a perspective and roadmap. Mol Psychiatry 28:3171–3181
5. Bao L, Brownlie EB, Beitchman JH (2016) Mental health trajectories from adolescence to adulthood: language disorder and other childhood and adolescent risk factors. Dev Psychopathol 28(2):489–504
6. Copeland WE, Wolke D, Shanahan L et al (2015) Adult functional outcomes of common childhood psychiatric problems: a prospective, longitudinal study. JAMA Psychiatry 72(9):892–899
7. Schlack R, Peerenboom N, Neuperdt L et al (2021) The effects of mental health problems in childhood and adolescence in young adults: results of the KiGGS cohort. J Health Monit 6(4):3–19
8. Pretorius C, Chambers D, Coyle D (2019) Young People's online help-seeking and mental Health difficulties: systematic narrative review. J Med Internet Res 21(11):e13873
9. Chein J, Albert D, O'Brien L et al (2011) Peers increase adolescent risk taking by enhancing activity in the brain's reward circuitry. Dev Sci 14:F1–F10
10. Blakemore SJ, Mills KL (2014) Is adolescence a sensitive period for sociocultural processing? Annu Rev Psychol 65:187–207
11. Dalsgaard S, Thorsteinsson E, Trabjerg BB et al (2019) Incidence rates and cumulative incidences of the full Spectrum of diagnosed mental disorders in childhood and adolescence, vol 77. JAMA Psychiatry, p 155
12. Dumontheil I (2016) Adolescent brain development. Curr Opin Behav Sci 10:39–44
13. Steinberg LA (2008) Social neuroscience perspective on adolescent risk-taking. Dev Rev 28:78–106
14. Casey BJ, Jones RM, Hare TA (2008) The adolescent brain. Ann N Y Acad Sci 1124:111–126
15. Crone EA, Dahl RE (2012) Understanding adolescence as a period of social–affective engagement and goal flexibility. Nat Rev Neurosci 13:636–650
16. Pfeifer JH, Allen NB (2021) Puberty initiates cascading relationships between neurodevelopmental, social, and internalizing processes across adolescence. Biol Psychiatry 89:99–108
17. Haidt J, Allen N (2020) Scrutinizing the effects of digital technology on mental health. Nature 578:226–227
18. Abraham A, Walker-Harding L (2022) The key social determinants of mental health: their effects among children globally and strategies to address them: a narrative review. Pediatr Med 5
19. Sawyer MS, Rima A, Bearinger H et al (2012) Adolescence: a foundation for future health. Lancet 379:1571–1676
20. Gordon RS Jr (1983) An operational classification of disease prevention. Public Health Rep 98(2):107–109
21. Eaton WW, Badawi M, Melton B (1995) Prodromes and precursors: epidemiologic data for primary prevention of disorders with slow onset. Am J Psychiatry 152(7):967–972
22. Haggerty RJ, Mrazek PJ (1994) Can we prevent mental illness? Bull N Y Acad Med 71(2):300–306
23. Patel V, Flisher AJ, Hetrick S et al (2007) Mental health of young people: a global public-health challenge. Lancet 369(9569):1302–1313
24. Vyas NS, Birchwood M, Singh SP (2014) Youth services: meeting the mental health needs of adolescents. Irish J Psychol Med 32:13–19
25. Patton GC, Romaniuk H, Mackinnon A et al (2014) The prognosis of common mental disorders in adolescents: a 14-year prospective cohort study. Lancet 383(9926):1404–1411
26. Rice SM, Purcell R, McGorry PD (2018) Adolescent and Young adult male mental Health: transforming system failures into proactive models of engagement. J Adolesc Health 62(3S):S9–S17
27. Marmot M, Friel S, Bell R et al (2008) Health CoSDo. Closing the gap in a generation: health equity through action on the social determinants of health. Lancet 372(9650):1661–1669
28. Schleidgen S, Klingler C, Bertram T et al (2013) What is personalized medicine: sharpening a vague term based on a systematic literature review. BMC Med Ethics 14:55
29. Shah J, Scott J (2016) Concepts and misconceptions regarding clinical staging models. J Psychiatry Neurosci 41(6):E83–E84
30. Allen D, Gillen E, Rixson L (2009) The effectiveness of integrated care pathways for adults and children in health care settings: a systematic review. JBI Libr Syst Rev 7(3):80–129
31. Stevens M (2011) The costs and benefits of early interventions for vulnerable children and families to promote social and emotional wellbeing: economics briefing. National Institute for Health and Care Excellence, London
32. Häfner H, Maurer K, Löffler W et al (1998) The ABC schizophrenia study: a preliminary overview of the results. Soc Psychiatry Psychiatr Epidemiol 33(8):380–386
33. Charlson FJ, Ferrari AJ, Santomauro DF et al (2018) Global epidemiology and burden of schizophrenia:

findings from the global burden of disease study 2016. Schizophr Bull 44:1195–1203
34. WHO (2023) Schizophrenia. https://bit.ly/3MONOkW. Accessed Sept 2023
35. Vacheron MN, Veyrat-Masson H, Wehbe E (2017) Quelle prise en charge du jeune présentant un premier épisode psychotique, quand la scolarité est mise à mal? L'Encephale 43:570–576
36. Häfner H, van Der Heiden W (1999) The course of schizophrenia in the light of modern follow-up studies: the ABC and WHO studies. Eur Arch Psychiatry Clin Neurosci 249(suppl.4):14–26
37. Woods SW, Walsh BC, Saksa JR et al (2010) The case for including attenuated psychotic symptoms in DSM-5 as syndrome as a psychosis risk syndrome. Schizophr Res 123(2–3):199–207
38. Harrison PJ, Weinberger DR (2005) Schizophrenia genes, gene expression, and neuropathology: on the matter of their convergence. Mol Psychiatry 10(1):40–68
39. Fusar-Poli P, Borgwardt S, Bechdolf A et al (2013) The psychosis high-risk state. A comprehensive state-of-the-art review. JAMA Psychiatry 70(1):107–120
40. Phillips LJ, Yung AR, McGorry MD (2010) Identification of young people at risk of psychosis: validation of personal assessment and crisis evaluation clinic intake criteria. Aust N Z J Psychiatry 34:S164–S169
41. Yung AR, Yuen HP, McGorry PD et al (2005) Mapping the onset of psychosis: the comprehensive assessment of at-risk mental states. Aust N Z J Psychiatry 39(11–12):964–971
42. Australian Clinical Guidelines for Early Psychosis (2010) Orygen Youth Research Centre
43. Miller TJ, McGlashan TH, Rosen JL et al (2003) Prodromal assessment with the structured interview for prodromal syndromes and the scale of prodromal symptoms: predictive validity, interrater reliability, and training to reliability. Schizophr Bull 29(4):703–715
44. Maurer K, Konnecke R, Shultze-Lutter F et al (2000) The early recognition inventory ERIraos: a two steps procedure for detection of "at-risk mental states". Schizophr Res 70(suppl):76–80
45. Raballo A, Meneghelli A, Cocchi A et al (2014) Shades of vulnerability: latent structures of clinical caseness in prodromal and early phases of schizophrenia. Eur Arch Psychiatry Clin Neurosci 264(2):155–169
46. Meneghelli A, Pisano A, Coronelli I et al (2013) Programma 2000. Un apripista con molte funzioni. Nuova Rassegna di Studi Psichiatrici, Rivista online di Psichiatria 8(20)
47. Riecher-Rössler A, Aston J, Ventura J et al (2008) The basel screening instrument for psychosis (BSIP): development, structure, reliability and validity. Fortschr Neurol Psychiatr 76(4):207–216
48. Schultze-Lutter F (2009) Subjective symptoms of schizophrenia in research and the clinic: the basic symptom concept. Schizophr Bull 35(1):5–8
49. Ziermans TB, Schothorst PF, Sprong M et al (2011) Transition and remission in adolescents at ultra-high risk for psychosis. Schizophr Res 126(1–3):58–64
50. Gross G, Huber G, Klosterkötter J et al (1987) Skala für die Beurteilung von Basisymptomen. In: BSABS; Bonn scale for the assessment of basic symptoms. Springer-Verlag, Berlin
51. Schultze-Lutter F, Klosterkötter J (2004) Schizophrenia prediction instrument, adult version—SPI-A. University of Cologne, Cologne
52. Schultze-Lutter F, Marshall M, Koch E (2012) Schizophrenia proneness instrument, child and youth version; extended English translation (SPI-CY EET). Giovanni Fioriti Editore, Roma
53. Parnas J, Møller P, Kircher T et al (2005) EASE: examination of anomalous self-experience. Psychopathology 38:236–258
54. Fusar-Poli P, De Micheli A, Patel R et al (2020) Real-world clinical outcomes two years after transition to psychosis in individuals at clinical high risk: electronic health record cohort study. Schizophr Bull 46(5):1114–1125
55. Fusar-Poli P, Hijazi Z, Stahl D et al (2018) The science of prognosis in psychiatry: a review. JAMA Psychiatry 75(12):1289–1297
56. Fusar-Poli P, Bonoldi I, Yung AR et al (2012) Predicting psychosis: meta-analysis of transition outcomes in individuals at high clinical risk. Arch Gen Psychiatry 69(3):220–229
57. Salazar de Pablo G, Radua J, Pereira J et al (2021) Probability of transition to psychosis in individuals at clinical high risk. An updated meta-analysis. JAMA Psychiatry 78(9):970–978
58. van Os J, Reininghaus U (2016) Psychosis as a transdiagnostic and extended phenotype in the general population. World Psychiatry 15:118–124
59. van Os J, Guloksuz S (2017) A critique of the "ultra-high risk" and "transition" paradigm. World Psychiatry 162:200–205
60. McGorry PD (2018) Beyond the "at risk mental state" concept: transitioning to transdiagnostic psychiatry. World Psychiatry 17(2):133–142
61. Davies C, Cipriani A, Ioannidis JP et al (2018) Lack of evidence to favor specific preventive interventions in psychosis: a network meta-analysis. World Psychiatry 17:196–209
62. van der Gaag M, Smit F, Bechdolf A et al (2013) Preventing a first episode of psychosis: meta-analysis of randomized controlled prevention trials of 12 month and longer-term follow-ups. Schizophr Res 149:56–62
63. Bechdolf A, Müller H, Stützer H et al (2017) PREVENT: a randomized controlled trial for the prevention of first-episode psychosis comparing cognitive-behavior therapy (CBT), clinical man-

agement, and aripiprazole combined and clinical management and placebo combined. Schizophr Bull 43(Suppl 1):56–77
64. McGorry PD, Nelson B, Markulev C et al (2017) Effect of ω-3 polyunsaturated fatty acids in Young people at ultrahigh risk for psychotic disorders: the NEURAPRO randomized clinical trial. JAMA Psychiatry 74:19–27
65. Rickwood D, Deane F, Wilson C et al (2005) Young people's help-seeking for mental health problems. Aust J Adv Ment Health 4(3):1–34
66. Gulliver A, Griffiths KM, Christensen H (2010) Perceived barriers and facilitators to mental health help-seeking in young people: a systematic review. BMC Psychiatry 10:113
67. McGorry PD, Killackey E, Yung A (2008) Early intervention in psychosis: concepts, evidence and future directions. World Psychiatry 7:148–156
68. Robinson DG, Schooler NR, Rosenheck RA et al (2019) Predictors of hospitalization with individuals with first-episode psychosis: data from a two-year follow-up in the RAISE-ETP study. Psychiatr Serv 70(7):569–577
69. Early Psychosis Guidelines Writing Group and EPPIC National Support Program (2016) Australian Clinical Guidelines for Early Psychosis, 2nd edition update. Orygen, The National Centre of Excellence in Youth Mental Health, Melbourne
70. Correll CU, Schooler NR (2020) Negative symptoms in schizophrenia: a review and clinical guide for recognition, assessment, and treatment. Neuropsychiatr Dis Treat 16:519–534
71. Petersen L, Jeppesen P, Thorup A et al (2005a) A randomised multicentre trial of integrated versus standard treatment for patients with a first episode of psychotic illness. BMJ 331:602
72. Kane JM, Robinson DG, Schooler NR et al (2016) Comprehensive versus usual community care for first-episode psychosis: 2-year outcomes from the NIMH RAISE Early Treatment Program. Am J Psychiatry 173:362–372
73. Srihari VH, Tek C, Kucukgoncu S et al (2015) First-episode services for psychotic disorders in the U.S. public sector: a pragmatic randomized controlled trial. Psychiatr Serv 66:705–712
74. Penn DL, Waldheter EJ, Perkins DO et al (2005) Psychosocial treatment for first-episode psychosis: a research update. Am J Psychiatry 162:2220–2232
75. Birchwood M, Todd P, Jackson C (1998) Early intervention in psychosis: the critical period hypothesis. Br J Psychiatry 172(S33):53–59
76. Birchwood M, Fiorillo A (2000) The critical period for early intervention. Psychiatr Rehabil Skills 4(2):182–198
77. McGorry PD (2015) Early intervention in psychosis—obvious, effective, overdue. J Nerv Ment Dis 203(5):310
78. Birchwood M, MacMillan F (1993) Early intervention in schizophrenia. Aust N Z J Psychiatry 27:374–378
79. Hoftman GD (2016) The burden of mental illness beyond clinical symptoms: impact of stigma on the onset and course of schizophrenia Spectrum disorders. Am J Psychiatry Resident J 11:2–14
80. Cassidy CM, Norman R, Manchanda R et al (2010) Testing definitions of symptom remission in first-episode psychosis for prediction of functional outcome at 2 years. Schizophr Bull 36:1001–1008
81. McGlashan TH (2008) Premorbid adjustment, onset types, and prognostic scaling: still informative? Schizophr Bull 34(5):801–805
82. Kendler KS, Lonn SL, Sundquist J et al (2015) Smoking and schizophrenia in population cohorts of Swedish women and men: a prospective correlative control study. Am J Psychiatry 172(11):1092–1100
83. Abdel-Baki A, Ouellet-Plamondon C, Salvat E et al (2017) Symptomatic and functional outcomes of substance use disorder persistence 2 years after admission to a first-episode psychosis program. Psychiatry Res 247:113–119
84. Khokhar JY, Dwiel LL, Henricks AM et al (2018) The link between schizophrenia and substance use disorder: a unifying hypothesis. Schizophr Res 194:78–85
85. Diaz-Caneja CM, Pina-Camacho L, Rodriguez-Quiroga A et al (2015) Predictors of outcome in early-onset psychosis: a systematic review. NPJ Schizophr 1:14005
86. Doyle R, Turner N, Fanning F et al (2014) First-episode psychosis and disengagement from treatment: a systematic review. Psychiatr Serv 65:603–611
87. Mascayano F, van der Ven E, Martinez-Ales G et al (2021) Disengagement from early intervention services for psychosis: a systematic review. Psychiatr Serv 72:49
88. Poletti M, Preti A, Raballo A (2022) Mind the (transition) gap: youth mental health-oriented early intervention services to overcome the child-adolescent vs. adult hiatus. Front Psych 13:965467
89. Pelizza L, Leuci E, Quattrone E et al (2023) Rates and predictors of service disengagement in adolescents with first episode psychosis: results from the 2-year follow-up of the Pr-EP program. Eur Child Adolesc Psychiatry 33:2217. https://doi.org/10.1007/s00787-023-02306-5
90. National Institute for Health and Care Excellence (NICE) (2013) Psychosis and schizophrenia in children and young people: recognition and management. NICE, London
91. Remington G, Kapur S, Zipursky RB (1998) Pharmacotherapy of first-episode schizophrenia. Br J Psychiatry Suppl 172(33):66–70
92. Abdel-Baki A, Ouellet-Plamondon C, Malla A (2012) Pharmacotherapy challenges in patients with first-episode psychosis. J Affect Disord 138(Supplement):S3–S14
93. Lieberman JA, Koreen AR, Chakos M et al (1996) Factors influencing treatment response and outcome of firstepisode schizophrenia: implications for

understanding the pathophysiology of schizophrenia. J Clin Psychiatry 57(suppl 9):5–9
94. Agid O, Arenovich T, Sajeev G et al (2011) An algorithm-based approach to first-episode schizophrenia: response rates over 3 prospective antipsychotic trials with a retrospective data analysis. J Clin Psychiatry 72(11):1439–1444
95. Keating D, McWilliams S, Schneider I et al (2017) Pharmacological guidelines for schizophrenia: a systematic review and comparison of recommendations for the first episode. BMJ Open 7:e013881
96. Lehman AF, Lieberman JA, Dixon LB et al (2004) American Psychiatric Association; steering committee on practice guidelines. Practice guideline for the treatment of patients with schizophrenia, second edition. Am J Psychiatry 161(suppl 2):1–56
97. Fankhauser MP (2013) Drug interactions with tobacco smoke: implications for patient care. Curr Psychiatr Ther 12(1):12–16
98. Robinson DG, Schooler NR, John M et al (2015) Prescription practices in the treatment of first-episode schizophrenia spectrum disorders: data from the national RAISE-ETP study. Am J Psychiatry 172(3):237–248
99. Fisher MD, Reilly K, Isenberg K et al (2014) Antipsychotic patterns of use in patients with schizophrenia: polypharmacy versus monotherapy. BMC Psychiatry 14(1):341
100. Barnes TR, Paton C (2011) Antipsychotic polypharmacy in schizophrenia: benefits and risks. CNS Drugs 2(5):383–399
101. Hasan A, Falkai P, Wobrok T et al (2013) WFSBP task force on treatment guidelines for schizophrenia. World Federation of Societies of biological psychiatry (WFSBP) guidelines for biological treatment of schizophrenia, part 2: update 2012 on the long-term treatment of schizophrenia and management of antipsychotic-induced side effects. World J Biol Psychiatry 14(1):2–44
102. International Early Psychosis Association Writing Group (2005) International clinical practice guidelines for early psychosis. Br J Psychiatry 187(suppl. 48):s120
103. Altamura AC, Aguglia E, Bassi M et al (2012) Rethinking the role of long-acting atypical antipsychotics in the community setting. Int Clin Psychopharmacol 27(6):336–349
104. Nandra KS, Agius M (2012) The difference between typical and atypical antipsychotics: the effects on neurogenesis. Psychiatr Danub 24(Suppl 1):S95–S99
105. Pietrini F, Albert U, Andrea Ballerini A et al (2019) The modern perspective for long-acting injectables antipsychotics in the patient-centered care of schizophrenia. Neuropsychiatr Dis Treat 15:1045–1060
106. Robinson DG, Woerner MG, Alvir JM et al (2002) Predictors of medication discontinuation by patients with first-episode schizophrenia and schizoaffective disorder. Schizophr Res 57(2–3):209–219
107. Morrison A (2013) Cognitive therapy for people experiencing psychosis. In: Read J, Dillon J (eds) Models of madness: psychological, social and biological approaches to psychosis. Routledge/Taylor & Francis Group, London, pp 319–335
108. Bird V, Premkumar P, Kendall T et al (2010) Early intervention services, cognitive–behavioural therapy and family intervention in early psychosis: systematic review. Br J Psychiatry 97:350–356
109. Hansen HG, Starzer M, Nilsson SF et al (2023) Clinical recovery and long-term Association of Specialized Early Intervention Services vs treatment as usual among individuals with first-episode schizophrenia Spectrum disorder: 20-year follow-up of the OPUS trial. JAMA Psychiatry 80(4):371–379
110. Petersen L, Nordentoft M, Jeppesen P et al (2005b) Improving 1-year outcome in first episode psychosis: OPUS trial. Br J Psychiatry 187(148):98–103
111. Alpi A, Cocchi A, Meneghelli A et al (2008) Lavorare con le famiglie negli esordi psicotici: un intervento strutturato per i caregiver. G Ital Med Lav Ergon 30(3):B62–B70
112. Eack SM, Hogarty GE, Cho RY (2010) Neuroprotective effects of cognitive enhancement therapy against gray matter loss in early schizophrenia: results from a 2-year randomized controlled trial. Arch Gen Psychiatry 67(7):674–682
113. Goulding SM, Chien VH, Compton MT (2010) Prevalence and correlates of school drop-out prior to initial treatment of nonaffective psychosis: further evidence suggesting a need for supported education. Schizophr Res 116:228–233
114. Carmona VR, Gómez-Benito J, Rojo-Rodes JE (2019) Employment support needs of people with schizophrenia: a scoping study. J Occup Rehabil 29(1):1–10
115. Duffy A, Goodday SM, Christiansen H et al (2023) The Well-being of children at familial risk of severe mental illness: an overlooked yet crucial prevention and early intervention opportunity. Nat Ment Health 1:534–541
116. Wiedemann A, Stochl J, Neufeld SAS et al (2022) The impact of the initial COVID-19 outbreak on young adults' mental health: a longitudinal study of risk and resilience factors. Sci Rep 12:16659
117. Torous J, Bucci S, Bell IH et al (2021) The growing field of digital psychiatry: current evidence and the future of apps, social media, chatbots, and virtual reality. World Psychiatry 20:318–335
118. Lewinsohn PM, Rohde P, Seeley JR (1996) Adolescent suicidal ideation and attempts: prevalence, risk factors, and clinical implications. Clin Psychol Sci Pract 3(1):25
119. Dahlsgaard KK, Beck AT, Brown GK (1998) Inadequate response to therapy as a predictor of suicide. Suicide Life Threat Behav 28(2):197–204
120. Bridge JA, Ruch DA, Sheftall AH (2023) Youth suicide during the first year of the COVID-19 pandemic. Pediatrics 151(3):e2022058375
121. Protecting Youth Mental Health (2021) The US surgeon General's advisory. https://www.hhs.gov/sites/

default/files/surgeon-general-youth-mental-health-advisory.pdf
122. Ayer L, Colpe LJ (2023) The key role of schools in youth suicide prevention. J Am Acad Child Adolesc Psychiatry 62(1):19–21
123. Griffin KW, Botvin GJ (2010) Evidence-based interventions for preventing substance use disorders in adolescents. Child Adolesc Psychiatr Clin N Am 19(3):505–526
124. Turner WC, Muck RD, Muck RJ (2004) Co-occurring disorders in the adolescent mental health and substance abuse treatment systems. J Psychoactive Drugs 36(4):455–462
125. Tomlinson KL, Brown SA, Abrantes A (2004) Psychiatric comorbidity and substance use treatment outcomes of adolescents. Psychol Addict Behav 18(2):160–169
126. Christie GIG, Cheetham A, Lubman DI (2020) Interventions for alcohol and drug use disorders in Young people: 10 key evidence-based approaches to inform service delivery. Curr Addict Rep 7:464–474

7 Gender Inequality and Women Mental Health: Where Do We Stand?

Cinzia Niolu, Emanuela Bianciardi, and Alberto Siracusano

Abstract

According to the World Health Organization (WHO), gender is one of the main determinants of health. Thus, there is an urgent need to understand and eliminate gender disparities in mental health, as gender equality is fundamental in science, medicine, and global health. Gender is a variable that influences several aspects of mental health, including the prevalence of mental disorders, clinical expression, disease course, response to treatment, and help-seeking attitudes. Depression is three times more frequent in women than in men, anxiety and panic disorders are twice as frequent in women than in men, bulimia three times, and anorexia nervosa 13 times. On the other hand, early-onset schizophrenia, substance use disorders, and neurodevelopmental disorders such as autism spectrum disorder and attention-deficit/hyperactivity disorder, are more prevalent in males. Gender differences in the pharmacokinetics and pharmacodynamics of drugs are responsible for their different efficacy and possible side effects. However, women are underrepresented in biomedical clinical studies. Indeed, an individual may respond to stimuli such as drugs based on circulating levels of sex hormones that fluctuate during the female reproductive cycle and are different in men and in people taking hormone treatments.

A neglected problem is paternal and maternal perinatal depression. The perinatal period is an extremely delicate passage in a woman's life. There is clear evidence that one in five women suffer from maternal mental disorders in the perinatal period and that relapses of major depressive disorder and bipolar episodes can frequently occur. It is also important to focus on the emotional well-being of co-parents in the perinatal period as it affects both of them and the mother and baby.

Many screening programs and interventions are developing to promote healthy parenting and family bonding, targeting mental health, medication counseling, and reducing neurodevelopmental risk factors in offspring.

Addressing gender inequality and incorporating gender differences into mental health and pharmacology are essential to establishing an effective and safer treatment strategy.

Keywords

Gender medicine · Women mental health · Perinatal depression · LGBTQI+ health · Gender inequality · Social determinants of health

C. Niolu · E. Bianciardi (✉) · A. Siracusano
Department of Systems Medicine, University of Rome Tor Vergata, Rome, Italy
e-mail: niolu@med.uniroma2.it; bianciardi@med.uniroma2.it; siracusano@med.uniroma2.it

A. Fiorillo, S. De Giorgi (eds.), *Social Determinants of Mental Health*, Sustainable Development Goals Series, https://doi.org/10.1007/978-3-031-70165-8_7

7.1 Gender Inequality

According to the World Health Organization (WHO), gender is a major determinant of health and mental illness as it influences "the different control that men and women have over socio-economic determinants of their mental health, their social position, status in society and their susceptibility to exposure to specific mental health risks" [1].

However, there is still little clarity on the definition of the term gender (Table 7.1). Gender refers to the social attributes, circumstances, and relationships associated with being male and female. These characteristics are constructed and learned socially. They are context specific and change with age. Gender determines what is expected, allowed, and appreciated in a woman or a man.

Gender equality is a human right, and it is indispensable to the economic development of the societies. Gender inequalities affect everyone—men, women, gender-non-conforming people—and cause excess mortality and morbidity worldwide.

Gender inequality becomes a health risk due to discriminatory values, norms, beliefs, and practices; different exposures and susceptibility to diseases, disabilities, and injuries; and biases in health systems and health research. At each of these level, inequality impacts health and society. At the social level, women have the socially prescribed role of caregiver and men of breadwinner; women are discriminated against in the workplace and have difficulty accessing top positions; moreover, interpersonal violence is more frequent against women and transgender and non-gender-binary people are also exposed to high risk of violence and minority stress.

There is an urgent need of understanding gender disparities in mental health, as gender equality is critical in science, medicine, and global health.

Decades of research have shown that mental disorders resulted from a combination of stress, environmental, neurobiological, and genetic factors. Therefore, attention to the impacts of social inequalities and gender disparities on mental health is compelling. It has been found that not only hormonal difference makes women more susceptible to common mental disorders, but also social factors such as patriarchal social structure and disadvantaged status of women that are internalized as personality traits. Financial dependence on male members, as well as a lack of support against physical, financial, emotional, and sexual abuse, plays a significant role in making women more vulnerable.

The structure of the brain and the response to stressful life events are different between females and males. For example, community pressure regarding gender-based stereotypical social roles may have a different impact on mental health responses in women and men. In a culture of inequality, women and men may approach competition in the workplace differently.

Table 7.1 Definitions of terms

Gender	Socially constructed norms that impose and determine roles, relationships, and positional power for all people across their lifetime. Gender interacts with sex, the biological and physical characteristics that define women, men, and those with intersex identities [2]
Sex	A person's biological status (chromosomal, hormonal, gonadal, and genital) as male or female. An individual's sex at birth (birth-assigned sex) is usually determined on the basis of genital appearance, with those present usually assuming that other components of sex are consistent with the newborn's genital sex [3]
Transgender	An umbrella term that is used to describe people whose gender is not the same as, or does not sit comfortably with, the sex they were assigned at birth [3]
Gender equality	Refers to the equal rights, responsibilities, and opportunities of women and men and girls and boys. Equality does not mean that women and men will become the same but that women's and men's rights, responsibilities, and opportunities will not depend on whether they are born male or female. The interests, needs, and priorities of both women and men are taken into consideration, recognizing the diversity of different groups of women and men [4]

In the medical field, women doctors are called by their professional title 49% of the time, compared to 72% of men. In a context where men are called by formal and professional titles and women are not, women are perceived as less important. Accordingly, women make less money and are underrepresented in leadership positions in medical schools and hospitals, despite having leadership aspirations similar to those of men [5].

Due to the social stereotype, patients cannot tolerate that a visit with a female doctor can last less than 10 min [6].

At least half of female medical students experienced gender inequality and sexual harassment, which are significantly related to burnout. Disparities are usually perpetrated in front of other colleagues and defined as harmless or well-intentioned by the authors [7].

Gender discrimination leads to low self-esteem and lower productivity. Women have fewer opportunities to access resources, education, and funding and are more often faced with unpaid work, with serious consequences for mental and physical health. On the other hand, although men face fewer barriers to career progression compared to women, they do not have support for fatherhood. Paternity leave use remains low due to poor compensation and cultural expectations [8].

Non-conforming gender is not considered a mental health problem. However, transgender people are more likely to experience mental health problems than the general population. In a large cohort study, adolescents and adults with gender dysphoria reported high rates of anxiety, eating disorders, depression, self-harm, and suicidal ideation [9]. Rates of suicidality and suicide attempts for transgender individuals are reported to range from 30% to 80%, with risk factors including past maltreatment, gender victimization, depression, substance abuse, and younger age. Among adolescents, the highest rate of suicide attempt is among transgender young men, followed by those identifying themselves as neither male nor female [10]. Transgender people experience what is called "minority stress," with negative health consequences. Transgender youth often face discrimination at home and school and drop out, leave home, or are expelled from home; their identity documents are often incongruent with their gender identity; they face discrimination in the workplace that often results in unemployment or underemployment; and they are at risk of economic poverty, especially if they drop out of school, cannot turn to social services, and are discriminated against in the workplace [11]. The U.S. National Transgender Discrimination Survey found that transgender people experience greater hiring discrimination than cisgender people and differential treatment once hired [12].

Transgender people also perceive stigma in health care settings; it has been reported that nearly half of transgender people avoid emergency rooms even in emergencies due to fear of discrimination and previous negative experiences [13]. Stigma and inequality can manifest in the denial of services (e.g., hormone treatments), gender insensitivity with use of incorrect pronouns (e.g., using "he" in reference to transgender woman), comments (for example, telling a transgender man that he is not "a real man"), avoidance of eye contact in the doctor–patient relationship, substandard care, keeping patients waiting for prolonged periods, verbal abuse, or forced cures like be forced to undergo psychiatric examination.

The social determinants of health (SDOH) framework have been used in gender equality studies. The SDOH model studies the conditions under which people are born, raised, worked, lived, and aged, as well as the social policies and social norms. The life course perspective and the SDOH framework were integrated to propose a model of mental illness in which individuals are embedded in gender inequality throughout life and in many domains of life, including family, community, education, workforce, and politics [14].

To measure and understand gender inequality in all these areas, indicators have been developed such as the Gender Inequality Index (GII), the Gender Empowerment Measure (GEM), the Gender Development Index (GDI), and the Global Gender Gap Index (GGGI) [15].

7.2 Gender Differences in Mental Health

According to the World Health Organization (WHO), the principle of equity does not only concern equal access to care, but also its appropriateness in relation to gender. There has been an increased recognition of gender differences in medicine, as demonstrated by the establishment of the "Gender, Women and Health" department (GWH) at the WHO and the inclusion of gender medicine among the objectives of the Equity Act. Women have gender-specific health problems, which concern pregnancy, menopause, genitourinary system, pelvic floor disorders, breast cancer, or uterine carcinoma. Many pathologies that affect both men and women can express themselves with peculiar characteristics and affect women with greater frequency and severity [16].

The National Institute of Health (NIH) indicates the "Women's Top 5 Health Concerns": women die of heart attacks more frequently than men, they are twice as likely to suffer from depression and anxiety, and they suffer more often from disorders of the osteoarticular and urogenital tract [17].

Gender is a variable that affects different aspects of mental health, including prevalence of mental disorders, clinical expression, course of the disease, response to treatment, and help-seeking attitudes [18]. Females and males present different risks of developing neurodegenerative diseases such as Alzheimer's disease, Parkinson's disease, amyotrophic lateral sclerosis, or Huntington's disease. Mental disorders affect women and men differently: the prevalence of depression in women is three times higher than in men, anxiety and panic disorders are twice as frequent in women than in men, bulimia three times, and anorexia nervosa 13 times. On the other hand, the autism spectrum disorders (ASD), the attention-deficit/hyperactivity disorder (ADHD), the early-onset schizophrenia, and substance use disorders are more prevalent in males. Finally, women make more suicide attempts while men have a higher risk of death by suicide [19]. The psychiatric and neurological disorders mentioned above, which present strong gender differences in their incidence, prevalence, symptom presentation, course, and therapeutic approach, have been associated, in different ways, with fetal antecedents, including maternal stress. The mechanisms through which the latter contributes to the development of mental disorder highlight a complex interaction between the maternal environment and its effects on the placenta at crucial moments of neurological development [20].

Maternal stress in the early stages of pregnancy induces sex-dependent epigenetic programming, thus influencing the evolutionary pathways of the child's brain, whether female or male. The various studies highlight the involvement of different mediators [21]. Among these are the mechanisms of inflammation, central and peripheral, through the action of cytokines, in particular interleukin-1 [22]. While social determinants are undoubtedly important, gender differences in brain development in the critical period of early life suggest that much of this differential risk may be caused by differential vulnerability of brain circuits during maturation.

The psychologist Simon Baron-Cohen argues that there are three types of normal human brains: "empathic" (type E), "systematic" (type S), and "balanced" (type B, which is a balance of types E and S). His central hypothesis is that men have an S-type brain, while the female brain is predominantly E-type [23].

Empathy involves the attribution of mental states to others and an appropriate affective response to the other's affective state. Empathic brain results from early neuronal maturation. Systematization is an inductive process that allows us to understand how a system works. By observing a situation repeatedly, the differences in certain variables within the event are quantified determining their correlation with the results. After confirming a reliable association model, the results can be predicted. Systematization arises from late neuronal maturation and has been implicated in the etiology of autism spectrum disorder.

Several neurobiological substrates of gender differences have been highlighted such as synaptogenesis, synaptic activation, increased sensory perceptual threshold, increased cerebral blood flow, and increased glucose metabolism in the central nervous system, which also influence the different sensitivity to pain [24]. The total volume of the brain is greater in men than in women: in women, there is more gray matter and less white matter in percentage. Functional imaging studies have demonstrated gender differences in many neurotransmitter systems, such as serotonin, dopamine, and gamma-aminobutyric acid (GABA) [25]. The innate and adaptive immune response is stronger in women, resulting in greater effectiveness of vaccines. Additionally, there is a difference in the risk of autoimmune diseases and immune-mediated conditions, such as organ rejection. Autoimmune diseases affect women more than men. The prevalence of multiple sclerosis has increased considerably over the past five decades, suggesting a role for gender-specific environmental exposures such as reduced vitamin D levels or increased female adiposity. In addition to differences in genetic architecture, gender differences arise from environmental factors that regulate epigenetic effect through DNA methylation, histone modifications, and RNA silencing. These mechanisms allow for flexible gene expression in response to the environment in a sex-specific manner. Gender differences in epigenetic processes are influenced by endogenous (e.g., hormones and enzymes) and environmental factors related to sociocultural differences such as diet, exercise, cigarette smoking, and environmental toxins.

Gender differences in pharmacokinetics and pharmacodynamics of drugs are responsible for different efficacy and side effects such as sexual dysfunctions [26]. The influences of endogenous and exogenous hormones on the disease and its interactions with other drugs taken by the person further contribute to differences in effectiveness. Women have a 1.5–1.7 times greater risk of developing adverse drug reactions; they are more likely to have chronic diseases and, therefore, take more medications, including hormones. Many drugs, such as antiretrovirals, antiepileptics, and antimicrobials, compromise the effectiveness of hormonal contraceptives, increasing the rate of unplanned pregnancies. In conclusion, understanding gender differences in pharmacology is essential to establish an effective and personalized therapeutic strategy.

7.3 Gender Difference in Preclinical and Clinical Studies

Including sex as a biological variable (SABV) in clinical studies represents an important contribution to improving treatments of mental disorders.

Sex differs from gender, which is a construct related to societal, social, and self-identity issues.

Research refers to the sex to describe genetic, structural, and gonadal differences between individuals. Women/females have XX chromosomes/vagina/ovaries, and men/males have XY chromosomes/penis/testes. Beyond this simple dichotomy, there are many naturally occurring intersex variations in the human population due to the developmental process, which can also alter brain structure and susceptibility to mental disorders. For instance, individuals with Klinefelter's syndrome suffer from hypogonadism and infertility and they have higher risk of developing mental disorder compared to the general population [27].

The literature on the differences in the physiology of males and females, in their response to the disease, with greater susceptibility to adverse drug reactions in women than men, is extensive. In addition, female hormones influence positively and negatively human diseases ranging from multiple sclerosis to cardiovascular disease.

However, women are underrepresented in biomedical studies. Neuroscience research has historically been conducted using males. Before the 1990s, research excluded women of reproductive age for fear of long-term effects on offspring. These fears were in response to side effects resulting from the use of thalidomide in pregnancy, which induced severe deformities in offspring in the 1950s–1960s.

Moreover, preclinical studies with non-human models to develop drugs for conditions, such as mood disorders, that are more common in women produce a significant discrepancy regarding the effectiveness of these treatments when used in women.

In 1992, the Office of Research on Women's Health at the National Institutes of Health (NIH) asked the Institute of Medicine (IOM) to establish the Committee on the Ethical and Legal Issues Relating to the Inclusion of Women in Clinical Studies. The Committee's charge was to: (1) consider the ethical and legal implications of including women, particularly pregnant women and women of childbearing potential, in clinical studies; (2) examine known instances of litigation regarding injuries to research subjects and describe existing legal liabilities and protections; and (3) provide practical advice on these issues for consideration by NIH, institutional review boards (IRBs), and clinical investigators.

The 16 Committee members had various backgrounds: bioethics, law, epidemiology and biostatistics, public health policy, obstetrics and gynecology, clinical research, pharmaceutical development, social and behavioral sciences, and clinical evaluative sciences. Although in 1993 the Food and Drug Administration (FDA) replaced its 1977 guidelines, which prohibited the inclusion of women of childbearing potential in early phases of most clinical drug trials, the IOM Committee issued its final report and recommendations, requiring the inclusion of women in clinical trials [28].

In 2016, following the recall of different drugs due to their adverse effects on women, the NIH mandated to include female person in preclinical studies and researchers to consider sex as a biological variable to obtain funding. Subsequently, many studies have explored whether sex differences exist.

Before the 2016, most preclinical studies investigated the effect of steroid hormones on the brain and behavior without considering sex as a genetic variable. It was found that steroid hormones, as androgens/estrogens, could shape the development of certain brain regions when exposure occurred during a sensitive period. This phenomenon can interact with the effectiveness of mental disorder treatments. Moreover, an individual may respond to stimuli such as drugs based on circulating levels of sex hormones that fluctuate during the female reproductive cycle and are different in men and in people taking hormone treatments. During pregnancy and breastfeeding, a woman's brain changes at macroscopic, microscopic, cellular, and molecular levels and, indeed, the maternal brain was described as an organ with perinatal plasticity [29]. The brain regions involved in the changes associated with peripartum may form "maternal circuits" and serve to prepare the woman for the challenges of motherhood, regulating the onset, maintenance, and maternal behaviors such as nest building, grooming, and protection of the young. These changes make the brain of a pregnant woman different from the brain during breastfeeding and that of a nulliparous woman and affect maternal mental health, the mother–child relationship, and, therefore, the development of the offspring. Stress during the perinatal period affects peripartum-associated brain plasticity, potentially contributing to physiological and psychological pathologies such as perinatal depression. Moreover, this evidence suggests the crucial role of hormones and glucocorticoids in the development of mental disorders in women. However, little is known about the role of biological sex and gender in psychopathology and how these differences determine incidence rates, symptom manifestation, or responses to treatment in lesbian, gay, bisexual, transgender, queer (or questioning) and intersex (LGBTQI+) people. Data on gender differences in mental health comes from studies that have not considered gender as a spectrum but have selectively focused on the male/female sexual binary, despite a large population of transgender and gender non-conforming individuals.

7.4 Perinatal Mental Health

The perinatal period begins at the time of conception, includes pregnancy and the postpartum phase, and lasts up to a year after giving birth. The perinatal period is an extremely delicate transition in women' life who face biological, neuroendocrine, psychological, social, and physical changes toward a unique and irreversible experience: the motherhood.

The term perinatal emphasizes the need to consider both maternal and child health in the context of a dyadic relationship, at a time when the risk for the mother of the onset or recurrence of mood disorders is high and begins the neurological development of the child. All these factors weigh on the development of the mother–child attachment relationship and the health of the unborn child.

Perinatal mental disorders are the commonest complication of childbearing and are associated with considerable cost in terms of maternal and childhood morbidity and mortality. In addition, there is a high-cost burden, estimated in the United Kingdom of 8.1 billion pounds. The 72% of this economic burden is attributable to subsequent childhood morbidity [30].

Pregnancy has long been considered a blessed time, when the mother-to-be is concentrated on her own well-being and on that of the child, without mental disorders. However, there is strong evidence that one in five women suffer from maternal mental health disorder in the perinatal period and the relapse of major depressive disorder and bipolar episodes may occur [31, 32], if therapy is interrupted and adequate management and treatment are not provided.

A "perinatal depression treatment cascade" was described; accordingly, less than 50% of women with perinatal depression are recognized, less than 15% are treated, less than 10% receive appropriate treatment, and less than 5% achieve clinical remission [33]. Somatic symptoms such as tiredness and fatigue, insomnia, and tearfulness may be attributed to hormonal changes during pregnancy and interfere with the detection of prenatal depression. Women with a history of sexual abuse present more somatic depressive symptoms during the prepartum period, and often develop fear of childbirth and tokophobia. Furthermore, maternal history of trauma, posttraumatic stress disorder, borderline personality disorder, and depression often overlap, confounding the diagnosis and hindering recognition of depression [34, 35]. This leaves even more women undiagnosed and untreated.

Pregnancy is a time during which physiological and psychological preparation for motherhood takes place. Daniel N. Stern described this change as the "maternal constellation," the change of psychic life in the representations of oneself as a daughter, a woman, a partner, and now a mother, meaning a process that is gradually structured over the 9 months of pregnancy thanks to the transformation of the body, fantasies, desires, and dreams and which integrates with the experience of the birth and growth of a child [36]. For some women, it is a difficult time as women feel unable to care for their newborn. Prenatal depression affects pregnant women, is also followed by postnatal depression in 50% of cases, and has negative effects on offspring.

The risk of prenatal depression is greatest when other environmental factors such as low socioeconomic status are added. The strongest risk factors are the woman's familiarity with depression, young age, poor social support, the quality of the relationship with the partner, and, above all, recent stressful events, childhood trauma, and domestic violence [37]. In particular, the risk of depression increases up to four times in cases of violence during pregnancy. The role of other vulnerability factors, such as attachment style and the relationship with one's parents, has recently been demonstrated, finding differences with respect to the onset of depression during pregnancy or postnatally [38, 39].

A neglected problem is the paternal perinatal depression that affected the 10% of the new father. Paternal depression is associated with an increased risk of developmental and behavioral problems in offspring [40]. Focusing on the emotional well-being of fathers in the perinatal period is important, as well as for their co-parents and children. Programs that recommend screening for maternal perinatal mental disorders should include investigations into the father's psychological state and, if his illness is recognized, it should be discussed and followed up with support and intervention if necessary.

High rates of anxiety symptoms reported in pregnant women suggested that anxiety is more prevalent than depression. A form of anxiety that has not received clinical attention is pregnancy-specific anxiety, the condition characterized by worries, concerns, and fears about pregnancy, childbirth, the health of the infant, and future parenting. This is considered to be distinct from generalized anxiety, as it occurs specifically during pregnancy and the anxiety thoughts are related to pregnancy-specific issues [41].

Epidemiology data showed that up to 20% of women suffer from anxiety disorder, 20% suffer from a specific phobia, panic disorder has a prevalence of 20%, and between 2 and 9% of women are affected by obsessive-compulsive disorder [42]. Moreover, it was documented that 65% of new parents reported experiencing intrusive thoughts, although for many these were fleeting and did not affect functioning [43].

People with non-conforming gender can and do become pregnant, but there are limited data regarding mental health outcomes. Prenatal care access barriers, minority stress and stigma, and prior or ongoing use of hormone may influence the risk of perinatal disorder. Gender-affirming hormone therapy significantly affects reproduction. In transgender women, estrogen suppresses gonadotropin levels resulting in reduction of testosterone, and low testosterone levels reduce the number and motility of spermatozoa. In transgender males, therapy with testosterone suppresses ovulation and causes amenorrhea, but the effects of testosterone on ovarian function can also be reversible with discontinuation of therapy. Nonetheless, a review showed that few patients (3–5%) choose to preserve fertility [44]. As in cisgender families, disorders related to peripartum period and parenting appear in homosexual families and those with non-binary parents. Feelings of anger over the discrimination suffered during parenting and the fear of losing the support of the community are highlighted because pregnancy can be interpreted as the desire to conform to the cisgender lifestyle, the guilt of growing up a child with a stigma, and, in the case of adoptions, adding one trauma to another [45].

7.5 Recommendations for the Field of Gender Mental Health

The recommendations made by the United States Preventive Services Task Force (USPSTF) stated that pregnant or postpartum women who are at increased risk for depression—based on subthreshold symptoms, history of depression, or socioeconomic and demographic factors including recent intimate partner violence or other negative life events—would benefit from counseling cognitive behavioral therapy (CBT) or interpersonal psychotherapy adapted for this purpose with grade B of evidence [46].

There is also increasing evidence on the depression prevention effects of parental interventions in the perinatal period. These are developed to promote healthy parenting and family bonding, targeting depressive symptoms, substance use counseling, and treatment and screening for risks to the development of a child.

Moreover, there are some characteristics of the maternity care context that should be considered, shifting the general focus to health rather than illness—the need to differentiate between peripartum-related manifestations and mental disorders. Including psychological well-being in maternal care is a mandatory approach for screening the prevention and interventions that we offer to women and, furthermore, can help address the associated stigma with the diagnosis of perinatal depression accentuating the barriers to treatment [47].

Finally, there is strong evidence that pre- and perinatal factors are major contributors to offspring mental health in adulthood [48].

Several strategies designed to support parents' mental health are effective and relevant in preventing negative mental health outcomes for their children. However, attention to pregnancy may not be early enough to prevent the intergenerational transmission of mental disorders (Fig. 7.1). Emerging evidence suggests that poor mental health in the preconception period may be associated with poor mother–infant bonding, an indicator of future mental health problems. These data underline the importance of preserving the

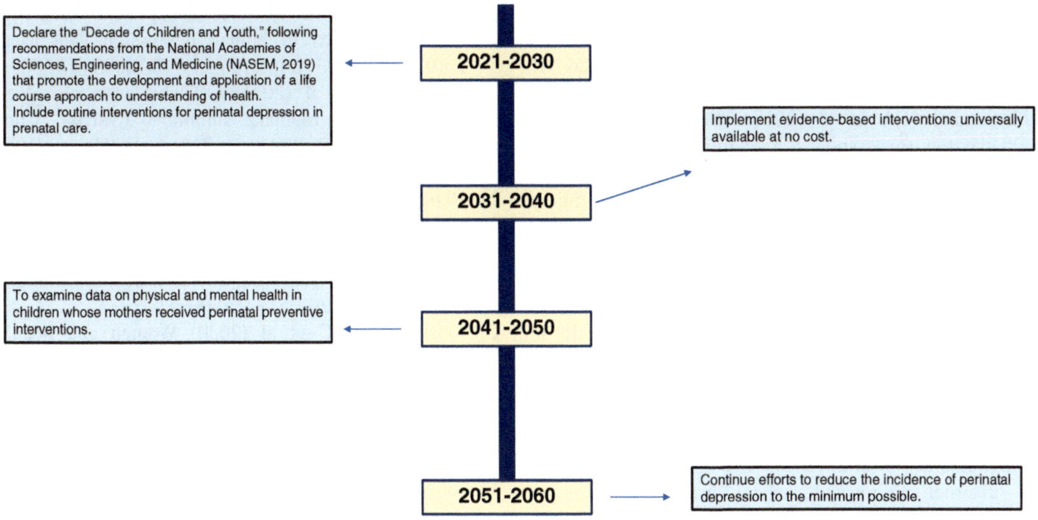

Fig. 7.1 The next 40 years of women mental health. (Adapted from the *Archives of Women's Mental Health journal*; [50])

mother–child relationship, promoting education on gender differences, and addressing gender inequality through interventions starting from childhood and adolescence.

Accordingly, the effects of gender inequality are proximally mediated through disempowerment of women and increased risk of intimate partner violence, which can be addressed through implementing laws that enshrine equality for women, such as in the workplace, and a range of strategies to prevent gender-based violence [49].

The WHO has published a series of comprehensive reports about mental health and has made a significant effort to collect the data that has permitted an exploration of the gender disparities in mental health. Furthermore, there is the need to be more inclusive of trans- and intersex individuals; further research is necessary to determine the functional role of sex differences and how they occur. We need to study women's specific conditions, including the impact of hormonal birth control across the lifespan, pregnancy, and menopause.

References

1. World Health Organization (2001) Mental health: a call for action by World Health Ministers. WHO, Geneva
2. Hawkes S, Buse K (2020) The politics of gender and global health. In: McInnes C, Lee K, Youde J (eds) The Oxford handbook of global health politics. Oxford University Press, Oxford. https://doi.org/10.1093/oxfordhb/9780190456818.013.4
3. Winter S et al (2016) Transgender people: health at the margins of society. Lancet 388(10042):390–400. https://doi.org/10.1016/S0140-6736(16)00683-8
4. United Nations (2002) Gender mainstreaming an overview. https://www.un.org/womenwatch/osagi/pdf/e65237.pdf
5. Rabinowitz LG (2018) Recognizing blind spots—a remedy for gender bias in medicine? N Engl J Med 378:2253–2255
6. Signani F (2017) How gender affects the relationship between physician and patient. Ital J Gender Spec Med 3(4):160–161. https://doi.org/10.1723/2924.29399
7. Kaye EC (2021) Misogyny in medicine. N Engl J Med 384(24):2265–2267. https://doi.org/10.1056/nejmp2104228
8. Shannon G et al (2019) Gender equality in science, medicine, and global health: where are we at and why does it matter? Lancet 393(10171):560–569. https://doi.org/10.1016/S0140-6736(18)33135-0
9. Wiepjes CM et al (2020) Trends in suicide death risk in transgender people: results from the Amsterdam cohort of gender dysphoria study (1972–2017). Acta Psychiatr Scand 141(6):486–491. https://doi.org/10.1111/acps.13164
10. Meyer IH et al (2021) Minority stress, distress, and suicide attempts in three cohorts of sexual minority adults: a U.S. probability sample. PLoS One 16:e0246827. https://doi.org/10.1371/journal.pone.0246827
11. Cruz TM (2014) Assessing access to care for transgender and gender nonconforming people: a consideration of diversity in combating discrimination. Soc Sci Med 110:65–73. https://doi.org/10.1016/j.socscimed.2014.03.032

12. Davidson S (2016) Gender inequality: nonbinary transgender people in the workplace. Cogent Soc Sci 2(1):1236511. https://doi.org/10.1080/23311886.2016.1236511
13. Samuels EA et al (2018) "Sometimes you feel like the freak show": a qualitative assessment of emergency care experiences among transgender and gender-nonconforming patients. Ann Emerg Med 71(2):170–182.e1. https://doi.org/10.1016/j.annemergmed.2017.05.002
14. Siracusano A, Ribolsi M (2018) La povertà vitale Disuguaglianza e salute mentale. Il Pensier, Rome
15. Milner A et al (2021) Gender equality and health in high-income countries: a systematic review of within-country indicators of gender equality in relation to health outcomes. Womens Health Rep 2(1):113–123. https://doi.org/10.1089/whr.2020.0114
16. Chimenti MS et al (2021) The burden of depressive disorders in musculoskeletal diseases: is there an association between mood and inflammation? Ann Gen Psychiatry 20:1–13. https://doi.org/10.1186/s12991-020-00322-2
17. Niolu C et al (2016) Insecure attachment style predicts low bone mineral density in postmenopausal women. A pilot study. Riv Psichiatr 51(4):143. https://doi.org/10.1708/2342.25118
18. Niolu C et al (2015) Predictors of poor adherence to treatment in inpatients with bipolar and psychotic spectrum disorders. Riv Psichiatr 50(6):285. https://doi.org/10.1708/2098.22686
19. GBD 2019 Mental Disorders Collaborators (2022) Global, regional, and national burden of 12 mental disorders in 204 countries and territories, 1990–2019: a systematic analysis for the global burden of disease study 2019. Lancet Psychiatry 9(2):137–150. https://doi.org/10.1016/S2215-0366(21)00395-3
20. Howerton CL et al (2013) O-GlcNAc transferase (OGT) as a placental biomarker of maternal stress and reprogramming of CNS gene transcription in development. Proc Natl Acad Sci U S A 110(13):5169–5174. https://doi.org/10.1073/pnas.1300065110
21. Bianciardi E et al (2023) The mother-baby bond: role of past and current relationships. Children 10:421
22. Viviani B et al (2014) Early maternal deprivation immunologically primes hippocampal synapses by redistributing interleukin-1 receptor type I in a sex dependent manner. Brain Behav Immun 35:135–143. https://doi.org/10.1016/j.bbi.2013.09.008
23. Baron-Cohen Simon S (2010) Empathizing, systemizing, and the extreme male brain theory of autism. Prog Brain Res 186(C):167–175. https://doi.org/10.1016/B978-0-444-53630-3.00011-7
24. Catanese MC, Vandenberg LN (2019) Low doses of 17α-ethinyl estradiol alter the maternal brain and induce stereotypies in CD-1 mice exposed during pregnancy and lactation. Reprod Toxicol 73:20–29. https://doi.org/10.1016/j.reprotox.2017.07.007
25. Labonté B et al (2017) Sex-specific transcriptional signatures in human depression. Nat Med 23(9):1102–1111. https://doi.org/10.1038/nm.4386
26. Jannini TB et al (2021) Off-label uses of selective serotonin reuptake inhibitors (SSRIs). Curr Neuropharmacol 20(4):693–712. https://doi.org/10.2174/1570159x19666210517150418
27. Bianciardi E, Orsaria P et al (2020a) Laparoscopic sleeve gastrectomy for morbid obesity and Klinefelter syndrome: clinical report on two patients, with long-term follow-up. Eat Weight Disord 26:1685. https://doi.org/10.1007/s40519-020-00951-2
28. Mastroianni AC et al (2020) Women and health research: a report from the institute of medicine. Kennedy Inst Ethics J 4(1):55–62
29. Hillerer KM et al (2014) The maternal brain: an organ with peripartal plasticity. Neural Plast 2014:574159. https://doi.org/10.1155/2014/574159
30. Harrison SE et al (2021) Prevalence and factors associated with postpartum posttraumatic stress in a population-based maternity survey in England. J Affect Disord 279:749–756. https://doi.org/10.1016/j.jad.2020.11.102
31. Meltzer-Brody S et al (2018) Postpartum psychiatric disorders. Nat Rev Dis Primers 4:18022. https://doi.org/10.1038/nrdp.2018.22
32. Wesseloo R et al (2016) Risk of postpartum relapse in bipolar disorder and postpartum psychosis: a systematic review and meta-analysis. Am J Psychiatry 173(2):117–127. https://doi.org/10.1176/appi.ajp.2015.15010124
33. Cox EQ et al (2016) The perinatal depression treatment cascade: baby steps toward improving outcomes. J Clin Psychiatry 77:1189. https://doi.org/10.4088/JCP.15r10174
34. Putnam K et al (2015) Heterogeneity of postpartum depression: a latent class analysis. Lancet Psychiatry 2:59. https://doi.org/10.1016/S2215-0366(14)00055-8
35. Robertson-Blackmore E et al (2013) Antecedent trauma exposure and risk of depression in the perinatal period. J Clin Psychiatry 74:e942. https://doi.org/10.4088/JCP.13m08364
36. Stern DN (1995) The motherhood constellation. A unified view of parent-infant psychotherapy. Routledge, New York
37. Bianciardi E et al (2021) Inflammatory markers of perinatal depression in women with and without history of trauma. Riv Psichiatr 56(5):237–245. https://doi.org/10.1708/3681.36671
38. Bianciardi E, Vito C et al (2020b) The anxious aspects of insecure attachment styles are associated with depression either in pregnancy or in the postpartum period. Ann Gen Psychiatry 19:51. https://doi.org/10.1186/s12991-020-00301-7
39. Terrone G et al (2023) Psychological characteristics of women with perinatal depression who require

psychiatric support during pregnancy or postpartum: a cross-sectional study. Int J Environ Res Public Health 20(8):5508. https://doi.org/10.3390/ijerph20085508
40. Gentile S, Fusco ML (2017) Untreated perinatal paternal depression: effects on offspring. Psychiatry Res 252:325–332. https://doi.org/10.1016/j.psychres.2017.02.064
41. Chandra PS, Nanjundaswamy MH (2020) Pregnancy specific anxiety: an under-recognized problem. World Psychiatry 19(3):336–337. https://doi.org/10.1002/wps.20781
42. Fairbrother N et al (2016) Perinatal anxiety disorder prevalence and incidence. J Affect Disord 200:148–155. https://doi.org/10.1016/j.jad.2015.12.082
43. Hudepohl N, Maclean JV, Osborne LM (2023) Perinatal obsessive–compulsive disorder: epidemiology, phenomenology, etiology, and treatment. Curr Psychiatry Rep 24(4):229–237. https://doi.org/10.1007/s11920-022-01333-4
44. Cartaya J, Lopez X (2018) Gender dysphoria in youth: a review of recent literature. Curr Opin Endocrinol Diabetes Obes 25(1):44–48. https://doi.org/10.1097/MED.0000000000000378
45. Lingiardi V, Nardelli N, Drescher J (2015) New Italian lesbian, gay and bisexual psychotherapy guidelines: a review. Int Rev Psychiatry 27(5):405–415. https://doi.org/10.3109/09540261.2015.1064875
46. Munoz RF (2019) Prevent depression in pregnancy to boost all mental health. Nature 574(7780):631–633
47. Alderdice F (2020) Supporting psychological well-being around the time of birth: what can we learn from maternity care? World Psychiatry 19(3):332–333. https://doi.org/10.1002/wps.20778
48. Mawson ER, Morris BJ (2023) A consideration of the increased risk of schizophrenia due to prenatal maternal stress, and the possible role of microglia. Prog Neuropsychopharmacol Biol Psychiatry 125(April):110773. https://doi.org/10.1016/j.pnpbp.2023.110773
49. Patel V et al (2023) Transforming mental health systems globally: principles and policy recommendations. Lancet 402(10402):656–666. https://doi.org/10.1016/S0140-6736(23)00918-2
50. Muñoz RF et al (2021) Leading the charge toward a world without depression: perinatal depression can be prevented. Arch Womens Ment Health 24(5):807–815. https://doi.org/10.1007/s00737-021-01160-1

Violence and Mental Health

8

Brunella Lagrotteria, Giovanna Paoletti, Corrado Villella, Alessia D'Andrea, Enrico Pompili, and Giuseppe Nicolò

Abstract

People diagnosed with psychiatric disorders are more likely to be both victims and perpetrators of violent conducts (Sariaslan et al., JAMA Psychiatry 77:359–367, 2020). Several studies (Witt et al., PLoS One 8(2):e55942, 2013) have found the correlation between different risk factors and violent behavior: history of violent victimization, male gender, low socioeconomic status, history of physical or sexual abuse in childhood, parents with criminal behavior and alcohol abuse, lack of insight, diagnosis of antisocial personality disorder and Cluster B, manic episodes, positive symptoms, history of substance abuse, and nonadherence to psychological and pharmacological treatments. People diagnosed with schizophrenia, bipolar disorder, depressive disorder, attention-deficit hyperactivity disorder (ADHD), antisocial personality disorder, substance use disorders and psychopathy are more likely to engage in violent behavior. Violent risk assessment in psychiatric patients takes into account a series of co-occurring factors of different nature (clinical, social, environmental) that are also distinguished into static and dynamic risk factors. The evaluation, prevention, and management of violent recidivism, therefore, involve the early identification of personal risk factors, through several assessment tools: BPRS, SCID-5-CV, SCID-5-PD, MMPI-2, PID 5, DERS, TAS-20, BIS-11, AIS, HARM-FV, HCR-20 V3, PCL-R. The prevention of aggression in the early stages involves interventions and techniques used in the immediacy to reduce the emotional reactions that lead to aggression; in the long term, the risk factors resulting from the assessment tools are considered to reduce or eliminate, when possible, the highlighted risk themselves and also psychopathological relapse. In forensic settings, the presence among staff of shared procedures aimed to prevent violent episodes is necessary. Various therapeutic de-escalation techniques are used, in order to manage aggressive behaviors.

B. Lagrotteria · G. Nicolò (✉)
Rome 5 Mental Health and Addiction Department, Third Centre of Cognitive Psychotherapy, LUMSA University of Rome, Rome, Italy
e-mail: brunella.lagrotteria@aslroma5.it; giuseppe.nicolo@aslroma5.it

G. Paoletti · C. Villella · A. D'Andrea · E. Pompili
Rome 5 Mental Health and Addiction Department, Rome, Italy
e-mail: giovanna.paoletti@aslroma5.it; corrado.villella@aslroma5.it; alessia.dandrea@aslroma5.it; enrico.pompili@aslroma5.it

A. Fiorillo, S. De Giorgi (eds.), *Social Determinants of Mental Health*, Sustainable Development Goals Series, https://doi.org/10.1007/978-3-031-70165-8_8

Keywords

Violent behavior · Forensic setting · Risk factors · Violent risk assessment De-escalation techniques

8.1 Introduction

World Health Organization defines violence as "the intentional use of physical force or power, threatened or actual, against oneself, another person, or against a group or community, that either results in or has a high likelihood of resulting in injury, death, psychological harm, maldevelopment, or deprivation." [1].

People diagnosed with a psychiatric disorder are more likely to be both victims or perpetrators of acts of violence. A Swedish population-based study found that persons living with psychiatric disorders were three to four times more likely than their siblings without psychiatric disorders to have been subjected to violence or to have perpetrated violence after the onset of their conditions [2].

8.2 Risk Factors

Witt and collaborators [3] conducted a systematic review and meta-regression analysis on 110 studies in order to clarify the association with protective risk factors for violence.

Violence was strongly associated with a history of being violently victimized, moderately associated with recent homelessness, a history of homelessness and being male. And slightly associated with non-white ethnicity and low socioeconomic status.

Violence was moderately associated with reporting childhood physical or sexual abuse, parental history of criminal involvement, and parental history of alcohol misuse.

It was significantly associated with criminal history, mostly with a history of assault, history of imprisonment, history of conviction for a violent offence, history of arrest for any offence, and of violent behavior.

Violence was strongly associated with lack of insight, and moderately associated with a diagnosis of antisocial personality disorder, with impulsivity and higher general symptoms score. Violence was associated with higher excitement scores and higher positive symptoms scores, while no association was found with negative symptoms, nor with neuropsychological factors.

It was also strongly linked with a history of substance misuse, with recent substance misuse, both from alcohol and for other drugs.

Nonadherence to psychological or pharmacological therapies was also associated with violence risk.

8.2.1 Schizophrenia

In people diagnosed with Schizophrenia, the odds ratio (OR) for the risk of committing homicide versus population controls is 19.5 (95% confidence interval [CI]: 14.7–25.8), even if the absolute lifetime risk is under 3%. [4]: a mediating role is played by comorbid substance misuse, a condition doubling the risk, and gender, with men at higher risk than women, as the results from a large Swedish study [5] show 11% of men and 3% of women had a 5-year incidence of violent conviction after fist diagnosis. Around 40% of individuals living with psychotic disorders who commit homicide do so during the first episode before treatment initiation [6].

8.2.2 Bipolar Disorder

Increased odds ratios for violence in people living with bipolar disorder vary between 2.2 and 8.9 across different studies, with a pooled OR of 4.6 (CI: 3.9–5.4) [7]. Absolute rates of violent crime are estimated at 8% in men and 2% in women with bipolar disorder; 701% of these crimes occur in the first 5 years after diagnosis [8]. Absolute risks are lower compared to those run by people living with schizophrenia spectrum disorders, partly because of differences of age and sex distributions associated with these disorders.

8.2.3 Depressive Disorders

People living with depressive disorders have a three times increased risk for violent offending compared to the general population, with an OR of 3.0 (95% CI: 2.8–3.3). Over a follow-up of 3 years after diagnosis, 3.7% of men and 0.5% of women had violent convictions [9].

8.2.4 ADHD

A meta-analysis of studies focusing on individuals diagnosed with attention-deficit hyperactivity disorder (ADHD) before the age of 18 years noted an increased OR of arrests related to violence of 3.6 (95% CI: 2.3–5.7) compared with controls [10]. Population surveys show that associations between ADHD and violence are moderated by comorbidities with other psychiatric and substance-related disorders [11]. An odds ratio of 2.7 (95% CI: 2.0–3.5) was still present after controlling for socioeconomic factors, substance misuse, and psychiatric comorbidities, as found in a Swedish sibling study [12]. Aldo for this condition, men are at higher risk, with 14.7% of men and 3.6% of women with ADHD convicted for a violent offence in a 4-year follow-up.

The increased risk for violence for people affected by autism spectrum disorder is accounted for by the association with ADHD or conduct disorder [13].

8.2.5 Personality Disorders

Among personality disorders, antisocial personality disorder leads to an increased risk for violence versus the general population, with an OR of 10.4 (95% CI: 7.3–14.0) [14]; however, one of the diagnostic criteria for this condition is the history of aggression and criminality from adolescence.

Alcohol and substance use disorders are the strongest risk factors for violence among other psychiatric conditions, with an odds ratio of 7.4 (95% CI: 4.3–12.7) [15].

Literature also reports as risk factor for violence the presence of psychopathy, criminal versatility (i.e., number and variety of violent crimes), and the interaction between environmental and genetic risk factors [16, 17].

8.3 Assessment

The assessment, prevention, and management of violent recidivism, therefore, require early identification of personal risk factors. In psychiatric–forensic settings, the purpose of assessing the risk of recidivism is multiple: to quantify the violent and antisocial conduct carried out; identify individual risk factors to plan personalized therapeutic-rehabilitative projects, taking in charge of these risk factors in order to reduce and/or eliminate them; to monitor any progress (therapeutic objectives achieved) or the level of severity and risk of violent recidivism, for the evaluation of psychiatric social dangerousness. The nature and variety of violence risk factors compel the clinician to perform a structured evaluation which, therefore, includes tools capable of detecting the current psychopathological conditions and the level of adherence to the treatment of the examined subject (i.e., acute symptoms, presence of hallucinations acoustic–verbal with imperative content, delusions of persecution, Cotardians, Capgrasians, oscillations of the thymic axis in both opposite polarities, the current use of substances of abuse and alcohol) and of specific tools for the risk of violence. It is also important, prior to the evaluation interview, to have as many sources of information as possible on the medical history of the subject being examined (information provided by family members, by mental health services previously in charge, prior assessments, reconstruction of the legal history) to collect a medical history that is as timely and detailed as possible, to overcome the risk of the examined lying or omitting information on life history. Equally important is to take into account any organic conditions that can interfere with mental conditions, such as intoxication conditions [18].

Violence risk assessment of persons living with psychiatric disorders takes into account the scientific evidence in the field of forensic psychiatry, i.e., the risk factors for violent recidivism reported by scientific literature. In fact, violent behavior results from a set of co-occurring factors of different nature (clinical, social, environmental); they are also differentiated into static risk factors (historical and non-modifiable) and dynamic risk factors (modifiable) [19, 20]. Static risk factors include previous criminal conduct, problems with the law, substance use, problems with the law experienced by the father figure and having suffered abuse and/or mistreatment in childhood [20]. Dynamic risk factors include frequent emotions of anger, meeting diagnostic criteria for schizophrenia, meeting diagnostic criteria for personality disorder, use of substances and alcoholism, poor work skills and unemployment, lack of family support, precarious economic conditions, poor education, and housing insecurity [20–25]. The psychiatric diagnoses most associated with the risk of violence are schizophrenia spectrum disorders and bipolar disorder [26], Cluster B personality disorders, and substance use [27, 28].

Below is a brief description of the tools for the evaluation of psychiatric patients at risk of violent conduct which comprehends tools for assessing the subjects' current psychopathological condition, personality and affectivity, and the risk of violence. The usefulness of risk assessment tools is greater if the employed tools meet psychometric validity characteristics and are concise. They have to be time-efficient, administered with consent and practical for risk management planning [29].

8.3.1 BPRS: Brief Psychiatric Rating Scale Version 4.0 ([30]; ad. it. [31])

Scale composed of 24 items that investigate symptomatic aspects. For each scale, definitions of symptoms, interview questions, and an operational definition of severity levels are specified: the scale is very useful for assessing the severity of psychotic disorders and severe depressive disorders. The scale integrates information from different sources, focusing not only on symptoms but also on patient behaviors. It can be repeated over time and allows monitoring of both clinical course and treatment outcomes.

8.3.2 SCID-5-CV: Structured Clinical Interview for DSM 5 Disorders (First et al. [32]; ad. it. [33])

It is used as a guide to investigate the main diagnoses of the DSM 5. The clinician version includes the diagnoses most frequently encountered in clinical contexts (depressive disorders, bipolar disorders, schizophrenia spectrum disorders and other psychotic disorders, substance-related disorders, anxiety disorders, obsessive-compulsive disorder, poststress disorder trauma, attention deficit hyperactivity disorder, and adjustment disorders).

8.3.3 SCID-5-PD: Structured Clinical Interview for DSM 5 Personality Disorders (First et al. [32]; ad it. [34])

The Structured Clinical Interview for DSM-5 Personality Disorders evaluates the 10 personality disorders and personality disorder with other specification.

8.3.4 MMPI-2: Minnesota Multiaxial Personality Inventory [35]

Self-report personality inventory includes 567 True/False items and different groups of scales (validity scales, basic clinical scales, supplementary scales, content scales, PSY-5 scales). In the psychiatric–forensic population, there are elevated scores in the Pd (psychopathic deviation), Pa (paranoia), Sc (schizophrenia), Ma (mania) scales; MAC-R (alcoholism), OH (overcontrolled hostility), APS (potential drug addiction), AAS (admission of drug addiction), Ho (hostility), Biz (bizarre thinking), Ang (anger), Cyn (cynicism), Asp (behaviors antisocial), AGGR (aggression), PSYC (psychoticism), DISC (impaired self-control), NEGE (negative emotionality/neuroticism), and INTR (introversion/low positive emotionality).

8.3.5 PID 5: Personality Inventory for DSM-5 [36]

The inventory measures maladaptive traits in five domains (negative affectivity, detachment, antagonism, disinhibition, and psychoticism). In psychiatric–forensic patients higher scores are observed in the domains that reveal the presence of externalizing factors and, therefore, at risk of violence such as the "Antagonism" dimension (manipulativeness, cunning, grandiosity, attention seeking, insensitivity) and "Disinhibition" (irresponsibility, impulsiveness, distractibility, tendency to take risks, perfectionistic rigidity).

8.3.6 DERS: Difficulties in Emotion Regulation Scale [37]

It measures specific patterns of emotional regulation. Emotional dysregulation is considered predictive of aggressive behavior and a risk factor for recidivism [38–41]. Nonacceptance of emotional responses, difficulty in adopting goal-oriented behaviors, difficulty in impulse control, lack of emotional awareness, limited access to emotional regulation strategies, and lack of emotional clarity ([42]) are the investigated areas.

8.3.7 TAS-20: Toronto Alexithymia Scale [43]

It is used to identify alexithymic subjects who present reduced awareness and emotional management. It detects three representative dimensions of the alexithymia construct: difficulty in identifying feelings, difficulty in communicating feelings to others, and externally oriented thinking. Poor awareness of one's emotions is the basis of emotional dysregulation, which in turn causes maladaptive behavior [44].

8.3.8 BIS-11: Barratt Impulsiveness Scale [45]

It is a self-administered scale used to evaluate impulsivity determined by a lack of control over thoughts and behaviors. It is able to discriminate between impulsive and nonimpulsive subjects, across three dimensions: motor impulsiveness, impulsiveness without planning and attentional impulsiveness.

8.3.9 AIS: Aggressive Incident Scale [46]

It is a scale of clinical and predictive utility for violent acts. It is used to record aggressive and violent actions of psychiatric patients; it is a tool that, therefore, allows the detection, reporting and recording of aggressive and/or violent behaviors, thus giving the possibility of identifying and keep record of clinically relevant information, such as the patients' aggressive behaviors, with a simple shared language within the team. The scale consists of a sheet on which recording the number of aggressive behavior in a month; these actions are then summed up each month with a cumulative data and the graphic representation of the recording of aggressive behavior. The AIS was introduced to meet different purposes: having available documentation of aggressive behavior and violence, improving communication among professionals thanks sharing on-site documentation, monitoring the escalation of aggressive and violent behavior of a particular patient, and then evaluating the path and therapeutic objectives possibly achieved. Furthermore, this scale, both in the assessment and monitoring phases of the therapeutic process, allows the clinician to design and implement effectively individualized therapeutic rehabilitation projects, i.e., personalized on the basis of the outcome of the initial assessment, therefore, considering therapeutic needs. This tool also promotes simple and shared team work communication on the possibility that there is a risk of violent acts. It presents a series of advantages: for example, it is easy to use, consisting of a single-digit scale for recording violent behavior (from 1 to 9), and codes to indicate the type of intervention implemented by the operator. Its user friendliness guarantees that all team members of a team use it with a common and shared language despite the fact that they may have different professional roles. This tool is also easily interpreted, immediate to read and decode, in the sense that by looking at a patient's weekly or monthly statement one immediately has a complete overview of the frequency of violent acts by the same patient. As already mentioned, another advantage is the possibility of assessing and managing the risk of violence during the decision-making process in team meetings. It is, therefore, important that every aggressive behavior is recorded in the scale and not overlooked, so that a trace remains and that every member of the team is informed of it. And again, the detection of aggressive actions is functional to the management of aggressive escalation; in fact, early identification allows the implementation of a series of de-escalation techniques that range from verbal ones to pharmacological tranquilization based on the level of intensity of the act itself, trying to prevent and avoid more violent episodes and protect operators and other patients. Considering the scores of the various AIS over time actually allows a more accurate assessment of the risk of aggression in a subject. As already mentioned, the scale is made up of two parts: one consists of a scale (with a score from 1 to 9) which is indicative of the intensity and, therefore, the severity of the behavior that is recorded (three-column table, in one it is reported the level of intensity, in the second column the type of accident, and in the third column the description of the same). The second part, instead, consists of a letter that corresponds to the way in which the team members intervene during the accident, whether the intervention took place or not, specifying its verbal or physical nature.

8.3.10 HARM-FV: Hamilton Anatomy of Risk Management—Forensic Version [46]

Tool used for the purpose to identify psychiatric patients who are offenders most at risk of violent recidivism, based on the presence of specific characteristics (risk factors). Designed in the hospital psychiatric field, specifically the forensic version of the instrument is used in psychiatric–forensic contexts, administered to psychiatric patients who have committed crimes, most of the time subjected to custodial security measures, in which an objective evaluation plays a fundamental role in the management of the patient himself, particularly in preventing and managing violent acts. It examines the risk of violence through a systematic assessment of six historical risk factors (1. History of violent crime; 2. History of nonviolent crime; 3. Major mental disorder—Psychosis, bipolar disorder; 4. Personality disorder; 5. Use of substances; 6. Cognitive deficits) and 10 dynamic factors (1. Adherence to the rules of the structure; 2. Insight; 3. Mood disorder that arose during hospitalization; 4. Persistent psychotic symptoms; 5. Impulses dyscontrol; 6. Absence/presence of social support; 7. Substance abuse during hospitalization; 8. Nonadherence to pharmacological treatment; 9. Antisocial attitude; 10. Abnormal response to stress). Major historical risk factors are considered the presence of personality disorders (especially antisocial and borderline personality disorders) which increase the risk of violent behavior and/or of legal relevance [47, 48], substance use (both historical and dynamic risk factor). The HARM-FV present risk factors include the AIS scale (Aggressive Incident Scale). The HARM-FV future risk factors part (with a score ranging from 1 to 3) refers to the possible need for professional support (after days and weeks) and the possibility of identifying potential victims considering the need of protection. The HARM-FV, as a medical history (life and illness history) tool for detecting personal risk factors, allows the creation of an individualized treatment plan in respect of personal risk factors emerging from the assessment.

An electronic version of the tool (eHARM) is also available to exploit the functionalities of data analysis to improve the assessment, monitoring, and management of risk in the clinical setting [49].

8.3.11 HCR-20 V3: Assessing Risk for Violence ([50]; ad. it. [51])

The HCR-20 is a semi-structured interview that assesses the risk of violent recidivism and crime in the judicial and forensic–psychiatric population; it is used to evaluate social dangerousness and estimate the risk of criminal recidivism. After the interview, the 20 items grouped into three types of risk factors are compiled: 10 historical factors (H—Historical) which concern the subject's clinical history in the past; 5 clinical factors (C—Clinical) relating to the clinical condition of the subject in the present and 5 future risk factors (R—Risk), therefore, relating the future risk factors to the subject's condition. The use of the tool integrated with clinical judgment allows us to conclude a judgment on the prevention of potential violent behavior. The identification of risk factors and protective factors of violent behavior allows and facilitates the prevention and management of the risk of aggressive relapses. The focus of the instrument is on physical violence, assessed through the analysis of the subject's past and present functioning, and by objectives and plans for the future. In psychiatric–forensic care contexts, it is used as a tool for the assessment, management, and prevention of the risk of violence within a project of care and protection of the psychiatric patient.

The HCR-20 can be used with individuals aged 18 or over; however, it can also be sometimes used with younger people (16 or 17 years old) if they have already been living independently for a period of time; similarly, it may not be useful to administer it to subjects over 18 years of age (19 or 20 years old) if they still live at home or depend on their parents. Generally, it is linked to legal or clinical needs (e.g., making decisions regarding the risk of violence within correctional, psychiatric, civil, forensic settings, for treatment plans that aim to reduce or eliminate such factors for the prevention of violent recidivism). The tool is, therefore, used in clinical and forensic fields to make decisions (e.g., placement, treatment, management of an individual by reducing the risk factors that have emerged). However, there are circumstances in which its application is not useful: for instance, in situations where there is an immediate need to make a decision to face an immediate risk of violence.

Regarding the attribution of scores, these are assigned from 0 (N—factor not present), 1 (P—factor probably present), to 2 (S—factor present); for each factor the level of relevance is indicated with a score from 0 to 2 (from B—low, M—medium, A—high). The scoring can assign a maximum score of 40 for both presence and relevance. The minimum significant score is considered a score equal to or greater than 27. There is also a separate version of the HCR-20 for women, which, however, differentiates the types of risk factors, there are 9 items, allowing the level of relevance for each item.

8.3.12 PCL-R 20: Psychopathy Checklist—Revised [16, 17] (ad. it. [52])

It is a semi-structured interview, considered a gold-standard tool [53] for the assessment of personality traits and behaviors connected to the construct of Psychopathy. This instrument provides both a dimensional and a categorical measures of psychopathic traits, which result from the adoption of a well-defined administration procedure and collateral investigations which involves the consultation of official documentation, the collection of collateral information regarding conduct, relationships with family, etc. The acquisition of this information is carried out prior to administration (due to the possibility that the interviewed subject may lie or omit a series of personal information) and analysis of the interview which investigates interpersonal, affective, and antisocial characteristics. It could be used in different clinical and forensic settings, in different ethnic, cultural and socioeconomic groups, for clinical, forensic and research purposes.

The acquisition of anamnestic and in particular legal information is aimed above all at evaluating and identifying moments in which the patient may not be sincere during the administration of the interview. PCL-R is made up of 20 items, divided into 4 components (1—interpersonal, 2—affective, 3—lifestyle, 4—antisocial) and 2 factors (factor 1—interpersonal/affective, given by the sum of components 1 and 2; and factor 2—social deviance, given by components 3 and 4). Each item is evaluated on a three-point ordinal scale (0, 1, 2); however, the value cannot be attributed to the item only on the basis of its title, but the description of the item itself must be respected for the purposes of attribution of the score (0 corresponds to "item does not apply to the subject; 1 to "partially present"; 2 is representative of the presence of the characteristic described by the item). The PCL-R provides a dimensional score, representative of how much a subject corresponds to the "psychopath prototype." Compared to the clinically significant reference scores, in the first edition of the PCL-R (1991) it was suggested to use a cutoff of 30 to classify an individual as a psychopathic; this cutoff provided excellent diagnostic efficiency: the cutoff of 30 was approximately one standard deviation above the mean for the sample of male criminals and forensic patients. Currently, this cutoff value is maintained [17], although several researchers doubted whether a single cutoff could really be representative of the same level of psychopathy in different populations (criminal, psychiatric, etc.). There are three score ranges indicative of the level of severity: a raw score (T points) between 33 and 40 corresponds to the "very high" level, a score between 25 and 32 is considered "high"; if between 17 and 24, it is considered a "moderate" level; a score between 9 and 16 is "low" and a score between 0 and 8 is considered "very low" [52]. The PCL-R, in addition to producing dimensional measurements, can be used to classify or diagnose patients for research or clinical purposes.

There is also a version for children under 18, the Hare Psychopathy Checklist: Youth Version (PCL-YV, it. ad. [54]).

8.3.13 The Dundrum Toolkit [55]

This instrument aims to guide a structured professional judgment in different stages of forensic psychiatric treatment, starting from pre-admission and ongoing during the whole program. The assessment involves a multiprofessional team and is divided in four sections focusing on security items, triage urgency items, program completion items, and recovery items.

8.4 Risk of Subjection to Violence

According to Sariaslan (cit), persons with psychiatric disorders are at increased risk of being subjected to violence compared to those without these conditions. Both men and women with a psychiatric disorder are more likely to be subjected to violence than their siblings without psychiatric disorders: This outcome was more common among people diagnosed with drug and alcohol use disorders, and remained statistically relevant for bipolar disorders, depression, personality disorders, anxiety disorders, while persons diagnosed with schizophrenia did not show higher risk of being subjected to violence compared to their siblings.

8.5 Prevention and Management of Aggressivity

The prevention of aggression in mental health can be distinguished into a short-term and long-term one; the first involves interventions and techniques used in the "here and now" to lower the levels of emotions that predispose to aggression (e.g., anger); the second considers the risk factors resulting from the assessment tools described to reduce or eliminate, when possible, risk factors for violence and psychopathological relapse; the latter intended as a risk factor for violent relapse. For the purposes of preventing the risk of aggression and for the safety and security of the clinician, it is also good to keep in mind that psychiatric patients at high risk of violent behavior are to be visited preferably in settings in which an entire team is present rather than in outpatient care settings where the clinician may be alone.

Several variables should be taken into consideration for the prevention and/or management of aggressive and violent conduct implying an evaluation at multiple levels: from evidence-based medicine techniques to reduce the risk of an escalation of potentially aggressive behavior, to the assessment of the characteristics of the environments and related specific risks, to the clinical evaluation of the person at risk of engaging in aggressive conduct. Risk prevention and management include the safety of other guests in the facility and the safety of staff.

In residential or outpatient care environments with a higher risk of aggressive behavior, such as emergency/urgent departments, facilities for psychiatric offenders (REMS), the presence of shared among staff procedures for the prevention of violent episodes. They are generally drawn up by the company risk manager.

Among the first steps for the healthcare team exposed to real or potential episodes of violence are debriefing meetings, in which the team itself evaluates the risk related to the individual case, employing both standardized tools and comparisons between the operators themselves; in the debriefing meeting, it is essential to proceed with the clinical evaluation of the person at risk of aggressive conduct and guarantee the safety of other users and staff.

For example, in the case of a patient who has engaged in aggressive behavior and must access a ward, both a preliminary assessment and an adequate intervention plan are necessary. In such cases, to guarantee safety, it would be recommended for the first interventions of the healthcare personnel to be assisted by the public force who usually accompanies the person to the ward following an aggressive action.

Furthermore, to proceed while ensuring maximum safety, it is best to protect other users/guests of the facility in spaces where the potentially aggressive person is not expected to access or in any case in separate spaces from the one destined for entry. It is necessary to keep in mind that a safe intervention is based on top by an adequate number of people involved. It is important that the team also decides which conductor will relate directly to the subject and what to say. Immediately after access, the team will have to observe the person considering different levels of intensity, based on what the situation requires:

- Extraordinary observation (Level 1): involves a slight increase in attention levels during the user's placement in the structure;
- Close surveillance (Level 2): involves checking every 15 minutes;
- Constant monitoring (Level 3): in such cases the constant presence of operators is expected for observation, guaranteeing privacy;
- Intensive control (Level 4): involves the continuous presence of operators and constant and direct observation.

The purpose of preventing violent acts implies considering the possible presence of various **aspects** and **risk factors**, including:

- *Factors that increase the risk of violence* (previous episodes of self- and/or hetero-directed violence; young age; male gender; any criminal record; any use of substances; antisocial personality traits or presence of impulsivity; poor adherence to treatments; belonging to groups prone to violence; vagrancy; direct contact with people with whom one is in conflict, linguistic and cultural diversity).
- *Type of violent action* (consider whether it occurred, potential and/or threatened; description and frequency of the threat, or differentiate whether it is simple, an idea without a plan to act vs. an action, whether it is spontaneous or elicited by triggering factors; evaluate the

type of risk, potential damage and severity of the action; possible presence and expression of feelings of guilt and/or remorse on the part of the person who committed the violence; motivation for the aggressive action; identify potential targets at risk and possible presence of a concrete plan; evaluate the possibilities that the subject has access to harm tools and the probability that harm will occur).
- *Clinical factors and status* (evaluate the psychic functions and the possibility that they act as triggering factors that cause aggressive behavior, e.g., paranoid delusions, hallucinations and disturbances of consciousness; in such cases it is essential to establish a good therapeutic alliance).
- *Possible suicidal risk* (since it is associated with hetero-aggressive behavior, it is important to consider the possible presence in the clinical history of interpersonal violence and/ or exposure to episodes of violence or mistreatment from early age).

In preventing the risk of violence, it is effective to consider the **characteristics of the spaces** and **personnel** that could represent factors potentially precipitating this risk. When assessing **structural characteristics,** it is important to plan an adequate reception space and to take into consideration a series of aspects of the structure itself: the lack of air, the absence of privacy, air conditioning, care for the environment, good visibility of all spaces of the structure, possible overcrowding. Easily accessible alarm systems are necessary in the structure and it is necessary to ensure that there are no blunt or potentially dangerous objects (e.g., large objects) in the space destined to the entry/reception of the subject. In regard to the **characteristics of the staff,** attention should be paid to critical issues such as: lack of clarity or definition of roles within the healthcare team, any unstructured department activities, hyper-involvement of staff members or an overly authoritarian climate, inadequate leadership, lack of training and competence of staff, lack of human, and instrumental resources.

The **management of an aggressive event in the team** includes three types of intervention, namely support for the victim of the aggression and sharing, management of relationships with the aggressor if he is still present in the structure, management of the team dynamics, and verification on the adequacy of the procedures adopted by the leadership. Debriefing meetings and clinical audits are necessary, during which it is important that the feelings elicited by the aggressive actions can be shared and that the incident can be considered as a moment of crisis and a growth opportunity that interests and involves the entire team, rather than the single staff member. It has to be prevented the risk of him having an experience of estrangement from his own work. In such cases, it is important to enhance and take advantage of the sensitivity and relational skills of the individual. During meetings, it is important to maintain a climate of collaboration, avoiding a judgmental attitude and the risk of a climate of revenge toward the aggressor.

During the meeting, the team must carefully evaluate the aggressive episode (evaluate the antecedents, i.e., events brought to the attention of the subject immediately preceding the aggressive response; know the aggressor's motivations and the circumstances surrounding the action; evaluate the content of the state mental and the ability to self-control the aggressive instances). The **evaluation following the aggressive behavior** involves an assessment of the aggressor (symptoms, behavioral strategies—for example, obtaining privileges, relationships with the main support group and imprinting on violent behavior), of the environment (adequacy of spaces, management of free time, the relationship with other users, quality and effectiveness of care), and of the team (leadership skills, communication and relational style, clarity of rules and roles shared by all team members). In particular, the main actions following the attack involve aspects relating to the victim (talking openly about the event, recognizing the impact and one's emotions over time, sense of helplessness and abandonment, blaming, returning to work, possible sense of indignation), the team (sharing what happened, empathic listening and sharing of emotions, support for the victim through a proactive and confident attitude towards the team's ability to manage the event, a nonjudgmental attitude based on support and growth common through the experience, provide support to the victim to process the experience, avoid comparisons and comments), and leadership (plan meetings, audits and debriefings in a structured way, provide individual listening spaces, plan the activities to be carried out in the days following the event, postpone the learning and experience that derives from such episodes to the entire team, examining the procedures together with the entire team, facilitate the victim's return to work, postpone the procedure of a possible administrative investigation is to the benefit of the victim and the entire team).

Furthermore, it is important to differentiate cases in which the origin of aggressive episodes has organic causes (the most common are head trauma, vascular lesions, meningitis, encephalitis, focal processes of the prefrontal cortex, temporal lobe epilepsy, neoplasms, dementia, delirium tremens, intoxication and/or withdrawal from substances of abuse and alcohol, serious metabolic and electrolyte imbalances); the possibility of such distinction is also linked to the place where the intervention is performed (giving the person access to the structure responsible for such diagnostic evaluations in the most immediate and safe way possible).

Regarding the **staff skills** that guarantee the prevention and management of violent acts, it is essential that mental health workers have knowledge of the theoretical bases of the cycle of aggression (in order to apply the most appropriate intervention techniques) and of the physical and behavioral signals that precede aggressive action. The latter include standing up, a red or purple face, high tone and volume of the voice, breathlessness, direct and prolonged eye contact, increased gestures, muscle tension, clenched fists, tense face and jaw muscles, increased agitation and progressive physical rapprochement with the interlocutor.

Staff knowledge and competence regarding the aggression cycle involve **two main aspects to recognize**: *psychomotor activation* (*arousal*) which causes physical, emotional, and psychological changes (activation of the cardiovascular system, central and peripheral nervous system, skeletal muscles, remodulation of communication and problem-solving skills, shift of attentional focus). The other aspect concerns the *cycle of aggression* and the *escalation phase*, that is, considering the five phases:

1. Presence of triggering factors;
2. The escalation phase characterized by the point of no return;
3. The actual crisis phase;
4. The recovery phase in which aggression tends to reduce (although further crises cannot be ruled out);
5. The postcritical depression phase.

8.6 De-Escalation Techniques

The therapeutic de-escalation techniques are aimed at limiting and/or reversing the natural cycle of aggression; however, it is important to take into consideration that, should the subject reach phase 3 (crisis) of the aggression cycle, these interventions will result ineffective. The alternative in such cases is the so-called rapid tranquilization, i.e., psychopharmacological interventions to be considered if the de-escalation techniques have not been successful.

Applying de-escalation techniques effectively requires the operator to have good listening skills, empathic understanding, problem solving, and maintaining calm and assertiveness.

It is useful to set the conversation on calm tones, lower your voice (sometimes it is enough to avoid escalation), speak slowly, appear confident, show calm, guarantee a listening space (even physical), maintain eye contact but avoid it being persistent, appear sincerely interested in finding the solution to the problem by avoiding discussions, and maintain a language that meets the abilities and cultural level of the interlocutor, not asking direct questions. It is useful to use downplaying strategies without trivializing or devaluing the interlocutor; to maximize the effectiveness of de-dramatization techniques and pay attention to the verbal and nonverbal dimensions of communication. The rules and techniques of verbal and nonverbal communication are displayed in Table 8.1.

Table 8.1 Rules and techniques of verbal and nonverbal communication

Verbal communication	Nonverbal communication	Communication techniques
Show up as early as possible	Avoid postures that evoke an attitude of closure or authority	Establish a relationship (ask for the name, do not use diminutives; in some cultures or in the case of elderly people address with "Sir/Madam")
Calm and clear tone of voice, modulating prosody Don't ask direct questions, but open ones Avoid too many references to your personal condition Don't anticipate answers Talk down	Adapt to the level of the interlocutor (sitting or standing); facial expressions consistent with the contents expressed Maintain eye contact, avoiding it being insistent and intimidating	Ask tangible questions to help focus on the problem; in cases where the person is not very agitated, explain the reason for the question For example: "*I would like to have some information so that I can help you better*"
Negotiation; active listening	Maintain a physical distance of at least 1 meter (increasing it 3 times in response to verbal aggression; reduce the distance as the aggressive response decreases) Avoid physical contact Position yourself to the side of the interlocutor (forming a right angle and at a distance of 3 meters) keeping your arms relaxed at your sides and feet slightly apart Be accessible with a calm tone of voice, suitable facial expressions (friendliness, acceptance, etc.), gestures of openness and welcome, and also let the interlocutor establish physical distance based on cultural and personal differences; Then use the so-called SOLER position: – **S** it squarely – **O** pen posture – **L** ean forward – **E**ye contact – **R** elaxation	Use short sentences with clear content (if the other person doesn't understand, simplify the question)
Focus the interlocutor's attention on the social impact of his behavior, but communicating to him that our presence is to help him and not punish or repress him		Finding agreement on something: positive language has a greater effect than negative one, active listening helps to establish a point of agreement in order to consolidate relationships and trust
Identify any trigger with the interlocutor		Speak to the person with respect, paying attention to the words, tone of voice, volume and rhythm of speech, nonverbal communication, using cordial words such as "You're welcome" and "Thank you"
Be willing to change your opinion		Don't improvise statements or descriptions about the person's character Avoid praising excessively so as not to risk not appearing credible (e.g., giving a compliment to someone you have just met, but using small reinforcements in the communication "I *see and appreciate that you are trying to lower your voice*" Use a warm and reassuring tone of voice Don't argue or openly oppose the interlocutor Offer the interlocutor alternative choices

8.6.1 De-Escalation Steps and Techniques

Step 1: Recognize anger. It implies attitudes that result into benefits for those who implement them such as catching others attention, avoiding what is not desired, having control on others and on the situation.

Step 2: Health workers recognize their state of mind. It involves constant awareness of one's own emotions, to prevent them from interfering ineffectively in the situation.

Step 3: Be in control of your emotional state. This is the case in which the operator who interacts with the patient feels angry; the operator must know and use emotion management techniques and ask for help if they are ineffective in the here and now.

Step 4: **Carry out a quick self-assessment** by asking yourself if you can control criticism or the necessity to point out others' mistakes, if you manage not to appear judgmental, if you manage to avoid conflict, if you have the ability at that moment to put yourself in the other person's shoes by trying to understand and take on other people's points of view and needs, if you manage to stay calm and protect other users and colleagues.

Step 5: Recognition of alarm signals by capturing and decoding the interlocutor's behavioral changes. It is useful to let the other person know that you have noticed the behavioral changes by talking about them openly, in order to reduce stress and frustration if the interlocutor does not feel understood.

Below are the main **de-escalation techniques:**

1. **Talk Down:** It consists of progressively decreasing one's tone of voice, which induces the other to lower the tone of their voice, adapting to each other. Lowering your voice can have the effect of reducing anger and aggressive behavior.
2. **Time Out:** It involves removing the person from the situation in which they demonstrate aggressive behavior, in order to be removed from the source of reinforcement/trigger, remaining in a quiet place free of activating stimuli as long as necessary. The purpose of this technique is the interruption of aggressive and/or negative behaviors, facilitating the subject's reflection; the health worker will appear confident, firm, and coherent, taking care not to appear punitive but instead intent on solving the problem. It is important to give the interlocutors confidence in their ability to regain control of their emotions and manage the crisis differently.
3. **Simple Listening:** Make yourself available to listen to the angry person so that you can vent tensions and frustrations.
4. **Active Listening**: It involves empathy, listening skills and the attempt to read the situation from the interlocutor's perspective; it is essential for the conductor to pay attention to his own nonverbal communication; it is important to convey to the interlocutor an actual desire for collaboration rather than resulting in an exchange and a hierarchical relationship (caregiver-patient). Active listening techniques involve five fundamental points:
   I. Introduce yourself, promote communication by greeting, introducing yourself and asking the other person's name;
   II. "I" Statements, using short statements to tell the other what you are seeing and feeling (e.g., "*I notice that you are angry*; *I can hear from your voice that you are angry*; *I am here to help you*," etc..);
   III. Reiterate;
   IV. Reflect;
   V. Reflect, paraphrase, and summarize.
5. **Recognition**: It consists in the attempt to identify the underlying emotions, the words with which the other expresses himself and the comments on the emotions themselves, so that understanding and sharing facilitate the resolution of the emotions.
6. **Tolerate Silence**: It facilitates reflection for the angry person; it is important for the conductor to recognize its usefulness, rather than feeling uncomfortable.
7. **Agree**: Despite the other person's anger, it is possible to find a point on which you agree with the person, sharing it in order to facilitate a constructive interaction.
8. **Apologize**: In case there may have been something unfair or a misunderstanding; sincere apologies are representative of an empathetic and prejudice-free availability.
9. **Invite Criticism**: It urges the angry person to express what made him angry with his interlocutor; initially it could increase anger; however, by reiterating it, it helps the person to vent verbally, reducing the risk of aggressive behavior.
10. **Develop a Plan**: This implies having a plan of effective strategies based on the progress

of the conversation with the angry person, so as not to find yourself unprepared for any worsening of the escalation.

11. **When Everything Is Ineffective**: In the event that de-escalation techniques are ineffective, it is essential to ensure the safety of other users and staff. We proceed with an ultimatum which must in any case be pursued in a coherent and resolute manner, also reporting the possible intervention of the police. It is clear that this strategy must be considered a last resort, especially considering the relational consequences with the person involved, using it only in conditions of extreme necessity and when previous interventions were not effective in reversing the escalation.

8.7 Pharmacological Interventions

Fazel et al. [56] using data from national Swedish registers demonstrated an association between antipsychotic drugs and reductions in the rates of violent crimes in the same people when they were on medication compared with when they were not. Similar findings were recorded for mood stabilizers in people living with bipolar disorder. The addition of antipsychotics to mood stabilizers was more effective than mood stabilizers alone, while the addition of mood stabilizers to antipsychotics had no effect. Furthermore, the use of depot antipsychotics drugs led to a reduction in rates of violence, and this relation is at least as strong as for orally administered antipsychotics. Clozapine was associated with a reduced rate of violent crime, but this decrease was not significant due to the small number of patient who received this drug. However, the American Psychiatric Associations [57] practice guidelines for schizophrenia suggest to prescribe clozapine for patients with schizophrenia considered at risk for aggressive behavior despite other treatments.

National institute for health and clinical excellence (NICE) guidelines for the management of violence and aggression recommend to define a pharmacological treatment strategy including the clarification of target symptoms; the likely timescale for response to medication; the total daily dose of medication, prescribed and administered, including p.r.n. medication; the number of and reason for any missed doses; the therapeutic response; and the emergence of unwanted effects. Further research is needed on pharmacological interventions in forensic psychiatry [58].

8.8 Nonpharmacological Strategies

It is difficult to draw firm conclusions about the effectiveness of nonpharmacological interventions to reduce the risk of violence in forensic psychiatric settings [59].

In an umbrella review by Wolf and colleagues [60] papers have included if used a rigid outcome measure (e.g., police- or hospital-recorded violence or reincarceration) and contained randomized or non-randomized controlled study. Five reviews met our inclusion criteria (n = 8876 patients in total), of which four received a GRADE rating of "low" or "very low". Three randomized trials (n = 636) reported that community-based therapeutic interventions can reduce reincarceration in drug-using offenders with co-occurring mental illnesses.

References

1. World Health Organization (2014) Global status report on violence prevention. World Health Organization, Geneva
2. Sariaslan A, Arseneault L, Larsson H, Lichtenstein P, Fazel S (2020) Risk of subjection to violence and perpetration of violence in persons with psychiatric disorders in Sweden. JAMA Psychiatry 77:359–367
3. Witt K, van Dorn R, Fazel S (2013) Risk factors for violence in psychosis: systematic review and meta-regression analysis of 110 studies. PLoS One 8(2):e55942
4. Fazel S, Langstrom N, Hjern A, Grann M, Lichtenstein P (2009b) Schizophrenia, substance abuse, and violent crime. JAMA 301(19):2016–2023
5. Fazel S, Zetterquist J, Larsson H, Langstrom N, Lichtenstein P (2014b) Antipsychotics, mood stabilizers, and risk of violent crime. Lancet 384:1206–1214

6. Nielsen O, Large M (2010) Rates of homicide during the first episode of psychosis and after treatment: a systematic review and meta-analysis. Schizophr Bull 36:702–712
7. Fazel S, Lichtenstein P, Frisell T, Grann M, Goodwin G, Langstrom N (2010) Bipolar disorder and violent crimes: time at risk reanalysis. Arch Gen Psychiatry 67:1325–1326
8. Webb RT, Lichtenstein P, Larsson H, Geddes JR, Fazel S (2014) Suicide, hospital presenting suicide attempts, and criminality in bipolar disorder: examination of risk for multiple adverse outcomes. J Clin Psychiatry 75:e809–e816
9. Fazel S, Wolf A, Chang Z, Larsson H, Goodwin GM, Lichtenstein P (2015) Depression and violence: a Swedish population study. Lancet Psychiatry 2:224–232
10. Erskine HE, Norman RE, Ferrai AJ et al (2016) Long term outcomes of attention deficit/hyperactivity disorder and conduct disorder: a systematic review and meta-analysis. J Am Acad Child Adolesc Psychiatry 55:841–850
11. Gonzales RA, Kallis C, Coid JW (2013) Adult attention deficit hyperactivity disorder and violence in the population of England: does comorbidity matter? PLoS One 8:e75575
12. Lundstrom S, Forsman M, Lasson H et al (2014) Childhood neurodevelopmental disorders and violent criminality: a sibling control study. J Autism Dev Disord 44:2707–2716
13. Heeramun R, Magnusson C, Gumpert CH et al (2017) Autism and convictions for violent crimes: population-based cohort study in Sweden. J Am Acad Child Adolesc Psychiatry 56:491–497.e2
14. Yu R, Geddes JR, Fazel S (2012) Personality disorders, violence and antisocial behavior: a systematic review and meta-regression analysis. J Personal Disord 26:775–792
15. Fazel S, Smith EN, Chang Z, Geddes JR (2018) Risk factors for interpersonal violence: an umbrella review of meta-analyses. Br J Psychiatry 213:609–614
16. Hare RD (1991) Manual for the Hare psychopathy checklist—revised. Multi-Health Systems, Toronto
17. Hare RD (2003) Hare psychopathy checklist revised (PCL-R). In: Technical manual, 2nd edn. Multi-Health Systems, Toronto, ON
18. Lagrotteria B, Alocci G, D'Andrea A, Paoletti G, Pascale F, Posteraro DE, Villella C, Nicolò G (2023) Valutazione del paziente psichiatrico autore di reato: valutazione clinico-forense, trattamenti personalizzati e "restituzione" all'Autorità Giudiziaria. In: Festa GM (ed) La Valutazione psicologica forense. Giunti Psychometrics, Florence
19. Douglas KS, Skeem JL (2005) Violence risk assessment. Getting specific about being dynamic. Psychol Public Policy Law 11:347–383
20. Ferracuti S (2008) I test mentali in psicologia giuridica forense. Centro Scientifico Editore, Torino
21. Bolanos AD, Mitchell SM, Morgan RD, Grabowski KE (2020) A comparison of criminogenic risk factors and psychiatric symptomatology between psychiatric inpatients with and without criminal justice involvement. Law Hum Behav 44(4):336–346
22. Draine J, Salzer MS, Culhane DP, Hadley TR (2002) Role of social disadvantage in crime, and homelessness among persons with serious mental illness. Psychiatr Serv 53(5):565–573
23. Elbogen EB, Johnson SC (2009) The intricate link between violence and mental disorder: results from the National Epidemiologic Survey on alcohol and related conditions. Arch Gen Psychiatry 66(2):152–161
24. Fazel S, Gulati G, Linsell L et al (2009a) Schizophrenia an violence: systematic review and meta-analysis. PLoS Med 6:e1000120
25. Markowitz FE (2011) Mental illness, crime, and violence: risk, context, and social control. Aggress Violent Behav 16(1):36–44
26. Volavka J (2013) Violence in schizophrenia and bipolar disorder. Psychiatr Danub 25(1):24–33
27. Dellazizzo L, Dugré JR, Berwald M, Stafford MC, Côté G, Potvin S, Dumais A (2018) Distinct pathological profiles of inmates showcasing cluster B personality traits, mental disorders and substance use regarding violent behaviors. Psychiatry Res 260:371–378
28. Howard R, Hasin D, Stohl M (2020) Substance use disorders and criminal justice contact among those with co-occurring antisocial and borderline personality disorders: findings from a nationally representative sample. Pers Ment Health 15:40
29. Chaimowitz G, Mamak M, Moulden H, Furimsky I, Olagunju A (2020) Implementation of risk assessment tools in psychiatric services. J Healthc Risk Manag 40(1):33–43
30. Ventura J et al (1993) Training and quality assurance with the brief psychiatric rating scale "the drift busters". Int J Methods Psychiatr Res 3:221
31. Morosini P, Casacchia M, Ventura J (1995) Brief Psychiatric Rating Scale (BPRS): versione 4.0 ampliata: manuale di istruzioni: [scale, definizioni operative dei livelli di gravità dei sintomi e domande dell'intervista]. Rivista di Riabilitazione Psichiatrica e Psicosociale 1:48–54
32. First MB et al. (2017) SCID-5-CV Starter Kit, Milano, Raffaello Cortina Editore
33. Fossati A, Borroni S (2017a) Intervista Clinica Strutturata per i disturbi del DSM 5. Versione per il Clinico. Raffaello Cortina Editore, Milan
34. Fossati A, Borroni S (2017b) Intervista Clinica Strutturata per i disturbi di Personalità del DSM 5. Raffaello Cortina Editore, Milan
35. Hathaway SR, McKinley JC (1995) MMPI-2. Minnesota multiphasic Inventory-2. Giunti O. S., Firenze
36. American Psychiatric Association APA (2015) The personality inventory for DSM-5 (PID-5), Italian edition. Raffaello Cortina Editore, Milano
37. Gratz KL, Roemer L (2004) Multidimensional assessment of emotion regulation and dysregulation:

development, factor structure, and initial validation of the difficulties in emotion regulation scale. J Psychopathol Behav Assess 26(1):41–54
38. Garofalo C, Holden CJ, Zeigler-Hill V, Velotti P (2016) Understanding the connection between self-esteem and aggression: the mediating role of emotion dysregulation. Aggress Behav 42:3–15
39. Loas G, Baelde O, Verrier A (2015) Relationship between alexithymia and dependent personality disorder: a dimensional analysis. Psychiatry Res 225:484–488
40. Nemiah JC, Sifneos PE (1970) Psychosomatic illness: a problem in communication. Psychitherapy & Psychosomatics 18:154–160
41. Roberton T, Daffern M, Bucks RS (2014) Maladaptive emotion regulation and aggression in adult offenders. Psychol Crime Law 20:933–954
42. Sighinolfi C, Norcini PA, Rocco CL, Marchetti I, Sica C (2010) Difficulties in emotion regulation strategies (DERS). Psicoterapia Cognitiva e Comportamentale 16(2):141–170
43. Bagby RM, Parker JDA, Taylor GJ (1994) The twenty-item Toronto alexithymia scale-I. Item selection and cross validation of the factor structure. J Psychosom Res 38:23–32
44. Jenkins AL, McCloskey MS, Kulper D, Berman ME, Coccaro EF (2014) Self-harm behavior among individuals with intermittent explosive disorder and personality disorders. J Psychiatr Res 60:125–131
45. Barratt ES, Stanford MS (1995) Impulsiveness, in personality characteristics of the personality disordered client. Wiley, New York
46. Chaimowitz G, Mamak M (2011) Companion guide to the aggressive incidents scale and the Hamilton anatomy of risk management. St. Joseph's HealthCare, Hamilton
47. Cooper ML, Wood PK, Orcutt HK, Albino A (2003) Personality and the predisposition to engage in risky or problem behavior during adolescence. J Pers Soc Psychol, 84:390–410.
48. Mauricio AM, Tein JY, Lopez FG (2007) Borderline and Antisocial Personality score sas mediators between attachment and intimate partner violence. Violence and Victims, 22:139–157
49. Mullally K, Mamak M, Chaimowitz GA (2018) La prossima generazione di valutazione e gestione del rischio: presentazione di eHARM. International Journal of Risk and Recovery 1(1):21–26
50. Douglas KS, Hart SD, Webster CD, Belfrage H (2013) HCR-20v3: assessing risk for violence—user guide, mental health, law, and policy institute. Simon Fraser University, Burnaby
51. Caretti V, Scarpa F, Ciappi S, Castelletti L, Catanesi R, Carabellese FF, Ferracuti S, Nava FA, Nicolò G, Paterniti R, Rivellini G, Schimmenti A (2019) HCR-20V3 Checklist per la Valutazione del Rischio di Recidiva di un Crimine Violento. Hogrefe Editore, Firenze
52. Caretti V, Manzi GS, Schimmenti A, Seragusa L (2014) Hare psychopathy checklist—revised (PCL-R), 2nd edn. Giunti O. S, Firenze
53. Edens JF, Skeem JL, Cruise KR, Cauffman E (2001) Assessment of "juvenile psychopathy" and its association with violence: a critical review. Behav Sci Law 19:53–80
54. Sabatello U, Abate L, Spissu L (2012) Hare psychopathy checklist: youth version. Giunti O.S, Firenze
55. Kennedy HG, O'Neill C, Flynn G, Gill P, Davoren M (2016) Dangerousness understanding, recovery and urgency manual (the Dundrum Quartet) V1.0.30. http://www.tara.tcd.ie/bitstream/handle/2262/76545/THE_DUNDRUM_TOOLKIT_DRAFT%20V1%200%2030%2012_05_16.pdf. Accessed 30 May 2016
56. Fazel S, Wolf A, Palm C, Lichtenstein P (2014a) Violent crime, suicide, and premature mortality in patients with schizophrenia and related disorders: a 38 year total population study in Sweden. Lancet Psychiatry 1:44–54
57. American Psychiatric Association (2020) Practice guidelines for the treatment of patient with schizophrenia, 3rd edn. American Psychiatric Association, Washington, DC
58. Reisegger A, Slamanig R, Winkler H et al (2021) Pharmacological interventions to reduce violence in patients with schizophrenia in forensic psychiatry. CNS Spectr:1–11. https://doi.org/10.1017/S1092852921000134
59. Slamaning R, Reisegger A, Winkler H et al (2021) A systematic review of non-pharmacological strategies to reduce the risk of violence in patients with schizophrenia spectrum disorders in forensic psychiatric settings. Front Psychiatry 12:618860
60. Wolf A, Whithing D, Fazel S (2017) Violence prevention in psychiatry: an umbrella review of interventions in general and forensic psychiatry. J Forensic Psychiatry Psychol 28:659–673

New Psychoactive Substances (NPS): A Rising Pandemic in the Mental Health Field?

9

Stefania Chiappini, Clara Cavallotto, Tommaso Piro, Francesco Maria Semeraro, Ilenia Rosa, Francesco Di Carlo, Mauro Pettorruso, and Giovanni Martinotti

Abstract

Known as "designer drugs" or "legal highs," new psychoactive substances (NPS), are a growing concern globally. These substances refer to synthetic or modified compounds designed, including synthetic cannabinoids, synthetic cathinones, synthetic opioids, and other compounds, mimicking the effects of traditional illicit drugs while avoiding legal restrictions. The chemical structures of NPS can change quickly, complicating efforts to understand their effects and risks. Although marketed as safe and legal, the use of NPS poses significant challenges to public health and mental health professionals, being a rising concern related to unknown risks, unpredictable and potentially severe physical and mental health consequences, including anxiety, paranoia, hallucinations, and toxicity-related overdose. Moreover, their easy availability, both online and in physical stores and their global distribution networks, can contribute to increased use. Efforts to address the accessibility of NPS often involve collaboration between law enforcement, regulatory agencies, and public health organizations. Strategies include updating and expanding legislation to cover a broader range of substances, enhancing international cooperation, and increasing public awareness about risks associated with these substances. It is important for health professionals, policymakers, and public to stay informed about the evolving NPS scenario and work together to implement effective prevention, education, and harm reduction measures.

Keywords

New psychoactive substances · Misuse
Addiction · Illicit drug · Abuse

S. Chiappini
UniCamillus International University of Medical Sciences, Rome, Italy

Psychopharmacology, Drug Misuse and Novel Psychoactive Substances Research Unit, School of Life and Medical Sciences, University of Hertfordshire, College Lane Campus, Hatfield, UK

C. Cavallotto · T. Piro · F. M. Semeraro · I. Rosa · F. Di Carlo · M. Pettorruso · G. Martinotti (✉)
G. D'Annunzio University, Chieti, Italy
e-mail: clara.cavallotto@laconchiglia.srl;

9.1 Epidemiology

The term "New Psychoactive Substances" (NPS) refers to psychoactive molecules not regulated by the United Nations Conventions on Narcotic Drugs and Psychotropic Substances issued in 1961 and 1971. However, they may pose a threat to public health comparable to substances included in these conventions [1].

A. Fiorillo, S. De Giorgi (eds.), *Social Determinants of Mental Health*, Sustainable Development Goals Series, https://doi.org/10.1007/978-3-031-70165-8_9

It is impossible to precisely quantify the amount of NPS available in the illicit market, as they are often, by definition, unrecognized by regulatory authorities. However, a measure can be derived from the quantity of identified substances and how they are distributed among the various categories of formulable NPS. In 2021, European Union (EU) member states confiscated a record quantity of 8.5 tons of NPS [2]. According to the European Monitoring Centre for Drugs and Drug Addiction (EMCDDA), from 2010 to 2022, at least 40 NPS have been identified every year and in certain instances, the number has reached as high as 100 NPS; among the various types of NPS, there is a clear prevalence of synthetic cannabinoids and synthetic cathinones [2]. Indeed, the 24 newly identified cannabinoids constitute more than half of the new substances reported for the first time to the EU's Rapid Alert System in 2022 [2]. Specifically, national estimates indicating NPS consumption among young adults (aged between 15 and 35 years) in the last year have ranging rates from 0.1% in Latvia to 5.1% in Romania (excluding gamma hydroxybutyrate/GHB and ketamine). The most recent European survey between 15 and 16 years old school children highlighted that in 2019 the lifetime use of NPS was, on average, 3.5%, while in several countries it exceeded 6%; specifically, the average lifetime consumption of synthetic cannabinoids and synthetic cathinones was, respectively, 3.1% and 1.1% [3]. The internet, encompassing online forums, chat rooms, and blogs, has become a primary information source for drugs in general, with a particular focus on NPS. Approximately 61% of young Europeans aged 15–24 commonly identify the Internet as their go-to platform for drug-related information [4, 5]. Users share their encounters with various substances, offering recommendations on sources and methods of delivery. Aggressive marketing tactics, such as enticing names, vibrant packaging, and free samples, target vulnerable young consumers, heightening the risk of early exposure to these substances [6, 7].

NPS, often lacking regulation, may gain popularity due to the misconception of low associated risks. Regrettably, there is a lack of thorough surveys regarding the spread of NPS. Emerging evidence indicates that the utilization of NPS often occurs unintentionally, coupled with their concurrent use with other substances. Moreover, there is an increasing body of evidence supporting the potentially severe psychiatric and physical consequences linked to the consumption of NPS [8, 9]. Potent and highly rewarding NPS are frequently associated with substance-related exogenous psychosis and will likely challenge and shape substance-related psychopathology for years to come [8].

9.2 Most Important Substances Involved

9.2.1 Synthetic Cathinones

Synthetic cathinones are often sold as "bath salts," due to their similar appearance to white powder or crystals to be added to bath water; actually, they are synthetic derivatives of the stimulant molecule cathinone (also known as benzoylethanamine, or β-keto-amphetamine), which is a monoamine alkaloid found in the shrub *Catha edulis* (khat) and is chemically similar to ephedrine, cathine, methcathinone, and other amphetamines [2]. Synthetic cathinones are sold in clandestine packaging to avoid detection by law enforcement. Methylenedioxypyrovalerone (MDPV) and mephedrone are the most important active compounds (Table 9.1), with effects similar to those of ecstasy. Street slang terms and product names include *drone, bubbles, meow-meow, MCAT, Ivory Wave, Vanilla Sky, Cloud 9, Red Dove, and White Rush.* Use is most prevalent among teens and young adults who wish to avoid drug detection while enjoying what used to be a "legal high." Before the US Drug Enforcement Administration acted to make bath salts illegal in September 2011, these substances were sold at gas stations, head shops (retail drug paraphernalia outlets), and record stores. Users still can purchase the products online. Typically, cathinones are inhaled, ingested orally ("bombed," meaning swallowed after being wrapped in cigarette paper), or injected. They act as inhibitors of the

Table 9.1 Most important clinical characteristics of new psychoactive substances (NPS)

Substance category	Types of substances	Pharmacology	Symptomatic effects and psychopathology	Short- and long-term effects	Intoxication treatment	De-addiction therapy
Synthetic cathinones	Mephedrone, MDPV, alpha-PVP, butylone, methedrone	Psychoactive, affecting dopamine, serotonin, and norepinephrine transporters	Euphoria, increased sociability, paranoia, hallucinations	*Short-term:* agitation, euphoria, hyperthermia, seizures; *Long-term*: cognitive deficits, addiction	Symptomatic treatment, benzodiazepines for seizures, hydration for hyperthermia	Cognitive-behavioral therapy, support groups, pharmacotherapy (antidepressants, mood stabilizers)
Synthetic cannabinoids	K2, spice, JWH-018, CP 47,497, HU-210	Mimic THC, bind to cannabinoid receptors	Anxiety, psychosis, paranoia	*Short-term*: tachycardia, agitation, paranoia; *Long-term*: psychotic symptoms, dependency	Supportive care, benzodiazepines for severe agitation, antipsychotics for psychosis	Psychotherapy, motivational interviewing, contingency management
Piperazine derivatives	BZP, TFMPP, MeOPP, MBZP, pFPP	Serotonin and dopamine receptor agonists	Anxiety, hallucinations, confusion	*Short-term*: agitation, euphoria, hyperthermia, seizures, gastrointestinal distress; *Long-term:* neurotoxicity, psychological issues	Symptomatic treatment for acute toxicity, antipsychotics for severe cases	Psychological counseling, support groups, selective serotonin reuptake inhibitors
Methoxetamine (MXE)	Slang terms: Mexxy, MKET, Roflcopter, Mexi, Minx	NMDA receptor antagonist, similar to ketamine	Dissociative effects, altered perception	*Short-term*: Tachycardia, hypertension; *Long-term*: Bladder toxicity, cognitive impairment	Supportive care, benzodiazepines for agitation, hydration	Psychotherapy, support groups, potential use of NMDA antagonists
New synthetic opioids	Fentanyl analogs, U-47700, Carfentanil, AH-7921, MT-45	Opioid receptor agonists	Euphoria, analgesia, respiratory depression	*Short-term*: nausea, sedation, respiratory depression and coma; *Long-term*: hyperalgesia, opioid dependence	Naloxone for overdose, supportive care for respiratory depression	Opioid substitution therapy (methadone, buprenorphine), counseling, 12-step programs
Designer benzodiazepines	Etizolam, flubromazolam, clonazolam, diclazepam, flualprazolam	GABA-A receptor modulators	Sedation, muscle relaxation, anxiolysis	*Short-term*: drowsiness, ataxia; *Long-term*: cognitive decline, dependence	Tapering protocols with long-acting benzodiazepines, symptomatic care for withdrawal	Psychotherapy, gradual tapering of doses, support groups

BZP benzylpiperazine, *GABA* gamma amino hydroxybutyric acid, *MBZP* methylbenzylpiperazine, *MDPV* 3,4-methylenedioxypyrovalerone, *MeOPP* 4-methoxyphenylpiperazine, *NMDA* N methyl-D-aspartate, *pFPP* p-fluorophenylpiperazine (pFPP), *TFMPP* trifluoromethylphenylpiperazine, *THC* tetrahydrocannabinol, *alpha-PVP* alpha-pyrrolidinovalerophenone serotonin transporter (SERT), noradrenaline transporter (NET), and dopamine transporter (DAT), leading to an elevation in the activity of these neurotransmitters at the synapse [10]. They induce an ecstasy-like empathic and entactogenic effects, along with amphetamine-like energizing and anorectic effects. Nonetheless, these effects are less intense and of shorter duration, with the risk of consumption of a large dose that can lead to delirium, hallucinations, and sympathomimetic effects (e.g., elevated pulse and blood pressure; diaphoresis; agitation; and, with long-term use, psychotic features) [11]. Patients' management includes supportive care. Benzodiazepines are useful for agitation and psychosis. Patients who have used amphetamines such as methylenedioxymethamphetamine (MDMA) may present with serotonergic symptoms, this constitutes a triad characterized by autonomic hyperactivity (tachycardia, diaphoresis, mydriasis, and hyperthermia), changes in mental status, and altered neuromuscular activity (myoclonus, and hyperreflexia, and muscle rigidity) [12]. The consumption of these substances by individuals struggling with severe mental illness can result in heightened aggressiveness, self-destructive behavior, and potentially leading to suicide. Numerous NPS are linked to self-harming behavior, and this association is particularly pronounced in the case of synthetic cathinones, however, the cause-and-effect relationship is not definitively understood [13].

9.2.2 Herbal Marijuana Alternatives and Synthetic Cannabinoids

Herbal marijuana alternatives (HMAs), such as *Spice* and *K2*, have been prominent as substances of abuse since the early 2000s in Europe, and later in the United States. Marketed as incense or potpourri, they are deceptively labeled *not for human consumption*, yet they are widely recognized as legal alternatives to marijuana [2, 14]. Indeed, these HMAs contain synthetic cannabinoids, compounds engineered to mimic tetrahydrocannabinol (THC), the active ingredient in marijuana, yet with a much higher affinity for cannabinoid receptors CB1 and CB2 in the central nervous system (CNS) and peripheral tissues. This elevated affinity contributes to their potent effects, significantly exceeding those of THC.

The cellular signaling of synthetic cannabinoids also differs significantly from that of THC. Indeed, while THC is a weak partial agonist at CB1 and CB2 receptors, synthetic cannabinoids and their metabolites often act as full agonists with high potency and efficacy. This difference in receptor affinity and efficacy contributes to the severe health risks associated with synthetic cannabinoids, including a greater potential for tolerance, dependence, and withdrawal compared to marijuana [15]. Moreover, synthetic cannabinoids may interact with non-cannabinoid systems like the serotonin system, potentially contributing to adverse effects, such as anxiety and psychosis [15]. The clinical effects of synthetic cannabinoids are diverse, often more severe than those observed with natural cannabis. They encompass CNS/psychiatric symptoms such as anxiety, paranoia, agitation, psychosis, and physiological effects like tachycardia, hypertension, and in some cases, severe outcomes like myocardial infarction and renal failure [16–18]. The treatment for synthetic cannabinoid toxicity is mainly supportive, as there is no specific antidote. Benzodiazepines, such as lorazepam or diazepam, are commonly used to manage agitation, anxiety, and convulsions. Supportive care might include cooling measures, hydration, sedation, and in severe cases, intubation. The management strategy is largely dictated by the patient's presenting symptoms and the severity of the toxicity (Table 9.1).

9.2.3 Piperazine Derivatives

Piperazine derivatives have emerged among NPS since the late 2000s, distinguished by their euphoric and stimulant properties [2]. Chemically, piperazine derivatives are broadly categorized into two primary classes: benzylpiperazines and phenylpiperazines. Each class is defined by the central structure of a heterocyclic piperazine ring, which is critical to its pharmacological activity. This piperazine core, bonded at the nitrogen atom to an aryl group, varies among different derivatives, significantly influencing their biological activity and potency. The pharmacodynamics of piperazine derivatives are intricately linked to their interaction with neurotransmitter systems, particularly serotonin (5-HT), dopamine (DA), and norepinephrine (NE). These compounds modulate the extracellular concentrations of these neurotransmitters, either by inhibiting their reuptake or by stimulating presynaptic receptors. This dual mechanism of action results in a spectrum of effects, ranging from stimulant to hallucinogenic, depending on the specific compound and its affinity for different neurotransmitter systems [18]. The pharmacological effects of BZP and its derivatives primarily involve amphetamine-like stimulation, e.g., piperazine blends, especially those combining N-benzylpiperazine (BZP) and 1-(3-trifluoromethylphenyl)piperazine (TFMPP), emulate the effects of MDMA. These compounds are commonly sold as tablets, capsules, or powders on the black drug market, in headshops, or through internet platforms. Blends containing up to four different piperazines are frequently consumed, often mixed with other drugs of abuse such as ecstasy or cocaine [19, 20]. Toxic effects include alertness, agitation, anxiety, psychosis, cardiac symptoms (like tachycardia), and in some cases, seizures and death [21, 22] (Table 9.1).

9.2.4 Methoxetamine

Methoxetamine (MXE) is an analog of ketamine ("special K"), sharing structural similarity with phencyclidine (PCP). MXE use is popular in the United Kingdom but has the potential for wider use via Internet sales (Table 9.1). Little is known about the users or specific patterns of abuse, other than that the drug can be injected intravenously. MXE has two major mechanisms of action, the first as an N-methyl-D-aspartate (NMDA) antagonist and the second as a monoamine reuptake inhibitor, with a strong affinity for the dopamine transporter (DAT) [12].

The clinical experience with MXE is limited to self-reporting and advertising. It was specifically formulated for the illicit market as an alternative to ketamine without urotoxic activity [23]. Users reported abusing the drug for its euphoric, hallucinogenic, and dissociative effects but may experience opioid effects such as respiratory depression, vomiting, diarrhea, anxiety, and paranoia [23]. Classically associated with ketamine, nystagmus may be observed. One case report describes a 19 years old who injected MXE intravenously and later presented with semi-stuporous mental status, agitation, ataxia, hypertension, and tachycardia [24]. Another case report of a 23 years old who injected MXE intravenously reported, several days after the restoration of his medical conditions, the persistence of visual and auditory hallucinosis, as if he was still on MXE "high" [25]. No specific management of MXE intoxication has been described at this time. However, similar management to that for ketamine, PCP, or opioid intoxication should be used. Suggested strategies may include supportive care, intravenous fluid resuscitation, benzodiazepines for agitation, and respiratory support [26].

9.2.5 New Synthetic Opioids

The emergence of new synthetic opioids (NSOs), including a variety of fentanyl derivatives, e.g., acetylfentanyl, acryloylfentanyl, alpha-methylfentanyl, butyrylfentanyl, and carfentanil, has become a prominent concern in the drug market worldwide [2, 27]. The clinical presentation and management of NSOs present a complex and concerning picture in the realm of substance abuse and overdose. They exert profound effects on the CNS, ranging from euphoria and analgesia to severe respiratory depression, coma, and death. Even non-fatal overdoses can result in debilitating outcomes, including seizures, motor paralysis, coma, and stroke to more chronic and progressive impairments like mental disorientation, amnestic syndromes, ataxia, gait disturbances, paraplegia, catatonia, and diminished motor and cognitive functions or psychosis secondary to hypoxic brain injury [18, 28] (Table 9.1). Additionally, withdrawal symptoms, including sweating, nausea, jaw tension, and intense psychic stress, have been noted, particularly in chronic users attempting detoxification. These symptoms are often severe due to the high dependency potential of NSOs. The standard treatment protocol for opioid overdose revolves around the restoration of spontaneous respiration. Naloxone, a mu-opioid receptor (MOR) antagonist, remains the first-line intervention. However, the heightened potency of synthetic opioids often requires escalated doses of naloxone for effective reversal. This has led to recommendations for increasing the standard doses administered by first responders in opioid overdose scenarios [27].

9.2.5.1 Designer Benzodiazepines

Designer benzodiazepines (BDZ) exhibit a structural resemblance to pharmaceutical BDZ. Frequently these molecules have undergone testing as potential drugs by pharmaceutical companies, but have not subsequently been approved as medicinal substances, at other times, these molecules are produced by starting with the structure of pharmaceutical BDZs and subsequently modifying them [29]. Pharmaceutical benzodiazepines are extensively utilized for their muscle relaxant, anxiolytic, hypnotic, and anticonvulsant properties. They are employed in the treatment of conditions such as anxiety, panic attacks, insomnia, seizures, and agitation. While generally considered safe, these drugs do carry the potential for serious side effects including dizziness, drowsiness, falls, confusion, respiratory depression, and coma [30]. BDZs, whether pharmaceutical or designer, function as allosteric modulators of the gamma amino butyric acid (GABA)-A, receptor. They bind to its α-subunits, amplifying its inhibitory effects on the CNS. These compounds are typically categorized based on the duration of their effects, ranging from minutes to days. Other times, they may be categorized based on their potency or on the onset time of their effects after administration [31]. Specifically, designer BDZ is characterized by an imbalanced profile, exhibiting more pronounced and specific effects. These effects include intense sedation accompanied by enduring amnesia, a sense of pleasure extending to euphoria, and disinhibition, among the numerous designer BDZs, notable examples include flubromazolam, clonazolam, deschloroetizolam, meclonazepam, and others [32] (Table 9.1). Their use as substances of abuse is linked both to their intrinsic abuse potential and their utilization as substances that enhance the effects of alcohol or balance the effects of cocaine. What makes designer BDZ appealing in the illicit market is evidently linked to the sensations of pleasure, euphoria, or drowsiness they can induce. Additionally, their rapid inducement of tolerance and the manifestation of withdrawal symptoms contribute to their attractiveness as substances of abuse. The primary issue associated with the consumption of designer BDZ is attributed to the wide range of potency, dose concentrations, and purity, exposing the consumer to an unpredictable risk of overdose and intoxication. This risk is particularly heightened for individuals who concurrently use other substances [29].

9.2.5.2 Misuse of Medications

The misuse of medications, particularly opioids and benzodiazepines, has been a longstanding issue, recently leading to significant public health challenges, including opioid epidemics, which refer to the widespread misuse and addiction to prescription opioids (painkillers, especially oxycodone, tramadol, etc.) and illicit opioids (such as heroin), and their consequent fatalities [33]. Overprescribing of opioids for pain management, coupled with factors like increased availability and misuse, contributed to a significant rise in opioid-related overdoses and deaths, the greatest increase being recorded with oxycodone [34, 35]. Misuse of medications refers to "any intentional improper or inappropriate use of prescription or over-the-counter drugs" [36]. This can include actions such as taking medication in higher doses than prescribed, using medication for non-medical purposes (e.g., recreational use), combining medications without consulting a healthcare professional or continuing to use the medication after the prescribed treatment period has ended or beyond its intended use. The following are some common patterns of non-medical medicine use:

1. some people with anxiety disorders and other mental health problems or pain may use medicines to self-medicate these symptoms without appropriate medical supervision or outside of accepted medical practice;
2. some people who have no medical reasons for using medicines use them for recreational or enhancement purposes, for example, to obtain a high, improve their physique, or facilitate concentration for long periods;
3. benzodiazepines or "Z-drugs" may also be used to increase the high, postpone opioid withdrawal, or reduce the adverse symptoms occurring after consuming stimulants (anxiety, depression, sleeplessness, etc.).

This type of polydrug use can also be considered a form of self-medication in people who use heroin and stimulants [37]. Although antiepileptic medications such as pregabalin and gabapentin, [37–40] and antipsychotic drugs such as olanzapine and quetiapine [37, 41, 42] have been reported as misuse for recreational purposes, the groups of medications that have most commonly been associated with concerns about their non-medical use in the EU include:

1. sedatives and hypnotics, including barbiturates, benzodiazepines, and benzodiazepine-like drugs such as the "Z-drugs" [37, 43, 44];
2. opioids, including pain relief medications and opioid agonist treatment medications; CNS stimulants prescribed to treat attention deficit and hyperactivity disorder (ADHD);
3. and over-the-counter drugs, mostly in association with alcohol and illicit drug use, including cough syrups containing codeine or dextromethorphan, some decongestants (e.g., pseudoephedrine), antidiarrheal drugs (e.g., loperamide) and certain antihistamines such as promethazine, chlorphenamine, and diphenhydramine [34, 37, 45, 46] (Table 9.1).

9.3 Prevention and Harm-Avoidance Strategies

The utilization of illicit drugs is linked to both chronic and acute health issues, exacerbated by various factors such as substance properties, administration methods, individual susceptibility, and the social environment in which drug consumption occurs. Persistent problems encompass issues like dependency and drug-induced infectious diseases, including drug overdose [2]. In this context, several harm reduction services have progressively become integrated into the mainstream healthcare provision for individuals engaging in drug use across Europe in the past two decades. Initially, the emphasis was on expanding the availability of opioid agonist treatment and needle and syringe programs as part of the response to high-risk drug use, particularly focusing on the injection of heroin and the HIV/AIDS epidemic. Over the last two decades, harm reduction approaches in some EU countries have broadened to include additional measures, such as supervised drug consumption rooms and take-home naloxone programs designed to mitigate fatal overdoses. In certain countries, there are also facilities for drug checking, established to assist individuals in understanding the composition of the illicit drugs they have purchased. Given the proliferation of synthetic stimulants and NPS in visually similar powders or pills on the illicit market, consumers may face an increasing risk of being unaware of the specific stimulant or combination of substances they are ingesting [2]. Certain indicators now suggest an increasing potential for synthetic opioids and synthetic stimulants to contribute to drug-related harms in Europe. Unintentional consumption of these substances, often present in powders or mixtures sold as other drugs, can result in poisonings and fatalities. Furthermore, the use of illicit stimulants and other substances can also be employed to facilitate group sexual encounters, particularly among men who have sex with other men and is known as chemsex. The drugs involved in *chemsex* can vary, encompassing stimulants such as methamphetamine, cocaine, and synthetic cathinones, as well as alcohol, depressants like GHB/GBL, and dissociatives like ketamine. High-risk consumption of these substances, including the parenteral use of drugs, exposes individuals to infectious diseases like HIV and HCV, as well as acute drug toxicity, fatal overdose, acute psychiatric complications, substance use disorder, and other psychiatric problems such as anxiety and depression. Providing effective harm reduction responses for individuals engaged in these high-risk behaviors remains a challenge, requiring the development of tailored harm reduction interventions (Table 9.2) [2]. However, some interventions continue to generate controversy, driven by factors such as their legal standing and the evolving body of evidence supporting their efficacy. Consequently, the adoption and implementation of these newer interventions exhibit disparities both within individual countries and across different nations. In addition, when present, these interventions are frequently concentrated in larger urban areas. In general, the extent of coverage and accessibility to harm reduction services, encompassing well-established and substantiated service models, differs significantly among EU countries. While certain harm reduction strategies may be met with controversy in certain European countries, the overarching concept that evidence-based measures to minimize harm play a crucial role in well-rounded drug policies is widely accepted [2].

9.3.1 Drug Monitoring Programs

Scientific evidence regarding the possible efficacy of drug checking services in altering behavior and mitigating drug-related harms is gradually surfacing [47, 48].

These services aim to prevent harm by allowing individuals to discover which chemicals are contained in the illicit substances they have purchased, and in some cases, they provide access to counseling or brief interventions. The analytical techniques used by these services range from sophisticated technologies capable of providing information on the potency and content of a wide

Table 9.2 Advancing effective approaches for addressing new psychoactive substances (NPS)

Prevention and harm-avoidance strategies	• Establishing and enhancing early warning capabilities to identify, assess, and communicate risks associated with particularly harmful substances. This is crucial for addressing the acute harms linked to NPS • Developing support and training initiatives to empower professionals within existing services, enabling them to recognize how their skills and competencies can be applied to address issues associated with NPS • Formulating practice guidelines for tackling problems related to new substances. These guidelines typically draw from responses to other drugs, encompassing areas such as drug education, professional training, and low-threshold services like needle and syringe programs. These responses should be tailored to the unique needs of various groups using new substances and the potential harms they may experience • Creating specific guidance on responding to the use of these substances in prisons and custodial settings • Fostering cultural competence within services to enhance service engagement and utilization • Providing education, including harm reduction measures, specifically tailored to new substances. This is particularly relevant for specific target groups and individuals already using drugs or at an increased risk of doing so • Incorporating school-based prevention activities related to new substances into generic prevention programs with evidence of effectiveness • Embracing multidisciplinary approaches and connecting various services to engage vulnerable groups that may not interact with traditional services (e.g., individuals engaged in chemsex or homeless populations) • Evaluating the development of responses to new substances to identify effective interventions capable of addressing the diverse challenges they present

Table 9.3 Future information needs for the drug monitoring system

New tools for the future	• Ensuring regular monitoring adapts to changes and contributes to the research knowledge cycle (including more current analysis, examination of new age groups and older cohorts, and an increase in qualitative research) to shape future research agendas • Augmenting routine monitoring with more proactive, timely, and targeted threat assessments • Investigating novel technologies such as automated data processing methods, bio-monitoring, and real-time data collection • Addressing ethical and data protection concerns associated with new monitoring methods and emerging information • Adopting a co-creation approach and involving information providers more actively in analysis and knowledge creation and sharing (information design)
Dissemination strategies	• Exploring the potential of innovative and digital communication methods for analyses, including user-friendly data platforms or dashboards • Enhancing the speed of reporting with a focus on real-time information • Strengthening messaging through consistent and reiterated communication, formulation of recommendations, and advocacy for evidence-based responses to counter disinformation and build trust • Providing training opportunities, particularly through e-learning, for key stakeholders such as professionals and policymakers • Customizing products to meet specific requests from stakeholders or cater to the needs of specialized customers • Designing information for impact and decision-making by more effectively integrating communication objectives into the planning of scientific work

variety of substances to methods that simply indicate the presence or absence of a particular drug. Current research has primarily concentrated on the dynamics between individuals and these services, exploring factors such as the willingness to use the services and behavioral intentions triggered by the receipt of drug-checking results (for example, disposing of harmful substances) [49, 50].

In this context, there have been limited assessments of the design and implementation of communications and alerts, either as independent initiatives within drug-checking services or as integral components of a comprehensive multiagency strategy. This is noteworthy because, like all interventions in the field of drugs, there exists the potential for unintended consequences and "communication backfire,"where communications may produce effects contrary to the intended outcomes (e.g., the targeted audience actively seeking out potent drugs). Consequently, it remains crucial to consistently incorporate research, monitoring, and evaluation into the activities of drug-checking services (Health risk communication strategies for drug checking services, a manual [2]) (Table 9.3).

9.4 Therapeutic Strategies and Telemedicine

Specialized treatment for harms related to NPS is not well established in most European countries. Additionally, there is limited demand in Europe for specialized drug treatment addressing issues arising from the use of new substances. Several factors may contribute to this, such as poor identification of use, a low prevalence of use, and limited instances of problematic use. It is also possible that many substances falling into this category are more linked to acute issues rather than chronic problems like dependence [2].

The poor identification of use might stem from underreported use or the misreporting of substances, particularly as individuals using these drugs might not be aware of what they are taking. Other contributing factors include a lack of suitable screening and monitoring instruments and low professional awareness of new substances. Despite these challenges, clinical guidelines are being established in certain European countries to address acute and chronic health harms. Moreover, there is an increasing focus on developing targeted education and prevention activities, along with initiating training and awareness-raising programs for professionals. Specific guidance for responding to the use of NPS in prisons and other custodial settings is also under development in certain countries [2].

Nevertheless, several ongoing experimental studies are exploring the potential utility of pharmacological interventions for cannabis-related problems. These interventions include the examination of THC and synthetic versions in combination with other psychoactive medications, such as antidepressants, anxiolytics, and mood stabilizers, among others. Despite that, the results thus far have been inconsistent, and an effective pharmacological approach for treating cannabis dependence has not been identified to date [2].

In this context, telemedicine, currently utilized across multiple branches of psychiatry (better known as telepsychiatry), is relevant [51]. The pandemic of coronavirus disease 2019 (COVID-19), along with increased technological adoption and revised regulations, has necessitated the incorporation of telepsychiatry into the care of addiction patients [52]. This approach is not only used to treat patients with addiction, but also to assess prognosis. In this regard, various factors play a crucial role:

1. trajectory of symptoms (whether they will improve, worsen or remain stable over time);
2. health-related factors influencing quality of life, such as the likelihood of developing complications and the severity of existing health issues;
3. the duration of abstinence;
4. strategies for preventing relapse;
5. accessibility and effectiveness of available therapies.

The results of recent studies suggest that the prognosis for addiction patients treated with telepsychiatry is comparable to that of in-person treatment [53, 54]. Although telepsychiatry offers some advantages and is a potential therapeutic strategy in this area it also presents challenges, which can be mitigated through specific approaches. Despite the unprecedented surge in the use of telepsychiatry during the pandemic, its future use will depend on various factors, including government regulations and the availability of secure, encrypted platforms to instill greater trust between clinicians and patients [55].

Authors' Contribution All authors have contributed to the chapter and approved its final version.

References

1. United Nations Office on Drugs and Crime (UNODC) (2014) World drug report 2014. UNODC, New York
2. European Monitoring Centre for Drugs and Drug Addiction (EMCDDA), (2023) European Drug Report 2023: trends and developments. https://www.emcdda.europa.eu/publications/european-drug-report/2023_en. Accessed 8 Dec 2023
3. Espad (2023) Results from the European School Survey Project on alcohol and other drugs. https://europa.eu/!Xy37DU. Accessed 6 Dec 2023
4. Eurobarometer (2009) Young people and drugs: analytical report. http://ec.europa.eu/public opinion/flash/fl 233 en.pdf. Accessed 5 Dec 2023
5. Schifano F, Leoni M, Martinotti G et al (2003) Importance of cyberspace for the assessment of the drug abuse market: preliminary results from the Psychonaut 2002 project. Cyberpsychol Behav 6(4):405–410. https://doi.org/10.1089/109493103322278790
6. Corazza O, Valeriani G, Bersani FS et al (2014) "Spice," "kryptonite," "black mamba": an overview of brand names and marketing strategies of novel psychoactive substances on the web. J Psychoactive Drugs 46(4):287–294. https://doi.org/10.1080/02791072.2014.944291
7. Schifano F, Deluca P, Agosti L et al (2005) New trends in the cyber and street market of recreational drugs? The case of 2C-T-7 ('Blue Mystic'). J Psychopharmacol 19(6):675–679. https://doi.org/10.1177/0269881105056660
8. Martinotti G, De Risio L, Vannini C et al (2021) Substance-related exogenous psychosis: a postmodern syndrome. CNS Spectr 26(1):84–91. https://doi.org/10.1017/S1092852920001479

9. Martinotti G, Negri A, Schiavone S et al (2020) Club drugs: psychotropic effects and psychopathological characteristics of a sample of inpatients. Front Psych 11:879. https://doi.org/10.3389/fpsyt.2020.00879
10. Schifano F, Vento A, Scherbaum N et al (2023) Stimulant and hallucinogenic novel psychoactive substances; an update. Expert Rev Clin Pharmacol 16(11):1109–1123. https://doi.org/10.1080/17512433.2023.2279192
11. Altun B, Çok I (2020) Psychoactive bath salts and neurotoxicity risk. Turk J Pharm Sci 17(2):235–241. https://doi.org/10.4274/tjps.galenos.2018.40820
12. Schifano F, Chiappini S, Miuli A et al (2021a) New psychoactive substances (NPS) and serotonin syndrome onset: a systematic review. Exp Neurol 339:113638. https://doi.org/10.1016/j.expneurol.2021.113638
13. Chiappini S, Mosca A, Miuli A et al (2021) New psychoactive substances and suicidality: a systematic review of the current literature. Medicina (Kaunas) 57(6):580. https://doi.org/10.3390/medicina57060580
14. Alves VL, Gonçalves JL, Aguiar J et al (2020) The synthetic cannabinoids phenomenon: from structure to toxicological properties. A review. Crit Rev Toxicol 50(5):359–382. https://doi.org/10.1080/10408444.2020.1762539
15. Schifano F, Orsolini L, Papanti D et al (2017) NPS: medical consequences associated with their intake. Curr Top Behav Neurosci 32:351–380. https://doi.org/10.1007/7854_2016_15
16. Martinotti G, Santacroce R, Papanti D et al (2017) Synthetic cannabinoids: psychopharmacology, clinical aspects, psychotic onset. CNS Neurol Disord Drug Targets 16(5):567–575. https://doi.org/10.2174/1871527316666170413101839
17. Orsolini L, Chiappini S, Papanti D et al (2019) The bridge between classical and "synthetic"/chemical psychoses: towards a clinical, psychopathological, and therapeutic perspective. Front Psych 10:851. https://doi.org/10.3389/fpsyt.2019.00851
18. Schifano F, Napoletano F, Chiappini S et al (2021b) New/emerging psychoactive substances and associated psychopathological consequences. Psychol Med 51(1):30–42. https://doi.org/10.1017/S0033291719001727
19. Kuropka P, Zawadzki M, Szpot P (2023) A review of synthetic cathinones emerging in recent years (2019-2022). Forensic Toxicol 41(1):25–46. https://doi.org/10.1007/s11419-022-00639-5
20. Soares J, Costa VM, Bastos ML et al (2021) An updated review on synthetic cathinones. Arch Toxicol 95(9):2895–2940. https://doi.org/10.1007/s00204-021-03083-3
21. Daziani G, Lo Faro AF, Montana V et al (2023) Synthetic Cathinones and neurotoxicity risks: a systematic review. Int J Mol Sci 24(7):6230. https://doi.org/10.3390/ijms24076230
22. Schifano F, Napoletano F, Arillotta D et al (2020) The clinical challenges of synthetic cathinones. Br J Clin Pharmacol 86(3):410–419. https://doi.org/10.1111/bcp.14132
23. Horsley RR, Lhotkova E, Hajkova K et al (2016) Detailed pharmacological evaluation of methoxetamine (MXE), a novel psychoactive ketamine analogue—behavioural, pharmacokinetic and metabolic studies in the Wistar rat. Brain Res Bull 126(1):102–110. https://doi.org/10.1016/j.brainresbull.2016.05.002
24. Hofer KE, Grager B, Müller DM et al (2012) Ketamine-like effects after recreational use of methoxetamine. Ann Emerg Med 60(1):97–99. https://doi.org/10.1016/j.annemergmed.2011.11.018
25. Moccia L, Tofani A, Mazza M et al (2019) Dorsolateral prefrontal cortex impairment in Methoxetamine-induced psychosis: an 18F-FDG PET/CT case study. J Psychoactive Drugs 51(3):254–259. https://doi.org/10.1080/02791072.2019.1578444
26. Craig CL, Loeffler GH (2014) The ketamine analog methoxetamine: a new designer drug to threaten military readiness. Mil Med 179(10):1149–1157. https://doi.org/10.7205/MILMED-D-13-00470
27. Edinoff AN, Martinez Garza D et al (2023) New synthetic opioids: clinical considerations and dangers. Pain Ther 12(2):399–421. https://doi.org/10.1007/s40122-023-00481-6
28. Armenian P, Vo KT, Barr-Walker J et al (2018) Fentanyl, fentanyl analogs and novel synthetic opioids: a comprehensive review. Neuropharmacology 134(Pt A):121–132. https://doi.org/10.1016/j.neuropharm.2017.10.016
29. Orsolini L, Corkery JM, Chiappini S et al (2020) 'New/designer benzodiazepines': an analysis of the literature and psychonauts'. Trip reports. Curr Neuropharmacol 18(9):809–837. https://doi.org/10.2174/1570159X18666200110121333
30. Stahl SM (2021) Essential psychopharmacology: Prescriber's guide, 6th edn. University Press, Cambridge
31. Stahl SM (2013) Stahl's essential psychopharmacology: neuroscientific basis and practical applications, 4th edn. University Press, Cambridge
32. Edinoff AN, Nix CA, Odisho AS et al (2022) Novel designer benzodiazepines: comprehensive review of evolving clinical and adverse effects. Neurol Int 14(3):648–663. https://doi.org/10.3390/neurolint14030053
33. Chiappini S, Mosca A, Miuli A et al (2022a) Misuse of anticholinergic medications: a systematic review. Biomedicine 10(2):355. https://doi.org/10.3390/biomedicines10020355
34. Chiappini S, Vickers-Smith R, Guirguis A et al (2022b) Pharmacovigilance signals of the opioid epidemic over 10 years: data mining methods in the analysis of pharmacovigilance datasets collecting adverse drug reactions (ADRs) reported to EudraVigilance (EV) and the FDA adverse event reporting system (FAERS). Pharmaceuticals 15(6):675. https://doi.org/10.3390/ph15060675

35. Kibaly C, Alderete JA, Liu SH et al (2021) Oxycodone in the opioid epidemic: high 'Liking', 'Wanting', and abuse liability. Cell Mol Neurobiol 41(5):899–926. https://doi.org/10.1007/s10571-020-01013-y
36. European Medicines Agency (EMA) (2017) Guideline on good pharmacovigilance practices (GVP)—Annex I (Rev 4) EMA/876333/2011 Rev 4. https://www.ema.europa.eu/en/documents/scientific-guideline/guideline-good-pharmacovigilance-practices-annex-i-definitions-rev-4_en.pdf. Accessed 5 Dec 2023
37. European Monitoring Centre for Drugs and Drug Addiction (EMCDDA) (2021) Non-medical use of medicines: health and social responses. https://www.emcdda.europa.eu/publications/mini-guides/non-medical-use-of-medicines-health-and-social-responses_en. Accessed 5 Dec 2023
38. Bonnet U, Scherbaum N (2017) How addictive are gabapentin and pregabalin? A systematic review. Eur Neuropsychopharmacol 27(12):1185–1215. https://doi.org/10.1016/j.euroneuro.2017.08.430
39. Chiappini S, Schifano F (2016) A decade of Gabapentinoid misuse: an analysis of the European medicines Agency's 'Suspected adverse drug Reactions' database. CNS Drugs 30(7):647–654. https://doi.org/10.1007/s40263-016-0359-y
40. Evoy KE, Morrison MD, Saklad SR (2017) Abuse and misuse of Pregabalin and gabapentin. Drugs 77(4):403–426. https://doi.org/10.1007/s40265-017-0700-x
41. Evoy KE, Humpert S, Torrez S et al (2023) Quetiapine and olanzapine misuse prevalence in a US general population sample. Ment Health Clin 13(2):25–35. https://doi.org/10.9740/mhc.2023.04.025
42. Vento AE, Kotzalidis GD, Cacciotti M et al (2020) Quetiapine abuse fourteen years later: where are we now? A systematic review. Subst Use Misuse 55(2):304–313. https://doi.org/10.1080/10826084.2019.1668013
43. Orsolini L, Chiappini S, Grandinetti P et al (2021) 'Z-trip'? A comprehensive overview and a case-series of zolpidem misuse. Clin Psychopharmacol Neurosci 19(2):367–387. https://doi.org/10.9758/cpn.2021.19.2.367
44. Schifano F, Chiappini S, Corkery JM et al (2019) An insight into Z-drug abuse and dependence: an examination of reports to the European medicines Agency database of suspected adverse drug reactions. Int J Neuropsychopharmacol 22(4):270–277. https://doi.org/10.1093/ijnp/pyz007
45. Chiappini S, Schifano F (2020) What about "pharming"? Issues regarding the misuse of prescription and over-the-counter drugs. Brain Sci 10(10):736. https://doi.org/10.3390/brainsci10100736
46. Schifano F, Chiappini S, Miuli A et al (2021c) Focus on over-the-counter drugs' misuse: a systematic review on antihistamines, cough medicines, and decongestants. Front Psych 12:657397. https://doi.org/10.3389/fpsyt.2021.657397
47. Betzler F, Helbig J, Viohl L et al (2020) Drug checking and its potential impact on substance use. Eur Addict Res 27(1):25–32. https://doi.org/10.1159/000507049
48. Wallace B, van Roode T, Pagan F et al (2020) What is needed for implementing drug checking services in the context of the overdose crisis? A qualitative study to explore perspectives of potential service users. Harm Reduct J 17(1):29. https://doi.org/10.1186/s12954-020-00373-4
49. Measham F, Turnbull G (2021) Intentions, actions and outcomes: a follow up survey on harm reduction practices after using an English festival drug checking service. Int J Drug Policy 95:103270. https://doi.org/10.1016/j.drugpo.2021.103270
50. Valente H, Martins D, Carvalho H et al (2019) Evaluation of a drug checking service at a large scale electronic music festival in Portugal. Int J Drug Policy 73:88–95. https://doi.org/10.1016/j.drugpo.2019.07.007
51. Gude J, Subhedar RV, Zhang MH et al (2021) Emerging needs and viability of Telepsychiatry during and post COVID-19 era: a literature review. Cureus 13(8):e16974. https://doi.org/10.7759/cureus.16974
52. Mohan A, Ambekar A (2020) Telepsychiatry and addiction treatment. Indian J Psychol Med 42:52–56. https://doi.org/10.1177/0253717620958169
53. Gliske K, Welsh JW, Braughton JE et al (2022) Telehealth services for substance use disorders during the COVID-19 pandemic: longitudinal assessment of intensive outpatient programming and data collection practices. JMIR Ment Health 9(3):e36263. https://doi.org/10.2196/36263
54. Zheng W, Nickasch M, Lander L et al (2017) Treatment outcome comparison between Telepsychiatry and face-to-face buprenorphine medication-assisted treatment for opioid use disorder: a 2-year retrospective data analysis. J Addict Med 11(2):138–144. https://doi.org/10.1097/ADM.0000000000000287
55. Kamma HK, Alabbas M, Elashahab M et al (2023) The efficacy of telepsychiatry in addiction patients: a systematic review. Cureus 15(4):e38133. https://doi.org/10.7759/cureus.38133

10 The Mental Health of LGBTQIA+ Population

Antonio Ventriglio, Gian Maria Galeazzi, Mattia Marchi, Federica Pinna, Manlio Converti, Francesco Amaddeo, Massimo Mirandola, and Andrea Fiorillo

Abstract

Sexuality and *gender identity* are crucial aspects of human personal identity and experience. Both significantly affect the individual self-perception, any personal belief, thinking, social being, and connections with the family and community. *Sexual variations* (e.g., LGBTQIA+: lesbian, gay, bisexual, transgender, queer, intersex, asexual) are common expressions of sexuality beyond the *binary* model based on the heteronormative conception. Also, *gender identity* may be not aligned with the sex assigned at birth (biological) and this may lead to specific health needs among persons requiring an affirmative trail of their own gender identity. Non-binary expressions of gender and sexuality are often associated with variable social stigma and oppression with consequent psychosocial distress and mental health issues (including depression, anxiety, adjustment disorders, eating disorders, substance abuse as well as non-suicidal self-injury) for variants people experiencing *minority stress*. *Minority stress* may include any experienced childhood adverse event, non-acceptance in the family, school, peers-group, and workplaces. Clinicians and psychiatrists need to consider these specific health

A. Ventriglio (✉)
Department of Clinical and Experimental Medicine, University of Foggia, Foggia, Italy
e-mail: a.ventriglio@libero.it

G. M. Galeazzi · M. Marchi
Department of Biomedical, Metabolic and Neural Sciences, University of Modena and Reggio Emilia, Modena, Italy

Dipartimento ad Attività Integrata di Salute Mentale e Dipendenze Patologiche, Azienda USL-IRCCS di Reggio Emilia, Reggio Emilia, Italy
e-mail: gianmaria.galeazzi@unimore.it

F. Pinna
Dipartimento di Scienze Mediche e Sanità Pubblica, Università degli Studi di Cagliari, Cagliari, Italy

M. Converti
ASL Napoli 2 Nord, Naples, Italy
e-mail: manlio.converti@aslnapoli2nord.it

F. Amaddeo
Department of Neurosciences, Biomedicine and Movement, University of Verona, Verona, Italy
e-mail: francesco.amaddeo@univr.it

M. Mirandola
WHO Collaborating Centre for Sexual Health and Vulnerable Populations, Epidemiology Unit—Infectious Diseases Division, Department of Diagnostics and Public Health, University of Verona, Verona, Italy
e-mail: massimo.mirandola@aovr.veneto.it

A. Fiorillo
Department of Psychiatry, University of Campania "Luigi Vanvitelli", Naples, Italy
e-mail: andrea.fiorillo@unicampania.it

A. Fiorillo, S. De Giorgi (eds.), *Social Determinants of Mental Health*, Sustainable Development Goals Series, https://doi.org/10.1007/978-3-031-70165-8_10

and mental health needs as well as psychotherapies should be focused on affirmative approaches. In addition, educational interventions aimed at contrasting social and cultural oppression should be encouraged in order to reduce the impact of minority stress on LGBTQIA+ people and their psychological burden.

Keywords

Sexuality · Sexual variations · Sexual diversity · LGBTQIA+ · Mental health Assessment · Interventions

10.1 Sexuality

Sexuality is a crucial part of our personal identity. It wholly affects the way individuals perceive themselves, satisfy themselves (or others), and may engage in a relationship with others [1]. Sexuality also characterizes personal activities such as pleasure, recreation, and procreation [1]. The individual sexuality may be considered as the result of the personal psychosexual development, culture, personal and family identity, early life events, relationships, religion, and societal influences [2]. Some authors also suggest the role of genetic and epigenetic in the modeling of personal sexual identity, encouraging further research in the field of *sexogenomics* [3]. Since sexuality is part of the personal identity, *sexual variations* equally affect the identity.

10.1.1 Sexual Variations

Sexual variation or *sexual diversity* is defined as any sexual orientation or behavior that differs from the *heteronormative* experience, including the individual preference for sexual and emotional relationships with persons of a particular sex [4]. The *heteronormative* model proposes the heterosexuality as the standard legitimate social and sexual relationship, thus, according to this conception, sexual variations might be seen as an "*abnormality*" [5]. However, over the last decade, sexual diversities have been gaining an increasing acceptance and are largely recognized as representative of human experience [6]. Sexual variations include heterosexuality, homosexuality, bisexuality, asexuality, transexuality, intersexuality, and pansexuality (omnisexuality) [6]. The acronym LGBTQIA (lesbian, gay, bisexual, transgender, queer, intersex, asexual) has been proposed through the decades for recognizing a set of sexual variants, with the term gay (G) proposed in 1869 by Kerbeny, lesbian and bisexual (L and B) in the '1980s', transgender (T) in the beginning of the '1990s' by Prince, and the terms queer (according to the Theory of Queer, proposed in 1996) and asexual (A) in the late 1990s [7]. Four components have been recognized in the description of sexual variations: (a) the self-identification label such as homosexual, bisexual, heterosexual; (b) the actual sexual behavior: depending on the current opportunities and relationships; (c) subjective sexual feelings such as fantasies and desires; (d) physiological genital and brain responses [7]. It is of relevance that these components are congruent with each other and the personal choice is congruent with fantasies, arousal, and the availability of partner. Sexual choices and self-identification may be also influenced by social and cultural factors as well as social and cultural contexts that significantly affect the integration of individuals on the base of their sexual orientation or variation [6].

The sexual identity may be related to the sexual behaviors and/or sexual orientation. Thus an individual may report a homosexual orientation and engage in homosexual relationships and behaviors. However, there may be a discordance between these factors with individuals self-defined homosexual but engaging in heterosexual relationships, mostly due to their social or cultural pressure as well as due to their bisexual fantasies and desires [6]. In fact, there may be an innate *sexual fluidity* in the experience of many individuals as well as multiple sexual identities may coexist [6]. In fact, the internal and external pressures due to gender, family, society, culture, and religion may modulate the public identity, which may be different from the self-perceived identity: all these factors may lead to a contrast between how individuals feel themselves, behave, and the way they are expected to behave [6]. Religion, in particular, may affect the sexual public attitudes on the basis of morality and may censor sexual practices [6]. Thus, in the clinical setting, it is important to differentiate what may be subjective sexuality from sexual public attitudes, as well as what may be considered as a sexual variation from sexual perversions (*Paraphilias*) [8].

Paraphilias, also known as sexual perversions, are based on a sexual arousal to unusual or atypical objects, behaviors, individuals, or situations. This definition may be highly controversial in the clinical setting. Once again, cultural and societal factors may determine the interpretation of such behaviors and sexual norms. The Diagnostic and Statistical Manual of Mental Disorders—fifth edition—text revised (DSM-5-TR; [9]), clarified that the perceived mental distress or the impairment in individual's functioning, caused by these fantasies and behaviors, may be considered as a threshold for the diagnosis of paraphilias. Eight paraphilic disorders are listed in the latest version of the DSM. Although these do not exhaust the list of possible paraphilic disorders, they are selected because relatively common, in relation to other paraphilic disorders, and some of them entail actions for their satisfaction that, because of their noxiousness or potential harm to others, are classified as criminal offenses. These are classified into two groups. The first group of disorders is based on *anomalous activity preferences*, further subdivided into *courtship disorders*, which resemble distorted components of human courtship behavior (*voyeuristic disorder*, *exhibitionistic disorder*, and *frotteuristic disorder*), and *algolagnic disorders*, which involve pain and suffering (*sexual masochism disorder* and *sexual sadism disorder*). The second group of disorders is based on *anomalous target preferences* and includes one directed at other humans (*pedophilic disorder*) and two directed elsewhere (*fetishistic disorder* and *transvestic disorder*) [9].

The International Statistical Classification of Diseases and Related Health Problems [10] classifies *paraphilic disorders* including the following: (a) exhibitionistic disorder; (b) voyeuristic disorder; (c) pedophilic disorder; (d) coercive sexual sadism disorder; (e) frotteuristic disorder; (f) other paraphilic disorder involving non-consenting individuals; (g) other paraphilic disorder involving solitary behavior or consenting individuals. The individual must have acted on the arousal pattern that involves consenting adults or solitary behaviors or must be exposed to risk and be markedly distressed by it.

Gender and Gender Identity: Gender and gender identity play a key role in the individual sexuality, and are strongly affected by social components. The intrinsic sense of being male, female, or an alternative gender (boy-girl, girl-boy, trans-gender, gender-queer, eunuch, a-gender) sets the stage for the *identity* development. Gender includes all the characteristics pertaining to masculinity and femininity and has been traditionally seen as binary [6]. Gender may correspond to biological sex or not. Also, *"the gender as a role"* is the expression of the individual own status with attitudes, including sexual ones, and the role in the society beyond the biological sex and social expectations.

Gender identity may be defined as how an individual experiences and acknowledgments his/her own gender [6]. All societies are based on the rough binary distinction between male and female genders and masculinity vs. femininity sex/gender model. However, biological sex, gender identity, and gender expression may be not congruent with each other [11]. Gender is a complex construct including biological sex, socially determined identity, acts, and self-identification. Beyond the binary dichotomy between masculinity and femininity, the concept of *gender spectrum* has been proposed, with the proposal to include individuals in a range of variations between male and female [12]. Also, the concept of *gender neutrality* has been proposed: neutrality includes traits, behaviors, fantasies, and desires of both genders [12].

Pansexuality: The sexual identity may be also based on a broader sexual orientation and attraction toward people of any sex and gender, also called pansexuality or omni-sexuality [13]. This condition is not based on the relevance of gender for the selection of sexual target, and pansexual individuals may be also defined as gender-blind. Also, pan-sexuality may be interpreted as an attraction virtually directed towards everything.

Sexual Fluidity: According to the models previously reported, we may intend that sexual identity as well as gender identity is flexible and may change over time. In fact, sexual self-identification and attraction may vary within a spectrum and change over the course of life [6, 14]. Kinsey et al. [15] argued that there may be a *sexual fluidity* in the self-recognizing as heterosexual or homosexual or predominantly heterosexual and homosexual. Also, sexual behaviors and attraction may change over the time on the base of situations and opportunities. According to Kinsey's model, gender and sexual orientation may be *flexible* over time, changing in a kind of sexual/gender *flux*: any personal attitude, sexual preference, and behavior as well as identity are plastic and modifiable (people may be accordingly labeled as heteroflexible, homoflexible; [15, 16]). In addition, Kanazawa [17] proposed that bisexuality may be intended as a transition phase, in the fluidity framework, followed by a change of orientation or identity in the middle-term. We may summarize that *fluidity* is based on the following three principles: (a) *Nonexclusivity* in sexual orientation and attraction; (b) *Change* over time and situations; (c) *Variance* among different phases, e.g., mostly "heterosexual," "strictly heterosexual" back and forth frequently, "bisexual" as well as "homosexual."

10.1.2 Prevalence of Sexual Variations

The data collection regarding the prevalence of sexual diversities may present a large degree of challenges. In fact, as discussed above, definitions and terminology are not universally agreed and measurements may be misleading. Also, sexual variations are not easily and openly disclosed because of the related social stigma and oppression.

Geary et al. [18] argued that some dimensions of sexuality such as identity, attraction, or behaviors may differently impact the prevalence of sexual variations and are poorly routinely collected in the healthcare settings, including the mental health assessment. Also, research studies in this field mostly include data regarding the LGBT (lesbian, gay, bisexual, and transgender) cluster, and details of each specific subgroup are missed. These biases in research may be also due to the lack of an *inclusive registry* that allows researchers to include a wide set of sexual variations in a standardized manner. In the last decade, there has been a growing interest in the use of inclusive registries above all in the data collection for research purposes [19].

Alfred Kinsey [15] published his book entitled *Sexual Behaviour in the Human Male,* reporting on sexual behaviors and characteristics of a large sample surveyed in the US general population: he described that 37% of men may report same-sex experiences in their life and sexual fluidity is more common among women.

Even if the sexual variations are common in all societies, heterosexuality is still recognized as the prevalent sexual identity by the 90–95% of the general population [18, 20]. In the UK, the estimated prevalence of homosexual identity among 16–75 years old aged subjects was 1.5% and bisexuality reached 1% [18]. These findings were considered as misleading since they were mostly based on the reported self-identity, whereas reports on sexual orientations concluded that 6.5% of subjects disclosed a same-sex attraction and 6.8% a same-sex experience.

Recently, Rahman et al. [21] surveyed 191,088 participants from 28 different countries (including Asia, Europe, North America, and Oceania) exploring their sexual identity and same-sex attraction: they described similar rates of LGBT identities among participants from all countries with no differences between Western and non-Western societies/cultures. As expected,

90–90.7% of individuals self-reported a heterosexual identity whereas 5.1–7.2% defined themselves as bisexual, 2.1 and 4.9% as lesbian and gay, respectively. Other evidence indicated an increase in prevalence in the last years likely as a result of a higher level of comfort with the sexual disclosure within some communities. For instance, Gates [22] described an increase from 2.7% to 5.4% of LGBT identities in the US General Social Survey, predominantly among the so-called *millennial generation* (or *Y generation*, including those citizens born between 1980s and 1990s). This trend may be explained by: (a) an increasing societal acceptance of non-heterosexual identity and behaviors, including homosexual relationships and marriage; (b) the decriminalization of homosexuality and the approval of legislation on gay marriage in many counties; (c) an increase in activism through the countries with a reduction of stigma and favorable attitudes toward homosexuality; (d) increased awareness on sexual variations through the social media (TV, social network and so on) [6].

10.2 Culture and Sexual Variations

Culture is a relevant factor in determining the expression of sexual behaviors, their social acceptance as well as the epidemiological recognition of them. Culture may also impact on sexuality and its related mental health issues, including diagnostic criteria and clinical assessments. Also, any experience of stigma, discrimination, and social oppression may be mediated by cultural and religious factors leading to variable degrees of societal and moral acceptance of non-heterosexual identities.

It is of note, that same-sex behaviors are still criminalized in 70 countries all over the world, as reported by the International Lesbian, Gay, Bisexual, Trans and Intersex Association (ILGA) in [23], including six United Nations member states proposing the death penalty for same-sex acts [24].

Roberts [25] reported findings from an anthropological analysis regarding the societal acceptance of same-sex behaviors in 87 countries over 30 years (1981–2012). She argued that the employment of the internet, social media, social networks as well as international travels have largely contributed to increase the acceptance of sexual variations in all countries regardless of their predominant cultures, religions, and legislative frameworks. Although all these factors represent a cultural revolution in the last decades, the cultures strongly based on religious principles reported a lower increase in the acceptance of sexual diversity [26]. Kite et al. [27] proposed a set of cross-cultural factors, which may be considered as associated with an increased social acceptance of the LGBT identities: (a) interpersonal exchanges with LGBT friends; (b) higher education level; (c) lower level of religious education or not being a religious practitioner; (d) women are generally more accepting than men.

10.2.1 Historical Notes

Three cultural models of homosexuality have been historically recognized [28]: the Greek model, the Melanesian model and the Western model.

In the Greek culture-based model, an older, even married, man was allowed to approach sexually or have a relationship with a younger boy (*eromenos*). The older man had the role to mentor him and training him into manhood. The young guy was educated as homosexual, in this relationship with the bisexual mentor, in order to become bisexual himself. Interestingly, beyond this educational exception, other homosexual relationships between adults were discouraged in the Greek culture.

The Melanesian model, adopted in the Papua New Guinea Islands, proposed three stages of the individual sexual life: (a) passive exclusive homosexuality; (b) active exclusive homosexuality; and (c) exclusive adult heterosexuality. Adolescents were expected to engage in fellatio with younger boys from the age of 7 years old within their puberty. This was a form of social obligation and duty to be performed until the marriageable age when they were expected to become heterosexual. Any homosexual behavior out of this range of age was considered deviant.

Finally, in the Western model, the homosexual relationships were possibly accepted also between adults.

Sexual variations and gender variants have been also described in the Orthodox Jews, the *Hijras* (eunuch) in India, the *kathoeys* (transgender) in Thailand, *Xanith* (transgender) in Oman, the Gallae (tansgender priests) in the Roman Empire, the *Mahu* ("in the middle" individuals) of Polynesia and the *two-spirits person* in native North America.

In conclusion, the association between culture and sexual variations is complex and relevant since culture may affect their expression, explanatory models, and consequent mental health issues, including diagnostic criteria and assessment [15].

10.3 Sexual Variations and Mental Health

10.3.1 Nosography

Historically, the engagement in same-sex relationships and behaviors were stigmatized and considered as "*demonic*" as well as related to "*insanity.*" Also, a model of sexual pathology explaining the clinical models of sexual variations was formulated in the Victorian era [29].

Freud in 1905 published his *Three Essays on the Theory of Sexuality* [30] and introduced the concept of sexual aberrations and variants, including "homosexuality" and "heterosexuality." Later, Drescher in 2015 published a report on the depathologization of homosexuality in the nosography based on the newer editions of the Diagnostic and Statistical Manual of Mental Disorders (DSM).

As specified by Drescher [31] and Suess Schwend [32], the inclusion of same-sex behaviors as a pathological issue occurred in 1948 in the International Classification of Diseases (ICD)-6. In fact, these behaviors were intended as part of a pathological personality (sexual deviations). In 1952, the American Psychiatric Association included homosexuality in the DSM as a "sociopathic personality disturbance." Later in 1965, in the ICD-8, the category "homosexuality" has been introduced as well as in the DSM-II (1968) it has been proposed as "sexual deviation." After the influence of gay activism and emerging scientific evidences, in 1973 the label "homosexuality" has been removed from the DSM III and proposed under the category "Sexual Orientation Disturbance." Professor Robert Spitzer [33] reformulated the concept of homosexuality and sexual orientation disturbance (SOD) proposing the differentiation between the normal sexual variant from other same sex attractions characterized by experienced distress or psychological disturbance. In 1975, the same sex attractions were reported in the ICD-9 including homosexuality even if it has been distinguished in normal variants and variants associated with a mental disorder.

In 1980, in the DSM-III, according to the emerging proposals, the diagnosis of "ego-dystonic" homosexuality has been introduced referring to those individuals presenting a same-sex attraction with subjective distress. In 1987, in the revised version of the DSM-III edition (DSM-III-R), the label of homosexuality was removed from the diagnostic categories and the ego-dystonic subtype was included under the label of sexual disorder not otherwise specified. Similarly, the removal of homosexuality was confirmed in the following editions of the manual DSM-IV (1994), DSM-IV-TR (2000), and DSM-5 (2013) as well as the ego-dystonic sexual orientation has been omitted in the ICD-11 (2018).

10.3.2 Epidemiology

A relevant higher rate of mental health issues has been described among subjects reporting sexual variations.

King et al. [34] published a systematic review of literature reporting a 1.5 times higher risk of mood disorders, anxiety disorders, and higher rates of lifetime suicides among LGBT groups. Also, it has been described as a significantly higher risk of substance abuse/misuse including cigarettes and alcohol [35]. More recently, Crowell [29] confirmed data available in the literature as well as from the National LGBT Alliance, both reporting an increased risk of developing mood and anxiety disorders, substance dependence and abuse as well as suicidal attempts and ideation among LGBT individuals. Alongside this mental health morbidity, they also are exposed to an increased risk of sexually transmitted infections due to unhealthy sexual behaviors [36]. Severe mental disorders (psychotic or bipolar disorders) as well as depression, anxiety, and post-traumatic stress disorder may reach an incidence of two-to-four times higher among LGBT than heterosexual population [36, 37]. Beyond these major mental health issues, it is well documented that individuals with sexual variants may also experience psychosocial distress characterized by worry, anxiety, and tension [38]. In fact, it has been largely described that part of the mental health burden among LGBT individuals is due to the minority stress and the lack of social policies in their favor. Hatzenbuehler et al. [39] reported data from a large US sample of the general population including 34.653 inhabitants and 577 LGBTs. The rate of mood and anxiety disorders as well as substance abuse were two times higher among LGBT (20.4%) than heterosexual individuals (10.2%) in those US states with any specific policy in defense of the homosexual community. Also, LGBT sample has shown two-to-five times higher risk of substance dependence (40.8% vs. 20.9%, above all alcohol misuse) and higher levels of multiple psychiatric comorbidities. The same authors in 2012 [40] reported that the introduction of social policies in support of the LGBT community, including the legalization of gay marriage, led to a reduction of psychiatric morbidity and promoted the access to mental health services among LGBT individuals. Also, lower rates of alcohol abuse and fewer risky sexual behaviors were observed in the same sample [41].

Interestingly, Crowell [29] reported an increased risk of homelessness among LGBT individuals: in this study, 20–40% of the interviewed homeless subjects disclosed a sexual variation and most of them reported have been rejected by their family and society.

Sex differences have been also described in the epidemiology of mental disorders among LGBT individuals with higher morbidity among women. The Longitudinal Study of the Health of Australian Women (LSHAW-study) reported that 38% of same-sex attracted females aged 22–27 years old presented symptoms of depression (vs. 19% of heterosexual females) as well as higher levels of anxiety (17.1% vs. 7.9%) [42]. Also self-harm and suicidal thoughts were higher among women and often related to violence or sexual harassment. Substance abuse rated higher among sexual variants than in the heterosexual female population: cigarette smoking (65% vs. 54%), risky alcohol use (7.0% vs. to 3.9%), marijuana use (58.2% vs. 21.5%), use of other illicit drugs (40.7% vs. 10.2%), and injecting drug use (10.8% vs. 1.2%) [43].

10.3.3 Leading Causes

The LGBT population is highly vulnerable to psychological distress and social inequalities. In particular, the condition of being/belonging to a minority group may play a key role. Thus, social factors leading to mental illness may include discrimination, social stigma, prejudice, lack of inclusion, lack of policies, social disadvantage, and inequalities [44]. Consequently, legislative and social changes are encouraged in order to increase their acceptability and reduce the social and legal inequalities affecting people reporting a sexual minority condition.

Minority Stress Theory: The minority stress theory was proposed to explain any experience of discrimination and violence reported by ethnic, cultural, and religious minorities. In 1995, Meyer [45] conceptualized the application of this explanatory model to better understand the social and psychological burden of non-heterosexual individuals. He proposed that LGBT individuals regularly experience ongoing stress, discrimination, and internalized negative attitudes about their own sexuality and behaviors, stigma at many levels of society. It has been already argued that both acute and chronic stress may contribute to poor mental and physical health, including the higher incidence of related stress as well as anxiety and depressive disorders [44, 46]. In a clinical setting, it may be useful to focus on the experience of being minority and the related internalized feelings of being "bad" or "wrong": psychological as well as practical support for the social and work involvement are encouraged.

Sexual Identity Formation: Cass [47] proposed and developed a theory regarding the formation of a nonheterosexual identity. This explanatory model has been based on six stages of development, all characterized by a step of acquisition and assumption of stability regarding the new identity and following changes in behaviors and social interactions. If any of these stages becomes problematic, health challenges or distress may occur with the following mental health issues. Her stages included: (a) identity confusion; (b) identity comparison; (c) identity tolerance; (d) identity acceptance; (e) identity pride; (f) identity synthesis. This process includes a change of self-perception switching from a negative view of being wrong and bad to a positive sense of a newer identity. In the clinical setting, the problematic steps within these stages should be assessed and considered as well as patient's experience of ambivalence, internalized homophobia, shame, and personal mastery.

Coming-out (of the closet) is a metaphor used to describe LGBT people's self-disclosure of their sexual orientation or their gender identity. The coming-out experience is a complex and crucial psychological process based on individual's self-acceptance of personal sexual identity and orientation and disclosure of the personal high sensitive information with selected others. It may lead to rejection in the family or friendly or societal contests and may be related to a relevant amount of psychological stress caused by possible judgment as well as discrimination and social exclusion [29]. In the clinical setting, it may be very helpful to support individuals next to their own coming-out in any stage of disclosure and self-acceptance. Also, the coming out process is a crucial construct in the framework of minority stress model by Meyer [45]. Institutions (e.g., schools, universities, health care services) should provide help and support in order to promote nd facilitate the coming-out as well as the identity concealment and disclosure (also labeled as *Visibility Concealment*) [48].

Internalized Homo/bi/trans-phobia: In 2010 a meta-analytic review of literature on the relationship between internalized homophobia/bi/trans-phobia and mental health among LGBTQIs, concluded that these constructs are significantly associated with the onset of internalizing mental disorders (e.g., depression, anxiety, stress/trauma-related disorders, obsessive-compulsive disorder, eating and dissociative disorders) [49]. Homophobia is defined as the individual inward direction of societal homophobic attitudes, including the internalization of negative attitudes leading to a conflict with the own self-regard, with a consequential self-denigration or identification with the beliefs of heterosexual aggressor [50].

10.4 The Italian Working-Group on LGBTQI Mental Health

In 2021, the *Italian Society of Social Psychiatry* chaired by Professor Andrea Fiorillo (Naples, Italy) promoted a research working-group in order to explore relevant topics in the field of LGBTQI mental health. The main findings and evidences are listed as follows:

(a) *Mental health for LGBTQI people: a policies' review* [51]: This review article aimed to search systematically and describe the international policies, guidelines, position statements, and recommendations regarding the protection and promotion of mental health rights for LGBTQI people. The authors provided a detailed list and description of documents gathered from the literature and official websites of various organizations (scientific and governmental) and concluded that more specific policies and pathways to care should be promoted in order to defend LGBTQI mental health rights and properly address their mental health needs.
(b) *Barriers in care pathways and unmet mental health needs in LGBTIQ+ communities* [52]: Findings reported that LGBTIQ individuals experience stigmatization and higher rates of

substance misuse and mental illness with relevant barriers in accessing health care services as well as a lack of specific tailored interventions.

(c) *Mental health in transgender individuals: A systematic review* [53]: the findings, in line with previous evidences, indicated that transgender individuals experience higher prevalence of mental health disorders than the general population with higher rates of substance abuse and suicide.

(d) *Self-harm and suicidality among LGBTIQ people: A systematic review and meta-analysis* [54]: this article included 50 studies comparing 3.735.601 controls and 87.252 LGBTIQ people. LGBTIQ people reported a higher risk of suicidal attempts (odds ratio [OR]: 4.36), suicidal ideation (OR: 3.76), and nonsuicidal self-injuries (OR:4.24), with higher rates of suicidality among bisexuals> gay-lesbian> transgender-intersex-queers.

(e) *Mental health and well-being of LGBTQ+ people during the COVID-19 pandemic* [55]: this article reported that LGBTQ people have reported feelings of worry about the future, negative emotions, and uncertainty during the course of COVID-19 pandemic. Also, they have experienced difficulties in the access to hormone therapy, health facilities as well as in living with family members not accepting their condition.

(f) *Microaggression toward LGBTIQ people and implications for mental health: A systematic review* [37]: This article reported that LGBTQI people experience a higher number of microaggressions (standardized mean difference [SMD]: 0.89; 95% CI [0.28, 1.50])—defined as the statements, actions, or incidents regarded as an instance of indirect, subtle, or unintentional discrimination against members of a minority group such as sexual minority, which were significantly associated with higher levels of depression, anxiety, suicide attempts, and alcohol abuse across the selected studies.

(g) *Mental health of transgender people in prison: a systematic review and meta-analysis* [56] reported on the relevant issue of the placement of transgender people in the prisons and their mental health needs. Thirteen studies were considered and compared 1255 transgenders with 174,314 controls: findings have shown that the transgender sample presented higher levels of depression, post-traumatic stress disorder and suicide attempts during the detention. Reduced access to gender-affirming treatments and heteronormative rules in the placement within the prison further compounded the challenges faced by this vulnerable population.

(h) *Ensuring equitable, inclusive and meaningful gender identity- and sexual orientation-related data collection in the healthcare sector: insights from a critical, pragmatic systematic review of the literature* [57]: Authors report that no gender identity- and sexual orientation-related data collection is routinely performed, if not for specific health or administrative/social purposes. It is suggested that implementing and ensuring equitable and inclusive socio-demographic data collection is of paramount importance since the LGBTI community suffers from a large number of communicable and non-communicable diseases.

10.5 Assessments

It is likely that LGBT individuals may experience stress or major mental health issues as well as may access to mental health services at any stage of their life. Mental health professionals need to be trained and equipped to cope with these specific psychological and mental health issues affecting this population.

The mental health professional may wear several heats and play many roles in the consultation setting as the following: (a) assessor, (b) diagnostician, (c) educator, (d) referrer, (e) psychotherapist, (f) advocate, (g) supporter, (h) counselor, (i) healer [1].

The aim of the therapeutic consultation should be to maximize the individual acceptance alongside the psychological well-being and quality of life. Any therapeutic intervention should be based on a correct and effective assessment of patient's health needs. The mental health professional should be comfortable with patient's personal view on sexuality and sexual behaviors and should help the patient to be opened and comfortable himself in telling about these personal experiences [1]. Strategies to lead patients to be fully opened on any issue, including communication skills, are essential in this clinical setting. Language and terms are also crucial and the therapist should be not afraid to use specific languages including those related to intimacy.

The personal, family, and clinical history should be collected in detail: particular interest must be accounted for the childhood and early life of patients and the social background in which they have been growing up. Any information should be collected with a non-judgmental attitude, providing empathic validation and avoiding any non-verbal message. Techniques of normalization should be very useful [1].

Life experiences of discrimination and social exclusion should be correctly collected and described. An early pathologization of life experiences should be avoided including the assignment of categorical diagnostic labels in the assessment phase: this will help the patient to be open, honest, and accurate in his/her narrative report [1].

The usage of the correct language is fundamental. Heterosexist languages or assumptions as well as stereotypes of terms leading to patients' discomfort should be avoided [1]. Examples of nonappropriate language may include the following questions: "are you married?"; Do you have a girlfriend (for homosexual males) or boyfriend (for homosexual females)?," "how many boys/girls have you dated?"; "do you have any children?"; "are you the top or bottom partner?"; "which role in sex do you prefer?"; etc.

The appropriate language may include a comfort set of questions like: "are you in a relationship?"; "Are you dating anybody currently"; use the blank of gender and not binary distinctions (male/female).

The employment of a careful and comfortable language will help the patient to open up with his/her history and intimate issues and would reduce his/her subjective feeling of being a minority [58].

As suggested by Cass [47], the assessment of all factors related to the "coming-out" is crucial.

Exploration and assessment should involve the self-acceptance and self-disclosure of the personal sexual and gender identity. The coming out process should be investigated in all its stages: (a) pre-coming out (characterized by no awareness or poor awareness of same-sex feelings and attraction); (b) coming out with selected life individuals; (c) exploration of sexual identity; (d) first same-sex relationships; (e) integration of public and private identities.

Cass proposed stages of homosexual identity formation in a theoretical model to be explored and assessed in the narrative report: (a) Identity confusion, first awareness of feelings or thoughts and behaviors (age 13–18); (b) Identity comparison with peers, accepting identity but inhibiting and normalizing the behaviors at heteronormative standards (age 13–18 years old); (c) Identity tolerance, accepting to be not the only one reporting these fantasies and desires (age 15–21); (d) Identity acceptance, accepting identity with a positive connotation and may start evaluating the coming-out (age 15–21); (e) Identity pride, enjoying the gay culture and self-image (age 18); (f) Identity synthesis, with an integration of private and public identity (age > 18).

The psychiatrist needs to help the patients with the exploration of various implications related to the coming-out in their life and personal comfort about them. All socio-cultural factors impacting on the process should be assessed and evaluated properly.

All clinical emerging issues related to the patient's personal history should be assessed and categorized according to the current nosography.

10.6 Interventions

10.6.1 Historical Approaches

In accordance with the previous models of pathologization of sexual variations, psychological and psychiatric interventions were proposed in order to *cure* the sexual deviance among LGBT people.

It has been proposed that psychotherapy, behavioral therapy, assertiveness or social skills training, hypnosis, group therapy, and intensive inpatient admissions might help the patient to change their sexual orientation into heteronormative behaviors and cognitions. These approaches are commonly known as "*reparative therapies*" or "*conversion therapies*" or "*Sexual Orientation Change Efforts.*" Based on old etiopathological explanatory models, these interventions were *totally unsuccessful* and patients did not reach any recovery to the heterosexual identity and many of them were coerced to intensive treatments including the hormonal therapies, lobotomy, electroconvulsive therapy or castration [29].

Conversion therapies did not collect any evidence of efficacy over the years and biological findings as well as newer etiological models of sexual orientations led to the concept that sexual variants are innate.

Graham [59] reviewed some other healing approaches based on spiritual leaders or so-called treatments causing physical and psychological harm: conversion techniques to induce pain, discomfort, and sometimes paralysis when individuals were aroused by homoerotic stimuli. All these approaches were largely associated with an increase in mental illness, self-harm, and suicides among LGBT.

Legal and political actions have been launched for contrasting the conversion therapies with a significant role of LGBT activism. In 2015 Obama's administration in the US released a White House statement in order to ban conversion therapies for sexual minorities [59]. Conversion therapies are also banned in those countries adopting ILGA policies and only three UN Member States did ban this practice [60].

Adamson et al. [61] performed an online survey including Europe, Latin America, Asia, Northern America, and Africa and reported that conversion therapy practices still occur around the world.

10.6.2 Current Practices

LGBT Affirmative Practice: Affirmative practice is a model of clinical care based on the conceptualization that sexual variations are part of a healthy human sexual experience. Affirmative approaches are based on principles of positive regard for LGBT subjects and the development of a therapeutic alliance or relationship characterized by dignity and self-worth.

Edwards-Leeper et al. [62] argued that clinicians should consider a holistic view of LGBT clients: considering the range of factors impacting the individual identity, environmental triggers, self-determination, and consciousness in order to promote an empowering process. Clinicians should also understand the complexities of sexual diversity, offer advocacy and validation, improve the quality of patients' care and promoting self-awareness, critical thinking, and personal insight. These approaches also aim to promote an LGBT-affirming environment contrasting the heterosexist movements and spreading LGBT culture and information.

Psychotherapies and Psychoeducation: Psychoeducation plays a key role in providing information and awareness about sexual identity, sexual variations, and related experiences [1, 63]. Psychotherapy will be employed for addressing patients' clinical needs with a supportive approach and providing suggestions for subjective well-being and environmental interactions [1]. Affirmative therapies also aim to encourage a positive self-sense of identity, a positive view of being lesbian, gay, bisexual, and transgender identities, and address negatively homophobia, transphobia, and heterosexism with their impact on patients' life.

Gay-affirmative therapist needs also: (a) to create an LGBT friendly clinical setting with specific reading material and information; (b) to use appropriate and affirming language (avoiding heteronormative assumptions); (c) to challenge heterosexist and homophobic social attitudes; (d) to challenge discrimination, cultural and religious instances implicated in the pathologization of sexual personal experience [1].

Often families, family members, as well as friends and life selected persons may be involved in the therapy and may need psycho-education in order to improve their parental and family support, which is essential for the subjective well-being in many cultures. Some other patients may need a workplace-related support as well [1]. Psychoeducation may be particularly important in reducing the level of minority stress and supporting the person during the coming-out process [63].

All clinical mental health issues including depression, anxiety, or substance use disorders should be assessed and treated properly and possible connections with the self-discomfort related to the individual sexual identity or integration into the public life should be addressed. Personal copying strategies oriented to resilience and recovery should be promoted. Also, for those people who seek gender-affirming treatments, a multidisciplinary approach should be offered in the clinical stting between psychotherapist, endocrinologist, and surgeon, on the basis of the treatment needs advanced by the person [1, 64].

Pharmacotherapies: Psychopharmacology will be employed when psychiatric issues come out from the initial assessment. In a combination approach with psychotherapy and psychoeducation, psychotropic agents may help in treating clinically significant anxiety, mood symptoms, or dysthymia that may affect patients reporting distress related to their own sexual variation. Psychotropic agent selection should take into account the possible concurrent treatments, such as hormonal therapies or antiviral treatments for any sexually transmitted disease (e.g., HIV) [1, 65].

10.7 Conclusions

Sexuality is a core part of personal identity and affects many processes in human life not only pleasure and procreation. Sexual variations are common in the general population and new conceptual frameworks promoting the sexuality spectrum model as well as sexual fluidity in the course of life have been affirming. Subjects reporting a sexual variation may experience subjective distress as well as social and cultural maladjustment. Most of personal discomfort and distress may be related to the condition of being minority (minority stress) and the coming-out process. Psychiatric morbidity and mental health issues should be carefully assessed and treated and new approaches based on affirmative therapies and psychotherapeutic interventions should be promoted to address any personal needs of LGBT individuals. Social policy and cultural interventions may also improve the acceptance level of sexual variations among societies and reduce the individual psychological burden in this population.

References

1. Kalra G, Ventriglio A, Foerster C, Bhugra D (2016) Sexual variation and mental health. In: Fiorillo A, Volpe U, Bhugra D (eds) Psychiatry in practice: education, experience, and expertise. Oxford University Press, Oxford, pp 457–474
2. Ventriglio A, Kalra G, Bhugra D (2018) Human rights and sexuality: sexual fluidity. Lancet Psychiatry 5(2):109–110. https://doi.org/10.1016/S2215-0366(18)30016-6
3. Bragazzi NL, Converti M, Crapanzano A, Zerbetto R, Siri A, Khamisy-Farah R (2023) The century-long quest for the gay gene: has the elephant given birth to a mouse? Towards sexogenomics. Available at SSRN: https://ssrn.com/abstract=4569915 or https://doi.org/10.2139/ssrn.4569915
4. Weiten W (1995) Motivation and emotion. In: Weiten W (ed) Psychology: themes and variations, 3rd edn. Brooks/Cole Publishing, Pacific Grove, CA, pp 375–415
5. Berlant L, Warner M (1998) Sex in public. Crit Inq 24(2):547–566
6. Ventriglio A, Bhugra D (2019) Sexuality in the 21st century: sexual fluidity. East Asian Arch Psychiatry 29(1):30–34
7. Mustanski BS, Chivers ML, Bailey JM (2002) A critical review of recent biological research on human sexual orientation. Annu Rev Sex Res 13:89–140
8. de Silva WP (1999) ABC of sexual health. Sexual variations. BMJ 318:654–656
9. American Psychiatric Association (2022) Diagnostic and statistical manual of mental disorders (DSM-5-TR®). American Psychiatric Association, Washington, DC
10. The World Health Organization (2021) International Statistical Classification of diseases and related health problems. ICD-11, 11th edn. WHO, Geneva
11. Eller JD (2015) Culture and diversity in the United States: so many ways to be American. Routledge, New York, p 137
12. Reimer D (2012) What does "Gender Neutral" look like?. The Gender Offender
13. Jones BE, Hill MJ (2002) Mental health issues in lesbian, gay, bisexual, and transgender communities. American Psychiatric Publishing, Washington, DC, p 95

14. Moleiro C, Pinto N (2015) Sexual orientation and gender identity: review of concepts, controversies and their relation to psychopathology classification systems. Front Psychol 6:1511
15. Kinsey AC, Pomeroy WR, Martin CE (1948) Sexual behavior in the human male. Am J Public Health 93:894–898
16. Baumeister RF (2000) Gender differences in erotic plasticity: the female sex drive as socially flexible and responsive. Psychol Bull 126:347–389
17. Kanazawa S (2017) Possible evolutionary origins of human female sexual fluidity. Biol Rev Camb Philos Soc 92:1251–1274
18. Geary RS, Tanton C, Erens B, Clifton S, Prah P, Wellings K, Mitchell KR, Datta J, Gravningen K, Fuller E, Johnson AM, Sonnenberg P, Mercer CH (2018) Sexual identity, attraction and behaviour in Britain: the implications of using different dimensions of sexual orientation to estimate the size of sexual minority populations and inform public health interventions. PLoS One 13:e0189607. https://doi.org/10.1371/journal.pone.0189607
19. The World Bank (2019) A set of proposed indicators for the LGBTI Inclusion Index. https://www.undp.org/sites/g/files/zskgke326/files/publications/ENGLISH_LGBTI_index_march2019.pdf
20. Bullough V (1974) Sexual deviance. University of Chicago Press, Chicago
21. Rahman Q, Xu Y, Lippa R, Vasey P (2020) Prevalence of sexual orientation across 28 nations and its association with gender equality, economic development and individualism. Arch Sex Behav 49:595–606
22. Gates GJ (2017) LGBT data collection amid social and demographic shifts of the US LGBT community. Am J Public Health 107(8):1220–1222
23. International Lesbian, Gay, Bisexual, Trans and Intersex Association (2019) Lucas Ramon Mendos, State-Sponsored Homophobia. ILGA World, Geneva. https://ilga.org/state-sponsored-homophobia-report-2019
24. Bhugra D, Killaspy H, Kar A, Levin S, Chumakov E, Rogoza D, Harvey C, Bagga H, Owino-Wamari Y, Everall I, Bishop A, Javate KR, Westmore I, Ahuja A, Torales J, Rubin H, Castaldelli-Maia J, Ng R, Nakajima GA, Levounis P et al (2022) IRP commission: sexual minorities and mental health: global perspectives. Int Rev Psychiatry 34(3–4):171–199
25. Roberts L (2019) Changing worldwide attitudes toward homosexuality: the influence of global and specific cultures, 1981-2012. Soc Sci Res 80:114–131
26. Mizan PA (2020) "Queer" across cultures: a decoding of the treatment of LGBTQ issues in countries with disparate cultures. Stud Indian Place Names 40(50):5129–5132
27. Kite ME, Togans LJ, Schultz TJ (2019) Stability or change? A cross-cultural look at attitudes toward sexual and gender identity minorities. In: Keith K (ed) Cross-cultural psychology: contemporary themese and perspectives, 2nd edn. https://doi.org/10.1002/9781119519348.ch20
28. Blackwood E (1986) The many faces of homosexuality: anthropological approaches to homosexual behavior. Harrington Press, New York
29. Crowell KA (2020) Sexual identity: development of the self in adolescent identity. In: Hupp S, Jewell JD (eds) The encyclopaedia of child and adolescent development. https://doi.org/10.1002/9781119171492.wecad456
30. Freud S (1962) Three essays on the theory of sexuality (trans. by J Strachey). Basic Books, New York. (1996). *Drei Abhandlungen zur Sexualtheorie*. Fischer: Frankfurt am Main. [reprint of the 1905 edition]
31. Drescher J (2015) Out of DSM: depathologising homosexuality. Behav Sci 5:565–575
32. Suess Schwend A (2020) Trans health care from a depathologization and human rights perspective. Public Health Rev 41:3. PMID: 32099728; PMCID: PMC7031999. https://doi.org/10.1186/s40985-020-0118-y
33. Spitzer RL (1981) The diagnostic status of homosexuality in DSM-III: a reformulation of the issues. Am J Psychiatry 138(2):210–215
34. King M, Semlyen J, Tai SS, Killaspy H, Osborn D, Popelyuk D, Nazareth I (2008) A systematic review of mental disorder, suicide, and deliberate self harm in lesbian, gay and bisexual people. BMC Psychiatry 8:70. https://doi.org/10.1186/1471-244X-8-70
35. Hagger-Johnson G, Taibjee R, Semlyen J et al (2013) Sexual orientation identity in relation to smoking history and alcohol use at age 18/19: cross-sectional associations from the longitudinal study of young people in England (LSYPE). BMJ Open 3:e002810. https://doi.org/10.1136/bmjopen-2013-002810
36. Pitonak M (2017) Mental health in non-heterosexuals: minority stress theory and related explanations frameworks review. Ment Health Prev 5:63–73
37. Marchi M, Travascio A, Uberti D, De Micheli E, Quartaroli F, Laquatra G, Grenzi P, Pingani L, Ferrari S, Fiorillo A, Converti M, Pinna F, Amaddeo F, Ventriglio A, Mirandola M, Galeazzi GM (2023b) Microaggression toward LGBTIQ people and implications for mental health: a systematic review. Int J Soc Psychiatry 70:23
38. Conron KJ, Mimiaga MJ, Landers SJ (2010) A populations-based study of sexual orientation identity and gender differences in adult health. Am J Public Health 100(10):1953–1960
39. Hatzenbuehler ML, Keyes KM, Hasin D (2009) State-level policies and psychiatric morbidity in lesbian, gay and bisexual populations. Am J Public Health 99:2275–2281
40. Hatzenbuehler ML, O'Cleingh C, Grasso C, Meyer K, Safren S, Bradford J (2012a) Effect of same sex marriage laws on health care use and expenditures in sexual minority men: a quasi-natural experiment. Am J Public Health 102:285–291
41. Hatzenbuehler ML, Pachanks JE, Wolff J (2012b) Religious climate and health risk behaviors in sexual minority youths: a population based study. Am J Public Health 102:657–671
42. McNair RP, Hegarty K (2010) Guidelines for the primary care of lesbian, gay, and bisexual people: a sys-

tematic review. Ann Fam Med 8(6):533–541. https://doi.org/10.1370/afm.1173
43. Hillier L, Hrrison L (2004) Homophobia and the production of shame: young people and same sex attraction. Cult Health Sex 6(1):79–94. https://doi.org/10.1080/1369105031000161156
44. National LGBTI Health Alliance (2020) The statistics at a glance: the mental health of lesbian, gay, bisexual, transgender and intersex people in Australia. National LGBTI Health Alliance, Sydney
45. Meyer IH (1995) Minority stress and mental health in gay men. J Health Soc Behav 36(1):38–56
46. Affuso G, Picone N, Costa PA, Bacchini D, De Angelis G, Esposito C, Aparicio-García ME (2023) Minority stress and mental health in gay and lesbian youth: a comparative study of Italy and Spain. Am J Orthopsychiatry 94:148. https://doi.org/10.1037/ort0000709
47. Cass V (1979) Homosexuality identity formation: a theoretical model. J Homosex 4:219–235
48. Beagan BL, Sibbald KR, Bizzeth SR, Pride TM (2023) Factors influencing LGBTQ+ disclosure decision-making by Canadian health professionals: a qualitative study. PLoS One 18(2):e0280558. https://doi.org/10.1371/journal.pone.0280558
49. Newcomb ME, Mustanski B (2010) Internalized homophobia and internalizing mental health problems: a meta-analytic review. Clin Psychol Rev 30(8):1019–1029. Epub 2010 Jul 24. https://doi.org/10.1016/j.cpr.2010.07.003
50. Allport G (1954) The nature of prejudice. Addison-Wesley, Reading, MA
51. Ventriglio A, Mirandola M, Galeazzi GM, Amaddeo F, Pinna F, Converti M, Fiorillo A, Italian Working-Group on LGBTQI Mental Health (2022) Mental health for LGBTQI people: a policies' review. Int Rev Psychiatry 34(3–4):200–214
52. Silveri G, Schimmenti S, Prina E, Gios L, Mirandola M, Converti M, Fiorillo A, Pinna F, Ventriglio A, Galeazzi GM, Sherriff N, Zeeman L, Amaddeo F, Italian Working Group on LGBTQI Mental Health (2022) Barriers in care pathways and unmet mental health needs in LGBTIQ + communities. Int Rev Psychiatry 34(3–4):215–229
53. Pinna F, Paribello P, Somaini G, Corona A, Ventriglio A, Corrias C, Frau I, Murgia R, El Kacemi S, Galeazzi GM, Mirandola M, Amaddeo F, Crapanzano A, Converti M, Piras P, Suprani F, Manchia M, Fiorillo A, Carpiniello B, Italian Working Group on LGBTQI Mental Health (2022) Mental health in transgender individuals: a systematic review. International review of psychiatry (Abingdon, England), 34(3-4), 292–359. https://doi.org/10.1080/09540261.2022.2093629
54. Marchi M, Arcolin E, Fiore G, Travascio A, Uberti D, Amaddeo F, Converti M, Fiorillo A, Mirandola M, Pinna F, Ventriglio A, Galeazzi GM, Italian Working Group on LGBTIQ Mental Health (2022) Self-harm and suicidality among LGBTIQ people: a systematic review and meta-analysis. Int Rev Psychiatry 34(3–4):240–256
55. Sampogna G, Ventriglio A, Di Vincenzo M, Del Vecchio V, Giallonardo V, Bianchini V, Fiorillo A (2022) Mental health and Well-being of LGBTQ+ people during the COVID-19 pandemic. Int Rev Psychiatry 34(3–4):432–438
56. Marchi M, Corbellini I, Vaccari E, Pingani L, Ferrari S, Amaddeo F, Converti M, Fiorillo A, Mirandola M, Pinna F, Ventriglio A, Galeazzi GM (2023c) Mental health of transgender people in prison: a systematic review and meta-analysis. Int Rev Psychiatry:1–15. https://doi.org/10.1080/09540261.2023.2287680
57. Bragazzi NL, Khamisy-Farah R, Converti M, Italian Working-Group on LGBTIQ Mental Health (2022) Ensuring equitable, inclusive and meaningful gender identity- and sexual orientation-related data collection in the healthcare sector: insights from a critical, pragmatic systematic review of the literature. Int Rev Psychiatry 34(3–4):282–291. https://doi.org/10.1080/09540261.2022.2076583
58. Kuyper L, Fokkema T (2011) Minority stress and mental health among Dutch LGBs: examination of differences between sex and sexual orientation. J Couns Psychol 58(2):222–233. https://doi.org/10.1037/a0022688
59. Graham TC (2019) Conversion therapy: a brief reflection on the history of the practice and contemporary regulatory efforts. Creighton Law Rev 149:419–425
60. Mendos LR (2019) ILGA world—the international lesbian, gay, bisexual, trans and intersex association state-sponsored homophobia: global legislation overview update. ILGA, Geneva
61. Adamson T, Wallach S, Garner A, Hanley M, Howell S (2020) The global state of conversion therapy—a preliminary report and current evidence brief. LGBT Foundation, Manchester
62. Edwards-Leeper L, Leibowitz S, Sangganjanavanich V, F. (2016) Affirmative practice with transgender and gender nonconforming youth: expanding the model. Psychol Sex Orientat Gend Divers 3(2):165–172
63. Iuso S, Petito A, Ventriglio A, Severo M, Bellomo A, Limone P (2022) The impact of psycho-education on school-children's homophobic attitudes. Int Rev Psychiatry 34(3–4):266–273. https://doi.org/10.1080/09540261.2022.2034603
64. Coleman E, Radix AE, Bouman WP, Brown GR, de Vries ALC, Deutsch MB, Ettner R, Fraser L, Goodman M, Green J, Hancock AB, Johnson TW, Karasic DH, Knudson GA, Leibowitz SF, Meyer-Bahlburg HFL, Monstrey SJ, Motmans J, Nahata L, Nieder TO et al (2022) Standards of Care for the Health of transgender and gender diverse people, version 8. Int J Transgender Health 23(Suppl 1):S1–S259. https://doi.org/10.1080/26895269.2022.2100644
65. Kelly TM, Daley DC (2013) Integrated treatment of substance use and psychiatric disorders. Soc Work Public Health 28(3–4):388–406. https://doi.org/10.1080/19371918.2013.774673

Promoting Mental Health in Low-Resource Settings: Focus on WHO Psychological Interventions

11

Corrado Barbui, Monica Bianca Bartucz, and Marianna Purgato

Abstract

In low-resource settings, marginalized communities, refugees, and impoverished populations encounter numerous risk factors that amplify psychological distress and elevate the susceptibility to mental disorders. These risk factors encompass poverty, inadequate healthcare access, heightened prevalence of infectious diseases, conflict, violence, displacement, and social and cultural obstacles. The World Health Organization (WHO) World Mental Health Report 2022 advocates for addressing these challenges by prioritizing individual autonomy and adopting person-centered interventions. These interventions, integrated into existing health and social services, aim to promote mental health and prevent mental disorder onset among vulnerable populations.

This chapter introduces a compendium of low-intensity psychological interventions aligned with the WHO's principles, specifically tailored or adapted to cater to diverse adversities faced by populations in low-resource settings. Through a systematic review and critical evaluation, we scrutinize the evidence base underpinning their effectiveness and analyze their feasibility and potential for widespread implementation.

By leveraging a person-centered approach, these interventions seek to empower individuals within vulnerable populations, offering support tailored to their unique circumstances while respecting their autonomy. Through this comprehensive approach, we aim to mitigate the impact of risk factors, bolster resilience, and foster mental well-being among populations confronting significant adversities in low-resource settings.

Keywords

Migrants · Refugees · Mental disorders
Psychosocial interventions · Prevention

11.1 Introduction

Low-resource settings are home to populations, including marginalized communities, refugees, and those living in poverty, who face numerous risk factors that may exacerbate psychological distress and increase the likelihood of developing mental disorders [1–4] (Charlson 2019, # 3186). These risk factors include poverty, limited access to healthcare, a high prevalence of infectious diseases, conflict, violence, displacement, and social

C. Barbui (✉) · M. B. Bartucz · M. Purgato
WHO Collaborating Centre for Research and Training in Mental Health and Service Evaluation, Section of Psychiatry, Department of Neurosciences, Biomedicine and Movement Sciences, University of Verona, Verona, Italy
e-mail: corrado.barbui@univr.it; monicabianca.bartucz@univr.it; marianna.purgato@univr.it

A. Fiorillo, S. De Giorgi (eds.), *Social Determinants of Mental Health*, Sustainable Development Goals Series, https://doi.org/10.1007/978-3-031-70165-8_11

and cultural challenges [5]. In an effort to tackle these risk factors and to protect the mental health of vulnerable population groups, the World Health Organization (WHO) World Mental Health Report 2022 proposes the development and implementation of interventions that prioritize the autonomy of individuals with mental health conditions, while adopting a person-centered approach [6]. These interventions should be integrated into existing health and social services, with a specific emphasis on promoting mental health and preventing the onset of mental disorders. In this chapter, we introduce a collection of low-intensity psychological interventions that adhere to these overarching principles, specifically designed or adapted by the WHO to cater to populations facing diverse adversities [7]. We systematically review and critically evaluate the evidence base supporting their effectiveness, while also analyzing their feasibility and potential for widespread implementation.

11.2 Risk Factors for Psychological Distress and Mental Disorders

Poverty is strongly associated with mental health problems due to chronic stress, inadequate living conditions, and limited access to essential resources [8]. Financial hardships can lead to feelings of helplessness, hopelessness, and social exclusion, increasing the risk of depression, anxiety, and other mental disorders. In low-resource settings, poverty also hinders the delivery of adequate mental healthcare, resulting in limited or nonexistent access to quality services [9, 10]. The lack of trained professionals, infrastructure, and resources further hampers the identification, diagnosis, and treatment of mental health conditions. Without early intervention and appropriate support, the severity and impact of mental health problems are exacerbated [6, 11].

Additionally, many low-resource settings are prone to conflict, violence, including armed conflicts, civil unrest, and natural disasters. These situations may all lead to internal displacement and migration. The psychosocial consequences of the exposure to humanitarian crises are trauma, loss of access to school and healthcare, forced family separation, violence, torture, insecure access to food and shelter, and disruption of social support networks, all of which contribute to an increased risk of mental health problems [12–15]. For example, individuals exposed to violence and displacement may develop post-traumatic stress disorder (PTSD), depression, and anxiety disorders [16, 17].

Moreover, people living in low-resource settings often face social and cultural challenges that impact their mental health. Stigmatization, discrimination, and cultural beliefs surrounding mental health discourage individuals from seeking help or openly discussing their concerns [18]. Lack of awareness, misconceptions, and inadequate education about mental health contribute to the under-recognition and under-treatment of mental health conditions in these settings [19, 20].

It is crucial to emphasize that these risk factors, which can determine or worsen psychological distress and elevate the chances of developing mental disorders, are applicable to low-resource settings, which may only partially align with the standard World Bank notion and criteria for defining low-income countries [21]. The categorization of countries solely based on income, such as low-income and middle-income countries, has been widely used for a long time to assess the economic status and development of nations. However, there has been a growing recognition among researchers and policymakers that the income-based classification may not accurately capture the true challenges and resource constraints faced by countries. It oversimplifies the complex realities of different countries. For example, some middle-income countries may have a high burden of disease, inadequate healthcare infrastructure, or limited access to essential resources like clean water and sanitation. Conversely, certain high-income countries may have resource constraints in specific sectors, such as healthcare or education, due to budgetary limitations or disparities in regional development [21]. This realization has led to the emergence of a more nuanced concept called low-resource settings, which recognizes that even countries classified as middle-income or high-income can experience significant resource constraints in certain sectors or regions [21]. This shift in perspective is crucial because it helps to focus attention on the specific resource limitations that hinder progress and development, regardless of a country's overall economic status. Consequently, risk factors like poverty, restricted healthcare access, a high prevalence of infectious diseases, conflict, violence, displacement, and social and cultural challenges can heighten psychological distress and susceptibility to the onset of mental disorders in countries at any level of economic development.

11.3 Protecting the Mental Health of Vulnerable Population Groups

In order to better support populations exposed to risk factors that can worsen psychological distress and increase the chances of developing mental disorders, several psychological interventions have been developed over the years. A growing body of randomized studies, followed by systematic reviews and meta-analyses, have documented their effectiveness in addressing various mental health outcomes [14, 22–30]. However, implementing these interventions in low-resource settings poses challenges due to the need for a well-trained clinical workforce with a mental health background, extensive training time, a monitoring and supervision infrastructure, and predominantly face-to-face individual delivery methods.

As these characteristics make them unlikely to be highly scaled-up, especially in low-resource settings, and their inability to effectively meet the needs of a large number of individuals while optimizing resource utilization, the WHO has developed a range of low-intensity psychological interventions for populations affected by diverse adversities [7]. These interventions have a key characteristic: they can be taught and administered by para-professional helpers, such as trained peers, workplace assistants, nurses, teachers, or psychosocial workers. This approach, known as task-shifting, involves transferring tasks from highly qualified healthcare workers to those with less extensive qualifications, thereby maximizing the efficient use of available resources [31].

The WHO psychological interventions are typically short in duration and follow well-defined protocols, enabling para-professional helpers to deliver them with fidelity. They have been designed to be applicable to a wide array of mental health problems, regardless of specific diagnoses, and can be easily adapted to different population groups, cultures, and languages. Moreover, the interventions and their implementation materials are openly accessible, and various delivery modalities can be employed, including the online version through mobile phones, laptops, or other devices.

As described in Table 11.1, available WHO psychological interventions may target the mental health needs of multiple age groups across various delivery models to reach diverse target populations [32–42]. They are short in duration, and their main aim is to reduce depression, anxiety, and psychological distress, and to improve functioning, coping with daily problems, well-being, and quality of life (Table 11.1).

Table 11.1 Main characteristics of WHO psychological interventions

Intervention	Theoretical framework	Target population	Format	Delivery	Sessions	Provider	Intervention manual available	Languages available
Problem Management Plus (PM+)	Based on Cognitive Behavioural Therapy	Adults with depression, anxiety, and stress	Individual or group	Face-to-face in person or online (synchronous)	Five	Trained lay facilitators	Yes	English, Arabic, Bengali, Chinese, English, French, Greek, Italian, Japanese, Kenyan, Korean, Kurdish/Badini, Portuguese, Russian, Serbian, Spanish, Tigrinya, Ukrainian, Urdu; Group: English, Urdu, Nepali, Portuguese, Spanish
Step-by-Step (SbS)	Based on Cognitive Behavioural Therapy	Adults with depression	Individual	Digital	Five	Mobile App	No	English, Arabic, Filipino
Self-Help Plus (SH+)	Based on Acceptance and Commitment Therapy	Adults in adversity	Group	Face-to-face in person	Five	Trained lay facilitators	Yes	English, Arabic, Juba, Spanish, Turkish, Ukrainian
Doing What Matters (DWM)	Based on Acceptance and Commitment Therapy	Adults in adversity	Individual	Digital	Five	Digital book and audio files	Yes	English, English versions adapted for the Caribbean and South Sudan, Juba, Arabic, Armenian, Chinese, Dari, Estonian, Farsi, Finnish, French, German, Georgian, Greek, Hungarian, Italian, Korean, Japanese, Lithuanian, Malay, Portuguese, Romanian, Russian, Spanish, Slovak, Tongan, Turkish, Ukrainian, Urdu, Vietnamese
Early Adolescent Skills for Emotions (EASE)	Based on Cognitive Behavioural Therapy	Young adolescents with depression, anxiety, and stress	Group	Face-to-face in person	7 sessions with young adolescents +3 sessions with caregivers	Trained lay facilitators	Yes	English, Arabic, Bengali, French, Italian, Turkish, Urdu

(continued)

Table 11.1 (continued)

Intervention	Theoretical framework	Target population	Format	Delivery	Sessions	Provider	Intervention manual available	Languages available
Sustainable Technology for Adolescents to Reduce Stress (STARS)	Based on Cognitive Behavioural Therapy	Young adolescents with depression, anxiety, stress	Individual	Digital	Ten	Chatbot	No	English
Thinking Healthy (TH)	Based on Cognitive Behavioural Therapy	Mothers exposed to psychosocial pressure	Individual	Face-to-face in person	16	Trained community health workers	Yes	English, Arabic, Bengali, French, Italian, Turkish, Urdu
Group Interpersonal Therapy (IPT-G)	Based on Interpersonal Psychotherapy	Adults with depression	Group	Face-to-face in person	Eight	Trained lay facilitators	Yes	English, Arabic, Chinese, Farsi, French, Russian, Spanish, Swahili

11.4 Evidence Base Supporting the Adoption of WHO Psychosocial Interventions

11.4.1 Methodological Considerations

The WHO planned to release psychosocial intervention manuals and implementation materials only when at least two high-quality randomized controlled trials (RCTs) have demonstrated their efficacy [7]. This policy, which aims at promoting the use of evidence-based interventions only, is ground-breaking considering the lack of specific standards about the type and quantity of evidence required before a new psychological intervention is made available for everyday use [43]. For interventions supported by experimental evidence of efficacy, the WHO called for further studies and research activities aiming at delineating how interventions may be scaled up into routine care, either in series with existing health and social care or in parallel with available services [7].

Notably, the term "scaling up" encompasses various research activities that use different methodologies to achieve diverse objectives [44]. The ultimate goal is to get evidence-based psychosocial interventions into routine and sustained use. As reported in Fig. 11.1, once psychosocial interventions have demonstrated effectiveness through randomized trials, real-world studies can be developed to assess how they should be adapted to local socio-cultural contexts and implemented into routine care. The term "implementation" refers to methods or techniques designed to enhance their adoption [44] (Fig. 11.1). Examples may include delivery modalities (individual, group, in-person, digital), reminders, interactive education, and others. Implementation outcomes may include acceptability, feasibility, fidelity, costs, sustainability, appropriateness, penetration, and adoption (see Table 11.2 for definitions of these terms). It is interesting to note that in order to achieve these goals, a combination of qualitative and quantitative methods may be utilized (Fig. 11.1) [45, 46]. Typically, qualitative approaches involving a wide range of stakeholders are used to identify barriers and facilitators to the adoption of a new intervention. Qualitative research can also aid in customizing a psychosocial intervention to a specific population and context, a process that is called adaptation. Quantitative approaches, or a mix of qualitative and quantitative approaches, are used to identify effective implementation strategies. Notably, these quantitative approaches may adopt a ran-

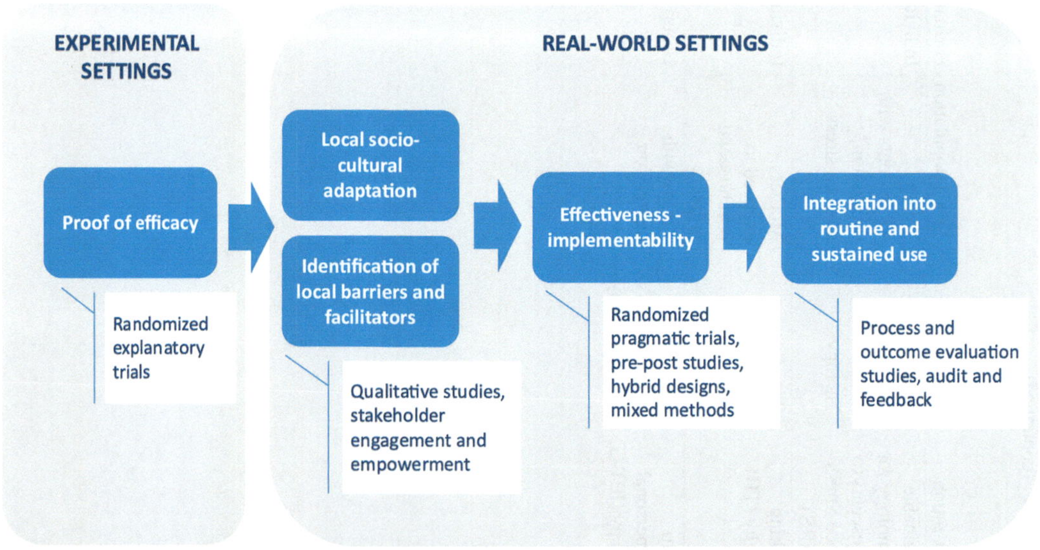

Fig. 11.1 Scaling up phases of psychological interventions

Table 11.2 Implementation outcomes definitions

Implementation outcome	Definition
Acceptability	The perception of stakeholders that the intervention is agreeable or satisfactory
Feasibility	The extent to which an intervention can be successfully carried out
Fidelity	The extent to which the intervention was implemented according to its original design
Implementation costs	The overall cost of delivery of an intervention
Sustainability	The maintenance of an intervention and its continued use
Appropriateness	The fit, relevance, or compatibility of the intervention for the setting, service provider or service user
Penetration	The integration of the intervention into a routine service or a measure of how many of those eligible are receiving it
Adoption	The process of putting an intervention to use

domized design, for example, aiming at the comparison of different implementation strategies, and may consider, as outcomes, both implementation indicators and clinical measures of improvement. The combination of implementation and effectiveness outcomes is referred to as hybrid design by Curran and colleagues [44], who proposed three types of hybrid studies: (1) testing effects of a clinical intervention on relevant outcomes while observing and gathering information on implementation; (2) dual testing of clinical and implementation interventions/strategies; and (3) testing of an implementation strategy while observing and gathering information on the clinical intervention's impact on relevant outcomes [44]. As a final step in the path from the generation of evidence to its uptake in practice, process and outcome evaluation studies, and audit and feedback initiatives, may be conducted to monitor the delivery and impact of interventions that have been adopted into sustained use (Fig. 11.1).

11.4.2 Studies Assessing WHO Psychosocial Interventions

The evidence base in support of WHO psychosocial interventions consists of 21 experimental studies that assessed their efficacy, 15 evaluations of local barriers and facilitators to implementation, 13 studies describing local socio-cultural adaptation, 33 hybrid effectiveness-implementation studies, and 4 evaluations of how interventions were integrated into routine care (Fig. 11.2). The distribution of these studies across scaling up phases and type of psychosocial intervention are graphically represented in Fig. 11.3. Box 11.1 presents the methodology that was employed to retrieve the included studies, and Box 11.2 includes the corresponding references.

The efficacy of Problem Management Plus (PM+) is supported by 19 randomized trials (3890 participants overall) that assessed both individual and group PM+. Interestingly, some trials that were conducted with the primary aim of assessing efficacy included implementation outcomes, or embedded into the trial design qualitative approaches to adapt PM+ to local context and target populations. In addition to studies with a specific focus on efficacy, a combination of qualitative and quantitative methods was used to assess a variety of implementation and effectiveness outcomes (Table 11.3). The target populations and settings mostly consisted of vulnerable participants, for example, refugees and women exposed to adversities, recruited in poor-resource settings (Table 11.3). Studies indicated that PM+ was feasible, safe, and acceptable to target populations. It also resulted in clinically meaningful improvements in psychological distress, general mental health, depression, and anxiety (Table 11.3). Notably, some studies have shown that the positive impact of PM+ remained evident during follow-up evaluations. One study evaluated the scaling up of PM+ into routine care. For SbS, the digital version of PM+, a randomized trial conducted in a population of adult Syrian refugees with moderate-to-severe depressive symptoms resettled in Lebanon found significant reductions in depressive symptoms and functional impairment at postintervention and 3-month follow-up (Table 11.3). Similar results were obtained by a second study conducted among people suffering from depression and impaired functioning in Lebanon (Table 11.3).

The efficacy of Self-Help Plus (SH+) is supported by three randomized trials (1795 participants overall). The digital version of SH+, called Doing What Matters (DWM), was studied in a randomized trial designed to assess feasibility and acceptability rather than efficacy. A second trial, conducted in a sample of adult health workers in Italy during the coronavirus disease 2019 (COVID-19) period, failed to show a significant reduction in the proportion of anxiety and PTSD symptoms at 6 months follow-up. However, there are currently several ongoing or recently completed efficacy trials for DWM. As for PM+, trials conducted with the primary aim of assessing efficacy included implementation outcomes, or embedded into the trial design qualitative approaches to study adaptation to target populations and implementation into local contexts. Overall, results suggested that SH+ was feasible, safe, and generally acceptable to target populations. It also resulted in clinically meaningful improvements in psychological distress, depression, and anxiety. Interestingly, two randomized trials, one conducted in Western Europe and another in Turkey, have recently assessed the preventative effect of SH+ in refugee populations [47, 48]. Both the Western European and Turkey studies showed evidence of an effect of SH+ in preventing the onset of mental disorders and reducing stress, but differences were observed between the studies. The effect was much more pronounced for the Turkey study, where efficacy (i.e., reducing the frequency of any mental disorder) was observed at 6 months, compared to the Western European study, where beneficial effects were only found immediately postintervention and not after 6 months [47, 48].

The Early Adolescent Skills for Emotions (EASE) intervention's effectiveness was evaluated in a trial with Syrian refugee children, adolescents, and adult caregivers in Jordan (Table 11.3). It randomized more than 470 participants and found a significant reduction in children internalizing problems after 3 months of follow-up. No significant results for children with externalizing problems and attention difficulties were observed (Table 11.3). Using quali-

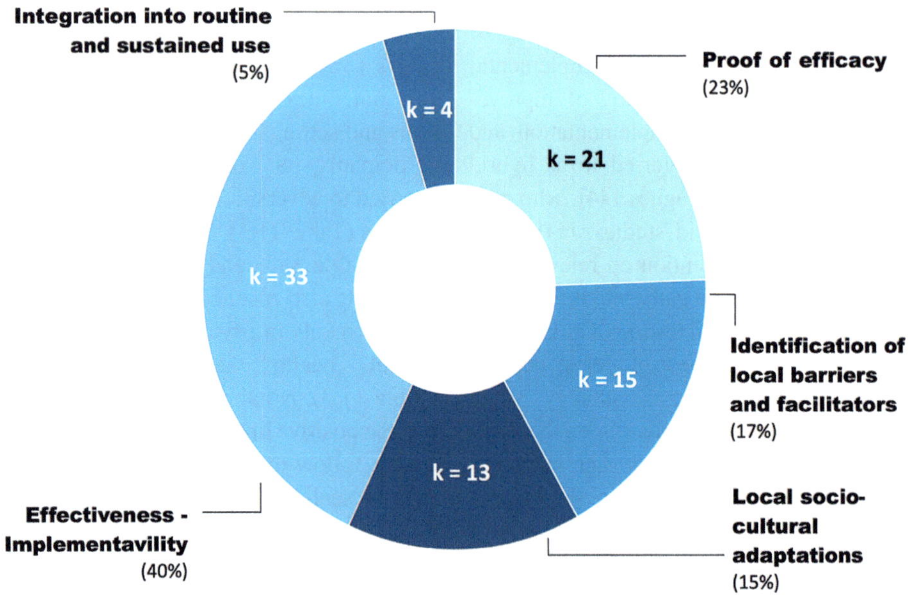

Fig. 11.2 The distribution of studies included in the systematic review across the scaling up phases of psychosocial interventions ($k = 52$)

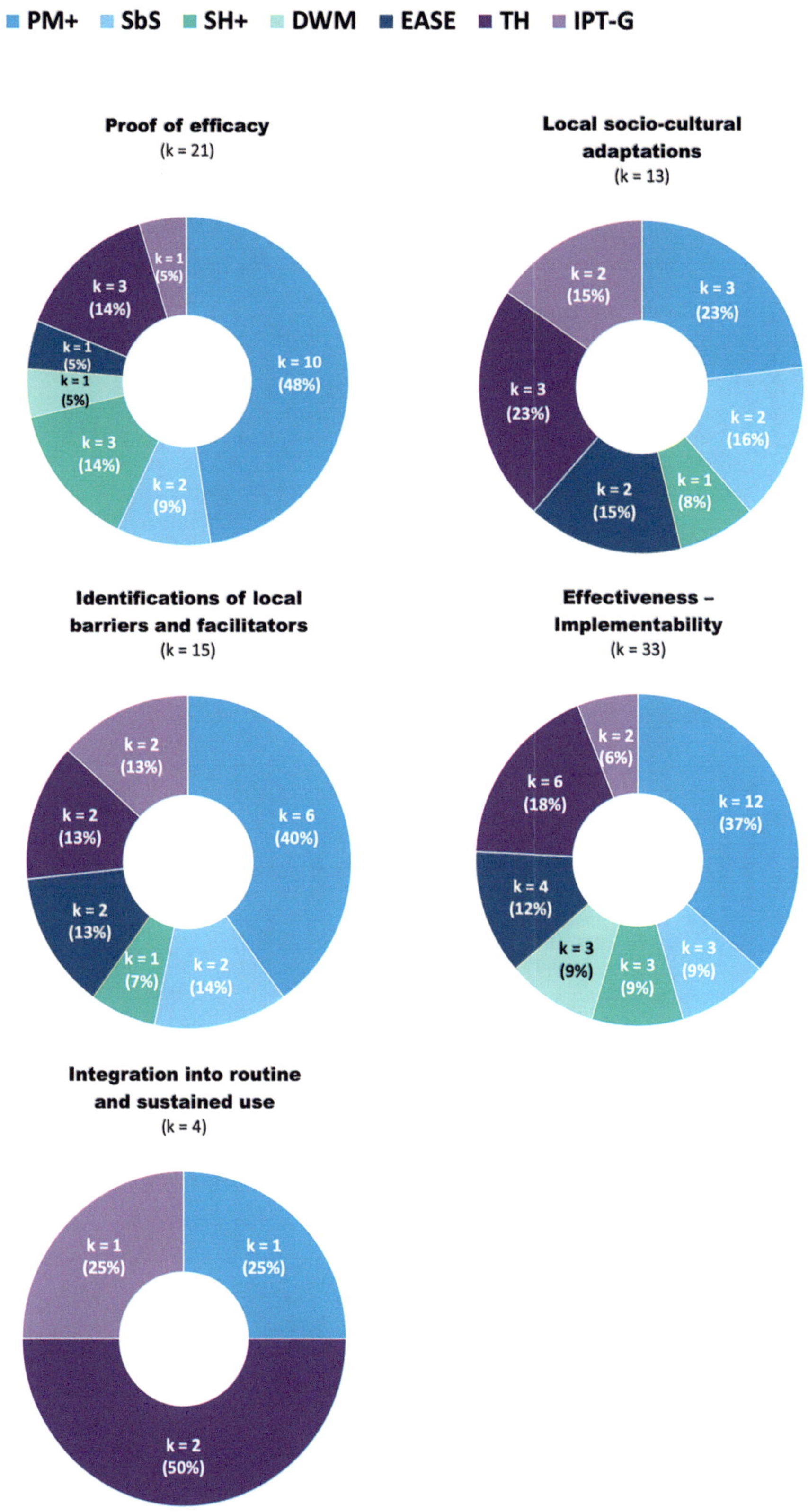

Fig. 11.3 The distribution of studies included in the systematic review across scaling up phases and type of psychosocial intervention ($k = 52$)

Table 11.3 Characteristics, primary outcome findings, and classification of completed studies

ID	Author	Intervention	Country of recruitment	Population	Design	N	Primary outcome findings	Classification
1	Dawson et al. (2016)	Individual PM+; in-person; guided	Kenya	Adult women affected by gender-based violence	RCT	56	PM+ was feasible, safe, and acceptable	Effectiveness—Implementability
2	Bryant et al. (2017)	Individual PM+; in-person; guided	Kenya	Adult women affected by gender-based violence	RCT	421	Significant improvement in psychological distress at post-test and at 3 months follow-up	Proof of efficacy
3	Rahman et al. (2016a)	Individual PM+; in person; guided	Pakistan	Adult patients from primary care centers	RCT	60	PM+ was feasible, safe, and acceptable	Effectiveness—Implementability
4a	Rahman et al. (2016b)	Individual PM+; in person; guided	Pakistan	Adult patients from primary care centers	RCT	346	Significant improvement in anxiety and depression symptoms at 3 months follow-up	Proof of efficacy
4b	Hamdani et al. (2020); same sample as Rahman et al. (2016b)	Individual PM+; in person; guided	Pakistan	Adult patients from primary care centers	RCT	346	PM+ was more expensive than EUC	Effectiveness—Implementability
5	Hamdani et al. (2021)	Individual PM+; in-person; guided	Pakistan	Adult outpatients from primary care centers	RCT	192	Significant reduction in anxiety symptoms between groups at 20 weeks follow-up. Significant differences for depressive symptoms only at postintervention	Proof of efficacy Integration into routine and sustained use

(continued)

Table 11.3 (continued)

ID	Author	Intervention	Country of recruitment	Population	Design	N	Primary outcome findings	Classification
6	Saraf et al. (2019)	Group PM+; in-person; guided	Pakistan	Adult entrepreneurs	RCT; mixed methods	235	No significant differences in the prevalence of depression and anxiety symptoms between groups at 3 months follow-up	Local socio-cultural adaptations Proof of efficacy Effectiveness—Implementability
7	Khan et al. (2019)	Group PM+; in-person; guided	Pakistan	Adult women Exposed to Adversity	cRCT; mixed methods	119	gPM+ was feasible, safe, and acceptable	Effectiveness—Implementability Identifications of local barriers and facilitators
8	Rahman et al. (2019)	Group PM+; in-person; guided	Pakistan	Adult women affected by gender-based violence	cRCT	612	Significant improvement in combined anxiety and depression symptoms at 3 months follow-up	Proof of efficacy
9	Sangraula et al. (2020)	Group PM+; in-person; guided	Nepal	Adults in humanitarian crises	RCT	121	PM+ was feasible, safe, and acceptable	Effectiveness—Implementability Identifications of local barriers and facilitators
10	Jordans et al. (2021)	Group PM+; in-person; guided	Nepal	Adults in humanitarian crises	cRCT	611	Significant improvement in psychological distress at 3 months follow-up	Proof of efficacy
11	Akhtar et al. (2021a)	Group PM+; in-person; guided	Jordan	Adult Syrian refugees	RCT	64	gPM+ was feasible, safe, and acceptable	Effectiveness—Implementability
12a	Bryant et al. (2022a)	Group PM+; in-person; guided	Jordan	Adult Syrian refugees	RCT	410	Significant improvement in depressive symptoms at 3 months follow-up. No significant results for anxiety symptoms	Proof of efficacy

(continued)

Table 11.3 (continued)

ID	Author	Intervention	Country of recruitment	Population	Design	N	Primary outcome findings	Classification
12b	Bryant et al. (2022b)	Group PM+; in-person; guided	Jordan	Adult Syrian refugees	RCT	410	No significant improvements in depressive and anxiety symptoms at 12 months follow-up	Proof o efficacy
13	Acarturk et al. (2022a)	Group PM+; in person; guided	Turkey	Adult Syrian refugees	RCT; mixed methods	46	gPM+ was feasible, safe, and acceptable	Effectiveness—Implementability Identifications of local barriers and facilitators
14	Spaaij et al. (2022)	Individual PM+; in-person; guided	Switzerland	Adult Syrian refugees	RCT; mixed methods	59	PM+ was feasible, safe, and acceptable	Effectiveness—Implementability Identifications of local barriers and facilitators
15	Dowrick et al. (2022)	Individual and Group PM+; in-person; guided	United Kingdom	Adult refugees and asylum seekers from Iran, Afghanistan, India, Iraq, Namibia, Nigeria, Pakistan, Yemen	RCT; mixed methods	105	The recruitment of participants was not finalized. The process of retention was found feasible	Effectiveness—Implementability Identifications of local barriers and facilitators Local socio-cultural adaptations
16	Perera et al. (2020)	Individual PM+; in person; guided	Colombia	Adult stakeholders working with Venezuelan migrants and refugees or Colombian returnees	Qualitative	6	Incorporation of culturally specific social activities and community support networks, inclusion of local common problems and explanatory models of distress, adaptation of pictures and terminology	Identifications of local barriers and facilitators Local socio-cultural adaptations

(continued)

Table 11.3 (continued)

ID	Author	Intervention	Country of recruitment	Population	Design	N	Primary outcome findings	Classification
17	Perera et al. (2022)	Individual PM+; in person; guided	Colombia	Adult Venezuelan migrants, refugees, or Colombian returnees	RCT; mixed methods	79	Significant improvement in well-being, personal problems, and quality of life at postintervention	Proof of efficacy Effectiveness—Implementability
18	Knefel et al. (2020)	Individual PM+; in-person; guided	Austria	Adult Afghan refugees and asylum seekers	RCT	88	Significant improvements in general mental health at postintervention	Proof of efficacy
19	de Graaff et al. (2020)	Individual PM+; in-person andonline; guided	Netherlands	Adult Syrian refugees	RCT; mixed methods	60	PM+ was feasible, safe, and acceptable	Effectiveness—Implementability
20	de Graaff et al. (2023)	Individual PM+; in-person and online; guided	Netherlands	Adult Syrian refugees	RCT	206	Significant improvement in depressive and anxiety symptoms at 3 months follow-up	Proof of efficacy
21	Abi Ramia et al. (2018)	SbS; digital; guided	Lebanon	Adult stakeholders and beneficiaries from Lebanon, Syria, Palestine	Qualitative	11	The feasibility of the intervention was debatable due to the low quality of the internet connection, busy lifestyle, and length of the sessions. Content and structural adaptations were recommended	Identifications of local barriers and facilitators Local socio-cultural adaptations
22	Burchert et al. (2018)	SbS; digital; optional guidance	Germany, Sweden, and Egypt	Adult Syrian refugees	Qualitative	128	The primary obstacles to implementation were acceptability, credibility, and technical requirements	Identifications of local barriers and facilitators

(continued)

Table 11.3 (continued)

ID	Author	Intervention	Country of recruitment	Population	Design	N	Primary outcome findings	Classification
23	Garabiles et al. (2019)	SbS digital; optional guidance	Philippines	Adult Filipino overseas workers	Qualitative	28	Incorporation of cultural values and destigmatizing content. Political or unacceptable content was removed. The text was simplified using both English and Filipino languages	Local socio-cultural adaptations
24	Heim et al. (2021)	SbS; digital; guided	Lebanon	Adult Syrian and Palestinian refugees and Lebanese citizens	RCT; mixed methods	138	SbS was feasible, safe, and acceptable	Effectiveness—Implementability
25	Cuijpers et al. (2022a)	SbS; digital; guided	Lebanon	Adult Syrian refugees	RCT	569	Significant reduction in depressive symptoms and functional impairment at post-test and 3 months follow-up	Proof of efficacy Effectiveness—Implementability
26	Cuijpers et al. (2022b)	SbS; digital; guided	Lebanon	Adults with moderate or severe depression	RCT	680	Significant reduction in depressive symptoms and functional impairment at post-test and 3 months follow-up	Proof of efficacy Effectiveness—Implementability
27	Tol et al. (2018a)	SH+; in-person; guided	Uganda	Adult Sudanese female refugees	Mixed methods	65	Adaptation to language, graphics, scheduling, and the roles of facilitators	Local socio-cultural adaptations Identifications of local barriers and facilitators Effectiveness—Implementability
28	Tol et al. (2018b)	SH+; in-person; guided	Uganda	Adult Sudanese female refugees	RCT; mixed methods	50	SH+ was feasible, safe, and acceptable	Effectiveness—Implementability

(continued)

Table 11.3 (continued)

ID	Author	Intervention	Country of recruitment	Population	Design	N	Primary outcome findings	Classification
29	Tol et al. (2020)	SH+; in-person; guided	Uganda	Adult Sudanese female refugees	cRCT	694	Significant improvement in psychological distress at postintervention and 3 months follow-up	Proof of efficacy
30a	Purgato et al. (2021)	SH+; in-person; guided	Western Europe	Adult refugees and asylum seekers from Afghanistan, Iraq, Nigeria, Pakistan, Syria,	RCT	459	No significant reduction in the frequency of mental health disorders at 6 months follow-up	Proof of efficacy
30b	Turrini et al. (2022); 12 months follow-up to Purgato et al. (2021)	SH+; in-person; guided	Western Europe	Adult refugees and asylum seekers from Afghanistan, Iraq, Nigeria, Pakistan, Syria,	RCT	246	No significant reduction in the frequency of mental health disorders at 12 months follow-up	Proof of efficacy
31a	Acarturk et al. (2022b)	SH+; in-person; guided	Turkey	Adult Syrian refugees	RCT	642	Significant reduction in the frequency of mental health disorders at 6 months follow-up	Proof of efficacy
31b	Park et al. (2022); same sample as Acarturk et al. (2022b)	SH+; in-person; guided	Turkey	Adult Syrian refugees	RCT	627	SH+ was cost-effective	Effectiveness—Implementability
32	Riello et al. (2021)	DWM (book + audio); digital; guided	Italy	Adult health workers in Italy during COVID	RCT	238	No significant reduction in the proportion of anxiety and PTSD symptoms at 6 months follow-up	Proof of efficacy Effectiveness—Implementability
33	Acarturk et al. (2022c)	DWM (book + audio); digital; guided	Turkey	Adult Syrian refugees and Turkish citizens	RCT	124	DWM was feasible and acceptable	Effectiveness—Implementability

(continued)

Table 11.3 (continued)

ID	Author	Intervention	Country of recruitment	Population	Design	N	Primary outcome findings	Classification
34	Lorenzo-Luaces et al. (2023)	DWM (book); digital; guided	USA	Adult general population	Single group assignment	141	DWM was feasible and acceptable	Effectiveness—Implementability
35	Brown et al. (2020)	EASE; in-person; guided	Lebanon and Jordan	Lebanese, Syrians, and Palestinian adolescents, adult caregivers, community members, and health professionals	Qualitative	40	Adaptations of the intervention contents (i.e., incorporation of examples of anger and bullying), and the intervention structure and delivery (i.e., reduced numbers of session contents, incorporation of more physical activities)	Identifications of local barriers and facilitators Local socio-cultural adaptations
36	Akhtar et al. (2021b)	EASE; in-person; guided	Jordan	Syrian refugee children and adult caregivers	RCT; mixed methods	59[a] 59b	EASE was feasible, safe, and acceptable	Effectiveness—Implementability
37	Bryant et al. (2022c)	EASE; in-person; guided	Jordan	Syrian refugee children and adolescents and adult caregivers	RCT	471a	Significant reduction in children internalizing problems at 3 months follow-up. No significant results for children externalizing problems and attention difficulties	Proof of efficacy
38	Brown et al. (2023)	EASE; in-person; guided	Lebanon	Syrian and Lebanese refugee adolescents and adult caregivers	RCT; mixed methods	67a 54b	EASE was feasible, safe, and acceptable	Effectiveness—Implementability Identifications of local barriers and facilitators Local socio-cultural adaptations
39	Fine et al. (2021)	EASE; in-person; guided	Tanzania	Burundian refugee adolescents and their caregivers	RCT; mixed methods	86a 68b	EASE was feasible, safe, and acceptable	Effectiveness—Implementability

(continued)

Table 11.3 (continued)

ID	Author	Intervention	Country of recruitment	Population	Design	N	Primary outcome findings	Classification
40	Hamdani et al. (2022)	EASE; in-person; guided	Pakistan	Adolescents in public schools and their caregivers	cRCT	59a	EASE was feasible, safe, and acceptable	Effectiveness—Implementability
41a	Rahman et al. (2008)	TH; in-person; guided	Pakistan	Adolescent and adult pregnant women	cRCT	903	No significant differences in infant weight and height at 6- and 12 months follow-up	Proof of efficacy
41b	Maselko et al. (2015); 7 years follow-up to Rahman et al. (2008)	TH; in-person; guided	Pakistan	Mother-child dyads	cRCT	584	No significant differences in child cognitive, socioemotional, and physical outcomes at 7 years follow-up	Proof of efficacy
42	Atif et al. (2017)	TH; in-person; guided	Pakistan and India	Women during or after 1 year of pregnancy and peer helpers	Mixed methods	44	TH was feasible, safe, and acceptable	Effectiveness—Implementability Identifications of local barriers and facilitators Local socio-cultural adaptations
43a	Sikander et al. (2019)	TH; in-person; guided	Pakistan	Adult pregnant women	cRCT	570	No significant reduction in depressive symptoms and remission of depression at 6 months postnatal	Proof of efficacy Effectiveness—Implementability
43b	Maselko et al. (2020); 3 years follow-up to Sikander et al. (2019)	TH; in-person; guided	Pakistan	Mother-child dyads	cRCT	1154	No significant reduction in depressive symptoms and remission of depression; no significant differences in child socioemotional skills at 3 years postnatal	Proof of efficacy

(continued)

Table 11.3 (continued)

ID	Author	Intervention	Country of recruitment	Population	Design	N	Primary outcome findings	Classification
44	Fuhr et al. (2019)	TH; in-person; guided	India	Adult pregnant women	RCT	280	Significant remission of depressive symptoms at 6 months. No significant differences in the severity of depressive symptoms	Proof of efficacy Effectiveness—Implementability
45	Tarannum et al. (2018)	TH; in-person; guided	Bangladesh	Adult pregnant women	RCT; mixed methods	70	TH was feasible, safe, and acceptable	Effectiveness—Implementability Identifications of local barriers and facilitators Local socio-cultural adaptations
46	Nisar et al. (2020)	TH; in-person; guided	China	Adolescent and adult pregnant women	Mixed methods	15	TH was feasible, safe, and acceptable	Effectiveness—Implementability Local socio-cultural adaptations Integration into routine and sustained use
47	Boran et al. (2023)	TH; in-person; guided	Turkey	Adult pregnant women	RCT; mixed methods	88	TH was feasible, safe, and acceptable	Effectiveness—Implementability Integration into routine and sustained use
48a	Bolton et al. (2003)	IPT-G; in-person; guided	Uganda	Adults with depressive symptoms	RCT	341	Significant improvement in depressive symptoms and functioning at 2 weeks postintervention	Proof of efficacy
48b	Bass et al. (2006)	IPT-G; in-person; guided	Uganda	Adults with depressive symptoms	RCT	216	Significant improvement in depressive symptoms and functioning at 6 months follow-up	Proof of efficacy

(continued)

Table 11.3 (continued)

ID	Author	Intervention	Country of recruitment	Population	Design	N	Primary outcome findings	Classification
49	Asrat et al. (2020)	IPT-G; in-person; guided	Ethiopia	HIV/AIDS-affected PLAWHA	Qualitative	18	IPT-G was seen as acceptable. Adaptation should focus on the incorporation of local explanatory models, selection of facilitators, selection of meeting spaces, and group structure	Identifications of local barriers and facilitators Local socio-cultural adaptations
50	Asrat et al. (2021)	IPT-G; in-person; guided	Ethiopia	Adolescents with depression	Mixed methods	31	IPT-G was feasible, safe, and acceptable	Effectiveness—Implementability
51	Rose-Clarke et al. (2020)	IPT-G; in-person; guided	Nepal	HIV/AIDS-affected PLAWHA	Qualitative	126	Incorporating therapy in secondary schools by school nurses and community members; enhancing parental involvement; reduce stigma; foster stronger relationships among group members	Identifications of local barriers and facilitators Local socio-cultural adaptations
52	Yator et al. (2021)	IPT-G; in-person; guided	Kenya	Community health workers and HIV+ postpartum adolescents	RCT; mixed methods	25	IPT-G was feasible, safe, and acceptable	Effectiveness—Implementability Integration into routine and sustained use

PM+ problem management plus, *SH+* self help plus, *DWM* doing what matters, *EASE* early adolescent skills for emotions, *TH* thinking healthy, *SbS* step by step, *IPT-G* group interpersonal therapy, *N* total number of participants recruited

[a]Total number of adolescents

[b]Total number of caregivers

tative and mixed methods approaches, evidence of the feasibility, safety, and acceptability of EASE has been accumulated (Table 11.3). For Sustainable Technology for Adolescents to Reduce Stress (STARS), a randomized controlled trial is currently ongoing in Jordan [39].

The beneficial effects of Thinking Healthy (TH) are less well-established (Table 11.3). The randomized trial conducted in Pakistan on more than 900 adolescent and adult pregnant women found no significant differences in infant weight and height at 6 and 12 months postpartum. However, mothers from the intervention were less likely to meet the criteria for depression at 6- and 12-month follow-up and they showed significant improvement in depressive symptoms, disability, functioning, and social support compared to the control group. Similarly, a randomized trial in India found significant remission of depressive symptoms at 6 months, but no differences in the severity of depressive symptoms in pregnant women. In contrast, a randomized trial conducted in Pakistan among 570 adult pregnant women showed no reduction in depressive symptoms and no remission of depression at 6 months and 3 years postpartum (Table 11.3). Qualitative and mixed-methods approaches showed that TH was feasible, safe, and acceptable.

For group interpersonal therapy (IPT), a randomized trial conducted with 341 adults with depressive symptoms in Uganda found that group IPT was effective in reducing symptoms of depression and improving functioning at 2 weeks postintervention and at 6 months follow-up (Table 11.3). However, given that it is an adaptation of an established intervention [49–52] studies have mainly focused on assessing feasibility, safety and acceptability in different populations, including adolescents with depression and people with HIV/AIDS (Table 11.3).

11.5 Practical Considerations for Action Planning

In this chapter, we delve into a compilation of low-intensity psychological interventions developed or adapted by the WHO. Aligned with the tenets laid out in the WHO WMHR 2022, these interventions place paramount importance on upholding the autonomy of individuals dealing with mental health challenges. They espouse a person-centered methodology, fostering a holistic approach that underscores mental health promotion and preventive measures within a public health framework.

These interventions, that can all be delivered through task-shifting, are uniquely suited for implementation in low-resource settings. Considering that the concept of low-resource settings is more appropriate than the concept of low- or middle-income countries, as even countries classified as middle-income or high-income may experience significant resource constraints in certain sectors or regions, these interventions may be appropriate for countries at any level of economic development.

This chapter described the main characteristics of the interventions, their content, delivery formats, the evidence base supporting their use in specific target populations, and the studies assessing how they may be successfully implemented in practice. What remains to be done in terms of research priorities? And what remains to be done by policymakers and service planners aiming to offer these interventions to vulnerable populations in different contexts?

In terms of research priorities, it is important to underline that evidence of efficacy for some interventions is substantial, while for others it is only initial. Individual and group PM+ are supported by large proof of efficacy studies, so future studies should be focused more on implementation and scaling up strategies rather than on efficacy. SH+ is also supported by randomized evidence showing promising results, even though uncertainty remains on its long-term beneficial effects, and on whether its online version, DWM may be similarly effective. Therefore, future randomized trials should be conducted to evaluate modalities for maintaining the effect over time, and to prove the efficacy of DWM. Studies with different target populations should be conducted to determine whether the effect of these interventions is specific to certain populations, such as refugees or migrants, or whether it can be generalized to populations exposed to different types of vulnerability. Research should also address the comparative effectiveness of these interventions against other forms of psychosocial support. For the remaining psychosocial interventions, both proof of efficacy studies and implementation research should be conducted, as further evidence is needed to better quantify and characterize their beneficial effects in different target populations and outcomes, and to inform how they should be implemented in routine care.

In terms of implications for policymakers aiming to scale up these interventions, the following steps might be followed:

1. Consider the target population and adapt the intervention accordingly. It is important to tailor the psychosocial intervention to the specific needs and characteristics of the target population. Policymakers should carefully assess the demographics, cultural norms, and unique challenges of the community or group for whom the intervention is intended. Adaptation may involve translating materials into local languages, considering cultural sensitivities, and incorporating feedback from local stakeholders. The goal is to ensure that the intervention is culturally relevant and responsive to the population it serves.
2. Identify local barriers and facilitators. Policymakers need to conduct a comprehensive assessment of the local context to identify factors that might hinder or facilitate the successful implementation of the intervention. Barriers may include logistical challenges, resource constraints, or community resistance. Facilitators could be existing community support systems, available infrastructure, or positive attitudes toward the intervention. Identifying these factors helps in planning strategies to overcome barriers and leverage facilitators.
3. Implement the intervention within a monitoring infrastructure. Establishing a robust monitoring infrastructure is crucial for tracking the progress and effectiveness of the intervention as it is scaled up. This infrastructure should include data collection mechanisms, reporting systems, and trained personnel. Monitoring allows policymakers to continuously assess how the intervention is being implemented, identify areas that need improvement or adjustment, and ensure that the intervention remains on track in achieving its intended outcomes.
4. Once the intervention is part of routing use, develop systems to evaluate process and outcome measures. Even after successful scaling up and integration into routine care, it is essential to maintain a commitment to evaluation. Policymakers should set up systems to regularly assess both the process and the outcomes of the intervention. Process evaluation involves monitoring how the intervention is being delivered, adherence to guidelines, and the fidelity of implementation. Outcome evaluation assesses the impact of the intervention on the target population, including changes in health, well-being, or other relevant outcomes. These evaluations help policymakers make informed decisions about the intervention's continued use, potential adjustments, or even discontinuation if it proves ineffective or unsustainable.

These steps should be considered by policymakers bearing in mind that interventions may be scaled up in parallel or in series with existing services. In the parallel approach, a new intervention is introduced alongside the existing services, creating a parallel track for addressing vulnerability to mental health challenges. This means that both the established services and the new intervention run concurrently, aiming to enhance coverage. By introducing parallel interventions, it may be possible to reach more individuals, ensuring that a broader spectrum of people can access the support they require. This approach often allows for a more targeted focus, as parallel interventions can be designed with specific, tailored goals in mind. They can address unique aspects of the problem or cater to a particular demographic that may not be adequately served by existing services alone. However, there are some challenges associated with parallel implementation. It can strain resources, as it necessitates separate funding, staffing, and infrastructure. This can lead to inefficiencies or duplication of efforts. Coordinating multiple programs running in parallel can be complex, potentially resulting in overlap, confusion, or competition between the existing services and the new intervention. Furthermore, if not carefully managed, parallel interventions may lead to fragmented care, where individuals receive disconnected support from various sources, resulting in a disjointed experience.

In contrast, the series approach involves introducing the new intervention sequentially, before or after individuals have received the existing social or healthcare services. This approach is generally viewed as a stepped-care approach, where individuals access the first step initially, and then, depending on the outcome, they may or may not progress to a second, more intense, step. One key advantage of implementing in series is resource efficiency. It maximizes the use of existing infrastructure and personnel before introducing new elements, minimizing duplication of resources. It also promotes streamlined care by building upon the foundation of existing services, ensuring a more integrated and coordinated support system. There is a clear pathway from one level of care to the next, creating a sense of continuity for individuals seeking assistance. However, there are potential downsides to this approach as well. Waiting until existing services have been exhausted can lead to delays in providing necessary help to individuals, especially in cases of urgent or emerging issues. The series approach may also be less adaptable to evolving needs or changing circumstances, and it may not accommodate specific, targeted interventions as effectively as the parallel approach. Additionally, if the demand for existing services is high, implementing in series could result in delays and backlogs in accessing necessary support, potentially leaving individuals without assistance for extended periods.

In conclusion, the choice between implementing an intervention in parallel with existing services or in series depends on several factors, including the nature of the problem, available resources, coordination capabilities, and desired outcomes. Striking the right balance between these two approaches, or even combining them effectively, can be the key to addressing complex issues, ensuring that individuals receive appropriate and timely support while optimizing resource allocation.

Box 11.1 Systematic Review Methodology

Identification and selection of studies

We performed a systematic review following the Preferred Reporting Items for Systematic Reviews and Meta-analyses (PRISMA) guidelines. A systematic search was conducted on 28 March 2023 to identify quantitative and qualitative studies assessing the efficacy, effectiveness, and feasibility of implementation, as well as the cultural adaptation process of interventions developed or endorsed by the World Health Organization (WHO). Psychosocial Interventions developed or adapted by the WHO that we targeted in our review are: Problem Management Plus (PM+) and its digital version, Step-by-Step (SbS); Self-Help Plus (SH+) and its digital version Doing What Matters (DWM); Early Adolescent Skills for Emotions (EASE); Sustainable Technology for Adolescents to Reduce Stress (STARS); Thinking Healthy (TH); Group Interpersonal Therapy (IPT-G).

We searched for relevant published studies in the Cochrane Library and PubMed databases using the following search string: ("world health organization"[MeSH Terms] OR "world health organization"[Title/Abstract]) AND ("psychosocial intervention"[MeSH Terms] OR "psychosocial intervention "[Title/Abstract] OR "psychological intervention "[Title/Abstract] OR "problem management plus"[Title/Abstract] OR "group problem management"[Title/Abstract] OR "pm"[Title/Abstract] OR "step by step"[Title/Abstract] OR "self help plus"[Title/Abstract] OR "sh"[Title/

Abstract] OR "DWM"[Title/Abstract] OR "early adolescent skills"[Title/Abstract] OR "EASE"[Title/Abstract] OR "sustainable technology for adolescents to reduce stress "[Title/Abstract] OR "thinking healthy"[Title/Abstract] OR "group interpersonal"[Title/Abstract]).

The inclusion criteria encompassed studies that report controlled clinical trials assessing the efficacy of the targeted psychosocial interventions, single-group implementation studies, and other quantitative or qualitative studies investigating the feasibility of these interventions, as well as those describing their cultural or contextual adaptation. In cases where multiple studies involved the same group of participants, we maintained all relevant studies but treated them as a singular entity. For instance, randomized controlled trials (RCTs) presenting primary outcomes and supplementary studies assessing follow-up data from identical participants were treated as a single study. Exclusion criteria comprised articles that merely described an intervention without conducting any form of qualitative or quantitative evaluation. We also omitted studies that solely focused on individual components of the intended interventions when integrated into other distinct or localized psychosocial programs.

For each included study, we extracted essential information, including the publication year, type of intervention, intervention format (i.e., group, individual), intervention delivery (i.e., in-person face-to-face, in-person online, digital), whether the intervention was guided or unguided (i.e., interventions were classified as guided if they were either entirely administered by a facilitator or if participants received minimal support from facilitators through phone calls or text messages.), country of recruitment, target population, participant developmental stage (i.e., children and adolescents, adults), sample size, study design (i.e., RCTs, single-group assignment, qualitative), primary outcome findings, and study classification (i.e., proof of efficacy, effectiveness-implementability, identifications of local barriers and facilitators, local socio-cultural adaptation, integration into routine and sustained use). This data was coded by one reviewer (MB) and cross-verified by a second reviewer (CB). We included 49 studies and 5 secondary analyses (See Table 11.3 for a description of the included studies, and Box 11.2 for references).

Box 11.2 References of studies included in the systematic review and summarized in Table 11.3

1. Dawson KS, Schafer A, Anjuri D et al (2016) Feasibility trial of a scalable psychological intervention for women affected by urban adversity and gender-based violence in Nairobi. BMC Psychiatry 16(1):410

2. Bryant RA, Schafer A, Dawson KS et al (2017) Effectiveness of a brief behavioural intervention on psychological distress among women with a history of gender-based violence in urban Kenya: a randomised clinical trial. PLoS Med 14(8):e1002371

3. Rahman A, Riaz N, Dawson KS et al (2016a) Problem Management Plus (PM+): Pilot trial of a WHO transdiagnostic psychological intervention in conflict-affected Pakistan. World Psychiatry 15(2):182

4. Rahman A, Hamdani SU, Awan NR et al (2016b) Effect of a multicomponent behavioral intervention in adults impaired by psychological distress in a conflict-affected area of Pakistan: a randomized clinical trial. JAMA 316(24):2609–2617

5. Hamdani SU, Huma ZE, Rahman A et al (2020) Cost-effectiveness of WHO Problem Management Plus for adults with mood and anxiety disorders in a post-conflict area of Pakistan: randomised controlled trial. Br J Psychiatry 217(5):623–629

6. Hamdani SU, Huma Z-e, Masood A et al (2021) Effect of adding a psychological intervention to routine care of common mental disorders in a specialized mental healthcare facility in Pakistan: a randomized controlled trial. Int J Ment Health Syst 15(1):1–12

7. Saraf P, Rahman T, Jamison JC (2019) Group-Based Cognitive Behavioral Therapy (CBT) training improves mental health of SME entrepreneurs: experimental evidence from conflict-affected areas of Pakistan. In: World Bank Policy Research Working Paper, p 8872

8. Khan MN, Hamdani SU, Chiumento A et al (2019) Evaluating feasibility and acceptability of a group WHO trans-diagnostic intervention for women with common mental disorders in rural Pakistan: a cluster randomised controlled feasibility trial. Epidemiol Psychiatr Sci 28(1):77–87

9. Rahman A, Khan MN, Hamdani SU et al (2019) Effectiveness of a brief group psychological intervention for women in a post-conflict setting in Pakistan: a single-blind, cluster, randomised controlled trial. Lancet 393(10182):1733–1744

10. Sangraula M, Turner EL, Luitel NP et al (2020) Feasibility of Group Problem Management Plus (PM+) to improve mental health and functioning of adults in earthquake-affected communities in Nepal. Epidemiol Psychiatr Sci 29:e130

11. Jordans MJD, Kohrt BA, Sangraula M et al (2021) Effectiveness of Group Problem Management Plus, a brief psychological intervention for adults affected by humanitarian disasters in Nepal: a cluster randomized controlled trial. PLoS Med 18(6):e1003621

12. Akhtar A, Giardinelli L, Bawaneh A et al (2021a) Feasibility trial of a scalable transdiagnostic group psychological intervention for Syrians residing in a refugee camp. Eur J Psychotraumatol 12(1):1932295

13. Bryant RA, Bawaneh A, Awwad M et al (2022a) Effectiveness of a brief group behavioral intervention for common mental disorders in Syrian refugees in Jordan: a randomized controlled trial. PLoS Med 19(3):e1003949

14. Bryant RA, Bawaneh A, Awwad M et al (2022b) Twelve-month follow-up of a randomised clinical trial of a brief group psychological intervention for common mental disorders in Syrian refugees in Jordan. Epidemiol Psychiatr Sci 31:e81

15. Acarturk C, Uygun E, Ilkkursun Z et al (2022a) Group problem management plus (PM+) to decrease psychological distress among Syrian refugees in Turkey: a pilot randomised controlled trial. BMC Psychiatry 22(1):8

16. Spaaij J, Kiselev N, Berger C et al (2022) Feasibility and acceptability of Problem Management Plus (PM+) among Syrian refugees and asylum seekers in Switzerland: a mixed-method pilot randomized controlled trial. Eur J Psychotraumatol 13(1):2002027

17. Dowrick C, Rosala-Hallas A, Rawlinson R et al (2022) The Problem Management Plus psychosocial intervention for distressed and functionally impaired asylum seekers and refugees: the PROSPER feasibility RCT. Public Health Res 10(10):1

18. Perera C, Salamanca-Sanabria A, Caballero-Bernal J et al (2020) No implementation without cultural adaptation: a process for culturally adapting low-intensity psychological interventions in humanitarian settings. Confl Heal 14:1–12

19. Perera C, Aldamman K, Hansen M et al (2022) A brief psychological intervention for improving the mental health of Venezuelan migrants and refugees: a mixed-methods study. SSM Ment Health 2:100109

20. Knefel M, Kantor V, Nicholson AA et al (2020) A brief transdiagnostic psychological intervention for Afghan asylum seekers and refugees in Austria: a randomized controlled trial. Trials 21(1):57

21. de Graaff AM, Cuijpers P, McDaid D et al (2020) Peer-provided Problem Management Plus (PM+) for adult Syrian refugees: a pilot randomised controlled trial on effectiveness and cost-effectiveness. Epidemiol Psychiatr Sci 29:e162

22. De Graaff AM, Cuijpers P, Twisk JWR et al (2023) Peer-provided psychological intervention for Syrian refugees: results of a randomised controlled trial on the effectiveness of Problem Management Plus. BMJ Ment Health 26(1)

23. Abi Ramia J, Harper Shehadeh M, Kheir W et al (2018) Community cognitive interviewing to inform local adaptations of an e-mental health intervention in Lebanon. Glob Ment Health 5:e39

24. Burchert S, Alkneme MS, Bird M et al (2018) User-centered App adaptation of a low-intensity E-mental health intervention for Syrian refugees. Front Psych 9:663

25. Garabiles MR, Harper Shehadeh M, Hall BJ (2019) Cultural adaptation of a scalable World Health Organization E-mental health program for overseas Filipino workers. JMIR Form Res 3(1):e11600

26. Heim E, Ramia JA, Hana RA et al (2021) Step-by-step: feasibility randomised controlled trial of a mobile-based intervention for depression among populations affected by adversity in Lebanon. Internet Interv 24:24

27. Cuijpers P, Heim E, Abi Ramia J et al (2022a) Effects of a WHO-guided digital health intervention for depression in Syrian refugees in Lebanon: a randomized controlled trial. PLoS Med 19(6):e1004025

28. Cuijpers P, Heim E, Abi Ramia J et al (2022b) Guided digital health intervention for depression in Lebanon: randomised trial. BMJ Ment Health 25(e1):e34–e40

29. Tol WA, Augustinavicius J, Carswell K et al (2018a) Translation, adaptation, and pilot of a guided self-help intervention to reduce psychological distress in South Sudanese refugees in Uganda. Glob Ment Health 5:e25

30. Tol WA, Augustinavicius J, Carswell K et al (2018b) Feasibility of a guided self-help intervention to reduce psychological distress in South Sudanese refugee women in Uganda. World Psychiatry 17(2):234

31. Tol WA, Leku MR, Lakin DP et al (2020) Guided self-help to reduce psychological distress in South Sudanese female refugees in Uganda: a cluster randomised trial. Lancet Glob Health 8(2):e254–ee63

32. Purgato M, Carswell K, Tedeschi F et al (2021) Effectiveness of self-help plus in preventing mental disorders in refugees and asylum seekers in Western Europe: a multinational randomized controlled trial. Psychother Psychosom 90(6):403–414

33. Turrini G, Purgato M, Tedeschi F et al (2022) Long-term effectiveness of Self-Help Plus in refugees and asylum seekers resettled in Western Europe: 12-month outcomes of a randomised controlled trial. Epidemiol Psychiatr Sci 31:e39

34. Acarturk C, Uygun E, Ilkkursun Z et al (2022b) Effectiveness of a WHO self-help psychological intervention for preventing mental disorders among Syrian refugees in Turkey: a randomized controlled trial. World Psychiatry 21(1):88–95

35. Park AL, Waldmann T, Kösters M et al (2022) Cost-effectiveness of the self-help plus intervention for adult syrian refugees hosted in Turkey. JAMA Netw Open 5(5):e2211489

36. Riello M, Purgato M, Bove C et al (2021) Effectiveness of self-help plus (SH+) in reducing anxiety and post-traumatic symptomatology among care home workers during the COVID-19 pandemic: a randomized controlled trial. R Soc Open Sci 8(11):210219

37. Acarturk C, Kurt G, Ilkkursun Z, Uygun E, Karaoglan-Kahilogullari A (2022c) "Doing what matters in times of stress" to decrease psychological distress during COVID-19: a randomised controlled pilot trial. Intervention 20(2):170

38. Lorenzo-Luaces L, Howard J, De Jesús-Romero R et al (2023) Acceptability and outcomes of transdiagnostic guided self-help bibliotherapy for internalizing disorder symptoms in adults: a fully remote nationwide open trial. Cognit Ther Res 47(2):195–208

39. Brown FL, Aoun M, Taha K et al (2020) The cultural and contextual adaptation process of an intervention to reduce psychological distress in young adolescents living in Lebanon. Front Psych 11:212

40. Akhtar A, Malik A, Ghatasheh M et al (2021b) Feasibility trial of a brief scalable psychological intervention for Syrian refugee adolescents in Jordan. Eur J Psychotraumatol 12(1):1901408

41. Bryant RA, Malik A, Aqel IS et al (2022c) Effectiveness of a brief group behavioural intervention on psychological distress in young adolescent Syrian refugees: a randomised controlled trial. PLoS Med 19(8):e1004046

42. Brown FL, Taha K, Steen F et al (2023) Feasibility randomised controlled trial of the early adolescent skills for emotions psychological intervention with young adolescents in Lebanon. BMC Psychiatry 23(1):131

43. Fine SL, Malik A, Guimond MF et al (2021) Improving mental health in low-resource settings: a feasibility randomized controlled trial of a transdiagnostic psychological intervention among Burundian refugee adolescents and their caregivers. Behav Res Ther 145:103944

44. Hamdani SU, Huma ZE, Tamizuddin-Nizami A et al (2022) Feasibility and acceptability of a multicomponent, group psychological intervention for adolescents with psychosocial distress in public schools of Pakistan: a feasibility cluster randomized controlled trial (cRCT). Child Adolesc Psychiatry Ment Health 16(1):47

45. Rahman A, Malik A, Sikander S, Roberts C, Creed F (2008) Cognitive behaviour therapy-based intervention by community health workers for mothers with depression and their infants in rural Pakistan: a cluster-randomised controlled trial. Lancet 372(9642):902–909

46. Maselko J, Sikander S, Bhalotra S et al (2015) Effect of an early perinatal depression intervention on long-term child development outcomes: follow-up of the Thinking Healthy Programme randomised controlled trial. Lancet Psychiatry 2(7):609–617

47. Atif N, Krishna RN, Sikander S et al (2017) Mother-to-mother therapy in India and Pakistan: adaptation and feasibility evaluation of the peer-delivered Thinking Healthy Programme. BMC Psychiatry 17(1):1–14

48. Sikander S, Ahmad I, Atif N et al (2019) Delivering the Thinking Healthy Programme for perinatal depression through volunteer peers: a cluster randomised controlled trial in Pakistan. Lancet Psychiatry 6(2):128–139

49. Maselko J, Sikander S, Turner EL et al (2020) Effectiveness of a peer-delivered, psychosocial intervention on maternal depression and child development at 3 years postnatal: a cluster randomised trial in Pakistan. Lancet Psychiatry 7(9):775–787

50. Fuhr DC, Weobong B, Lazarus A et al (2019) Delivering the Thinking Healthy Programme for perinatal depression through peers: an individually randomised controlled trial in India. Lancet Psychiatry 6(2):115–127

51. Tarannum R (2018) A pilot randomised controlled trial of a peer-based low-intensity psychosocial intervention for reducing depressive symptoms in pregnant women in rural Bangladesh. Doctoral dissertation, Victoria University

52. Nisar A, Yin J, Yiping N et al (2020) Making therapies culturally relevant: translation, cultural adaptation and field-testing of the Thinking Healthy Programme for perinatal depression in China. BMC Pregnancy Childbirth 20(1):368

53. Boran P, Dönmez M, Barış E et al (2023) Delivering the Thinking Healthy Programme as a universal group intervention integrated into routine antenatal care: a randomized-controlled pilot study. BMC Psychiatry 23(1):14

54. Bolton P, Bass J, Neugebauer R et al (2003) Group interpersonal psychotherapy for depression in rural Uganda: a randomized controlled trial. JAMA 289(23):3117–3124

55. Bass J, Neugebauer R, Clougherty KF et al (2006) Group interpersonal psychotherapy for depression in rural Uganda: 6-month outcomes: randomised controlled trial. Br J Psychiatry 188(6):567–573

56. Asrat B, Lund C, Ambaw F, Schneider M (2020) Adaptation of the WHO group interpersonal therapy for people living with HIV/AIDS in Northwest Ethiopia: A qualitative study. PLoS One 15(8):e0238321

57. Asrat B, Lund C, Ambaw F, Schneider M (2021) Acceptability and feasibility of peer-administered group interpersonal therapy for depression for people living with HIV/AIDS—a pilot study in Northwest Ethiopia. Pilot Feasibility Stud 7(1):1–15

58. Rose-Clarke K, Pradhan I, Shrestha P et al (2020) Culturally and developmentally adapting group interpersonal therapy for adolescents with depression in rural Nepal. BMC Psychol 8(1):83

59. Yator O, Kagoya M, Khasakhala L, John-Stewart G, Kumar M (2021) Task-sharing and piloting WHO group interpersonal psychotherapy (IPT-G) for adolescent mothers living with HIV in Nairobi primary health care centers: a process paper. AIDS Care 33(7):873–878

References

1. Turrini G, Purgato M, Ballette F, Nose M, Ostuzzi G, Barbui C (2017) Common mental disorders in asylum seekers and refugees: umbrella review of prevalence and intervention studies. Int J Ment Health Syst 11:51
2. Lund C, De SM, Plagerson S et al (2011) Poverty and mental disorders: breaking the cycle in low-income and middle-income countries. Lancet 378(9801):1502–1514
3. Lund C (2015) Poverty, inequality and mental health in low- and middle-income countries: time to expand the research and policy agendas. Epidemiol Psychiatr Sci 24(2):97–99
4. Bauer A, Baltra RA, Pabon MA et al (2021) Examining the dynamics between young people's mental health, poverty and life chances in six low- and middle-income countries: protocol for the CHANCES-6 study. Soc Psychiatry Psychiatr Epidemiol 56(9):1687–1703
5. Lund C, Brooke-Sumner C, Baingana F et al (2018) Social determinants of mental disorders and the sustainable development goals: a systematic review of reviews. Lancet Psychiatry 5(4):357–369
6. World Health Organization (2022) World mental health report: transforming mental health for all. World Health Organization, Geneva. https://www.who.int/publications/i/item/9789240049338
7. World Health Organization (2017) Scalable psychological interventions for people in communities

affected by adversity. World Health Organization, Geneva. https://www.who.int/publications/i/item/WHO-MSD-MER-17.1
8. Lund C, Breen A, Flisher AJ et al (2010) Poverty and common mental disorders in low and middle income countries: a systematic review. Soc Sci Med 71(3):517–528
9. World Health Organization (2014) Social determinants of mental health. World Health Organization, Geneva. https://www.who.int/publications/i/item/9789241506809
10. Marbin D, Gutwinski S, Schreiter S, Heinz A (2022) Perspectives in poverty and mental health. Front Public Health 10:975482
11. World Health Organization (2021) Comprehensive mental health action plan 2013–2030. World Health Organization, Geneva. https://www.who.int/publications/i/item/9789240031029
12. Charlson F, van Ommeren M, Flaxman A, Cornett J, Whiteford H, Saxena S (2019) New WHO prevalence estimates of mental disorders in conflict settings: a systematic review and meta-analysis. Lancet 394(10194):240–248
13. Purgato M, Uphoff E, Singh R, Thapa Pachya A, Abdulmalik J, van Ginneken N (2020) Promotion, prevention and treatment interventions for mental health in low- and middle-income countries through a task-shifting approach. Epidemiol Psychiatr Sci 29:e150
14. Uphoff E, Robertson L, Cabieses B et al (2020) An overview of systematic reviews on mental health promotion, prevention, and treatment of common mental disorders for refugees, asylum seekers, and internally displaced persons. Cochrane Database Syst Rev 9:CD013458
15. Barbui C, Purgato M, Acarturk C et al (2022) Preventing the mental health consequences of war in refugee populations. Epidemiol Psychiatr Sci 31:e24
16. IASC (2020) IASC Guidance on operational considerations for multisectoral mental health and psychosocial support programmes during the COVID-19 pandemic. Inter-Agency Standing Committee, New York. https://interagencystandingcommittee.org/iasc-reference-group-mental-health-and-psychosocial-support-emergency-settings/iasc-guidance-operational-considerations-multisectoral-mental-health-and-psychosocial-support
17. Ceccarelli C, Prina E, Muneghina O et al (2022) Adverse childhood experiences and global mental health: avenues to reduce the burden of child and adolescent mental disorders. Epidemiol Psychiatr Sci 31:e75
18. Henderson C, Noblett J, Parke H et al (2014) Mental health-related stigma in health care and mental health-care settings. Lancet Psychiatry 1(6):467–482
19. Kemp CG, Jarrett BA, Kwon CS et al (2019) Implementation science and stigma reduction interventions in low- and middle-income countries: a systematic review. BMC Med 17(1):6
20. Heim E, Kohrt BA, Koschorke M, Milenova M, Thronicroft G (2018) Reducing mental health-related stigma in primary health care settings in low- and middle-income countries: a systematic review. Epidemiol Psychiatr Sci 29:1–10
21. van Zyl C, Badenhorst M, Hanekom S, Heine M (2021) Unravelling 'low-resource settings': a systematic scoping review with qualitative content analysis. BMJ Glob Health 6(6):e005190
22. Singh V, Kumar A, Gupta S (2022) Mental health prevention and promotion—a narrative review. Front Psych 13:898009
23. Prina E, Ceccarelli C, Abdulmalik JO et al (2023) Task-sharing psychosocial interventions for the prevention of common mental disorders in the perinatal period in low- and middle-income countries: a systematic review and meta-analysis. Int J Soc Psychiatry 69:1578
24. Mutamba BB, van Ginneken N, Smith Paintain L, Wandiembe S, Schellenberg D (2013) Roles and effectiveness of lay community health workers in the prevention of mental, neurological and substance use disorders in low and middle income countries: a systematic review. BMC Health Serv Res 13:412
25. Le LK, Esturas AC, Mihalopoulos C et al (2021) Cost-effectiveness evidence of mental health prevention and promotion interventions: a systematic review of economic evaluations. PLoS Med 18(5):e1003606
26. Knettel BA, Knippler E, Martinez A et al (2023) A scoping review of counseling interventions for suicide prevention in Africa: few studies address this life-saving aspect of mental health treatment. J Affect Disord 328:183–190
27. Carter H, Araya R, Anjur K, Deng D, Naslund JA (2021) The emergence of digital mental health in low-income and middle-income countries: a review of recent advances and implications for the treatment and prevention of mental disorders. J Psychiatr Res 133:223–246
28. Turrini G, Tedeschi F, Cuijpers P et al (2021) A network meta-analysis of psychosocial interventions for refugees and asylum seekers with PTSD. BMJ Glob Health 6(6):e005029
29. Turrini G, Purgato M, Acarturk C et al (2019) Efficacy and acceptability of psychosocial interventions in asylum seekers and refugees: systematic review and meta-analysis. Epidemiol Psychiatr Sci 28:376–388
30. Barbui C, Purgato M, Abdulmalik J et al (2021) Efficacy of interventions to reduce coercive treatment in mental health services: umbrella review of randomised evidence. Br J Psychiatry 218(4):185–195
31. World Health Organization (2008) Task shifting: rational redistribution of tasks among health workforce teams. Global recommendations and guidelines. World Health Organization, Geneva. https://iris.who.int/handle/10665/43821?&locale-attribute=pt
32. World Health Organization (2018) Problem Management Plus (PM+): individual psychological help for adults impaired by distress in communities exposed to adversity. World Health Organization, Geneva. https://www.who.int/publications/i/item/WHO-MSD-MER-16.2

33. Dawson KS, Bryant RA, Harper M et al (2015) Problem Management Plus (PM+): a WHO transdiagnostic psychological intervention for common mental health problems. World Psychiatry 14(3):354–357
34. Carswell K, Harper-Shehadeh M, Watts S et al (2018) Step-by-Step: a new WHO digital mental health intervention for depression. Mhealth 4:34
35. Epping-Jordan JE, Harris R, Brown FL et al (2016) Self-Help Plus (SH+): a new WHO stress management package. World Psychiatry 15(3):295–296
36. World Health Organization (2021) Self-help plus (SH+). a group-based stress management course for adults. World Health Organization, Geneva. https://www.who.int/publications/i/item/9789240035119
37. World Health Organization (2021) Doing what matters in times of stress. World Health Organization, Geneva. https://www.who.int/publications/i/item/9789240003927
38. Dawson KS, Watts S, Carswell K et al (2019) Improving access to evidence-based interventions for young adolescents: Early Adolescent Skills for Emotions (EASE). World Psychiatry 18(1):105–107
39. Hall J, Jordan S, van Ommeren M et al (2022) Sustainable technology for adolescents and youth to reduce stress (STARS): a WHO transdiagnostic chatbot for distressed youth. World Psychiatry 21(1):156–157
40. Rahman A, Malik A, Sikander S, Roberts C, Creed F (2008) Cognitive behaviour therapy-based intervention by community health workers for mothers with depression and their infants in rural Pakistan: a cluster-randomised controlled trial. Lancet 372(9642):902–909
41. World Health Organization (2015) Thinking healthy. A manual for psychosocial management of perinatal depression. World Health Organization, Geneva. https://www.who.int/publications/i/item/WHO-MSD-MER-15.1
42. World Health Organization (2016) Group interpersonal therapy (IPT) for depression. World Health Organization, Geneva. https://www.who.int/publications/i/item/WHO-MSD-MER-16.4
43. Purgato M, Cuijpers P, Barbui C (2021) Regulatory requirements for psychological interventions. Lancet Psychiatry 8(3):174–176
44. Curran GM, Bauer M, Mittman B, Pyne JM, Stetler C (2012) Effectiveness-implementation hybrid designs: combining elements of clinical effectiveness and implementation research to enhance public health impact. Med Care 50(3):217–226
45. Proctor E, Silmere H, Raghavan R et al (2011) Outcomes for implementation research: conceptual distinctions, measurement challenges, and research agenda. Adm Policy Ment Health 38(2):65–76
46. Proctor EK, Landsverk J, Aarons G, Chambers D, Glisson C, Mittman B (2009) Implementation research in mental health services: an emerging science with conceptual, methodological, and training challenges. Adm Policy Ment Health 36(1):24–34
47. Purgato M, Carswell K, Tedeschi F et al (2021) Effectiveness of self-help plus in preventing mental disorders in refugees and asylum seekers in Western Europe: a multinational randomized controlled trial. Psychother Psychosom 90(6):403–414
48. Acarturk C, Uygun E, Ilkkursun Z et al (2022) Effectiveness of a WHO self-help psychological intervention for preventing mental disorders among Syrian refugees in Turkey: a randomized controlled trial. World Psychiatry 21(1):88–95
49. Cuijpers P, Geraedts AS, van Oppen P, Andersson G, Markowitz JC, van Straten A (2011) Interpersonal psychotherapy for depression: a meta-analysis. Am J Psychiatry 168(6):581–592
50. Cuijpers P, Donker T, Weissman MM, Ravitz P, Cristea IA (2016) Interpersonal psychotherapy for mental health problems: a comprehensive meta-analysis. Am J Psychiatry 173(7):680–687
51. Bolton P, Bass J, Neugebauer R et al (2003) Group interpersonal psychotherapy for depression in rural Uganda: a randomized controlled trial. JAMA 289(23):3117–3124
52. Bolton P, Bass J, Betancourt T et al (2007) Interventions for depression symptoms among adolescent survivors of war and displacement in northern Uganda: a randomized controlled trial. JAMA 298(5):519–527

12 Migration, Mental Health, and Human Rights

Marina Lalatta Costerbosa and Ilaria Tarricone

Abstract

This chapter focuses on the impact of people's migratory histories on the development of psychotic disorders in order to outline, firstly, a paradigm for social psychiatry. It will then attempt to identify a possible legal response to the demand for justice implicit in this reconstruction. This chapter aims to provide the link between the condition of migrancy and the onset of psychoses, and to discuss one of the fundamental legal–moral questions arising today from the migratory phenomenon: the notion of human dignity and its relationship to fundamental rights.

Keywords

Hannah Arendt · Human dignity · Human rights · Migrants · Psychotic disorders

M. Lalatta Costerbosa
Department of Philosophy and Communication Studies, University of Bologna, Bologna, Italy
e-mail: marina.lalatta@unibo.it

I. Tarricone (✉)
Department of Medical and Surgical Sciences, University of Bologna, Bologna, Italy
e-mail: Ilaria.tarricone@unibo.it

12.1 Introduction

The subject we will deal with in this section is enormous and the debate around the questions of justice that specifically involve migrants is endless. Inevitably, we must begin by delimiting the area of the reflections we propose. We will concentrate on the impact of people's migratory histories on the development of psychotic disturbances in order to outline, firstly, a paradigm for social psychiatry. We will then attempt to identify a possible legal response to the demand for justice implicit in our reconstruction. Our central theme will be, initially, the link between the condition of migrancy and the onset of psychoses. Subsequently, we will discuss one of the fundamental legal–moral questions arising today from the migratory phenomenon: the infringement of migrants' dignity and the denial of their fundamental rights.

12.2 Risk of Psychosis among Migrants

Over the years, mounting evidence has shown that migrants have a higher risk of psychotic disorders than do natives without a history of migration. A recent meta-analysis [1] found that in European countries the relative risk (RR) of psychosis among first- and second-generation migrants of non-European origin is three times

A. Fiorillo, S. De Giorgi (eds.), *Social Determinants of Mental Health*, Sustainable Development Goals Series, https://doi.org/10.1007/978-3-031-70165-8_12

higher than among native counterparts Migrants of European provenance had a lower, but still significantly increased risk. The multinational study by the EUropean Network of National Schizophrenia Networks Studying Gene-Environment Interactions (EU–GEI) group [2, 3] found that the incidence risk ratio (IRR) of psychotic disorders among migrants or ethnic minorities varied by study catchment site and was lowest in Valencia (IRR = 0.70, 95% confidence interval [CI] = 0.32–1.53) and highest in Paris (IRR = 2.47, 95% CI = 1.66–3.69). The IRR of psychosis among migrants and ethnic minorities, from site to site, was higher where the IRR of psychosis among the reference population (natives) was higher and vice versa. Overall, the IRR of psychosis was higher for migrants from non-Western countries (pooled IRR = 2.12, 95%CI = 1.88–2.40) than migrants from Western countries (pooled IRR = 1.09, 95%CI = 0.91–1.32). Those with the highest IRR were from sub-Saharan Africa (IRR = 3.23, 95%CI = 2.66–3.93). In a study conducted by Tarricone et al. [4], rates of psychosis were found to be considerably elevated in internal migrants as well (IRR = 1.93, 95%CI = 1.19–3.13).

12.2.1 Possible Explanations of the Phenomenon

One of the first hypotheses to explain this phenomenon was that of a higher incidence of psychosis in the countries of origin. Nevertheless, studies conducted in Jamaica [5], Trinidad [6], Barbados [7], Surinam [8], India, and China [9] failed to demonstrate this hypothesis.

Odegaard [10] proposed the hypothesis of "selective migration," meaning that the individuals carrying the highest risk of psychosis were more likely to migrate. This hypothesis was refuted by subsequent studies [11, 12]. Notwithstanding the aforementioned limitations, however, some evidence seems to support a mechanism of positive selection (the so-called "healthy migrant effect"). Also, host countries with strict immigration policies may tend to reinforce such a mechanism.

Some authors have suggested that the increased rates of psychosis in migrants could be due to misdiagnosis [13, 14]. Again, the hypothesis failed to be supported by later evidence: for instance, a study comparing diagnoses formulated by British and Jamaican psychiatrists on the same group of patients did not find differences in the rates of psychotic disorder diagnosis [15]. Nevertheless, in the light of the potential negative effect of a wrong diagnosis, it is of fundamental importance not to introduce such biases in epidemiological studies.

Another possible explanation is substance-induced psychosis. However, evidence as to the possible greater risk of substance-induced psychosis among migrants proves to be heterogeneous and inconclusive: due to the lack of conclusive evidence, Selten et al. [1, 16] conclude that abuse of psychotropic substances does not play a major role in explaining the excess of psychosis in migrants. In a multicentric study conducted in Italy none of the migrants recruited was diagnosed with substance-related psychosis [17].

Finally, some authors have highlighted the possible role of exposure to biological risk factors before, during, and after migration. These include infections, obstetric complications, and vitamin D deficiency. Again, the evidence supporting the role of these factors in populations of migrants is weak or limited [8, 18–20].

Taken together, the available data suggest that the excess of psychosis among migrants cannot be explained only in terms of genetic vulnerability, biological predisposition, or exposure to negative biological factors, nor by incorrect diagnoses. At the other hand these negative results suggest that the factors that most influence the mental health of migrants should be social in first place. Among the main etiopathogenic models taking into account the social determinants of psychosis, it is worth citing the "neuro-sociodevelopmental model" proposed by Morgan et al. [21, 22]. According to this model, exposure to social stressors (social adversities and childhood abuse), before or during migration, may interact with genetic susceptibility or other factors which can impair the neurodevelopment (perinatal infections, obstetric complications, etc.) generating a liability to psychosis. The cumulative effect of further stressors or environmental adversities, including substance use, may then lead to full-blown psychosis.

Another hypothesis is that of "social defeat," which is defined as "the long-term experience of a subordinate position or outsider status" [23, 24]. The prolongated experience of "social defeat" is believed to lead to sensitization of the mesolimbic dopaminergic system, which is linked to psychosis. Neurobiological evidence derived from animal models [25] and from a Canadian study conducted on migrants (healthy volunteers, subjects at clinical high risk of psychosis, and patients with schizophrenia) [26] would seem to support this hypothesis.

12.2.2 Vulnerability Factors in Migrants

A history of migration across the three stages (pre-migration, migration, and post-migration) may itself significantly contribute to the excess of psychosis in migrants, given the exposure to adversity and social disadvantages which, cumulatively, may lead to a 14-fold increase in the odds of psychosis [27]. Tarricone et al. [27] tried to disentangle the timing of the social disadvantages across the three phases of migration over a sample of first-generation migrants recruited from six different countries, finding an increase of about 1.5 in the odds of first-episode psychosis for each additional disadvantage (on a scale from 1 to 3) in the pre-migratory phase (OR = 1.61, 95%CI = 1.06–2.44) and about twofold for each additional disadvantage (range 1 to 3) in the post-migratory phase (OR = 1.89, 95%CI = 1.02–3.51). This study adds further evidence that the most significant risk factors for the onset of psychosis in migrants lie in the post-migration phase. Previous studies had already identified a pre-eminent role for the post-migration social disadvantages, such as difficulties of integration in the host society [28, 29], higher levels of perceived discrimination [30–32], reduced "social capital" [33, 34], mismatch between expectations prior to migration and achievements once resettled in a new country [35], and a worse quality of general health [17, 36]. In their study, Tarricone and colleagues claim that effective social and public health strategies should be adopted to address the social drivers of high rates of psychosis among migrants [27].

12.2.3 Resilience Factors in Migrants

Resilience factors may counterbalance the negative effects of migration-related stressors and protect the individuals from the development of psychosis. Among the factors that may exert a protective effect, the literature available to date lists: age of migration [37], family network (with gender specificities) [38], premorbid levels of psychosocial functioning [17], proficiency in the host country main language [39], and living in high-ethnic density neighborhoods [40].

Concerning age of migration, a meta-analysis has shown that those who migrate after age of 18 have a significantly lower risk of psychosis compared to those who migrate during childhood or adolescence [37]. This suggests that the effects of international migration stressors may have a greater impact on a brain that is still under development. Thus, migrant children deserve special attention and require specific intervention to promote their resilience and prevent psychosis onset.

A recent study found a significant association between family networks during migration and post-migration psychosis, and the association was influenced by gender [38]: for females it was protective to migrate with the family or to rejoin it, while for males this represented a risk factor. This is probably due to the difference in terms of perceived role and expectations about the migration. Males might feel the burden of having to care and support their families and perceive this as a strong post-migration stress (risk was higher when they also had dependent children). On the other hand, it is known that women encounter more difficulties to enter the labor market, risking obtaining exploitative jobs, and to integrate into the new society [41–43]; for this reason, they may have more benefit from a supportive family network.

There is evidence to support that migrants diagnosed with psychotic disorders may have higher levels of premorbid functioning and better occupational outcomes than native counterparts [17, 44]. In a multicentric Italian study [17], many migrants with first-episode psychosis presented with a "high functioning portrait": that is to say, they were highly educated, employed, and in a past or current stable affective relationship. This is in contrasts with common findings among natives with psychosis from the same country [45, 46]. Adjunctively, another study from Tarricone et al. [44] found that 12 months after the onset of first-episode psychosis, migrants were more likely than natives to have resumed studies or work activity. The personal resources are an important factor of resilience, and migrants diagnosed with psychosis should receive support and rehabilitative treatments to maintain adequate psychosocial functioning.

Recent findings from an EU-GEI study 39 highlighted the role of the linguistic distance (expressed as a combination of one's language proficiency and distance on a language tree between one's first language and the majority language in the country of arrival). Migrant with greater linguistic distance had significantly increased odds of psychosis. Language proficiency is pivotal for the integration in the new country and seems essential to promote resilience with respect to migrants' mental health.

Finally, there is established evidence that migrants living in neighborhoods with high ethnic density have lower psychosis risk [37], possibly due to reduced social stress, better social support, and increased social capital.

12.3 Matters of Injustice

Now that we have outlined the relevant role of social factors on migrants mental health, we will attempt to examine it in terms of the arguments involved. We will try, that is, to counter the validity of the arguments that are frequently advanced to justify and legitimize, in democratic contexts, practices of brutal rejection and social marginalization. Practices that—as we have seen—put at serious risk the health, and even the lives, of those involved.

However, we circumscribe it, any reflection on the present conditions of migrants in democratic countries must bring us face to face with the history of this same migrancy, an old, ugly story that rears its head every day. Ours is a world where there are a very few rich states and a majority of poor ones, states at peace and states at war—if we also include the so-called "low intensity conflicts," 59 wars are currently ongoing. It is a world where 6.5 million children in Syria, 2.7 in Afghanistan, and 2.2 in southern Sudan have had to abandon their homes to flee from war. A world where a destiny such as this awaits one child in four—almost 700 million children, nearly a third of the (registered) children on the planet. A world in which the decision to exercise what Johnson Carens, in his book *Ethics of Immigration*, aptly summarized as "discretional control of immigration" [47], plays a crucial role in maintaining the "privileges" of those living in the more advantaged states, the privileges of the most fortunate. Moreover, in spite of the reality of the migratory phenomena in the Mediterranean and from countries battered by war, by "wars without end," this provides a daily excuse for further crimes within the crime, suffered by civilians, by child–soldiers, by pregnant mothers, by people compelled by desperation to flee from war, hunger, cold and drought.

A further preliminary consideration must be added to this desolate portrait of the present moment.

The injustice implicit in this radical and painful condition of inequality that affects fundamental needs, survival, education, work, and health in the fullest and broadest sense, is exacerbated because it is dealt with by implementing new forms of legal–political and moral injustice—there is a close linkage between these latter.

Attention must be drawn, in fact, to the numerous breaches of international laws on human rights. Such as failure to recognize the status of refugee, formally envisaged in Europe as early as 1951, according to the protections as of the "Geneva Refugee Convention." Not to speak of the flouting of the basic rights of human beings to life and freedom of movement, rights that are concretely imperilled daily. Without forgetting the failure to apply the 1989 "Convention on the Rights of the Child." Breached, moreover, are the principles underlying the democratic constitutions, such as that of Italy which recites, under Article 10, that "The Italian legal system conforms to the generally acknowledged provisions of international law" and, more specifically, that "The legal status of foreigners shall be regulated by law in compliance with international provisions and treaties." This prescription is further clarified in the following paragraph, where we read a passage decisive for our argument: "Foreigners who, in their own country, are denied the actual exercise of the democratic freedoms guaranteed by the Italian Constitution shall have the right of asylum in the territory of the Italian Republic, in accordance with the conditions set forth by law."

12.4 Dangerous Reactions

How is it possible that, in a democratic state governed by the rule of law, the status quo is defended and, indeed, proposals are made to harshen further the procedures already in place?

Unashamedly demagogic explanations are part of the daily agenda, addressed to the instincts and "guts" of citizens who are often anguished, at times indifferent, and not always new to discriminatory, even racist, ideas. It is not rare to hear speeches of hatred camouflaged as political theories, resulting in increased hatred and a willingness to apply discrimination with a clean conscience.

We will not pursue these arguments here, since they are not serious, but self-serving and populist. The consequences they generate, obviously, are serious.

We will stop to consider two other even more dangerous possible reactions.

A first reaction to the migration question sees *the abandonment of the democratic order of the country*, a structural distancing from the constitutional coordinates of a country governed by law.

A first possibility, therefore, is to follow the example of, for instance, the Hungarian state that introduced, in 2017, an anti-migrant law, known as the anti-Soros law. Strongly wished for by the Prime Minister Viktor Orbàn, this envisages, in addition to closure of the borders, the introduction of a so-called "crime of solidarity," which makes it illegal even for humanitarian organizations, as well as for individuals, to give aid and protection to minors and their migrant or refugee relatives. The Parliament of Budapest pushed through this law, and defended it, in spite of condemnation by the EU and without regard for the humanitarian scandal on the border between Serbia and Hungary. This is an abdication of democracy, conferring primacy on national cultural rights at the expense of universal human rights. In place of these rights, that is to say, not complementary to them.

The second possible response is that of those who wish to repulse migrants, denying them access and condemning them to "clandestinity" (which is made a criminal offence), *in deference to the very principles of democracy*. They would protect dignity by denying dignity; they would defend rights by denying them. This solution apparently remains within constitutional parameters, but it is in reality all the more insidious for that reason.

This is to put into practice the argument that there is a balance between human dignity and human dignity. "Würde gegen Würde," to use the German phrase. We recall this, because it is a theme that appears in more than one writer central to the continental debate that even advocates the relegalization of torture, as proposed in the last 20 years (and more precisely, after the tragic event of 11 September 2001) by legal scholars and academics in several democratic countries.

The dignity of the citizen, that cannot be exposed to the risk of insecurity (of their lives or their cultural identity), of being defrauded of their traditional values, attacked, threatened or robbed, has to win against the dignity of the potential criminal and so that (note the stereotype applied) of the foreigner who is not a tourist or an entrepreneur, but a migrant.

This reasoning follows a logic that is more apparent than real.

Dignity, in this case, is not understood in the modern sense, in the sense that, from Kant onwards, has characterized the culture of a state governed by law, which assigns dignity to every human being *as such*.

With an implicit regressive gesture, it is surreptitiously reinterpreted according to *premodern* theoretical coordinates; it is defined in quantitative terms, becoming a principle subject to gradation in proportion to the conduct in act. A sort of *ex post* recognition, a prize to be attained on merit, and which can therefore always be withdrawn. This is the thesis sustained by, among others, Avishai Margalit in her *Decent Society* [48]. Thus, proceeding along this slippery slope, the argument reaches the conclusion that, to defend the human dignity of the many, we must sacrifice that of the few. The axiological gap must be filled, unless we wish to question the very sense and reason of the social pact, with respect to which the state must appear able to protect the security of its members. To defend the human dignity of the majority of citizens, we must sacrifice that of the minority, of the migrants. We must balance, weight, and compare the quantities.

The second line of reasoning aimed at proving that repressive policies toward migrants may be compatible with a democratic state concerns rights; the balance between fundamental rights according to a logic of weighting between different fundamental rights. To protect the fundamental rights of some citizens, we may infringe these same rights for others, namely migrants. The guarantee of fundamental rights must be defended even at the cost of their *relativization*.

It is not by chance that this second argument is among those most frequently produced in the current discussion on whether or not torture is justifiable even in a democracy. In reality, here too, what is lost is the non-negotiable recognition of fundamental rights, the relativization of which inevitably takes us outside the boundary of a democratic state governed by the rule of law.

12.5 Democracy at Stake

With regard to the first response to the migrancy question (that of Hungary, for example), we can only hold up our hands in horror. This response is an abandonment of democracy and of a state governed by the rule of law, because it negates the universal recognition of human rights. It opens up a political terrain without constitutional guarantees for the dignity and liberty of the individual. From the democratic angle, this option is self-disqualifying, since it proclaims itself de facto anti-democratic.

The second response is, in a certain sense, even more insidious from a political point of view, because it is by nature invasive and sinuous.

We would like to concentrate on this, in order to refute the correctness of its arguments as well as, in this case too, its democratic credentials.

How can the universal value of human dignity and the recognition of individual rights be so shaky and expendable without consequences for the survival of democracy in a state?

The reasoning differs partly between the two cases (the dignity-against-dignity argument and the balancing-of-fundamental-rights argument).

The concept of dignity is somewhat undermined by the ambivalence of the concept, which indicates both the ancient *dignitas* of Cicero, deserved on the strength of what the person has done, and the modern idea that it is a human condition as such.

Human dignity, in the modern concept, is by its very nature antagonistic to any concept of balancing and graduality [49, 50]. We should therefore reject the all-too-frequent attempts to attribute characteristics to the modern concept of human dignity that could be tolerated only in ancient times, in the Middle Ages and in the early modern period: characteristics that are hierarchical, anti-equalitarian, and merit based [51].

The result of such deceptive arguments is to debase and substantially nullify the fundamental universal value of human dignity, while the inevitable and foreseeable downward slide set in motion by this path makes a mockery of the concept.

It is claimed, to all effects, that the recognition of an individual's dignity is something he or she must deserve. That the individual may have complete, much, little or scarcely no human dignity, according to his or her conduct. It is argued that the individual must earn the *status*, the "rank" of dignity, that being human is not in itself a sufficient condition for having it. It is asked—and the implicit answer is "no"—if even a delinquent, a terrorist or a migrant should be recognized as having dignity.

But this is to overturn the theoretical and moral meaning of the modern idea of dignity, the meaning underlying our international and constitutional laws. This is a denial of human dignity that is attempted, furthermore, by making use of its own terminology, emptied of its real meaning and refilled with counterfeit content.

Independently of any empirical verification, independently of any other consideration, dignity is something that must be recognized to every human being as such, and whatever flouts that dignity should be intolerable for every morally responsible person.

Concerning rights, we find a convincing explanation in the pages of an essay written many years ago. I refer to the words of the German philosopher Hannah Arendt, active in the later twentieth century and well known for her pioneering analysis of totalitarian regimes in *The Origin of Totalitarianism* and for her book *Eichmann in Jerusalem. A Report on the Banality of Evil*, dedicated to the trial of the Nazi hierarch Adolf Eichmann [52].

The question of rights and the problems attached to their protection became clear to Arendt when she came dramatically face to face with the condition of statelessness.

The stateless were, for her, those who "once they had left their state," "became stateless," "deprived of their human rights," "rightless, the scum of the earth" [53] (ch. 9). Their condition became radically transformed, Arendt continued: "It turned out that the moment human beings lacked their own government and had to fall back upon their minimum rights, no authority was left to protect them and no institution was willing to guarantee them" [53] (ch. 9, § II). "The rights of man, supposedly inalienable, proved to be unenforceable – even in countries whose constitutions were based on them – whenever people appeared who were no longer citizens of any state" [53] (ch. 9, § II). Thus, during the Second World War, Arendt observed, "stateless people were invariably in a worse position than foreign *enemies* who were still protected indirectly by their governments through international treaties" [53] (ch. 9, § II).

What emerges is the retrospective effect, also in legal terms, assumed by the condition of belonging. "The calamity of the rightless is not that they are deprived of life, liberty, and the pursuit of happiness, or of equality before the law and freedom of opinion ... but that they no longer belong to any [recognized] community. Their plight is not that they are not equal before the law, but that no law exists for them; not that they are oppressed but that nobody wants even to oppress them" [53] (ch. 9, § II).

The question here is not the importance of belonging to a community for the recognition of personal autonomy, but the consequences of the total loss or lack of this belonging.

"We become aware of the existence of a right to have rights [...] and of a right to belong to some kind of organized community only"—a tremendous de facto truth—"when millions of people emerge who had lost and could not regain these rights because of the new global political situation" [53] (ch. 9, § II).

What is at play is not the discrimination of a politically recognized community, but the condition of not belonging to any community; and this, not for individuals who find they have to live and move in such a condition, but for the rest of the world, for nations that are unable to see these individuals because they have fallen into a condition of moral and legal invisibility.

"The decisive factor," Arendt concluded, "is that these rights and the human dignity they bestow should remain valid and real if only a single human being existed on earth; they are independent of human plurality and should remain valid even if a human being is expelled from the human community" [53] (ch. 9, § II), [52].

12.6 Conclusion

In conclusion, how can we attempt to defend rights and dignity? How can we deal with the premises, with the existential condition of people who face for this reason the probable manifestation of psychic unease and even psychotic disturbances?

First of all, since widespread political responsibilities are interwoven with murky processes aimed at influencing and forming public opinion, it is necessary to unmask the false arguments, purge the democratic process of unwanted accretions and throw a spotlight on the snares implicit in the concept of dignity and in the power to guarantee rights only to those counted as citizens. The challenge of migrants, of *people on the move*, is a challenge to democracy. For many of these are people who no longer have a land of their own, because it has been overturned, battered, or has become arid and sterile. It is the challenge already perceived 70 years ago by Arendt when she reasoned (with thoughts that make horrific reading today) on the condition of the stateless person, of the person without a recognized country, or the citizen of a country that no longer exists: destitute, destroyed and under attack.

Who will defend these people's rights now, those rights that pertain to a dignity they are entitled to because they are human beings? We should be able to reply: all democratic countries, because a democratic country must be able to recognize the right to have rights.

References

1. Selten JP, Van Der Ven E, Termorshuizen F (2019) Migration and psychosis: a meta-analysis of incidence studies. Psychol Med 50(2):303–313. https://doi.org/10.1017/S0033291719000035
2. European Network of National Networks studying Gene-Environment Interactions in Schizophrenia (EU-GEI), van Os J, Rutten BP et al (2014) Identifying gene-environment interactions in schizophrenia: contemporary challenges for integrated, large-scale investigations. Schizophr Bull 40(4):729–736. https://doi.org/10.1093/schbul/sbu069.49
3. Termorshuizen F, Van Der Ven E, Tarricone I et al (2022) The incidence of psychotic disorders among migrants and minority ethnic groups in Europe: findings from the multinational EU-GEI study. Psychol Med 52(7):1376–1385. https://doi.org/10.1017/S0033291720003219
4. Tarricone I, Boydell J, Kokona A et al (2016) Risk of psychosis and internal migration: results from the Bologna First Episode Psychosis study. Schizophr Res 173(1–2):90–93. https://doi.org/10.1016/j.schres.2016.02.032
5. Hickling FW, Rodgers-Johnson P (1995) The incidence of first contact schizophrenia in Jamaica. Br J Psychiatry 167(2):193–196. https://doi.org/10.1192/bjp.167.2.193
6. Bhugra D, Hilwig M, Hossein B et al (1996) First-contact incidence rates of schizophrenia in Trinidad and one-year follow-up. Br J Psychiatry 169(5):587–592. https://doi.org/10.1192/bjp.169.5.587.53
7. Mahy GE, Mallett R, Leff J, Bhugra D (1999) First-contact incidence rate of schizophrenia on Barbados. Br J Psychiatry 175(1):28–33. https://doi.org/10.1192/bjp.175.1.28
8. Selten JP, Slaets J, Kahn R (1998) Prenatal exposure to influenza and schizophrenia in Surinamese and Dutch Antillean immigrants to The Netherlands. Schizophr Res 30(1):101–103. https://doi.org/10.1016/S0920-9964(97)00105-9.55
9. Baxter AJ, Charlson FJ, Cheng HG, Shidhaye R, Ferrari AJ, Whiteford HA (2016) Prevalence of mental, neurological, and substance use disorders in China and India: a systematic analysis. Lancet Psychiatry 3(9):832–841. https://doi.org/10.1016/S2215-0366(16)30139-0
10. Odegaard O (1932) Emigration and insanity. Acta Psychiatr Neurol Scand Suppl 4:1–206. 57
11. Van Der Ven E, Dalman C, Wicks S et al (2015) Testing Ødegaard's selective migration hypothesis: a longitudinal cohort study of risk factors for non-affective psychotic disorders among prospective emigrants. Psychol Med 45(4):727–734. https://doi.org/10.1017/S0033291714001780
12. Cantor-Graae E, Selten J-P (2005) Schizophrenia and migration: a meta-analysis and review. Am J Psychiatry 162(I):12–24. https://doi.org/10.1021/jf1031026
13. Fernando S (1991) Mental health, race and culture. Macmillan Education UK, London. https://doi.org/10.1007/978-1-349-21644-4
14. Littlewood R, Lipsedge M (1997) Aliens and alienists: ethnic minorities and psychiatry, 3rd edn. Routledge, London
15. Hickling FW, McKenzie K, Mullen R, Murray R (1999) A Jamaican psychiatrist evaluates diagnoses at a London psychiatric hospital. Br J Psychiatry 175(September):283–285. https://doi.org/10.1192/bjp.175.3.283
16. van der Ven E, Veling W, Tortelli A et al (2016) Evidence of an excessive gender gap in the risk of psychotic disorder among North African immigrants in Europe: a systematic review and meta-analysis. Soc Psychiatry Psychiatr Epidemiol 51(12):1603–1613. https://doi.org/10.1007/s00127-016-1261-0
17. Tarricone I, D'Andrea G, Storbini V et al (2021) First-episode psychosis and migration in Italy: results from a study in the Italian Mental Health Services (Pep-Ita Study). J Immigr Minor

Health 23(3):519–527. https://doi.org/10.1007/s10903-021-01168-w
18. Selten JP, Van Vliet K, Pleyte W, Herzog S, Hoek HW, Van Loon AM (2000) Borna disease virus and schizophrenia in Surinamese immigrants to The Netherlands. Med Microbiol Immunol 189(2):55–57. https://doi.org/10.1007/PL00008256
19. O'Neill SM, Curran EA, Dalman C et al (2016) Birth by caesarean section and the risk of adult psychosis: a population-based cohort study. Schizophr Bull 42(3):633–641. https://doi.org/10.1093/schbul/sbv152
20. Huibers MHW, Visser DH, Deckers MML, Van Schoor NM, Van Furth AM, Wolf BHM (2014) Vitamin D deficiency among native Dutch and first- and second-generation non-Western immigrants. Eur J Pediatr 173(5):583–588. https://doi.org/10.1007/s00431-013-2198-x
21. Morgan C, Charalambides M, Hutchinson G, Murray RM (2010) Migration, ethnicity, and psychosis: toward a sociodevelopmental model. Schizophr Bull 36(4):655–664. https://doi.org/10.1093/schbul/sbq051
22. Morgan C, Knowles G, Hutchinson G (2019) Migration, ethnicity and psychoses: evidence, models and future directions. World Psychiatry 18(3):247–258. https://doi.org/10.1002/wps.20655
23. Selten JP, Van Der Ven E, Rutten BPF, Cantor-Graae E (2013) The social defeat hypothesis of schizophrenia: an update. Schizophr Bull 39(6):1180–1186. https://doi.org/10.1093/schbul/sbt134
24. Selten J, Cantor-Graae E (2005) Social defeat: risk factor for schizophrenia? Br J Psychiatry 187(2):101–102. https://doi.org/10.1192/bjp.187.2.101
25. Hammels C, Pishva E, De Vry J et al (2015) Defeat stress in rodents: from behavior to molecules. Neurosci Biobehav Rev 59:111–140. https://doi.org/10.1016/j.neubiorev.2015.10.006
26. Egerton A, Howes OD, Houle S et al (2017) Elevated striatal dopamine function in immigrants and their children: a risk mechanism for psychosis. Schizophr Bull 43(2):293–301. https://doi.org/10.1093/schbul/sbw181
27. Tarricone I, D'Andrea G, Jongsma HE et al (2021) Migration history and risk of psychosis: results from the multinational EU-GEI study. Psychol Med:1–13. https://doi.org/10.1017/s003329172000495x
28. Kirkbride JB, Morgan C, Fearon P, Dazzan P, Murray RM, Jones PB (2007) Neighbourhood-level effects on psychoses: re-examining the role of context. Psychol Med 37(10):1413–1425. https://doi.org/10.1017/S0033291707000499
29. Van Os J, Hanssen M, Bijl RV, Vollebergh W (2001) Prevalence of psychotic disorder and community level of psychotic symptoms: an urban-rural comparison. Arch Gen Psychiatry 58(7):663–668. https://doi.org/10.1001/archpsyc.58.7.663
30. Berg AO, Melle I, Rossberg JI et al (2011) Perceived discrimination is associated with severity of positive and depression/anxiety symptoms in immigrants with psychosis: a cross-sectional study. BMC Psychiatry 11:77. https://doi.org/10.1186/1471-244X-11-77
31. Cooper C, Morgan C, Byrne M et al (2008) Perceptions of disadvantage, ethnicity and psychosis. Br J Psychiatry 192(3):185–190. https://doi.org/10.1192/bjp.bp.107.042291
32. Misra S, Gelaye B, Williams DR et al (2021) Perceived major experiences of discrimination, ethnic group, and risk of psychosis in a six-country case−control study. Psychol Med:1–9. https://doi.org/10.1017/S0033291721000453
33. Allardyce J, Gilmour H, Atkinson J, Rapson T, Bishop J, McCreadie RG (2005) Social fragmentation, deprivation and urbanicity: relation to first-admission rates for psychoses. Br J Psychiatry 187:401–406. https://doi.org/10.1192/bjp.187.5.401
34. Kirkbride JB, Jones PB (2011) The prevention of schizophrenia—what can we learn from ecoepidemiology? Schizophr Bull 37(2):262–271. https://doi.org/10.1093/schbul/sbq120
35. Reininghaus UA, Morgan C, Simpson J et al (2008) Unemployment, social isolation, achievement– expectation mismatch and psychosis: findings from the ÆSOP Study. Soc Psychiatry Psychiatr Epidemiol 43(9):743–751. https://doi.org/10.1007/s00127-008-0359-4
36. Tarricone I, Atti AR, Salvatori F et al (2009) Psychotic symptoms and general health in a socially disadvantaged migrant community in Bologna. Int J Soc Psychiatry 55(3):203–213. https://doi.org/10.1177/0020764008093445
37. Anderson KK, Edwards J (2020) Age at migration and the risk of psychotic disorders: a systematic review and meta-analysis. Acta Psychiatr Scand 141(5):410–420. https://doi.org/10.1111/acps.13147
38. Dykxhoorn J, Hollander AC, Lewis G, Dalman C, Kirkbride JB (2019) Family networks during migration and risk of non-affective psychosis: a population-based cohort study. Schizophr Res 208:268–275. https://doi.org/10.1016/j.schres.2019.01.044
39. Jongsma HE, Gayer-Anderson C, Tarricone I et al (2021) Social disadvantage, linguistic distance, ethnic minority status and first-episode psychosis: results from the EU-GEI case-control study. Psychol Med 51(9):1536–1548. https://doi.org/10.1017/S003329172000029X
40. Schofeld P, Thygesen M, Das-Munshi J et al (2017) Ethnic density, urbanicity and psychosis risk for migrant groups—a population cohort study. Schizophr Res 190:82–87. https://doi.org/10.1016/j.schres.2017.03.032
41. Llácer A, Victoria Zunzunegui M, del Amo J, Mazarrasa L, Bolůmar F (2007) The contribution of a gender perspective to the understanding of migrants' health. J Epidemiol Community Health 61:4–10. https://doi.org/10.1136/jech.2007.061770
42. Milewski N, Struffolino E, Bernardi L (2018) Migrant status and lone motherhood—risk factors of female labour force participation in Switzerland.

Springer, Cham, pp 141–163. https://doi.org/10.1007/978-3-319-63295-7_7
43. Riaño Y, Baghdadi N (2007) Understanding the labour market participation of skilled immigrant women in Switzerland: the interplay of class, ethnicity, and gender. J Int Migr Integr 8(2):163–183. https://doi.org/10.1007/s12134-007-0012-1
44. Tarricone I, Morgan C, Boydell J et al (2017) Occupation and first episode psychosis in Northern Italy: better outcomes for migrants. Early Interv Psychiatry 11(6):522–525. https://doi.org/10.1111/eip.12325
45. Tarricone I, Mimmi S, Paparelli A et al (2012) First-episode psychosis at the West Bologna Community Mental Health Centre: results of an 8-year prospective study. Psychol Med 42(11):2255–2264. https://doi.org/10.1017/S0033291712000335
46. Lasalvia A, Bonetto C, Tosato S et al (2014) First-contact incidence of psychosis in North-Eastern Italy: influence of age, gender, immigration and socioeconomic deprivation. Br J Psychiatry 205(2):127–134. https://doi.org/10.1192/bjp.bp.113.134445
47. Carens J (2013) The ethics of immigration. Oxford University Press, Oxford
48. Margalit A (1998) The decent society (trans. Goldblum N). Harvard University Press, Cambridge, MA
49. Kant I (2008) Fundamental principles of the metaphysics of morals [1785] (trans: Kingsmill Abbott Th). Cosimo, New York
50. Arendt H (1998) The human condition [1958]. The University of Chicago Press, Chicago
51. Waldron J (2019) Human dignity: a pervasive value. NYU School of Law, Public Law Research Paper 20-46. https://ssrn.com/abstract=3463973
52. Arendt H (2006) Eichmann in Jerusalem. A report on the banality of evil [1963]. Penguin Books, New York
53. Arendt H (2017) The origin of totalitarianism [1951]. Penguin Books, New York

Radicalization and Mental Health

13

Corrado De Rosa, Andrea Fiorillo, Valeria Del Vecchio, Pierluigi Catapano, Davide Guadagno, Antonio Volpicelli, and Gaia Sampogna

Abstract

The recent increase in global conflicts has been associated with the phenomenon of the active participation of civilians into the conflicts, including "foreign fighters," often driven by complex motivations beyond economic gain. This phenomenon can be explained by the radicalization process, a multi-step process leading individuals to adopt extreme ideological beliefs that can manifest in mass violence. Different models of radicalization, including the Pyramid Model and the Two Pyramid Model, have been described, illustrating the gradient from sympathizers to terrorists, with the latter representing the apex of radical commitment. This chapter explores the changing landscape of radicalization in Europe, emphasizing the rise of "home-grown" terrorists and the shifting methods of recruitment facilitated by the internet. These changes have led to younger and more vulnerable individuals being drawn into radical ideologies. The focus will be on the specific case of foreign fighters, highlighting their historical presence in conflicts and the recent interest due to their involvement in the Middle East, particularly with jihadist groups like Daesh. The Russo-Ukrainian War has also attracted foreign fighters, with thousands joining both pro-Russian and pro-Ukrainian forces. Finally, we will underscore the need for strategies that aim to prevent radicalization and mitigate the associated security risks.

Keywords

Foreign fighter · Russo-Ukrainian War
Radicalization · Mental disorders
Interventions

13.1 Background

In recent years, the international scene has been increasingly marked by the outbreak of conflicts, driven by economic, geopolitical, and ideological reasons. A new phenomenon has been witnessed, that is the direct involvement in the war of civilians, choosing to fight without being formally compelled to do so. Additionally, there are those who, despite not belonging to the affected population nor being citizens of the country involved in the conflict, decide to join the fight and are defined foreign fighters. The phenomenon of foreign fighters—i.e., individuals who join insurgencies abroad and whose primary motivation is ideological or religious rather than financial—is quite recent.

C. De Rosa · A. Fiorillo · V. Del Vecchio · P. Catapano · D. Guadagno · A. Volpicelli · G. Sampogna (✉)
Department of Psychiatry, University of Campania "L. Vanvitelli", Naples, Italy
e-mail: andrea.fiorillo@unicampania.it; gaia.sampogna@unicampania.it

A. Fiorillo, S. De Giorgi (eds.), *Social Determinants of Mental Health*, Sustainable Development Goals Series, https://doi.org/10.1007/978-3-031-70165-8_13

From 1980 to mid-2010 between 10,000 and 30,000 such fighters took part in armed conflicts in the Muslim world. Since the Arab Spring protests turned into a fully fledged civil war in Syria, the phenomenon has acquired an entirely new dimension. The new surge of jihadism is not restricted to Syria and Iraq, since the Syrian conflict has attracted more foreign fighters than any other recent or current conflict.

The process of recruitment of foreign fighters is complex and can be analyzed from multiple points of view. In particular, a crucial role is played by radicalization, defined as a process by which individuals adopt political, social, and religious ideation that leads to the initiation of mass violence acts [1, 2]. Also, according to Khosrokhavar, radicalization is a "process by which an individual or a group adopts a violent form of action, directly linked to an extremist ideology with a social or religious political content that undermines the established political, social or cultural order".

According to recent reviews, no specific factors leading to radicalization have been identified: radicalized individuals come from different backgrounds, origins, family beliefs, social status, or gender [3–5].

Several models have been proposed for interpreting the process of radicalization, including the pyramid model of radicalization and the two pyramids model. The former emphasizes that only a few individuals are likely to commit an act of violence after going through a whole step-by-step process [1, 6]. This model describes radicalization as the gradient that separates terrorists from sympathizers. The basis of the pyramid is made up of all those who sympathize with the terrorists' goals/aims. From the basis to the apex, higher levels of the pyramid are associated with decreasing numbers of radicalized people, but increasing radicalization of beliefs, attitudes, and behaviors. In Northern Ireland, for example, the basis of the pyramid of support for the Irish Republican Army (IRA) was made up of those who were in favor of "Brits out." In the United States, the basis of the pyramid of support for antigovernment action is represented by the 40% of Americans, agreeing with the statement that "the federal government has become so large and powerful as to pose an imminent threat to the rights and liberties of ordinary people" [1]. The number of subjects sharing extreme ideologies is high and their ideas are deeply radicalized. However, there is a difference between radicalized individuals who commit violent acts as part of a radical group and individuals, the so-called "lone wolves," who become radicalized more quickly and for whom the pyramidal model does not apply [7]. According to recent studies, "lone wolves" represent a minority of terroristic individuals and are more likely to suffer from mental disorders.

Various predisposing factors might explain why certain individuals are more likely than others to move through the stages of the pyramidal process of radicalization, such as depressive symptoms suicidal thoughts [8, 9], or feelings of injustice or humiliation [10] (Table 13.1). Others insist on notions of identity and belonging, emphasizing that being part of a radical group and embracing a cause provides a comforting sense of "searching for meaning" around a commitment that has an "empowering effect" on the radicalized individual [5, 11, 12]. Moments of "existential fragility" have also been identified as elements of vulnerability that can promote radical commitment [13]. The radical group effect, together with the strong influence of leaders on individuals throughout the radicalization process, also plays a role [14]. Literature reviews suggest that environmental, political, religious, social, and cultural contexts are important, making it difficult to compare radicalization from one context to another [5, 6].

The two-Pyramids Model proposed by McCauley and Moskalenko [15] is an innovative model, distinguishing between the radicalization of beliefs and the radicalization of actionable

Table 13.1 Risks factor for radicalization process

• Depressive symptoms or suicidal thoughts
• Feelings of injustice or humiliation
• Notions of identity and belonging
• Searching for meaning
• Existential fragility

extremism, aligning with arguments presented by Borum and Fein [16], emphasizing the need to differentiate between the development of extremist ideologies and the commencement of violence or extremist behavior [15].

The differentiation is critical, as the psychological journey from holding extremist views to taking extremist action varies substantially. The prevailing research within social psychology highlights the weak association between one's attitudes and subsequent behaviors [17]. Further studies underscore the disparity between contemplation and execution of severe actions, such as the contemplation of suicide versus actual suicide attempts or the prevalence of homicidal thoughts versus their execution.

The differentiation of ideological and behavioral radicalization is conceptualized in the two-pyramids: (1) the Opinion Pyramid, which is constituted by "neutral individuals" who are indifferent, "sympathizers" (who support causes non-violently), "justifiers" (who advocate for violence in defense of a cause), and those who feel morally compelled to commit violence for their cause. This progression is not linear, and individuals can move among different levels non-sequentially; (2) the Action Pyramid considers individuals by their level of political action, from "inert" individuals to "activists" who participate in lawful actions, "radicals" engaging in unlawful actions, and "terrorists" who commit illegal and harmful acts against civilians. The transition between these levels is also non-linear. For example, although there are thousands with radical opinions, actual instances of jihadist terrorists in Western countries like the United States and United Kingdom are very low and often driven by personal reasons, such as personal revenge, escape, or love rather than ideological jihadist ideas.

The Two Pyramids model suggests that many people may hold radical ideologies, but only a few take radical actions, which often stem from personal factors or group dynamics rather than pure ideological reasons [18]. This highlights the complexity of the radicalization process and the need to understand both individual and group factors leading to extremist behavior.

13.2 Radicalization in Europe

With the emergence of "home-grown" terrorists, born and raised in Europe, who have adopted the ideology of violent radical Islamism, the phenomenon of terroristic acts has recently changed. The methods of recruitment and action have also changed, giving rise to new models of radicalization. According to Sageman (2008) and Khosrokhavar [19], since 2000s and 2010s, a new model of radicalization has emerged due to the increasing use of the Internet by jihadist movements, with radical groups being today less organized and less centralized than previous hierarchical organizations, such as al-Qaeda. This new model includes the following characteristics: the groups are small (up to three individuals), discrete (less proselytizing), younger, and composed of more vulnerable individuals who have been influenced by recruiters. Since 2010, radicalized individuals in Europe are younger than before (often teenagers) and that the number of young women involved is increasing.

13.3 The Foreign Fighters

Foreign fighters are militants who fight someone else's war and who, unlike mercenaries, choose to enlist for reasons that go beyond economic gain [20]. For more than 100 years, foreign fighters have been often present in conflict zones [16].

The phenomenon of foreign fighters has gained considerable attention due to the large number of individuals who have traveled in recent years to Iraq and Syria to join jihadist groups, especially Daesh (formerly known as ISIS). This phenomenon has increased with the involvement of foreign fighters in terrorist activities in European countries, as witnessed by the Franco-Belgian cell responsible for the attacks in Paris and Brussels during 2015–2016 [21]. Although most studies have focused on foreign fighters joining jihadist groups, another significant conflict, the Russo-Ukrainian War, has drawn a substantial number of foreign fighters as well. Foreign fighters have played a role in both phases of the conflict (2014–2021 and 2022–

present), with over 17,000 people joining the armed parties in Ukraine by 2021, many of whom were Russian or Russian-speaking. In February 2022, the Russian invasion was associated with a mass recruitment of foreign fighters, with Ukraine reporting over 20,000 volunteers from 52 countries signing up through its official website, and Russia claiming 16,000 fighters from the Middle East [22]. Foreign fighters pose significant security risks, particularly given the current rise in right-wing political violence, which some have labeled as a "fifth wave" of terrorism. However, the travel of far-right foreign fighters to Ukraine has not been evaluated at the EU level to the same extent as those going to Iraq and Syria [23].

Murauskaite [24] analyzed the reasons for joining Ukrainian War and grouped foreign fighters in four categories: (1) veterans with historical grievances; (2) disillusioned ideologues; (3) armed opposition; and (4) battle chasers. Each category, with the exception of the armed opposition, includes both pro-Russian and pro-Ukrainian fighters and, more generally, people with left and right-wing political convictions of varying extremity [24].

13.4 Radicalization and Mental Disorders

According to a systematic review, caution should be used for identifying a link between mental health/mental disorders and radicalization. Evidence to date is limited and available studies have several methodological limitations [2].

Bhui et al. (2014) have evaluated the role of depressive symptoms in a sample of Muslim participants living in the United Kingdom. They found that participants who were most sympathetic to violent protest had the highest scores for depressive symptoms [25]. However, a linear relationship with depressive symptoms was not found in any of the clusters that captured participants with different degrees of sympathy for violent protest (the most condemning group, the intermediate group, and the most sympathetic to violence). The role of depressive symptoms was examined also in the study by Coid et al. [26], who found that both pro-British and anti-British attitudes were linearly associated with violence but were negatively associated with depressive symptom scores. A study conducted on Palestinian refugees highlighted that greater support for religious-political violence was associated with loss of family members and feelings of injustice in the Israeli-Palestinian conflict [27]. Other studies did not confirm the association between depression and radicalization [28].

These discrepancies may be due to several factors. First, the relationship between depressive symptoms and radicalization has been investigated in different samples, recruited with different methodological approaches, and used different instruments to assess depressive symptoms. Second, the cross-sectional design of many studies does not allow for causal inference. Finally, it has long been suggested that depression may present in a variety of clinical forms that cannot be fully assessed with single instruments. Furthermore, sub-threshold depressive symptoms are also common in different mental disorders, including personality disorders, that may contribute to violent behaviors.

13.5 Lone Wolf Terrorists

Studies focused on lone wolf terrorists [7, 29] have found consistent evidence that this kind of terrorists, often socially isolated, may report higher prevalence rates of some mental disorders compared with group terrorists and the general population. Up to 43% of lone wolf terrorists have a history of mental illness, although not linked with any specific disorder [7, 30].

The prevalence of mental disorders is higher in sample of lone-wolf compared to terroristic group/organization, highlighting that recruiters tend to reject individuals with a history of mental disorder [31]. In particular, schizophrenia (8.5%), depression (7.2%), unspecified personality disorder (6.5%), bipolar disorder (3.9%), posttraumatic stress disorder (3.3%), autism spectrum disorder (3.3%), and delusional disorder (2.0%)

are the most frequent diagnoses in lone-actor terrorists [32].

Moreover, Corner and Gill [7] found no significant differences in pre-terrorist offending rates between those with or without a history of mental illness; raising the issue of whether terrorist acts are the first manifestation of a mental illness.

Although available studies on lone wolf have several methodological limitations, mental health of lone wolf warrants further investigation.

13.6 Personality Traits and Radicalization

During the 1970s and 1980s, studies on psychopathology and terrorist engagement focused on personality traits and disorders. Various studies supporting psychopathic and personality-level explanations were conducted without proper clinical diagnostic procedures and with clear methodological limitations. The relationship between mental disorders, personality traits, and extreme violence remained elusive due to study designs and data limitations [33, 34].

Nowadays, borderline, narcissistic, and antisocial personality disorders are most frequently represented in samples of terrorists. Those diagnosed with anti-social personality disorder present with persistent disregard for, and violation of, the rights of others, disrespect toward others' feelings, indifference and lack of remorse about their negative actions. Individuals with narcissistic personality disorder are marked by grandiosity, lack of empathy, and pathological need for admiration; individuals with borderline personality disorder present identity disturbance, difficulties in controlling anger, impulsivity, and instability in personal relationships. Other personality-driven explanations suggested that early life and family influences serve as a factor for terrorist engagement [35, 36]. However, these studies lacked empirical evidence and rigorous clinical diagnostic procedures, relying instead on autobiographies, biographies, and second-hand case studies.

Recent studies have focused on individuals sharing ideology of terrorist group, highlighting the role of many personal, contextual and social factors in determining the development of the terroristic behavior. For example, Feddes et al. [37] investigated the effects of resilience training on violent intentions and attitudes toward ideology-based violence in Muslim immigrant young people. The training significantly increased levels of agency, and there were marginal increases in self-esteem, empathy, perspective taking and narcissism; moreover, after the training, attitudes toward ideology-based violence and violent intentions were significantly lower. In particular, higher levels of empathy were associated with less positive attitudes toward ideology-based violence.

Identity fusion, right-wing authoritarianism, and group identification were significant predictors of in-group defensiveness in a study on university students and football hooligans [33]. The strongest predictors of acceptance of violent change were both right-wing and left-wing authoritarianism. Similarly, Laor et al. [38] found that both poles of political extremism are associated with high levels of ideological and morbid transcendence in a sample of Israeli Jewish participants. In addition, right-wing extremists have higher perceived threats to physical existence and national identity. Left-wing extremists report higher levels of perceived threats to moral integrity.

Soliman et al. [34] examined several cognitive, behavioral, and personality traits in relation to radicalization susceptibility in Egyptian adults. They found that the most important predictors of radicalization include rational decision-making, a dependent decision-making style, cognitive complexity, uncertainty, and an analytical cognitive style. Radicalization is also associated with paranoid personality disorder, antisocial personality disorder, and schizotypal personality disorder.

13.7 A Multidisciplinary Approach to Radicalization and Foreign Fighters

Those who become radicalized and join terrorist groups are typically ordinary individuals. They generally do not suffer from mental disorders, rather they are fanatical. They usually are not psychopaths, and apart from the isolated cases of "lone wolf" terrorists, they do not suffer from any mental disorder [39]. Given the complexity of the topic of radicalization, the various components of the process, including social, neuroscientific, psychological, and biological perspectives, should be considered [40].

13.8 Social Approach

Hyper-prosocial behaviors—extreme cooperative traits—are more likely to evolve during intergroup conflicts. Evidence shows that groups with a higher prevalence of prosocial individuals tend to collaborate better, passing these traits to future generations. Optimal conditions for such traits to flourish include intense competition among small groups [41].

Research also shows that humans tend to help or harm others based on perceived similarities, leading to strong in-group cooperation and out-group discrimination. This "like-me" psychology promotes tolerance and collaboration within groups but can result in ostracism or aggression toward those who are different or nonconforming. Both altruistic and violent behaviors have evolved through natural selection and are equally biologically important [42, 43].

Humans have the capacity for extreme sociality and, paradoxically, intense ruthlessness, often dehumanizing out-group members to justify aggression. From an evolutionary perspective, the aggression escalation toward out-groups may be an unintended consequence of selection for stronger in-group cooperation. Evolutionary patterns indicate that favoritism toward one's own group coupled with hostility toward others are successful survival strategies [44, 45].

Human behavior is strongly influenced by social contexts and others' behaviors. Milgram [46] found that two-thirds of participants were willing to administer lethal shocks to a person under authority pressure. Similarly, in the Zimbardo's prison experiment, a third of volunteer "guards" became abusive toward "prisoners." These studies highlight the role of situational factors and group dynamics in driving ordinary people to violence [46, 47]. However, the resistance of some individuals to engage in such acts despite pressure outlines the role of personality dispositions. The consistency of these obedience levels over the past 50 years suggests the enduring impact of these social influences [48]. Various personal traits can predict an individual's propensity to deliver high-intensity shocks in modified scenarios of the Milgram obedience experiment [49]. Functional neuroimaging studies suggest that empathy may play a role in how individuals obey authority. During a virtual reality version of the Milgram experiment, scans showed that individuals had heightened activity in brain areas such as the ventrolateral prefrontal cortex and amygdala when they observed virtual avatars experiencing pain [50], suggesting that violent behaviors can be due to the damage of these cerebral structures.

In order to identify social mechanisms underlying the process of radicalization, the Significance Quest Theory (SQT) has been developed as an analytical framework for violent extremism. According to this model, violent extremism is the product of a quest for significance triggered by a need for significance (need) and nourished by subscription to a radical ideology (narrative) and affiliation with a radical network (network) [51]. The Significance Quest Theory offers a framework for understanding how certain victimization narratives, especially those centered on the infringement of sacred values, may act as risk factors contributing to radicalization [51, 52].

13.9 Neuroscientific Approach

The complex relationship between the brain and behavior requires a collaborative, multidisciplinary effort. Social neuroscience stands at the intersection of these efforts, exploring the biological underpinnings of social systems, processes, and behaviors, and examining how these biological factors interact with social dynamics at various levels of organization [53].

In the field of political psychology, a multilevel interdisciplinary approach, combining the study of brain functioning with the analysis of beliefs, values, motivations, and emotions underlying political position, is very frequently adopted [54].

Current evidence indicates a robust connection between the structure and function of the brain and the psychological mechanisms influencing political attitudes. Variations in neurocognitive architecture and activity are indeed associated with a range of social and psychological dynamics that evolve over time [54].

A functional neuroimaging study recently found that when participants are faced with sacred values they would not trade for material benefits, there is an increased activity in the ventrolateral prefrontal cortex and in the left temporoparietal junction [55].

13.10 Psychological Approach

According to the psychological approach, cognitive theories explain the process of learning and thinking and are essential for understanding the development of extreme beliefs through psychological and social factors. Behaviorism, which focuses on observable behaviors and external reinforcements, has shaped educational and policy approaches to radicalization, but it has been considered an oversimplistic approach for such a complex phenomenon [56].

Cognitive flexibility is a psychological characteristic crucial in the process of radicalization [57]. People with low cognitive flexibility and lack of tolerance for ambiguity are prone to fall under the influence of extremists with ideological, political, or religious agendas, offering oversimplified perspectives. In fact, a positive correlation between cognitive inflexibility and tendencies toward authoritarian aggression, racism, and ethnocentrism has been found [9]. Rigid thinking and strong personal beliefs can act as barriers to unwelcome information, leading to intolerance. Extremism is not limited to any one ideology or religion [58].

Psychological factors, such as personal uncertainty, perceived injustice, group threat, and perceived immorality can lead to "hot cognition" with emotions influencing thinking and potentially leading to radical beliefs [59]. Low self-esteem and strong group identification can foster a sense of unfairness, driving defensive, or radical behaviors [58].

The psychoanalytic theory states that personality develops in distinct stages of life, with unresolved stages potentially leading to fixations and psychological issues [60, 61]. Since harmful violent thoughts and actions are labelled as "abnormal," this approach has been criticized, since not all extremists can be considered "psychologically abnormal".

13.11 Biological Approach

Executive functions, including cognitive flexibility, are based in specific brain areas of the prefrontal cortex and are necessary in the choice of actions when faced with conflicting internal objectives [62]. In particular, cognitive control and motivation are jointly regulated through bidirectional connections between the medial prefrontal cortex and the lateral prefrontal cortex, where control signals are graded along an anterior-posterior axis [63]. Zhong et al. [64] found a link between damage to the dorsolateral prefrontal cortex and the adoption of fundamentalist beliefs, a connection that is influenced by cognitive flexibility and the personality trait of openness [64].

A study involving around 1.3 million individuals, both adoptees and non-adoptees, revealed a higher propensity for engaging in violent criminal behavior in adoptees if there was a history of criminal violence in their biological parents [65].

Children who have experienced maltreatment and possess alleles linked to reduced activity of monoamine oxidase A (MAO-A) show a greater tendency to exhibit antisocial behavior by growing up [66]. This pattern is not confirmed in children with a genetic profile resulting in high MAO-A activity. These results show the complex interplay between genetic predispositions to violence and environmental influences. In addition to MAO-A, several neurotransmitter systems have been associated with aggressive antisocial behavior, including the serotonergic hypofunction [67]. An acute dose of a selective serotonin-reuptake inhibitor, which enhances serotonergic activity, led to healthy volunteers being more likely to accept unfair offers in the Crockett et al. study [68].

Neuroimaging studies reveal a heightened activity in the orbitofrontal cortex and a stronger connection to the temporoparietal junction when individuals imagine committing unjustified (like shooting civilians) versus justified (like shooting enemy soldiers) acts of killing [69].

Specific brain circuits seem to be involved in observing and imaging violent acts. Studies focusing on agency—the sense of control over one's actions and their outcomes—asking participants to imagine themselves as either the aggressor or the victim found that imagining oneself as the aggressor decreases the amygdala activity, reduces amygdala-ventromedial prefrontal cortex connectivity, and increases activity in the secondary visual cortex, posterior thalamus, and striatum. These neural changes, particularly the reduced activation in the ventromedial prefrontal cortex, align with brain response to patterns previously reported in studies on imagined aggression [70].

Increased activity in the thalamus and striatum along with decreased activity in the ventromedial prefrontal cortex has been associated with a pleasure response to aggression and a reduced ability to regulate aggressive impulses [71–73].

13.12 The Impact of Social Determinants on Radicalization Process

The social determinants of health are non-medical factors that influence health outcomes. These include the conditions in which people are born, grow, work, and live as well as a broader set of factors shaping the conditions of daily life. Among these forces and systems are economic policies, development agendas, social norms, social policies, racism, climate change, and political systems [74].

Several reviews have confirmed that there is no pre-determined path that leads to radicalization [3–5]. Socioeconomic status, ethnicity, education, deprivation, religious affiliation, poverty, and the quest for personal significance might play a role in the radicalization process. However, these elements are not sufficiently specific, necessary, or adequate to be recognized as fundamental causes [9, 75].

Understanding the interplay between discrimination, social cohesion, and violence can offer insights into how certain interpersonal and structural factors contribute to the risk of individuals engaging in terrorism or becoming violently radicalized [76].

Discrimination at the individual and institutional levels correlates with poor health outcomes and disparities [77]. Discrimination acts as a unique uncontrollable and unpredictable stressor and being perceived as a threat can reduce social cohesion and social capital, which are key to community health and violence prevention [78].

Social cohesion is the solidarity and connectedness within groups, social capital includes the elements of social structures—like trust, reciprocity, and mutual aid—that empower individuals and enable joint action. It includes the tangible benefits from social networks, such as support, information, and social credentials. Social capital forms networks by bringing similar people together (bonding) and connecting diverse individuals (bridging). Social capital's influence on social cohesion is related to the broader socio-political and economic context [79]. Social cohesion can improve health through sharing health knowledge, improving access to services, and providing emotional support and respect.

13.13 Intervention Strategies and Implications for Mental Health Professionals

Given the political and social impact of the phenomenon of radicalization, there is the need to identify possible preventive and intervention strategies (Table 13.2). In particular, primary prevention may involve building community cohesion and inclusion, while second-

Table 13.2 Levels of prevention strategies according to the WHO framework

		Target population	Type of intervention
Intervention strategies	Primary prevention	The overall population, encompassing law enforcement professionals, victims, and local societies	Programs focused on building community capacity/cohesion and feelings of inclusion
	Secondary prevention	Individuals or collectives flagged as vulnerable to radicalization or involvement in violent extremism and/or terrorist actions	Programs aimed to reduce vulnerability or risk of radicalization
	Tertiary prevention	Individuals or collectives (including those radicalized prior to any criminal justice involvement) or individuals or groups that have participated in acts of violent extremism and/or terrorist actions	Programs oriented to deradicalize convicted extremists

Adapted from World Health Organization [80]

ary prevention focuses on reducing the vulnerability to radicalization. Tertiary prevention includes deradicalization programs for convicted extremists [81]. Public security officers as well as legal system are essential for the promotion of de-radicalization [82, 83]. The complexity of radicalization and terrorism has led to a multi-agency approach involving information sharing, community outreach, intelligence gathering, and training programs. An example is the WORDE program, which includes community education, referral networks, and participation in community activity [84].

Mental health professionals can play a significant role in all these different levels of intervention. In particular, their involvement is particularly crucial in tertiary prevention, which focused on people already radicalized.

Deradicalization is an effort to eliminate radical thinking by promoting an understanding of inclusive, friendly, moderate, and peaceful values within the context of diversity and pluralism [85]. Deradicalization programs require collaboration among various stakeholders, including government institutions, religious organizations, non-governmental organizations, civil society, and program participants [86].

Several programs designed for the individual deradicalization process are available. The model proposed by Taskarina and Nuri in Indonesia [87] includes activities for re-educate, resocialize, and economically empower those previously involved in terrorism, with the ultimate aim of fostering nationalism and societal integration.

The Indonesian program is divided into inside-prison and outside-prison deradicalization, targeting various aspects of rehabilitation, education, and social reintegration. The inside-prison program targets terrorists in jails from admission to release, involving identification, assessment, rehabilitation, re-education, nationalism, civic education, and conflict management. The outside-prison program involves social reintegration and targets not only ex-terrorists, but also suspected communities surrounding ex-convicts.

Long-term deradicalization programs within correctional facilities face challenges due to non-ideal prison conditions, such as overcapacity, which may further increase the levels of radicalization of prisoners. In-prison deradicalization efforts should also target the prison environment itself, including general prisoners and local officers, to strengthen the values of peace and non-violence. The obstacles align with criticisms of peacemaking criminology regarding practical level issues and the need for individual transformation to overcome the motivations behind criminal offenses, especially terrorist acts.

A multidisciplinary approach involving criminology, sociology, psychology and psychiatry is needed for developing effective strategies. Despite the comprehensive nature of these programs, there is ongoing debate about their success and the risk of recidivism among terrorists [88].

13.14 Conclusions

Understanding the process of radicalization requires a multidisciplinary approach due to its complexity. The escalation of conflicts driven by economic, geopolitical, and ideological forces has resulted in civilians participating in combat activities.

Moreover, the interplay between mental health and radicalization is intricate, with personality traits, mental disorders, and cognitive processes playing a significant role in developing extremist beliefs and behaviors. Social factors, including discrimination, lack of social cohesion, and social capital, are critical in increasing an individual's vulnerability to the radicalization process. Intervention strategies including primary, secondary, and tertiary preventive approaches can play a significant role in the deradicalization program.

References

1. McCauley C, Moskalenko S (2008) Mechanisms of political radicalization: pathways toward terrorism. Terror Polit Violence 20:415–433. https://doi.org/10.1080/09546550802073367
2. Misiak B, Samochowiec J, Bhui K, Schouler-Ocak M, Demunter H, Kuey L, Raballo A, Gorwood P, Frydecka D, Dom G (2019) A systematic review on the relationship between mental health, radicalization and mass violence. Eur Psychiatry 56:51–59. https://doi.org/10.1016/j.eurpsy.2018.11.005
3. Fekih-Romdhane F, Chennoufi L, Cheour M (2016) Les terroristes suicidaires : qui sont-ils ? Ann Méd-Psychol Rev Psychiatr 174:274–279. https://doi.org/10.1016/j.amp.2015.10.026
4. McCauley C, Leuprecht C, Hataley T, Winn C, Biswas B (2011) Tracking the war of ideas: a poll of Ottawa Muslims. Terror Polit Violence 23:804–819. https://doi.org/10.1080/09546553.2011.596774
5. McGilloway A, Ghosh P, Bhui K (2015) A systematic review of pathways to and processes associated with radicalization and extremism amongst Muslims in Western societies. Int Rev Psychiatry 27:39–50. https://doi.org/10.3109/09540261.2014.992008
6. Moyano M, Trujillo HM (2014) Intention of activism and radicalism among Muslim and Christian youth in a marginal neighbourhood in a Spanish city / Intención de activismo y radicalismo de jóvenes musulmanes y cristianos residentes en un barrio marginal de una ciudad española. Rev Psicol Soc 29:90–120. https://doi.org/10.1080/02134748.2013.878571
7. Corner E, Gill P (2015) A false dichotomy? Mental illness and lone-actor terrorism. Law Hum Behav 39:23–34. https://doi.org/10.1037/lhb0000102
8. Merari A, Diamant I, Bibi A, Broshi Y, Zakin G (2009) Personality characteristics of "self martyrs"/"suicide bombers" and organizers of suicide attacks. Terror Polit Violence 22:87–101. https://doi.org/10.1080/09546550903409312
9. Victoroff J (2005) The mind of the terrorist: a review and critique of psychological approaches. J Confl Resolut 49:3–42. https://doi.org/10.1177/0022002704272040
10. Victoroff J, Quota S, Adelman JR, Celinska B, Stern N, Wilcox R, Sapolsky RM (2010) Support for religio-political aggression among teenaged boys in Gaza: part I: psychological findings. Aggress Behav 36:219–231. https://doi.org/10.1002/ab.20348
11. Mccauley C, Scheckter S (2008) What's special about U.S. Muslims? The war on terrorism as seen by Muslims in the United States, Morocco, Egypt, Pakistan, and Indonesia. Stud Confl Terror 31:1024–1031. https://doi.org/10.1080/10576100802400193
12. Kruglanski AW, Chen X, Dechesne M, Fishman S, Orehek E (2009) Fully committed: Suicide bombers' motivation and the quest for personal significance. Political Psychology 30(3):331–357.
13. Kruglanski AW, Bélanger JJ, Gelfand M, Gunaratna R, Hettiarachchi M, Reinares F, Orehek E, Sasota J, Sharvit K (2013) Terrorism—a (self) love story: redirecting the significance quest can end violence. Am Psychol 68:559–575. https://doi.org/10.1037/a0032615
14. Moghaddam FM (2005) The staircase to terrorism: a psychological exploration. American psychologist 60(2):161–169.
15. McCauley C, Moskalenko S (2017) Understanding political radicalization: the two-pyramids model. Am Psychol 72:205–216. https://doi.org/10.1037/amp0000062
16. Borum R, Fein R (2017) The psychology of foreign fighters. Stud Confl Terror 40:248–266. https://doi.org/10.1080/1057610X.2016.1188535
17. Wicker AW (1969) Attitudes versus Actions: The Relationship of Verbal and Overt Behavioral

Responses to Attitude Objects. Journal of Social Issues 25:41–78
18. Leuprecht C, Hataley T, Moskalenko S, McCauley C (2010) Narratives and counter-narratives for global Jihad: opinion versus action. In: Kessels EJAM (ed) Countering violent extremist narratives. National Coordinator for Counterterrorism (NCTb), Breda, pp 58–71
19. Khosrokhavar F (2017) Radicalization: Why Some People Choose the Path of Violence. New Press 1–192
20. Rasmussen NJ (2015) Countering violent Islamist extremism: the urgent threat of foreign fighters and homegrown terror [WWW Document]. https://www.odni.gov/index.php/nctc-newsroom/nctc-speeches-testimonies-and-interviews/3081-countering-violent-islamist-extremism-the-urgent-threat-of-foreign-fighters-and-homegrown-terror. Accessed 27 Dec 23
21. Mullins S (2019) Jihadist infiltration of migrant flows to Europe: perpetrators, modus operandi and policy implications. Palgrave Macmillan, Cham. https://doi.org/10.1007/978-3-030-13338-2
22. Murauskaite EE (2022) Foreign fighters in Ukraine: what concerns should really be on the agenda? [WWW Document]. russiamatters.org. https://www.russiamatters.org/analysis/foreign-fighters-ukraine-what-concerns-should-really-be-agenda. Accessed 18 Nov 23
23. Kaunert C, MacKenzie A, Léonard S (2023) Far-right foreign fighters and Ukraine: a blind spot for the European Union? New J Eur Crim Law 14:247–266. https://doi.org/10.1177/20322844231164089
24. Murauskaite EE (2020) Foreign fighters in Ukraine: assessing potential risks. Vilnius Inst Policy Anal 28
25. Bhui K, Everitt B, Jones E (2014) Might depression, psychosocial adversity, and limited social assets explain vulnerability to and resistance against violent radicalisation? PLoS One 9:e105918. https://doi.org/10.1371/journal.pone.0105918
26. Coid JW, Bhui K, MacManus D, Kallis C, Bebbington P, Ullrich S (2016) Extremism, religion and psychiatric morbidity in a population-based sample of young men. Br J Psychiatry 209:491–497. https://doi.org/10.1192/bjp.bp.116.186510
27. Victoroff J, Quota S, Adelman JR, Celinska B, Stern N, Wilcox R, Sapolsky RM (2011) Support for religio-political aggression among teenaged boys in Gaza: part II: neuroendocrinological findings. Aggress Behav 37:121–132. https://doi.org/10.1002/ab.20376
28. Bhui K, Warfa N, Jones E (2014) Is violent radicalisation associated with poverty, migration, poor self-reported health and common mental disorders? PLoS One 9:e90718. https://doi.org/10.1371/journal.pone.0090718
29. Gill P, Horgan J, Deckert P (2014) Bombing alone: tracing the motivations and antecedent behaviors of lone-actor terrorists. J Forensic Sci 59:425–435. https://doi.org/10.1111/1556-4029.12312
30. Bhui K, James A, Wessely S (2016) Mental illness and terrorism. BMJ 354:i4869. https://doi.org/10.1136/bmj.i4869
31. Dom G, Schouler-Ocak M, Bhui K, Demunter H, Kuey L, Raballo A, Frydecka D, Misiak B, Gorwood P, Samochowiec J (2018) Mass violence, radicalization and terrorism: a role for psychiatric profession? Eur Psychiatry 49:78–80. https://doi.org/10.1016/j.eurpsy.2018.01.001
32. Corner E, Gill P, Mason O (2016) Mental health disorders and the terrorist: a research note probing selection effects and disorder prevalence. Stud Confl Terror 39:560–568. https://doi.org/10.1080/1057610X.2015.1120099
33. Besta T, Szulc M, Jaśkiewicz M (2015) Political extremism, group membership and personality traits: who accepts violence?/Extremismo político, pertenencia al grupo y rasgos de personalidad: ¿Quién acepta la violencia? Rev Psicol Soc 30:563–585. https://doi.org/10.1080/02134748.2015.1065085
34. Soliman A, Bellaj T, Khelifa M (2016) An integrative psychological model for radicalism: evidence from structural equation modeling. Personal Individ Differ 95:127–133. https://doi.org/10.1016/j.paid.2016.02.039
35. Ferracuti S, Bruno F (1981) Psychiatric Aspects of Terrorism in Italy (From Mad, the Bad, and the Different, P 199-213, Israel L Barak- Glantz et al, ed. - See NCJ-84231)
36. Kent I, Nicholls W (1977) The psychodynamics of terrorism. Mental Health & Society. 4(1–2):1–8.
37. Feddes AR, Mann L, Doosje B (2015) Increasing self-esteem and empathy to prevent violent radicalization: a longitudinal quantitative evaluation of a resilience training focused on adolescents with a dual identity. J Appl Soc Psychol 45:400–411. https://doi.org/10.1111/jasp.12307
38. Laor N, Yanay-Shani A, Wolmer L, Khoury O (2010) A trauma-like model of political extremism: psycho-political fault lines in Israel. Ann N Y Acad Sci 1208:24–31. https://doi.org/10.1111/j.1749-6632.2010.05693.x
39. Horgan J (2014) The psychology of terrorism, revised and updated second edition. Political violence. Routledge, Taylor & Francis Group, Abingdon
40. Decety J, Pape R, Workman CI (2018) A multilevel social neuroscience perspective on radicalization and terrorism. Soc Neurosci 13:511–529. https://doi.org/10.1080/17470919.2017.1400462
41. Boyd R, Richerson PJ (2009) Culture and the evolution of human cooperation. Philos Trans R Soc B Biol Sci 364:3281–3288. https://doi.org/10.1098/rstb.2009.0134
42. Hare B (2017) Survival of the friendliest: Homo sapiens evolved via selection for prosociality. Annu Rev Psychol 68:155–186. https://doi.org/10.1146/annurev-psych-010416-044201
43. Kurzban R, Burton-Chellew MN, West SA (2015) The evolution of altruism in humans. Annu Rev

Psychol 66:575–599. https://doi.org/10.1146/annurev-psych-010814-015355
44. Choi J-K, Bowles S (2007) The coevolution of parochial altruism and war. Science 318:636–640. https://doi.org/10.1126/science.1144237
45. Kteily N, Hodson G, Bruneau E (2016) They see us as less than human: metadehumanization predicts intergroup conflict via reciprocal dehumanization. J Pers Soc Psychol 110:343–370. https://doi.org/10.1037/pspa0000044
46. Milgram S (1963) Behavioral study of obedience. J Abnorm Soc Psychol 67:371–378. https://doi.org/10.1037/h0040525
47. Banuazizi A, Movahedi S (1975) Interpersonal dynamics in a simulated prison: a methodological analysis. Am Psychol 30:152–160. https://doi.org/10.1037/h0076835
48. Doliński D, Grzyb T, Folwarczny M, Grzybała P, Krzyszycha K, Martynowska K, Trojanowski J (2017) Would you deliver an electric shock in 2015? Obedience in the experimental paradigm developed by Stanley Milgram in the 50 years following the original studies. Soc Psychol Personal Sci 8:927–933. https://doi.org/10.1177/1948550617693060
49. Bègue L, Beauvois J, Courbet D, Oberlé D, Lepage J, Duke AA (2015) Personality predicts obedience in a Milgram paradigm. J Pers 83:299–306. https://doi.org/10.1111/jopy.12104
50. Cheetham M (2009) Virtual milgram: empathic concern or personal distress? Evidence from functional MRI and dispositional measures. Front Hum Neurosci 3. https://doi.org/10.3389/neuro.09.029.2009
51. Pemberton A, Aarten PGM (2018) Narrative in the study of victimological processes in terrorism and political violence: an initial exploration. Stud Confl Terror 41:541–556. https://doi.org/10.1080/1057610X.2017.1311110
52. Kruglanski AW, Gelfand MJ, Bélanger JJ, Sheveland A, Hetiarachchi M, Gunaratna R (2014) The psychology of radicalization and deradicalization: how significance quest impacts violent extremism. Polit Psychol 35:69–93. https://doi.org/10.1111/pops.12163
53. Cacioppo JT, Berntson GG, Decety J (2010) Social neuroscience and its relationship to social psychology. Soc Cogn 28:675–685. https://doi.org/10.1521/soco.2010.28.6.675
54. Jost JT, Nam HH, Amodio DM, Van Bavel JJ (2014) Political neuroscience: the beginning of a beautiful friendship. Polit Psychol 35:3–42. https://doi.org/10.1111/pops.12162
55. Berns GS, Bell E, Capra CM, Prietula MJ, Moore S, Anderson B, Ginges J, Atran S (2012) The price of your soul: neural evidence for the non-utilitarian representation of sacred values. Philos Trans R Soc B Biol Sci 367:754–762. https://doi.org/10.1098/rstb.2011.0262
56. Benevento A (2023) The necessity to recognize processes of radicalization from a socio-cultural perspective. Integr Psychol Behav Sci 57:1418–1434. https://doi.org/10.1007/s12124-021-09620-0
57. Hogg MA, Kruglanski A, Van Den Bos K (2013) Uncertainty and the roots of extremism. J Soc Issues 69:407–418. https://doi.org/10.1111/josi.12021
58. Jordan CH, Spencer SJ, Zanna MP (2005) Types of high self-esteem and prejudice: how implicit self-esteem relates to ethnic discrimination among high explicit self-esteem individuals. Personal Soc Psychol Bull 31:693–702. https://doi.org/10.1177/0146167204271580
59. Kunda Z (1999) Social cognition: Making sense of people. The MIT Press 1–150
60. Craib I (1989) Psychoanalysis and social theory: the limits of sociology, 1. publ edn. Harvester Wheatsheaf, New York
61. Kristeva J, Roudiez LS, Kristeva J (1991) Strangers to ourselves, European perspectives. Columbia Univ. Press, New York
62. Miyake A, Friedman NP, Emerson MJ, Witzki AH, Howerter A, Wager TD (2000) The unity and diversity of executive functions and their contributions to complex "frontal lobe" tasks: a latent variable analysis. Cognit Psychol 41:49–100. https://doi.org/10.1006/cogp.1999.0734
63. Kouneiher F, Charron S, Koechlin E (2009) Motivation and cognitive control in the human prefrontal cortex. Nat Neurosci 12:939–945. https://doi.org/10.1038/nn.2321
64. Zhong W, Cristofori I, Bulbulia J, Krueger F, Grafman J (2017) Biological and cognitive underpinnings of religious fundamentalism. Neuropsychologia 100:18–25. https://doi.org/10.1016/j.neuropsychologia.2017.04.009
65. Hjalmarsson R, Lindquist MJ (2013) The origins of intergenerational associations in crime: lessons from Swedish adoption data. Labour Econ 20:68–81. https://doi.org/10.1016/j.labeco.2012.11.001
66. Caspi A, McClay J, Moffitt TE, Mill J, Martin J, Craig IW, Taylor A, Poulton R (2002) Role of genotype in the cycle of violence in maltreated children. Science 297:851–854. https://doi.org/10.1126/science.1072290
67. Moore TM, Scarpa A, Raine A (2002) A meta-analysis of serotonin metabolite 5-HIAA and antisocial behavior. Aggress Behav 28:299–316. https://doi.org/10.1002/ab.90027
68. Crockett MJ, Clark L, Hauser MD, Robbins TW (2010) Serotonin selectively influences moral judgment and behavior through effects on harm aversion. Proc Natl Acad Sci 107:17433–17438. https://doi.org/10.1073/pnas.1009396107
69. Molenberghs P, Gapp J, Wang B, Louis WR, Decety J (2016) Increased moral sensitivity for outgroup perpetrators harming ingroup members. Cereb Cortex 26:225–233. https://doi.org/10.1093/cercor/bhu195
70. Pietrini P, Guazzelli M, Basso G, Jaffe K, Grafman J (2000) Neural correlates of imaginal aggressive behavior assessed by positron emission tomography

in healthy subjects. Am J Psychiatry 157:1772–1781. https://doi.org/10.1176/appi.ajp.157.11.1772
71. Decety J, Michalska KJ, Akitsuki Y, Lahey BB (2009) Atypical empathic responses in adolescents with aggressive conduct disorder: a functional MRI investigation. Biol Psychol 80:203–211. https://doi.org/10.1016/j.biopsycho.2008.09.004
72. Decety J, Porges EC (2011) Imagining being the agent of actions that carry different moral consequences: an fMRI study. Neuropsychologia 49:2994–3001. https://doi.org/10.1016/j.neuropsychologia.2011.06.024
73. Murray EA (2007) The amygdala, reward and emotion. Trends Cogn Sci 11:489–497. https://doi.org/10.1016/j.tics.2007.08.013
74. CDC (2022) Social determinants of health [WWW Document]. Cent. Dis. Control Prev. https://www.cdc.gov/about/sdoh/index.html. Accessed 18 Nov 23
75. Roy O (2017) Jihad and death: the global appeal of Islamic State, Comparative politics and international studies series. Hurst & Company, London
76. Alcalá HE, Sharif MZ, Samari G (2017) Social determinants of health, violent radicalization, and terrorism: a public health perspective. Health Equity 1:87–95. https://doi.org/10.1089/heq.2016.0016
77. Rousseau C, Jamil U, Bhui K, Boudjarane M (2015) Consequences of 9/11 and the war on terror on children's and young adult's mental health: a systematic review of the past 10 years. Clin Child Psychol Psychiatry 20:173–193. https://doi.org/10.1177/1359104513503354
78. Husband C, Alam Y (2011) Social cohesion and counter-terrorism: a policy contradiction? 1st edn. Bristol University Press. https://doi.org/10.2307/j.ctt9qgv8v
79. Cheong PH, Edwards R, Goulbourne H, Solomos J (2007) Immigration, social cohesion and social capital: a critical review. Crit Soc Policy 27:24–49. https://doi.org/10.1177/0261018307072206
80. World Health Organization. Global action plan for the prevention and control of noncommunicable diseases 2013–2020. https://www.who.int/publications/i/item/9789241506236
81. Sydes M, Hine L, Higginson A, McEwan J, Dugan L, Mazerolle L (2023) Criminal justice interventions for preventing radicalisation, violent extremism and terrorism: an evidence and gap map. Campbell Syst Rev 19:e1366. https://doi.org/10.1002/cl2.1366
82. Mazerolle L, Eggins E, Cherney A, Hine L, Higginson A, Belton E (2020) Police programmes that seek to increase community connectedness for reducing violent extremism behaviour, attitudes and beliefs. Campbell Syst Rev 16:e1111. https://doi.org/10.1002/cl2.1111
83. Jones C, Narag RE (2019) Inmate radicalisation and recruitment in prisons, Routledge advances in sociology. Routledge, London/New York
84. Williams MJ, Horgan JG, Evans WP (2016) Evaluation of a multi-faceted, U.S. Community-based, Muslim-led CVE program | Office of Justice Programs [WWW Document]. Httpswwwojpgovncjrsvirtual-Libr.-Multi-Facet.-Us-Community-Based-Muslim-Led-Cve-Program. https://www.ojp.gov/ncjrs/virtual-library/abstracts/evaluation-multi-faceted-us-community-based-muslim-led-cve-program. Accessed 30 Dec 23
85. Subagyo A (2021) The implementation of the pentahelix model for the terrorism deradicalization program in Indonesia. Cogent Soc Sci 7:1964720. https://doi.org/10.1080/23311886.2021.1964720
86. Muhammad A, Hiariej E (2021) Deradicalization program in Indonesia radicalizing the radicals. Cogent Soc Sci 7:1905219. https://doi.org/10.1080/23311886.2021.1905219
87. Taskarina L, Nuri WV (2021) Dreaming of the peaceful ways: an evaluation of the Indonesian deradicalisation program. Tech Soc Sci J 25:687–700. https://doi.org/10.47577/tssj.v25i1.5092
88. Wozniak JF (2002) Toward a theoretical model of peacemaking criminology: an essay in honor of Richard Quinney. Crime Delinquency 48:204–231. https://doi.org/10.1177/0011128702048002002

14 Promotion of Physical Health and Healthy Lifestyle Behaviors in Patients with Mental Disorders

Mario Luciano, Bianca Della Rocca, Matteo Di Vincenzo, Claudia Toni, Gaia Sampogna, and Andrea Fiorillo

Abstract

The increased prevalence of cardiovascular and metabolic diseases, such as obesity, dyslipidemia, diabetes mellitus, and metabolic syndrome, has resulted in a significantly lower life expectancy for patients with severe mental disorders (SMD), namely major depression, bipolar disorders, and schizophrenia and other psychotic disorders. The adoption of unhealthy lifestyle behaviors (such as poor eating and physical activity habits, heavy smoking, alcohol or drug abuse, and reduced access to screening programs and checkup visits for physical illnesses) is primarily to blame for the high rates of comorbidity between mental and physical illnesses. Additional contributing factors include some characteristics of mental disorders, such as a decline in cognitive functioning, patient's reluctance to attend checkup visits, the neglect of physical health needs by patients and their caregivers, and the metabolic side effects of several psychotropic drugs. The need to improve the physical healthcare provided to people with SMD through medical screenings, monitoring, and regular checkups, as well as the need to provide psychosocial interventions aimed at modifying risk factors—i.e., unhealthy lifestyle behaviors—has been recently pointed out. Additionally, changes to the healthcare system and delivery of care could be required to address the issue of poor medical healthcare offered to these patients. In this chapter we will provide; (1) an overview of the most frequent comorbidities reported by patients with severe mental illnesses; (2) recommendations for the monitoring of their physical health; and (3) a description of the efficacy of behavioral lifestyle interventions to improve physical health of SMD people.

Keywords

Comorbidities · Mental disorders · Physical health · Life expectancy · Lifestyle Mortality · Promotion · Behavioral interventions

14.1 Introduction

In the last decades, life expectancy is rising globally, although the number of years lived without an illness has not increased [1]. Along with an increase of life expectancy,

M. Luciano (✉) · B. Della Rocca · M. Di Vincenzo · C. Toni · G. Sampogna · A. Fiorillo
Department of Psychiatry, University of Campania "Luigi Vanvitelli", Naples, Italy
e-mail: mario.luciano@unicampania.it; andrea.fiorillo@unicampania.it

A. Fiorillo, S. De Giorgi (eds.), *Social Determinants of Mental Health*, Sustainable Development Goals Series, https://doi.org/10.1007/978-3-031-70165-8_14

comorbidity rates of general population have increased significantly. The presence of physical illnesses is associated with a significant reduction of quality of life and impairments in personal and social functioning and autonomy [2, 3]. Comorbidity, i.e., the simultaneous presence of two or more illnesses, is significantly increased, even among young people [4].

It has been anticipated that the number of people with comorbidities will increase in the years to come, due to several factors, including the aging of the population [5], the tendency to adopt unhealthy lifestyle behaviors, climate changes, and environmental pollution. Comorbidity is not just the combination of two diseases that develop independently and progress according to their regular course. The prognosis of all diseases will worsen if two or more diseases are present at the same time. This will also increase the quantity (and severity) of consequences and make the treatment of each disease more challenging and potentially less effective. Even worse, one of the concomitant disorders is frequently disregarded.

When it comes to the comorbidity between physical and mental disorders, the situation becomes worse. In fact, compared to the general population, people with severe mental disorders (SMD)—namely affective and schizophrenia spectrum disorders—show significant higher rates of physical disorders, compared to the general population, with a worse prognosis and increased premature mortality [6, 7]. According to available estimates, people with serious mental disorders have a life expectancy loss of at least 10–25 years, mainly due to cardiovascular, metabolic, and infectious diseases [8–10]. In this chapter, we will provide; (1) an overview of most frequent comorbidities reported by patients with severe mental disorders (SMD); (2) recommendations for monitoring physical health of people with SMD; and (3) a description of the efficacy of behavioral lifestyle intervention to improve physical health of people with SMD.

14.2 Physical Comorbidities of Patients with SMD

14.2.1 Obesity and Metabolic Syndrome in Patients with SMD

People with SMD and comorbid obesity have a significantly reduced life expectancy and are more likely to develop a number of general medical conditions, such as type 2 diabetes mellitus (relative risk, RR, >3), cardiovascular disease (CVD) (RR >2–3), dyslipidemia (RR >3), hypertension (RR >2–3), respiratory problems (RR >3), abnormalities in reproductive hormones (RR >1–2), and cancer (RR >1–2) [11, 16, 28].

A growing body of research suggests that people with SMD are more likely than the general population to be overweight (defined as a body mass index [BMI] of 25–29.9), obese (defined as a BMI of 30 or higher), and to present abdominal obesity, which are associated with a greater risk of acute cardiovascular events, even in the early stages of illness and/or when not taking any medication. However, the risk of obesity varies depending on the diagnosis of SMD [11]. In fact, compared to the general population, the risk of obesity is up to 1.5 times higher in people with major depressive disorder (MDD) or bipolar disorder (BD) and up to more than 4 times higher in people with schizophrenia spectrum disorder [12].

In addition, the prevalence of metabolic syndrome ranges from 29.4% to 67.9%, with prevalence rates 1.58 times higher in people with mental disorders compared to the general population [13]. About 81.7% of people with SMD who are referred to mental health centers have untreated lipid abnormalities and 63.9% have untreated glycemic abnormalities, demonstrating that physical health is frequently disregarded in this population.

Use of psychotropic drugs is another important cause of obesity in patients suffering from SMD

[11]. Weight gain is a common side effect of antipsychotics (AP), affecting between 15% and 72% of patients receiving acute and maintenance treatment for schizophrenia. Several reviews and meta-analyses have supported a hierarchy for the risk of weight gain associated with AP. Clozapine and olanzapine cause the most weight gain, whereas quetiapine and risperidone have an intermediate risk. Ziprasidone, amisulpride, asenapine, and aripiprazole have negligible effects on weight. Chlorpromazine and thioridazine are examples of so-called low-potency conventional AP medicines that carry a higher risk than high-potency medications like haloperidol [14–16]. No medication, however, should be considered completely weight-neutral because all APs significantly increase weight gain in AP-naive or first-episode patients.

Although mood stabilizers have a considerable impact on weight gain, compared to antipsychotics, their use is less frequently associated to obesity. Lithium causes weight gain more frequently than placebo, with 77% of patients reporting an average increase of 4–6.3 kg, probably because of increased appetite, hypothyroidism, and nephrogenic diabetes insipidus. Also, up to 50% of patients taking valproate experience weight gain, which is dose-independent [17, 18].

The risk of weight gain is modest with antidepressants (AD). In patients with MDD, long-term use (>6 months) and polypharmacy of antidepressants, such as mirtazapine, amitriptyline, paroxetine, can cause weight gain of up to 2.7 kg. However, the impact of antidepressants on weight gain can differ from a person to another, especially in the long-term [12].

The significant interindividual heterogeneity of medication-induced weight gain raises the possibility that genetic variables play a role in weight gain susceptibility.

14.2.2 Cardiovascular Disorders in Patients with SMD

Cardiovascular diseases (CVD) are one of the leading causes of premature death among individuals with SMD, significantly reducing total life expectancy by 17.4% and 22.0% for men and women, respectively. Patients with schizophrenia or bipolar illness have a two- to threefold higher risk of CVD [19]. The etiology of this excess CVD is multifactorial, and the different causes can be grouped in three major categories: genetic causes, modifiable lifestyle factors, and iatrogenic causes [20]. These three categories are, however, in constant interplay. In fact, genome-wide association studies have identified several genetic variants associated with severe mental disorders and CVD risk factors, such as body mass index, type 2 diabetes, total cholesterol, high-density lipoprotein cholesterol, systolic blood pressure, diastolic blood pressure, and coronary artery disease [13]. These pre-existing factors are worsened by the incredibly high rates of smoking, unhealthy diet, and lack of physical exercise, which are particularly frequent in patients with SMD [21–25]. In fact, these patients, especially those suffering from depression, often have a sedentary and lonely lifestyle, with a 50% increased risk of CVD compared to the general population [26]. It has been reported that a diagnosis of depressive disorder is an independent risk factor for the increased morbidity and mortality due to coronary heart disease [20].

Iatrogenic causes can be further subdivided into non-pharmacological and pharmacological causes. The former is mostly due to the fact that physical health of patients with SMD is often neglected by healthcare providers due to negative stereotypes and diagnostic overshadowing [27]. This is made worse by the so-called internalized stigma (i.e., the subjective perception of devaluation, marginalization, secrecy, shame, and withdrawal) perceived by the patients themselves. Perceiving stigmatizing attitudes in healthcare providers increases reluctancy of patients with SMD to seek medical attention for both physical and mental disorders [28]. Additionally, internalized stigma results in social withdrawal, which may decrease physical health checkup visits and consequently increase the risk of cardiovascular illnesses and excess mortality [29].

As regards pharmacological-related factors, APs have a direct effect on CVD risk, along with the above-mentioned weight gain- and obesity-related mechanisms [30, 31]. Available studies found that the development of insulin-resistance could be directly influenced by atypical AP antagonism on D2 receptors [32]. Higher AP dosages are associated with a higher risk of coronary heart disease and cerebrovascular accident death [33]. While selective serotonin reuptake inhibitors (SSRIs) seem to be safe for cardiac adverse events, with minimal reported cardiac side effects, tricyclic ADs increase the likelihood to have unfavorable cardiac events [34], frequently causing orthostatic hypotension, slowed cardiac conduction, increased arrhythmias, and heart rate increase.

Moreover, some psychotropic drugs pose SMD patients at higher risk of sudden cardiac death [35, 36]. Both conventional and atypical APs are associated with a similar dose-related elevated risk of sudden cardiac death in patients receiving AP monotherapy. Similarly, large epidemiological studies have reported that tricyclic AD have a dose-dependent higher risk of sudden cardiac mortality [37]. Sudden cardiac events can be due to the fact that the majority of AP and some AD may cause QTc prolongation. There is a consensus that QTc values >500 ms, or an absolute increase of 60 ms compared with drug-free baseline, is a risk factor for the onset of torsade de pointes and ventricular fibrillation, which are associated with sudden cardiac death. Overall, patients on AP have higher rates of cardiac arrest or ventricular arrhythmias than controls. No occurrences of torsade de pointes have been linked to the use of SSRIs, even though these medications cause QTc prolongation, and no case of torsade de pointes has been documented in people taking lithium.

The complicated interactions between genes, environment, and mental diseases make it difficult for those with severe mental illnesses to manage their physical comorbidities effectively. Screening SMD patients for cardiovascular disorders is, therefore, of crucial importance.

14.2.3 Infectious Diseases in Patients with SMD

Patients with SMD are more likely to develop a number of chronic viral infections, including the most dangerous human immunodeficiency virus (HIV), tuberculosis (TB), and hepatitis C [11].

The prevalence of HIV positivity in patients with SMD is higher than in the general population [38–40], which is attributable to several factors, including a higher rate of substance abuse, sexual risky behaviors (such as unprotected sex or exchanging sex for drugs and money), and lack of awareness about HIV-related issues [11]. Between 5% and 7% of people with a history of mental illness have HIV infection [19]. Even though patients with schizophrenia are less sexually active than nonpsychotic people, they are more likely to have risky sexual behaviors. Additionally, many patients with SMD are unaware of the negative consequences of HIV infection. The long-term outcome of schizophrenia with comorbid HIV infection is poorer [19]; in fact, between 0.2% and 15% of individuals with HIV-spectrum illness experience new-onset psychosis. Whichever condition manifests first (HIV or schizophrenia), its co-occurrence is linked to higher morbidity and mortality than each illness alone. Also, HIV patients are more likely to experience depressive symptoms than HIV-negative people [41].

Moreover, some antiretroviral treatments have significant psychiatric side effects, and HIV directly affects the central nervous system, which causes cognitive and behavioral problems. Patients with SMD being treated with both AP and antiretroviral drugs simultaneously are at a particularly high risk for developing metabolic syndrome and CVD due to the metabolic abnormalities to which both drugs are associated.

People with SMD have a noticeably higher rates of hepatitis virus infection than the general population. Hepatitis C virus infection affects about 20–25% of people with SMD. Drug use and dysfunctional sexual habits are the most frequent transmission pathways for people with SMD. Therefore, hepatitis C virus infection should be routinely screened for and treated in patients with SMD and substance use disorders, in order to reduce its morbidity and mortality.

Furthermore, the coronavirus disease 2019 (COVID-19) pandemic has posed a significant direct threat to the physical health of the general population. Once more, growing clinical evidence shows that COVID-19 mortality is higher in patients with SMD [42]. Several systematic reviews and meta-analyses [43–46] revealed that having pre-existing mental problems is linked to a higher COVID-19-related mortality risk than controls, even after adjusting for sex, age, and other confounders. Such risk has been shown to increase even more with the higher use of psychotropic medications [47], particularly APs, which seem to increase the susceptibility to pneumonia and pneumonia-related mortality risk through some of their side-effects, such as sedation, hypersalivation, and impaired swallowing. Additionally, clozapine might also suppress the immune functioning, while risperidone induces dysregulation in the adaptive and inflammatory immune processes increasing the risk of respiratory illnesses [48–50]. Also, valproate is associated with an increased risk of respiratory infections [51].

Secondly, like the general population, older people with SMD (>60 years) are susceptible to COVID-19. However, patients in this age range appear to have an extra mortality from COVID-19 [52]. It was reported that people with SMD have a four times higher risk of death from COVID-19 when compared to the general population of the same age [53].

The increased COVID-19-related mortality risk may also be partially explained by the aforementioned higher physical comorbidity burden in patients with SMD compared to non-psychiatric patients (CVD, hypertension, diabetes, chronic obstructive pulmonary disease) [54–56]. Individual immunity in this vulnerable population can be improved by encouraging a healthy lifestyle, consistent exercise, nutritious eating, and adequate sleep, in addition to pathogen exposure reduction [57].

Finally, both people with schizophrenia and depression carry a twofold increased risk of developing tuberculosis (TB) compared to the general population. The comorbidity between tuberculosis and severe mental illness is very complex. In fact, tuberculosis is strongly associated with a number of severe mental illness risk factors, including HIV, diabetes, homelessness, poverty, and alcohol and drug abuse. Additionally, due to a lack of standard infection control measures or the fact that these institutions are overcrowded, patients living in long-term care facilities are more likely to contract several infectious diseases, including tuberculosis.

14.3 Increased Mortality in Patients with SMD

The increased mortality rates in people with SMD are in part due to the long-standing separation of psychiatry from other branches of medicine and to the lack of attention to comorbidities during undergraduate and postgraduate training of psychiatrists and other medical specialists [58]. For a long time, the prevalence of comorbidity has been underestimated by healthcare professionals and—on the other hand—patients have been reluctant to speak to psychiatrists about their physical health problems.

However, factors contributing to the reduced life expectancy of patients with SMD can be grouped in three categories: factors related to the patient, to the clinician, and to the healthcare system. Despite the fact that equal access to and provision of healthcare should be viewed as a fundamental human right, people with SMD have difficulties in accessing to an adequate care for physical diseases and in receiving high-quality treatments due to a confluence of patient, provider, treatment, and system factors.

Patient-related factors are related to their reluctance to seek for adequate medical attention due to symptoms directly attributable to their mental disorders, including the presence of cognitive impairment, social isolation, depressive symptoms, and suspiciousness. For this same reason, SMD patients tend to adopt unhealthy behaviors, such as sedentary lifestyle, heavy smoking, poor physical activity, unhealthy diet and alcohol, and drug abuse. Psychiatric symptoms and their adverse consequences (reduced social networks, low educational level, poor housing, lack of family support, poverty, and unemployment) also increase the difficulty in adhering to medical advice and in following required changes in lifestyle habits. Therefore, SMD patients might be less able than other patients to interpret physical signs and communicate their needs to physicians and to take care of themselves [6].

This increases the responsibility of psychiatric professionals to be in the forefront of patients' physical healthcare. In fact, psychiatrists tend to focus on mental rather than on physical health and are more prone to interpret physical complaints as psychosomatic symptoms and might have a lack of knowledge regarding medical issues, leading to rare physical examinations of SMD patients.

On the other hand, SMD patients receive less medical attention than those with physical illnesses, as a consequence of several factors, including poor communication with patients [59], stigmatizing attitudes among healthcare professionals not directly involved in mental healthcare toward patients suffering from SMD [60–63], and lack of collaboration between psychiatrists and other physicians [64].

The need to improve the physical healthcare provided to people with SMD through medical screenings, monitoring, and regular checkups, as well as the need to provide psychosocial interventions aimed at modifying risk factors—i.e., unhealthy lifestyle behaviors—has been recently pointed out [65]. Additionally, changes to the healthcare system and delivery of care could be required to address the issue of poor medical healthcare offered to patients with SMD.

The lack of integrated healthcare systems, due to their high costs, together with the underfunding of mental healthcare, contributes to the fragmentation of the physical and mental health systems, which reflects on the higher rate of comorbidities and mortality of this population of patients.

14.4 Monitoring Guidelines

Psychiatrists and primary care physicians should play an active role in ensuring that patients with mental illness are not disadvantaged in the screening and monitoring for physical diseases. Regular checkup should include the assessment and management of cardiovascular risk factors and diabetes as part of routine care of patients with SMD. However, a multidisciplinary team including cardiologists, diabetologists, and other specialists should be established in order to provide the best available integrated treatments to patients with comorbidities [20]. Physical health checkups that should be regularly performed in patients with SMD are summarized in Table 14.1.

Most of these physical health monitoring tests are simple, affordable, and easy to use and can be included in the healthcare systems in both developed and developing countries. Furthermore, some of these measurements (e.g., body weight and blood pressure) can be performed also by other health professionals with a minimal impact on physicians. The assessment of patients' lifestyle habits, such as smoking, diet, and physical activity, should be included in the screening and assessment of patients' physical health. Moreover, given the importance of each component of the metabolic syndrome in predicting the morbidity and mortality for CVD, diabetes, cancer, and other diseases, these parameters should be checked at baseline and regularly monitored.

In order to monitor obesity, the risk of metabolic syndrome, and CVD, psychiatrists should encourage their patients to track and chart their own weight at each visit, and they should monitor and chart BMI and weight circumference (WC), regardless of the prescribed medications. According to prospective studies in individuals with impaired glucose tolerance, WC is a better predictor of type 2 diabetes than body mass index (BMI) [66]. WC is also a stronger indicator than

Table 14.1 Clinical information to be monitored in patients with SMD

– Weight gain and obesity (body mass index, BMI, waist circumference)
– Blood pressure
– Dietary intake
– Activity level and exercise
– Use of tobacco and alcohol or other substances
– Fasting blood levels of glucose
– Fasting blood levels of lipids, especially triglycerides and high-density lipoprotein (HDL)-cholesterol
– Prolactin levels (if indicated by reproductive system and/or sexual symptoms)
– Cardiovascular disease (CVD) risk and electrocardiographic (ECG) parameters

Table 14.2 Outcomes and time-point assessments of the LIFESTYLE Trial

	Baseline	3 months	6 months	12 months	Yearly
Personal and family history	**X**				
Diet, exercise, smoking	X	X	X	X	X
Weight	X	X	X	X	X
Waist circumference	X	X	X	X	X
ECG	X				X
Blood pressure	X	X	X	X	X
Fasting plasma glucose	X	X	X	X	X
Lipid profile	X		X	X	X

BMI for systolic blood pressure, HDL cholesterol, or triglycerides [67].

The other criteria of the metabolic syndrome—i.e., blood pressure, fasting plasma glucose, and fasting lipid profile—should also be evaluated.

In SMD patients, high blood pressure is frequently overlooked [20]. Given that the measurement of blood pressure is inexpensive, and that hypertension is a significant risk factor for CVD, blood pressure should be checked frequently, if not at every visit. Patients with blood pressure between 120 and 130 mmHg or between 80 and 85 mmHg should be considered as prehypertensive, and they should change their lifestyle habits to prevent heart disease.

According to available recommendations, patients' individual CVD risk should be determined based on their age, sex, presence, or absence of diabetes mellitus (DM), smoking behavior, systolic blood pressure, total cholesterol, or the ratio of total cholesterol to HDL-cholesterol. In order to evaluate the overall heart health state of individuals with SMD, baseline ECG monitoring must be performed. However, it may not be easy to obtain an ECG in a psychiatric setting or in an acute medical setting. In these situations, patients should be asked about heart risks, including family history of early cardiac death, personal history of a heart murmur, prior prescription of cardiac medications or antihypertensives, or episodes of simple syncope in the past, before receiving any psychotropic medication. As a rule, it is advisable that every patient get their ECG checked before starting any medication, especially in people with clinical risk factors for arrhythmias. ECG monitoring can then be repeated based on the cardiologist's recommendation.

In order to identify high-risk individuals and ensure early identification of changes in metabolic markers, it is advisable to monitor all patients on any drug at baseline and every 3 months [68]. Unless patients have a particularly high risk of negative health outcomes, most guidelines recommend screening and monitoring at baseline, 3 months, 12 months, and annually (Table 14.2) [20, 69, 70].

14.5 How to Address Physical Comorbidities in Patients with SMD

Many patients with SMD are either unaware of the need for change or lack the information and abilities needed to change their lifestyle behaviors. Using efficient behavioral interventions, psychiatric specialists, medical professionals, nurses, and other multidisciplinary team members can inform and encourage individuals with SMD to address their lifestyle choices, such as smoking, nutrition, and exercise.

Patients with SMD, as well as their family members and caregivers, should learn about healthy behaviors and get psychoeducational materials to improve their lifestyle habits. Population-based research has shown that lifestyle choices can be easily measured and improved by using specific psychoeducational lifestyle interventions, which can be defined as programs that promote improved behavioral outcomes without the employment of any pharmacological aid [71]. They are usually cost-effective and do not need to be administered by a specialist nor require specific training. Many of such interventions are already available and tested for efficacy in randomized controlled trials (RCTs).

Lifestyle interventions include a range of programs incorporating a variety of approaches, such as health education and cognitive behavioral therapy (CBT). Additionally, they may incorporate practical elements like engaging in physical activities. They can be provided in different settings, such as in-person, over the phone, or online, both in individual and group settings.

Systematic reviews have shown that lifestyle interventions significantly improve anthropometric measures such as waist circumference, body weight, and body mass index (BMI), as well as physical activity and dietary outcomes such as fruit consumption [72]. Additionally, lifestyle modifications are linked to a lower risk of all-cause mortality, type 2 diabetes, metabolic syndrome, and cardiovascular disease [73].

Similarly, a recent review on the effectiveness of lifestyle interventions for individuals with SMD in community or outpatient settings found statistically significant improvements in three primary outcomes: weight, physical activity, and diet [73]. Additionally, the effectiveness of these behavioral approaches has been assessed also with respect to analytical blood parameters (i.e., blood levels of insulin, triglycerides, total cholesterol, and fasting glucose) [71, 74]. However, the majority of these studies had short follow-ups (up to 3 months), and therefore the long-term efficacy of these approaches cannot be evaluated yet. Notably, no research has explicitly examined how lifestyle modifications affect complex cardiovascular indices—like the Framingham and HOmeostasis Model Assessment of Insulin Resistance (HOMA-IR), which are more accurate indicators of cardiometabolic risk. The psychosocial well-being, quality of life, and symptom severity, particularly those associated with psychosis, depression, and anxiety, are all positively impacted by lifestyle interventions [75]. However, it has to be said that up to 64% of studies were rated at high risk of bias due to important methodological flaws, including the randomization process, lack of blinding, missing data, imprecise outcome reporting, small sample sizes, statistical heterogeneity, and absence of active controls [72].

In order to promote the physical health of people with SMD, our study group developed a behavioral lifestyle group intervention, which proved to be effective in a randomized controlled trial carried out with 400 patients with bipolar disorders, major depression, or schizophrenia spectrum disorder. Our experimental intervention (Table 14.3) was developed in accordance with the World Health Organization's [76, 77], the European Association for the Study of Diabetes' [78], the European Society of Cardiology's, and the European Psychiatric Association's [20] recommendations for the management of physical health in individuals with mental disorders.

Small groups of 5–10 patients received the intervention every 7–10 days for 6 months, according to the modules provided in Table 14.3. Each module included the following elements: (a) provision of information on the risks and advantages of each lifestyle choice; (b) training

Table 14.3 Program of the LIFESTYLE psychosocial group intervention

Starting session: Introduction of the intervention, aims, purposes, presentation of participants, and definition of personal healthy lifestyle goals
Module 1: Diet, information on health food, principles, and benefits of healthy eating
Module 2: Physical activity, how to increase routine physical activity
Module 3: Smoking habits, information on the dangers of smoking, craving, difficulties for quitting smoking and consequences of long-term abuse of nicotine
Module 4: Medication adherence, strategies for improving adherence, medical consequences of non-adherence
Module 5: Risky behaviors, sexually transmitted disorders, substance, and alcohol abuse
Module 6: Promotion of regular circadian rhythm, problems related to irregular daily activities
At the end of each meeting, a 20-min session of moderate physical activity (i.e., walking) is implemented with all participants

on practical strategies for reducing unhealthy behaviors; and (c) identification of personal goals, motivational support, and problem-solving training. A 20-min session of moderate physical activity was scheduled at the end of each meeting. Fresh fruits and healthy snacks were offered to participants during the meetings.

Patients who received the intervention reported higher weekly walking hours and higher weekly physical activity levels [74, 79, 80]. The inclusion of a walking session at the conclusion of each meeting encouraged patients to modify their sedentary behavior already during the groups and allowed them to share experiences, challenges, and potential solutions toward a more active and healthier lifestyle. Moreover, patients reported an improvement in eating habits, with increased intake of fruit and vegetables and a reduced consumption of junk food [79].

Patients receiving the LIFESTYLE intervention had a significant reduction in BMI, body weight, and waist circumference both at the end of the intervention [79] and after 6 months [74], and an improvement in the HOMA index at follow-up [74].

The LIFESTYLE intervention is particularly innovative and easy to use in routine care of patients with severe mental disorders due to several characteristics that might be considered when developing such interventions.

These include the presence of a motivational interview, which is a crucial strategy to support behavioral changes over time, a comprehensive approach to healthy living, with a focus on almost all aspects of healthy lifestyle behaviors, such as diet, sedentary behavior, physical activity, tobacco use, risky sexual behavior, and regularization of circadian rhythms. Finally, the group format allowed patients to share experiences and difficulties beyond those related to the disorders themselves (i.e., symptoms and pharmacological side effects).

14.6 Conclusions

The physical health of patients with SMD remains an urgent issue that needs to be addressed through systemic and individual actions [16]. A multidisciplinary approach, including monitoring and screening for the most frequent diseases and providing supportive interventions including the improvement of patients' cognitive and social functioning and lifestyle, is crucial.

There is still much to learn about factors underpinning the effectiveness of lifestyle interventions. Available studies report that interventions are more effective in improving patients' physical health when they incorporate both dietary and physical activity components, when they provide tailored interventions and include personalized goal settings, and when they incorporate a motivational component [19, 81]. Implementation issues are also a critical point for the provision of these interventions in routine care of patients with SMD. In fact, only a few studies have assessed the cost-effectiveness of lifestyle interventions clinical practice and their scalability in routine settings. Additionally, patients' individual experiences about these approaches, as well as their satisfaction with care, will need to be taken into account.

Finally, considering the complex interplay between mental and physical factors contributing to the reduced life expectancy of patients with SDM, a multilevel approach is needed, in which the different stakeholders establish workforces for the long-term management of physical and mental health conditions, including policymakers, psychiatrists, other medical specialists, carers, and users with mental disorders.

References

1. Thornicroft G (2011) Physical health disparities and mental illness: the scandal of premature mortality. Br J Psychiatry 199:441–442
2. Adriaanse MC, Drewes HW, van der Heide I, Struijs JN, Baan CA (2016) The impact of comorbid chronic conditions on quality of life in type 2 diabetes patients. Qual Life Res 25:175–182
3. Sarkadi A, Ådahl K, Stenvall E, Richard S, Batti H, Gavra P et al (2018) Teaching Recovery Techniques: evaluation of a group intervention for unaccompanied refugee minors with symptoms of PTSD in Sweden. Eur Child Adolesc Psychiatry 27:467–479
4. Sartorius N (2018) Comorbidity of mental and physical disorders: a key problem for medicine in the 21st century. Acta Psychiatr Scand 137:369–370

5. Bloom DE, Luca DL (2016) The global demography of aging. In: Handbook of the economics of population aging. Elsevier, Amsterdam, pp 3–56
6. Momen NC, Plana-Ripoll O, Agerbo E, Christensen MK, Iburg KM, Laursen TM et al (2022) Mortality associated with mental disorders and comorbid general medical conditions. JAMA Psychiatry 79:444–453
7. Teh WL, Cetty L, Jeyagurunathan A, Devi F, Roystonn K, Tang C et al (2021) Comorbid physical illnesses in adult outpatients with psychotic disorders: risk factors, psychological functioning, and quality of life outcomes. Soc Psychiatry Psychiatr Epidemiol 56:1633–1643
8. Tan XW, Lee ES, Toh MPHS, Lum AWM, Seah DEJ, Leong KP et al (2021) Comparison of mental-physical comorbidity, risk of death and mortality among patients with mental disorders—a retrospective cohort study. J Psychiatr Res 142:48–53
9. Soundy A, Wampers M, Probst M, De Hert M, Stubbs B, Vancampfort D (2013) Physical activity and sedentary behaviour in outpatients with schizophrenia: a systematic review and meta-analysis. Int J Ther Rehabil 20:588–595
10. Kisely S, Crowe E, Lawrence D (2013) Cancer-related mortality in people with mental illness. JAMA Psychiatry 70:209–217
11. De Hert M, Correll CU, Bobes J, Cetkovich-Bakmas M, Cohen DAN, Asai I et al (2011) Physical illness in patients with severe mental disorders. I. Prevalence, impact of medications and disparities in health care. World Psychiatry 10:52–77
12. Mazereel V, Detraux J, Vancampfort D, van Winkel R, De Hert M (2020) Impact of psychotropic medication effects on obesity and the metabolic syndrome in people with serious mental illness. Front Endocrinol 11:1–10
13. Rødevand L, Bahrami S, Frei O, Lin A, Gani O, Shadrin A et al (2021) Polygenic overlap and shared genetic loci between loneliness, severe mental disorders, and cardiovascular disease risk factors suggest shared molecular mechanisms. Transl Psychiatry 11:3
14. Leucht S, Burkard T, Henderson J, Maj M, Sartorius N (2007) Physical illness and schizophrenia: a review of the literature. Acta Psychiatr Scand 116:317–333
15. Bobes J, Rejas J, Garcia-Garcia M, Rico-Villademoros F, García-Portilla MP, Fernández I et al (2003) Weight gain in patients with schizophrenia treated with risperidone, olanzapine, quetiapine or haloperidol: results of the EIRE study. Schizophr Res 62:77–88
16. De Hert M, Dobbelaere M, Sheridan EM, Cohen D, Correll CU (2011) Metabolic and endocrine adverse effects of second-generation antipsychotics in children and adolescents: a systematic review of randomized, placebo controlled trials and guidelines for clinical practice. Eur Psychiatry 26:144–158
17. Vancampfort D, Wampers M, Mitchell AJ, Correll CU, De Herdt A, Probst M et al (2013) A meta-analysis of cardio-metabolic abnormalities in drug naïve, first-episode and multi-episode patients with schizophrenia versus general population controls. World Psychiatry 12:240
18. Bahrami S, Steen NE, Shadrin A, O'Connell K, Frei O, Bettella F et al (2020) Shared genetic loci between body mass index and major psychiatric disorders: a genome-wide association study. JAMA Psychiatry 77:1
19. Sampogna G, Di Vincenzo M, Della Rocca B, Mancuso E, Volpicelli A, Perris F et al (2022) Physical comorbidities in patients with severe mental disorders: a brief narrative review on current challenges and practical implications for professionals. Riv Psichiatr 57:251–257
20. De Hert M, Dekker JM, Wood D, Kahl KG, Holt RIG, Möller HJ (2009) Cardiovascular disease and diabetes in people with severe mental illness position statement from the European Psychiatric Association (EPA), supported by the European Association for the Study of Diabetes (EASD) and the European Society of Cardiology (ESC). Eur Psychiatry 24:412–424
21. Mitchell AJ, Vancampfort D, De Hert M, Stubbs B (2015) Do people with mental illness receive adequate smoking cessation advice? A systematic review and meta-analysis. Gen Hosp Psychiatry 37:14–23
22. Stubbs B, Firth J, Berry A, Schuch FB, Rosenbaum S, Gaughran F et al (2016) How much physical activity do people with schizophrenia engage in? A systematic review, comparative meta-analysis and meta-regression. Schizophr Res 176:431–440
23. Vancampfort D, Firth J, Schuch F, Rosenbaum S, De Hert M, Mugisha J et al (2016) Physical activity and sedentary behavior in people with bipolar disorder: a systematic review and meta-analysis. J Affect Disord 201:145–152
24. Schuch F, Vancampfort D, Firth J, Rosenbaum S, Ward P, Reichert T et al (2017) Physical activity and sedentary behavior in people with major depressive disorder: a systematic review and meta-analysis. J Affect Disord 210:139–150
25. Dipasquale S, Pariante CM, Dazzan P, Aguglia E, McGuire P, Mondelli V (2013) The dietary pattern of patients with schizophrenia: a systematic review. J Psychiatr Res 47:197–207
26. Whooley MA, De Jonge P, Vittinghoff E, Otte C, Moos R, Carney RM et al (2008) Depressive symptoms, health behaviors, and risk of cardiovascular events in patients with coronary heart disease. JAMA 300:2379
27. Lord O, Malone D, Mitchell AJ (2010) Receipt of preventive medical care and medical screening for patients with mental illness: a comparative analysis. Gen Hosp Psychiatry 32:519–543
28. De Hert M, Cohen D, Bobes J, Cetkovich-Bakmas M, Leucht S, Ndetei DM et al (2011) Physical illness in patients with severe mental disorders. II. Barriers to care, monitoring and treatment guidelines, plus recommendations at the system and individual level. World Psychiatry 10:138–151
29. Phelan M, Stradins L, Morrison S (2001) Physical health of people with severe mental illness: can be

improved if primary care and mental health professionals pay attention to it. BMJ 322:443
30. Scheen AJ, De Hert MA (2007) Abnormal glucose metabolism in patients treated with antipsychotics. Diabetes Metab 33:169–175
31. Nasrallah HA (2008) Atypical antipsychotic-induced metabolic side effects: insights from receptor-binding profiles. Mol Psychiatry 13(1):27–35
32. García-Tornadú I, Ornstein AM, Chamson-Reig A, Wheeler MB, Hill DJ, Arany E et al (2010) Disruption of the dopamine D2 receptor impairs insulin secretion and causes glucose intolerance. Endocrinology 151:1441–1450
33. Osborn DPJ, Levy G, Nazareth I, Petersen I, Islam A, King MB (2007) Relative risk of cardiovascular and cancer mortality in people with severe mental illness from the United Kingdom's general practice research database. Arch Gen Psychiatry 64:242–249
34. Sowden GL, Huffman JC (2009) The impact of mental illness on cardiac outcomes: a review for the cardiologist. Int J Cardiol 132:30–37
35. Kauppila JP, Pakanen L, Porvari K, Vähätalo J, Holmström L, Haukilahti MAE et al (2023) Use of psychotropic medication in victims of sudden cardiac death with nonischemic heart disease. Cardiology 148:134–137
36. Ray WA, Chung CP, Murray KT, Hall K, Stein CM (2009) Atypical antipsychotic drugs and the risk of sudden cardiac death. N Engl J Med 360:225
37. Cohen HW, Gibson G, Alderman MH (2000) Excess risk of myocardial infarction in patients treated with antidepressant medications: association with use of tricyclic agents. Am J Med 108:2–8
38. Sacks M, Dermatis H, Looser-Ott S, Burton W, Perry S (2006) Undetected HIV infection among acutely ill psychiatric inpatients. Am J Psychiatry 149:544–545. https://doi.org/10.1176/ajp1494544
39. Henning MP, Krüger C, Fletcher L (2012) HIV seropositivity in recently admitted and long-term psychiatric in-patients: prevalence and diagnostic profile. Afr J Psychiatry (Johannesbg) 15:47–53
40. Maj M (1990) Psychiatric aspects of HIV-1 infection and AIDS. Psychol Med 20:547–563
41. Lofgren SM, Bond DJ, Nakasujja N, Boulware DR (2020) Burden of depression in outpatient HIV-infected adults in sub-Saharan Africa; systematic review and meta-analysis. AIDS Behav 24:1752–1764
42. De Hert M, Mazereel V, Stroobants M, De Picker L, Van Assche K, Detraux J (2022) COVID-19-related mortality risk in people with severe mental illness: a systematic and critical review. Front Psychiatry 12:798554
43. Vai B, Mazza MG, Delli Colli C, Foiselle M, Allen B, Benedetti F et al (2021) Mental disorders and risk of COVID-19-related mortality, hospitalisation, and intensive care unit admission: a systematic review and meta-analysis. Lancet Psychiatry 8:797–812
44. Fond G, Nemani K, Etchecopar-Etchart D, Loundou A, Goff DC, Lee SW et al (2021) Association between mental health disorders and mortality among patients with COVID-19 in 7 countries: a systematic review and meta-analysis. JAMA Psychiatry 78:1208–1217
45. Liu L, Ni SY, Yan W, Lu QD, Zhao YM, Xu YY et al (2021) Mental and neurological disorders and risk of COVID-19 susceptibility, illness severity and mortality: a systematic review, meta-analysis and call for action. EClinicalMedicine 40:101111
46. Toubasi AA, AbuAnzeh RB, Tawileh HBA, Aldebei RH, Alryalat SAS (2021) A meta-analysis: the mortality and severity of COVID-19 among patients with mental disorders. Psychiatry Res 299:113856
47. Barcella CA, Polcwiartek C, Mohr GH, Hodges G, Søndergaard K, Niels Bang C et al (2021) Severe mental illness is associated with increased mortality and severe course of COVID-19. Acta Psychiatr Scand 144:82–91
48. Shinn AK, Viron M (2020) Perspectives on the COVID-19 pandemic and individuals with serious mental illness. J Clin Psychiatry 81:20com13412
49. Kuo CJ, Yang SY, Liao YT, Chen WJ, Lee WC, Shau WY et al (2013) Second-generation antipsychotic medications and risk of pneumonia in schizophrenia. Schizophr Bull 39:648
50. Haga T, Ito K, Sakashita K, Iguchi M, Ono M, Tatsumi K (2018) Risk factors for pneumonia in patients with schizophrenia. Neuropsychopharmacol Rep 38:204
51. Landén M, Larsson H, Lichtenstein P, Westin J, Song J (2021) Respiratory infections during lithium and valproate medication: a within-individual prospective study of 50,000 patients with bipolar disorder. Int J Bipolar Disord 9:4–9
52. Maripuu M, Bendix M, Öhlund L, Widerström M, Werneke U (2021) Death associated with coronavirus (COVID-19) infection in individuals with severe mental disorders in Sweden during the early months of the outbreak—an exploratory cross-sectional analysis of a population-based register study. Front Psych 11:609579
53. De Picker LJ, Yolken R, Benedetti F, Borsini A, Branchi I, Fusar-Poli P et al (2021) Viewpoint | European COVID-19 exit strategy for people with severe mental disorders: too little, but not yet too late. Brain Behav Immun 94:15
54. Wang QQ, Xu R, Volkow ND (2021) Increased risk of COVID-19 infection and mortality in people with mental disorders: analysis from electronic health records in the United States. World Psychiatry 20:124–130
55. Nemani K, Li C, Olfson M, Blessing EM, Razavian N, Chen J et al (2021) Association of psychiatric disorders with mortality among patients with COVID-19. JAMA Psychiatry 78:380–386
56. Reilev M, Kristensen KB, Pottegård A, Lund LC, Hallas J, Ernst MT et al (2020) Characteristics and predictors of hospitalization and death in the first 11 122 cases with a positive RT-PCR test for SARS-CoV-2 in Denmark: a nationwide cohort. Int J Epidemiol 49:1468–1481
57. Kim SW, Su KP (2020) Using psychoneuroimmunity against COVID-19. Brain Behav Immun 87:4–5

58. Fiorillo A, Sartorius N (2021) Mortality gap and physical comorbidity of people with severe mental disorders: the public health scandal. Ann General Psychiatry 20:52
59. Colton CW, Manderscheid RW (2006) PEER REVIEWED: congruencies in increased mortality rates, years of potential life lost, and causes of death among public mental health clients in eight states. Prev Chronic Dis 3:1–14
60. Fleischhacker WW, Cetkovich-Bakmas M, De Hert M, Hennekens CH, Lambert M, Leucht S et al (2008) Comorbid somatic illnesses in patients with severe mental disorders: clinical, policy, and research challenges. J Clin Psychiatry 69:3409
61. Kane JM (2009) Creating a health care team to manage chronic medical illnesses in patients with severe mental illness: the public policy perspective. J Clin Psychiatry 70:3921
62. Nasrallah HA, Meyer JM, Goff DC, McEvoy JP, Davis SM, Stroup TS et al (2006) Low rates of treatment for hypertension, dyslipidemia and diabetes in schizophrenia: data from the CATIE schizophrenia trial sample at baseline. Schizophr Res 86:15–22
63. Druss BG, Bradford WD, Rosenheck RA, Radford MJ, Krumholz HM (2001) Quality of medical care and excess mortality in older patients with mental disorders. Arch Gen Psychiatry 58:565–572
64. Hassan S, Heinkel S, Burton A, Blackburn R, McCloud T, Ross J et al (2020) A qualitative study exploring the barriers and facilitators of implementing a cardiovascular disease risk reducing intervention for people with severe mental illness into primary care contexts across England: the "PRIMROSE" trial. BMC Health Serv Res 20:1–15
65. Fiorillo A, Luciano M, Pompili M, Sartorius N (2019) Editorial: reducing the mortality gap in people with severe mental disorders: the role of lifestyle psychosocial interventions. Front Psych 10:1–3
66. De Vegt F, Dekker JM, Jager A, Hienkens E, Kostense PJ, Stehouwer CDA et al (2001) Relation of impaired fasting and postload glucose with incident type 2 diabetes in a Dutch population: The Hoorn Study. JAMA 285:2109–2113
67. Wahrenberg H, Hertel K, Leijonhufvud BM, Persson LG, Toft E, Arner P (2005) Use of waist circumference to predict insulin resistance: retrospective study. BMJ 330:1363
68. Waterreus AJ, Laugharne JDE (2009) Screening for the metabolic syndrome in patients receiving antipsychotic treatment: a proposed algorithm. Med J Aust 190:185–189
69. Mackin P, Bishop DR, Watkinson HMO (2007) A prospective study of monitoring practices for metabolic disease in antipsychotic-treated community psychiatric patients. BMC Psychiatry 7:1–6
70. van Winkel R, De Hert M, Van Eyck D, Hanssens L, Wampers M, Scheen A et al (2006) Screening for diabetes and other metabolic abnormalities in patients with schizophrenia and schizoaffective disorder: evaluation of incidence and screening methods. J Clin Psychiatry 67:19038
71. Mucheru D, Hanlon MC, McEvoy M, Thakkinstian A, MacDonald-Wicks L (2019) Comparative efficacy of lifestyle intervention strategies targeting weight outcomes in people with psychosis: a systematic review and network meta-analysis. JBI Database System Rev Implement Rep 17:1770–1825
72. Bradley T, Campbell E, Dray J, Bartlem K, Wye P, Hanly G et al (2022) Systematic review of lifestyle interventions to improve weight, physical activity and diet among people with a mental health condition. Syst Rev 11:1–31
73. Sampogna G, Luciano M, Del Vecchio V, Giallonardo V, Palummo C, Andriola I et al (2021) Stili di vita nei pazienti con disturbi mentali gravi: quali opportunità per il trattamento? Riv Psichiatr 56:261–271
74. Luciano M, Sampogna G, D'Ambrosio E, Rampino A, Amore M, Calcagno P et al (2023) One-year efficacy of a lifestyle behavioural intervention on physical and mental health in people with severe mental disorders: results from a randomized controlled trial. Eur Arch Psychiatry Clin Neurosci 274:903
75. Højlund M, Andersen K, Ernst MT, Correll CU, Hallas J (2022) Use of low-dose quetiapine increases the risk of major adverse cardiovascular events: results from a nationwide active comparator-controlled cohort study. World Psychiatry 21:444
76. Helwig NE, Hong S, Hsiao-wecksler ET (2013) Global action plan for the prevention and control of noncommunicable diseases 2013–2020. World Health Organization, Geneva
77. Schrag PG (2019) Global action: nuclear test ban diplomacy at the end of the cold war. Global action. Cambridge University Press, Cambridge, pp 1–232
78. Rydén L, Grant PJ, Anker SD, Berne C, Cosentino F, Danchin N et al (2013) ESC guidelines on diabetes, pre-diabetes, and cardiovascular diseases developed in collaboration with the EASD: The Task Force on diabetes, pre-diabetes, and cardiovascular diseases of the European Society of Cardiology (ESC) and developed in collaboration with the European Association for the Study of Diabetes (EASD). Eur Heart J 34:3035–3087
79. Luciano M, Sampogna G, Amore M, Bertolino A, Dell'Osso L, Rossi A et al (2022) Improving physical activity and diet in patients with severe mental disorders: results from the LIFESTYLE multicentric, real-world randomized controlled trial. Psychiatry Res 317:114818
80. Luciano M, Sampogna G, Amore M, Andriola I, Calcagno P, Carmassi C et al (2021) How to improve the physical health of people with severe mental illness? A multicentric randomized controlled trial on the efficacy of a lifestyle group intervention. Eur Psychiatry 64:e72
81. De Rosa C, Sampogna G, Luciano M, Del Vecchio V, Pocai B, Borriello G et al (2017) Improving physical health of patients with severe mental disorders: a critical review of lifestyle psychosocial interventions. Expert Rev Neurother 17:667–681

15 Pollution and Climate Changes as Environmental Determinants of Poor Mental Health

Alfonso Tortorella and Giulia Menculini

Abstract

During the last decades, the uncontrolled urbanization process, together with the increase of anthropogenic activities, led to a significant increase in phenomena such as global warming and pollution. Human health is significantly threatened by these events and growing attention has been paid to their effects on mental health. Different mechanisms mediate the association between climate change and the possible development of psychiatric conditions, such as the occurrence of natural disasters that represent a major risk factor for post-traumatic and mood disorders. Moreover, such events may critically impact social determinants of mental health, contributing to inequality in food and water access, increasing social disparities, and disrupting social networks. Climate change also influences urbanization processes by causing ecomigration phenomena, and may as well determine higher pollution levels. As for the latter, air pollution has been confirmed as a crucial environmental determinant of mental health, leading to the development of psychiatric disorders and to the exacerbation of pre-existing conditions, also on the basis of neuroinflammatory pathway that may activate in response to pollutant exposure. Not only air, but also noise and light pollution cause a detrimental effect on mental health, acting through different mechanisms that involve the disruption of circadian rhythms as well as biological pathways related to inflammation and oxidative stress. In this chapter, an overview of the role of climate change and different sources of pollution as determinants of mental health is provided, and specific attention is also paid to the possible mechanisms through which these factors may act.

Keywords

Climate change · Global warming
Urbanization · Pollution · Mental health
Psychiatric disorders

During the last decades, the growing and uncontrolled urbanization process, together with extreme climate changes, contributed to the development of urban surroundings where human health is seriously threatened. Nowadays, more than 50% of the world population lives in cities and it is expected that by 2050 this number will rise further, with urban settings reaching 500,000

A. Tortorella (✉) · G. Menculini
Section of Psychiatry, Department of Medicine and Surgery, University of Perugia, Perugia, Italy
e-mail: alfonso.tortorella@unipg.it; giulia.menculini@unipg.it

A. Fiorillo, S. De Giorgi (eds.), *Social Determinants of Mental Health*, Sustainable Development Goals Series, https://doi.org/10.1007/978-3-031-70165-8_15

inhabitants or more [1]. A number of environmental phenomena, e.g., by overheating, extreme climate events, and air pollution, impact citizens' wellbeing in indoor and outdoor environments [2]. Together with climate change-related phenomena, such as air pollution and urban heat island, further sources of pollution related to noise and artificial light compromise human well-being.

According to the World Health Organization (WHO) estimates, 24% of the deaths every year are attributable to the environment, and in the near future climate change could be responsible for 250,000 additional deaths per year [3]. Physical health has been demonstrated to be critically influenced by environmental factors [4], while fewer attention has been paid to the effect of these determinants on mental health. During the last years, a growing body of evidence supported the relationship between environmental factors, particularly climate change and pollution, and poor mental health [5–7]. It has now become clear that ecological determinants can both affect the development of psychiatric disorders, also impairing neurodevelopmental trajectories, and act as a trigger for the exacerbation of already-existing conditions. This complex interplay, which becomes evident mainly, but not solely, in urban areas, lays the foundation on both biological, e.g., physiological mechanisms activated by the exposure to pollutants, and socioeconomic, e.g., increased disparities in environmental wealth, factors [8]. Indeed, the urban dimension has rapidly been changing due to a series of complex factors, such as its fast expansion, the subsequent increase in the number of inhabitants, and the inequity in access to health resources and public services between various city areas, enforcing social disparities [9]. The heterogeneity of urban spaces, together with the variety of anthropogenic sources of pollutants, cause a diversified personal exposure into the same city, which means that environmental conditions widely change across different areas. To note, not only outdoor but also indoor environmental conditions should be considered in this perspective, since most of the global population spends a significant amount of time indoors [10]. These peculiar characteristics of the urban environment should then be studied into the more general framework of climate change, which influences mental health both directly and acting through its influence on specific psychosocial factors. The growing complexity of these phenomena requires a multidisciplinary response aimed at considering environmental determinants among possible risk factors for mental health issues, thus prompting target prevention and treatment strategies under a personalized medicine perspective, empowering environmental resilience, and sustainable development. In this chapter, we will unravel the complex relationship between environmental determinants and mental health, overviewing the possible role of climate change and different types of pollution in the development and worsening of psychiatric conditions.

15.1 Mental Health in the Climate Change Era

Climate change is dramatically impacting our planet, leading to potentially catastrophic consequences on our societies and representing a major threat to human health. This spreading phenomenon results from different factors, some of which—e.g., solar irradiation—are independent from human actions, while the majority of them is strictly linked to anthropogenic activities, particularly greenhouse gas emission and deforestation [5].

Global warming is considered to be responsible for a number of extreme weather events and natural disasters, such as floods, hurricanes, and tornados, which are likely to increase during the next decades with immediate consequences at a global level. Indeed, human lives are threatened during natural calamities, but such events also lead to reduction in food and water, especially in rural areas, and may force populations to migrate [11]. In this scenario, we may assist to a decrease of biodiversity and to major changes in specific animal populations, such as insects causing vector-borne diseases [12]. Indeed, apart from natural disasters, the WHO also estimates an increase in deaths up to 250,000 per year due to diseases that are potentially linked to this event, for example, infectious ones, with critical impact on health costs [3]. Moreover, global warming affects the livability of cities, since higher temperatures within urban areas may cause urban heat islands and affect precipitation patterns, also leading to extreme temperatures that have negative consequences on citizens' well-being [13].

In this scenario, mental health is seriously impacted by climate change-related phenomena acting at different levels. Global warming and specific variations in atmospheric conditions, e.g., the increase in humidity levels, are at least co-responsible for extreme weather events and natural disasters [5]. These calamities underpin the exposure to life-threatening circumstances and can be considered as potentially traumatic, leading to acute stress that may occur both during and after the event. This predisposes to the development of a full-blown post-traumatic stress disorder (PTSD), particularly if specific individual, psychosocial, and event-related risk factors co-occur [14–16]. Despite the development of PTSD is the most frequent consequence of the exposure to these events, a number of further psychiatric symptoms can manifest in the aftermath of such disasters, among which the most frequent are represented by affective manifestations ranging from isolated anxiety and depressive symptoms to generalized anxiety and major depressive disorder. Suicidal ideation has also been reported to increase after the occurrence of different types of natural disasters [17]. Even if the above-mentioned psychopathological manifestations do not occur, milder psychological reactions can present after the exposure to natural calamities. Such reactions are represented by different levels of distress linked with uncertainty and sense of vulnerability, which may in the end predispose to the development of psychiatric disorders. Hence, people may observe changes in the environment they were used to, leading to feelings of uncertainty about the future, but also to the more concrete need for reorganizing their daily habits and access to specific resources [5]. A wider sense of passivity and powerlessness may also occur, which hampers the achievement of a satisfying life quality and could also contribute to lower overall functioning. Indeed, the perception of negative climate conditions, as it could manifest during a drought, facilitates the occurrence of poor faith in the future, together with feelings of resignation and helplessness, which also increase the risk for the later development of depression [18]. In the long-term, natural disasters lead to highly-impacting socio-economic consequences [19]. Indeed, areas that are mostly hit by these events are often forced to face the lack of resources in terms of food and drinkable water, and the access to healthcare may as well be inequal. In this context, social disparities are likely to be exacerbated and create an environment where mental health matters could more easily grow, also as a consequence of conflicts arising from the lack of resources [20]. Heightened uncertainty about the future also reduces attitudes towards other people and may result in increased episodes of aggression, possibly facilitated by high temperatures that may also determine hyperarousal states where tendencies towards violence are reinforced [21]. Families could be displaced and face the issue of separation, which adds to concerns for safety of the loved ones and, possibly, feelings of responsibility for providing support to others [17]. Physical separation from home environment also leads to the need for reshaping personal identity and social connections, both in the familiar context and externally. The disruption of the social environment and the exacerbation of pre-existing economic and familiar issues may contribute to an increase in domestic violence episodes, as well as substance and alcohol abuse [22, 23]. Moreover, the decreased livability of natural environments could promote forced migration due to climate reasons (*ecomigration*) [20, 24]. On one hand, migration has been largely demonstrated to represent an independent risk factor for the development of psychiatric disorders, due to several determinants associated with potentially traumatic experiences lived before migration [25], with the migration process itself [26], as well as to adjustment issues in a new cultural context [27, 28]. This lays the foundations for the occurrence of severe psychiatric disorders, particularly post-traumatic spectrum, mood, and psychotic disorders [29]. On the other hand, since migration is more likely to occur from rural, under-developed areas, to urban ones, this may reinforce uncontrolled urbanization processes that critically impact pollution and climate situation at a global level. The psychological consequences of natural disasters are particularly relevant among vulnerable populations. Among these, extreme age groups are prone to mental health issues in the climate change era. Particularly, young people are more sensitive to climate changes and seem to experience more severe consequences after natural calamities, with possible long-lasting effects on their central nervous system [23]. Moreover, they can also be affected by worries faced by their caregivers and be impacted significantly by the impairment of their social support and educational networks [30].

Apart from natural disasters, further events that may be classified as extreme weather events have a profound impact on mental health. Heat waves and the urban heat island phenomenon can directly cause distress and have been linked to higher risk of developing psychiatric disorders [31], particularly mood disturbances and anxiety [32], also resulting in higher number of admissions [33, 34]. Higher outdoor temperatures were also associated with suicidal behaviors and completed suicide [35]. Mild conditions of sensitivity to weather variations, such as meteoropathic ones, may be exacerbated by higher temperature; similarly, well-established diseases, e.g., seasonal swing patterns, could display an increment in their incidence following climate change. To note, seasonal patterns are also frequently observed in affective disorders, with consequences on relapses that could be extremely influenced by abrupt weather variations [36]. Moreover, higher mortality rates due to high temperatures were detected among subjects suffering from psychiatric conditions, especially schizophrenia spectrum disorders, which have been pointed out as risk factor for heat-related deaths [37, 38]. Extreme heat may influence the central nervous system through different pathways. Indeed, it has been demonstrated that high temperatures may influence mood by modifying dopamine and serotonin production, as well as altering thermoregulation mechanisms [39, 40]. Indirect mechanisms should also be highlighted, like those linked to the disruption of biological rhythms, which may be significantly influenced by the exposure to high temperatures and subsequently alter mood states.

To note, new expressions of climate-related psychological distress are also emerging in this complex scenario. Overall, the perception of incapability in front of a specific situation leads to stress, which predisposes to the development of psychiatric symptoms, such as depression and anxiety, as well as to risky behaviors [41]. Climate-related stress should thus be considered as a tangible risk factor for poor mental health. Beyond this, specific psychological constructs were coined in the context of the climate crisis.

- *Solastalgia*, defining a profound sense of loss of connection with the surrounding environment, manifesting itself when changes in the lived landscape become evident [42]. It is characterized not only by desolation and emotional pain, but also by disorientation and uncertainty. Solastalgia may occur gradually, even in front of progressive environmental changes and not only after natural disasters, and does not necessarily depend on the direct experience of loss. As a consequence of this psychological state, people may encounter major difficulties in adapting themselves to the new environment and this could lead to higher risk of developing psychiatric disorders, such as depression.
- *Eco-anxiety* refers to anxiety that is being developed as a response to the current ecological crisis. It is not necessarily due to the direct exposure to climate change-related events, but could also occur as a consequence of being aware of the ongoing emergency [43]. The main manifestations of eco-anxiety include feeling deeply worried and experiencing hopelessness and sense of guilt and impotence, but this form of distress may also facilitate the development of sleep and mood disorders.
- *Climate* or *ecological grief* is associated with ecological losses, confirming that the ecosys-

tems are changing, but can also be due to the loss of environmental identity or with the fear of future losses due to climate reasons [44]. Ecological grief usually manifests with a profound sense of despair, loss, and hopelessness [20]. Despite climate grief can also lead to adaptive consequences, most times it occurs together with feelings of sadness and frustration and, in some cases, can even exacerbate physical pain [45].

Climate-related psychological distress is rapidly increasing, but its different manifestations are not yet being evaluated on large scale, since the issues of climate change and global warming mainly refer to a general population rather than to a personal dimension, so it has been argued that individuals are not significantly affected by these topics, which are usually considered with some form of psychological distance [17]. This could also underpin the substantial lack of structured initiatives to reduce the climate impact of anthropogenic actions, both at an individual and community level. Such actions should rely on a number of possible behaviors, among which the increase of urban green, the promotion of public transportation, and the use of clean energy. Not only may these behaviors help reducing global warming, but they could also contribute to healthier lifestyle, promoting physical health together with mental health. Under this perspective, wider actions of promotion should be implemented on large scale to increase consciousness about the detrimental consequences of climate change on global health and subsequently promote actions involving policy makers and different professions.

15.2 The Effects of Pollution on Mental Health

The increase in pollutants level represents one among the main consequences of uncontrolled urbanization, significantly contributing to the climate crisis as well. In the urban environment, heterogeneous sources of pollutants undermine the global health of citizens, whose overall exposure may be linked to the higher prevalence of psychiatric disorders in these areas. Despite anthropogenic sources of pollutants vary between different parts of the city, these possibly represent the major threat to human health in these context, also considering indoor sources of pollutants.

15.2.1 Air Pollution and Mental Health

Air pollution, namely the contamination of outdoor and indoor environment by chemical, physical, or biological agents that modify the composition of the atmosphere, represents a threatening problem for human health worldwide. Sources of air pollutants are mainly due to anthropic activities, such as industrial and traffic emissions, household biomass, plastic waste, combustion of fossil fuels, and are diffuse in both developed and under-developed countries with a higher impact on the latter. Even low concentrations of pollutants can be harmful and contribute to the onset of a number of noncommunicable diseases, such as respiratory, cardiovascular, neoplastic, and neurocognitive ones [46]. On these bases, collaborative initiatives were built to reduce the impact of pollution, which is also listed as a goal in the Sustainable Development Agenda. The WHO set minimal levels of air pollutants (particulate matter, ozone, nitrogen dioxide, and sulfur dioxide) in order to assist governments and policymakers in reducing the impact of scarce air quality. Despite this, according to the latest estimates 99% of the global population lives in areas where the WHO guidelines for air quality are not met [47].

The impact of air pollution on mental health has gained growing interest during the last years, with evidence concerning both short- and long-term effects relying on a number of direct and indirect mechanisms. The exposure to air pollution has an effect on the central nervous system, activating pathways of oxidative stress and neuroinflammation, as demonstrated at first in animal models where air pollutants caused depression-like syndromes [48]. Pollutants reach specific brain regions via the olfactory nerve or passing the blood–brain barrier after being inhaled and migrate to the systemic circulation [49]. The production of proinflammatory molecules can then be induced by air pollutants both in the lung and in the central nervous system, where they trigger the activation of astroglia and microglia, with subsequent production of cytokines (tumor necrosis factor-α (TNF-α), interleukin-1β (IL-1β), and interferon (IFN-γ). The upregulation of cytokines and chemokines also happens in specific brain areas, e.g., hippocampus, and is associated with the secretion of glucocorticoids [50]. The activation of the hypothalamic–pituitary axis and the subsequent increase in glucocorticoid concentrations represents another key mechanism contributing to pollutant-related psychiatric symptoms. Indeed, changes in glucocorticoid concentrations influence brain structure and function and also act on mood regulation [51]. Furthermore, oxidative stress pathways are stimulated by exposure to air pollutants, with subsequent neurotoxicity. This may result in changes in neurotransmitter gene expression in specific brain regions associated with internalizing disorders, particularly frontolimbic ones such as amygdala, hippocampus, and prefrontal cortex [52–54], altering gray matter volumes and white matter microstructure in these areas [55, 56].

The exposure to pollutants increases the risk of developing psychiatric disorders both in the short- and long-term, with a higher risk demonstrated for anxiety and depression [57–61], but also bipolar and psychotic disorders [62–65]. Moreover, pollutants can be involved in the development of suicidal behaviors [66], with a possible cumulative effect [67]. One relevant issue underlined by several studies is the effect of air pollutants even at low concentrations, below the current WHO limit values [65, 68]. Evidence concerning these associations is anyway limited by the heterogeneity of the study designs and by major difficulties in establishing causal relationships in this field, since the development of psychiatric disorders requires a multifactorial framework. As for suicide risk, for instance, the association with pollutant levels is possibly due to both *proximal* and *distal* mediators, since air pollution influences a number of suicide-related factors, such as external temperature and psychosocial stressors [69]. In addition, the possible development of psychiatric disorders represents itself a major risk factor for suicidal behaviors.

Another issue that may link air pollution and poor mental health is represented by the risk for developing physical illnesses, such as neoplastic ones, due to the exposure to environmental pollution. Indeed, physical and mental health are closely intertwined, so that medical diseases can influence the subsequent emergence of psychiatric disorders and vice versa [70]. Moreover, air pollution has been associated with poor life quality and low socio-economic status, psychological distress, circadian rhythm alterations and, in the case of indoor pollution, reduced cognitive performance, all representing further risk factors for the development of psychiatric symptoms [70–73].

Apart from the effects of air pollution on the development of clear-cut psychiatric conditions, it has been underlined that pre-existing psychiatric disorders can also by exacerbated by pollutant exposure. This is demonstrated by a growing body of literature highlighting the increase in psychiatric emergency accesses as a possible effect of air pollutants, such as ozone and particulate matter [74, 75]. A similar trend was demonstrated for outpatient visits [76] and number of hospitalizations for psychiatric disorders [77–79]. To note, the reduction in pollutant concentrations following restrictive measures for the containment of the Coronavirus disease 2019 (COVID-19) pandemic appeared to be associated with a reduction in hospital admissions [80]. The exacerbation of psychiatric disorders as a consequence of ambient pollution exposure was hypothesized to underpin pathophysiological mechanisms associated with oxidative stress and the reduction in antioxidative pathways [81]. Furthermore, specific risk factors, e.g., those related to sex and age, were demonstrated to increase the strength of this association with a higher vulnerability of special populations, such as elderly subjects [82]. Moreover, as already mentioned for climate change-related mental health issues, children and adolescent also represent vulnerable populations when it comes to the effects of air pollution [83, 84]. Indeed, the action of air pollutants on ongoing brain development processes may seriously affect the emergence of psychological distress and psychiatric disorders [85], the latter more frequently occurring for the first time during youth, with worse functional outcomes [86]. Noteworthy, environmental exposure to pollutants has possibly been linked to the emergence of neurodevelopmental diseases, such as autism spectrum disorders and related conditions [87–89]. Moreover, air pollution demonstrated a significant association with the development of affective disorders during youth, particularly depression with anxious features, also increasing the risk of suicidal behaviors [90]. These disturbances were associated with neuroimaging alterations involving the cortico-striato-thalamo-cortical circuitry, underlying clinical changes in cognitive and emotional regulation.

Despite the relationship between air pollution and mental health needs to be further clarified, the growing body of literature focusing on this topic underlines a strong association, which was demonstrated for all the main pollutants and even in case of low concentrations. This reinforces intensely the need for supporting actions oriented towards the reduction in pollutant concentrations, with a strong multidisciplinary commitment to improve air quality all around the globe.

15.2.2 Noise Pollution and Mental Health

During recent years, noise pollution has been confirmed to be associated with a number of medical conditions, e.g., cardiovascular and respiratory diseases [91–93]. In urban areas, different sources of noise can be identified, such as those related to road, railway, and aircraft traffic, with highly detrimental effects on human health. Despite social costs of noise-related health effects are still understudied, a recent document from the European Commission reports noise pollution to cause 69,000 hospital admissions and 15,900 cases of premature deaths every year [94]. Additionally, 22 million people living in Europe display high levels of noise annoyance, and 6.5 million people report chronic sleep disturbances caused by noise exposure [95]. Despite the exposure to traffic noise has been pointed out as the cause of 1.5 million years of healthy life lost [96], a progressive increase in the number of people exposed to high noise levels, especially in urban environments, was documented [97].

Studies on noise pollution are not as numerous as those focusing on air pollution, but a growing number of reports depicted the influence of high noise exposure on mental health, underlining the association with poor outcomes [98, 99]. Particularly, the exposure to different sources of noise increase the incidence of clear-cut psychiatric disorders, such as depressive and anxiety disorders and can influence the emergence of specific psychopathological features or increase perceived psychological stress, reducing health-related quality of life [100].

Similarly to what demonstrated for air pollution, noise acts through different mechanisms causing damage at a central nervous system level [101]. Such mechanisms may differ depending on the source of noise and on its characteristics [102]. The increase in corticosteroid hormones, inflammation, and oxidative stress [103] seems to be activated by noise, with possible effects on prefrontal regions function. Indeed, the prolonged exposure to high levels of noise may cause chronic stress, with subsequent activation of the sympathetic adrenal–medullary axis. The latter provides warning signals to the cortex and influences networks involving prefrontal and limbic areas, which are involved in cognition and emotional regulation [104]. It has also been demonstrated that the disruption of sleep-wake rhythms is a crucial mediator of noise-related psychiatric issues. Indeed, the alterations of sleep-wake patterns induce a pro-oxidative environment predisposing to neuroinflammation [105–107]. To note, exposure to noise and subsequent noise annoyance are also associated with medical diseases, e.g., atrial fibrillation [108, 109]. Among noise-related psychiatric symptoms, the most studied were anxiety and depression. Cohort and case–control studies demonstrated that the incidence of these conditions was higher in case of prolonged exposure to noise coming from different sources, suggesting that noise pollution could act as an independent risk factor for affective disorders [60, 110, 111]. Similarly, an increase in bipolar disorder risk was detected, especially in vulnerable populations such as those at genetic risk [112]. Levels of noise appeared to affect mood symptom severity as well, with an addictive effect [60, 110, 111, 113]. The number of hospitalizations due to depression and anxiety, as well as the daily number of suicides, also appeared to be influenced by noise pollution [114]. Further psychopathological features that resulted to be more represented in contexts where subjects were exposed to high levels of noise were aggressiveness, hostility, and anger [115]. It should also be underlined that people who suffer from serious mental illnesses show higher noise sensitivity, which means that noise exposure may trigger specific psychopathological features in these vulnerable population [116].

Circadian rhythms are also significantly affected by noise. Particularly, traffic noise was associated with sleep disturbances, with a dose-response relationship [117]. Poor sleep quality leads to subsequent cognitive and behavioral symptoms during daytime. Moreover, the link between noise pollution and sleep disturbances may itself act as a risk factor for developing subsequent psychiatric conditions, such as mood disorders. Circadian rhythm alterations play a significant role in the of these conditions and can also influence relapse rates, impacting overall functioning and outcomes. Sleep patterns also affect neurotransmission, particularly serotoninergic—since melatonin is synthesized from serotonin—which may explain further mediation processes between noise, circadian rhythm disturbances, and the development of mood alterations [118]. To note, noise pollution also influenced the prescription of hypnotics and anxiolytics [119, 120], as well as antidepressants [121]. Mental health outcomes are possibly associated not only with measured noise levels but also with perceived noise, as demonstrated by a growing body of research conducted during the last years [122–124].

This may depend on the fact that exposure to noise affects psychological well-being and health-related quality of life, apart from the development of clear-cut psychiatric disorders. Indeed, specific psychological features, such as noise annoyance, were demonstrated to significantly affect overall quality of life [125–129], possibly acting as a mediator of poor mental health [130, 131]. Noise annoyance affects emotional regulation, influencing daily activities as well as the development of distress and negative responses, e.g., discontent and anger [98]. Annoyance may develop as a consequence of exposure to noise on the basis of individual characteristics, such as personality traits oriented towards higher levels of neuroticism [125, 131], also enhancing noise sensitivity. This latter psychological construct refers to subjects who experience higher stress and psychological annoyance related to high levels of noise pollution, especially in the urban environment [132]. Sensitivity to noise may lead to higher severity of psychopathology [133–135].

When it comes to special populations, it has been underlined that youths, and particularly children, are highly sensitive to the effects of road traffic noise on sleep duration and quality [136]. Furthermore, noise exposure during childhood is also associated with psychiatric disturbances, particularly hyperactivity/inattention issues, as well as with abnormal conduct and peer relationships [137, 138]. This suggests that when youths are exposed to noise sources specific symptom clusters should always be screened due to the specific vulnerability of this population, possibly depending on limited capacity to react adaptively to environmental stressors. To note, circadian rhythms and chronotype preference are still under development during childhood and adolescence and the biological clock could thus be more sensitive to environmental stressors with subsequent changes in melatonin secretion [139–141]. As already stated for air pollution, it should then be underlined that noise levels are usually high in densely populated urban areas, where a number of other risk factors linked to mental health can be identified, such as reduced access to urban green and lack of physical activity, causing overall environmental discomfort [142].

As a consequence of what has been elucidated so far, noise pollution has to be considered as a major risk factor for poor mental health, despite this association still needs to be fully unraveled and specific pathophysiological mechanisms still need to be clarified. The lowering of noise levels should always be considered in the context of urban planning, so that initiatives and environmental measures aimed at reducing noise pollution need to be improved, with adequate transport planning and sound insolation measures for indoor environments. Special attention should also be dedicated to noise annoyance as a possible mediator of poor mental health after noise exposure, possibly identifying subjects who are at risk for developing higher levels of this noise-related feature.

15.2.3 Light Pollution and Mental Health

According to the world atlas of artificial sky luminance, it has been estimated that more than 80% of the global population (over 90% in Europe and the United States) lives in areas polluted by artificial light [143], with highest intensity of the phenomenon occurring in urban centers. Different spectral characteristics of artificial light present distinct effects on skyglow, e.g., 4000K white LED is significantly more polluting than low temperature lighting [143, 144]. The exposure to artificial light at night (ALAN) has been estimated to increase annually by 3–6% in past decades and continues to extend with more than 2% growth every year [144]. Despite this, appropriate legislation on the topic is lacking in most countries and preventive measure are scant. Moreover, due to technology advances individuals are now routinely exposed to artificial light through the use of laptop, tablet, and smartphone screens, which emit short wavelength light [145].

ALAN affects human health and well-being with both direct and indirect mechanisms, due to its effects on the secretion of melatonin that is regulated by the conditions of external illumination and is sensitive to different wavelengths. Indeed, after two hours of exposure to monochromatic light at 460 nm during the evening, the significant suppression of melatonin may occur, whilst the exposure to wavelength of 550 nm did not show similar effects [144]. Hence, a strong inhibitory effect has mainly been demonstrated for short wavelengths and color temperature of about 6500K.

Changes in melatonin release underpin the disruption of circadian rhythms, but also in further physiological processes, such as metabolism, hormone synthesis, and immune regulation [146]. Melatonin has been demonstrated to exert anxiolytic actions, both in animal models and in different clinical conditions [147]. The suppression of this hormone contributes to the development or worsening of endocrine and metabolic disruptions, possibly facilitating the occurrence of obesity [148]. The immune system disruption contributes to higher susceptibility to viral infections, as demonstrated by Italian studies depicting higher number of COVID-19 cases in areas with higher levels of light pollution [149].

The effects of light pollution on mental health seemed to be mainly mediated by alterations in circadian rhythms, particularly sleep-wake cycle. Indeed, sleep quality is an important determinant of mental health and is strongly linked to the environment where subjects live. Despite there are few studies quantifying the effect of light pollution on overall sleep quality, studies conducted on both adult and children populations demonstrated that higher exposure to ALAN, such as those happening in urban rather than rural areas, was associated with reduced sleep quality and duration, higher sleep latency, and with the emergence of sleep disorders [150–152]. Moreover, increasing exposure to ALAN seemed to be associated with greater prescription of hypnotic drugs, mainly in elderly populations [153]. To note, sleep disturbances may also be exacerbated by the exposure to pre-awake artificial light [154]. Artificial lighting can be highly represented in indoor conditions, e.g., individuals may be likely to fall sleep with bedroom of television lights on. Lights-on sleep was associated with a number of sleep alterations, decreased slow-wave sleep and increased arousal index. Spectral analysis also revealed that theta power during REM sleep and slow oscillation, delta, and spindle power during non-rapid eye movement (NREM) sleep were decreased in these conditions [155]. Apart from sleep disorders, the emergence of affective disturbances was linked with ALAN exposure. Particularly, the exposure to light pollution, both outdoors and indoors, was associated with a higher incidence of unipolar depression and bipolar disorders, as well as specific phobias and other anxiety disorders [140, 154, 156]. The neurobiological mechanisms through which ALAN may contribute to mood and affective disturbances rely on the disruption of circadian rhythmicity, as well. This is also supported by the evidence that people who experience seasonal variations in day length or those who suffer from jet lag and work regularly at night are more likely to develop depressive symptoms and mood changes. Preliminary evidence is also available for what concerns the possible higher risk of suicidal behaviors [153]. Sleep-wake cycle disruptions and artificial light pollution could also trigger relapses of affective episodes in subjects who suffer from bipolar disorders, which can be easily derived by the effects of sleep deprivation in inducing mania [157, 158]. It has also been hypothesized that light pollution blocks nocturnal production of melatonin, which may disrupt the rhythmicity of steroid hormone secretion with possible effects on the emergence of mania [159].

Apart from psychopathological manifestations, features of psychological distress were associated with ALAN, with significant influence of subjective risk perception concerning light pollution [145, 160]. Moreover, subjects who perceived higher levels of outdoor light pollution had poorer sleep quality, as well as higher symptoms of distress, compared to those who did not [145]. This could be explained by the fact that poor sleepers and people with high levels of psychological distress may experience hyper-arousal and pay higher attention to their sleeping environment. Moreover, they could have a higher light sensitivity towards and be thus more vulnerable to the effects of ALAN on sleep.

The effects of light pollution on mental health still need to be explored in depth, also identifying homogeneous means for measuring artificial night, in order to unravel its association with mental health outcomes. Among these, the role of circadian rhythm disruption remains central, suggesting that proper sleep hygiene and healthy behaviors including the promotion of regular biological rhythms could represent a highly protective factor for the development of psychiatric symptoms as a consequence of ALAN exposure. Further risk factors for higher risk perception in response to light pollution should also be identified, so that sensitive populations may benefit from targeted preventive measures.

15.3 Final Remarks

The relationship between climate change, pollution, and mental health underpins the complex interplay of several factors and lies on interactive processes. These may lead to the development of different manifestations, ranging from mild forms of psychological distress to the emergence of psychiatric disorders. The further clarification of the possible mechanisms and risk factors leading to the development of psychiatric disorders in the climate change era may help implementing preventive strategies that should include a comprehensive rethinking of the urban environment. In addition, health policies should take into account a wide range of factors, such as different kinds of pollutants, urban green cover, and social determinants. Furthermore, health policies should encourage behavioral strategies oriented towards lowering stress levels and improving circadian rhythms with an overall positive effect on mental health. Such interventions should specifically focus on vulnerable populations, particularly children and adolescents, who may strongly benefit from actions aimed at developing and strengthening environmental resilience.

References

1. United Nations Department of Economic and Social Affairs (2016) The world's cities in 2016. Statistical papers—United Nations (Ser. A), population and vital statistics report, New York (US)
2. Sarkar C, Webster C (2017) Urban environments and human health: current trends and future directions. Curr Opin Environ Sustain 25:33–44
3. World Health Organization (2023) World Health Organization. https://www.who.int. Accessed 29 Sep 2023

4. Watts N et al (2021) The 2020 report of The Lancet Countdown on health and climate change: responding to converging crises. Lancet 397(10269):129–170. https://doi.org/10.1016/S0140-6736(20)32290-X
5. Cianconi P, Betrò S, Janiri L (2020) The impact of climate change on mental health: a systematic descriptive review. Front Psych 11:74. https://doi.org/10.3389/fpsyt.2020.00074
6. Marazziti D et al (2021) Climate change, environment pollution, Covid-19 pandemic and mental health. Sci Total Environ 773:145182. https://doi.org/10.1016/j.scitotenv.2021.145182
7. Ventriglio A et al (2020) Environmental pollution and mental health: a narrative review of literature. CNS Spectr 26:51. https://doi.org/10.1017/S1092852920001303
8. Berry HL, Bowen K, Kjellstrom T (2010) Climate change and mental health: a causal pathways framework. Int J Public Health 55(2):123–132. https://doi.org/10.1007/S00038-009-0112-0
9. Menculini G et al (2021) The influence of the urban environment on mental health during the COVID-19 pandemic: focus on air pollution and migration—a narrative review. Int J Environ Res Public Health 18(8):3920. https://doi.org/10.3390/IJERPH18083920
10. Riva A et al (2022) Can homes affect well-being? A scoping review among housing conditions, indoor environmental quality, and mental health outcomes. Int J Environ Res Public Health 19(23):15975. https://doi.org/10.3390/IJERPH192315975
11. Crane K et al (2022) Climate change and mental health: a review of empirical evidence, mechanisms and implications. Atmosphere 13(12):2096. https://doi.org/10.3390/ATMOS13122096
12. Mojahed N, Mohammadkhani MA, Mohamadkhani A (2022) Climate crises and developing vector-borne diseases: a narrative review. Iran J Public Health 51(12):2664–2673. https://doi.org/10.18502/IJPH.V51I12.11457
13. University Corporation for Atmospheric Research (2023) Urban heat island. https://scied.ucar.edu. Accessed 29 Sep 2023
14. Gifford E, Gifford R (2016) The largely unacknowledged impact of climate change on mental health. Bull At Sci 72(5):292–297. https://doi.org/10.1080/00963402.2016.1216505
15. Golitaleb M et al (2022) Prevalence of post-traumatic stress disorder after flood: a systematic review and meta-analysis. Front Psych 13:890671. https://doi.org/10.3389/FPSYT.2022.890671
16. Huang W et al (2023) Health effects of cyclones: a systematic review and meta-analysis of epidemiological studies. Environ Health Perspect 131(8):86001. https://doi.org/10.1289/EHP12158
17. American Psychiatric Association (2017) Mental health and our changing climate: impacts, implications, and guidance. American Psychiatric Association, Washington, DC
18. Gronlund CJ et al (2019) Assessing the magnitude and uncertainties of the burden of selected diseases attributable to extreme heat and extreme precipitation under a climate change scenario in Michigan for the period 2041-2070. Environ Health 18(1):40. https://doi.org/10.1186/S12940-019-0483-5
19. Saeed SA, Gargano SP (2022) Natural disasters and mental health. Int Rev Psychiatry 34(1):16–25. https://doi.org/10.1080/09540261.2022.2037524
20. Sri A et al (2023) Global mental health and climate change: a geo-psychiatry perspectiv. Asian J Psychiatr 84:103562. https://doi.org/10.1016/J.AJP.2023.103562
21. Miles-Novelo A, Anderson CA (2019) Climate change and psychology: effects of rapid global warming on violence and aggression. Curr Clim Chang Rep 5:36–46
22. Epstein A et al (2020) Drought and intimate partner violence towards women in 19 countries in sub-Saharan Africa during 2011-2018: a population-based study. PLoS Med 17(3):e1003064. https://doi.org/10.1371/JOURNAL.PMED.1003064
23. Fernandez A et al (2015) Flooding and mental health: a systematic mapping review. PLoS One 10(4):e0119929. https://doi.org/10.1371/JOURNAL.PONE.0119929
24. Chersich MF et al (2018) Impacts of climate change on health and wellbeing in South Africa. Int J Environ Res Public Health 15(9):1884. https://doi.org/10.3390/IJERPH15091884
25. Mesa-Vieira C et al (2022) Mental health of migrants with pre-migration exposure to armed conflict: a systematic review and meta-analysis. Lancet Public Health 7(5):e469–e481. https://doi.org/10.1016/S2468-2667(22)00061-5
26. Bürgin D et al (2022) Impact of war and forced displacement on children's mental health-multilevel, needs-oriented, and trauma-informed approaches. Eur Child Adolesc Psychiatry 31(6):845–853. https://doi.org/10.1007/S00787-022-01974-Z
27. Brance K, Chatzimpyros V, Bentall RP (2023) Increased social identification is linked with lower depressive and anxiety symptoms among ethnic minorities and migrants: a systematic review and meta-analysis. Clin Psychol Rev 99:102216. https://doi.org/10.1016/J.CPR.2022.102216
28. Montemitro C et al (2021) Language proficiency and mental disorders among migrants: a systematic review. Eur Psychiatry 64(1):e49. https://doi.org/10.1192/J.EURPSY.2021.2224
29. Patanè M et al (2022) Prevalence of mental disorders in refugees and asylum seekers: a systematic review and meta-analysis. Global Ment Health (Camb) 9:250–263. https://doi.org/10.1017/GMH.2022.29
30. Banks DM, Weems CF (2014) Family and peer social support and their links to psychological distress among hurricane-exposed minority youth. Am J Orthopsychiatry 84(4):341–352. https://doi.org/10.1037/ORT0000006

31. Li D et al (2023a) Climatic and meteorological exposure and mental and behavioral health: a systematic review and meta-analysis. Sci Total Environ 892:164435. https://doi.org/10.1016/J.SCITOTENV.2023.164435
32. Padhy SK et al (2015) Mental health effects of climate change. Indian J Occup Environ Med 19(1):3–7. https://doi.org/10.4103/0019-5278.156997
33. Hansen A et al (2008) The effect of heat waves on mental health in a temperate Australian city. Environ Health Perspect 116(10):1369–1375. https://doi.org/10.1289/EHP.11339
34. Peng Z et al (2017) Effects of ambient temperature on daily hospital admissions for mental disorders in Shanghai, China: a time-series analysis. Sci Total Environ 590–591:281–286. https://doi.org/10.1016/j.scitotenv.2017.02.237
35. Thompson R et al (2023) Ambient temperature and mental health: a systematic review and meta-analysis. Lancet Planet Health 7(7):e580–e589. https://doi.org/10.1016/S2542-5196(23)00104-3
36. Medici CR et al (2016) Seasonal variations in hospital admissions for mania: examining for associations with weather variables over time. J Affect Disord 205:81–86. https://doi.org/10.1016/J.JAD.2016.06.053
37. Cornwall W (2023) Schizophrenia pinpointed as a key factor in heat deaths. Science 379(6637):1079. https://doi.org/10.1126/SCIENCE.ADH8294
38. Wang X et al (2014) Acute impacts of extreme temperature exposure on emergency room admissions related to mental and behavior disorders in Toronto, Canada. J Affect Disord 155(1):154–161. https://doi.org/10.1016/J.JAD.2013.10.042
39. Basu R et al (2018) Examining the association between apparent temperature and mental health-related emergency room visits in California. Am J Epidemiol 187(4):726–735. https://doi.org/10.1093/AJE/KWX295
40. Noelke C et al (2016) Increasing ambient temperature reduces emotional well-being. Environ Res 151:124–129. https://doi.org/10.1016/J.ENVRES.2016.06.045
41. Neria Y, Shultz JM (2012) Mental health effects of Hurricane Sandy: characteristics, potential aftermath, and response. JAMA 308(24):2571. https://doi.org/10.1001/JAMA.2012.110700
42. Albrecht G et al (2007) Solastalgia: the distress caused by environmental change. Australas Psychiatry 15 Suppl 1:S95. https://doi.org/10.1080/10398560701701288
43. Kurth C, Pihkala P (2022) Eco-anxiety: what it is and why it matters. Front Psychol 13:981814. https://doi.org/10.3389/FPSYG.2022.981814
44. Comtesse H et al (2021) Ecological grief as a response to environmental change: a mental health risk or functional response? Int J Environ Res Public Health 18(2):1–10. https://doi.org/10.3390/IJERPH18020734
45. Cianconi P et al (2023) Eco-emotions and psychoterratic syndromes: reshaping mental health assessment under climate change. Yale J Biol Med 96(2):211–226. https://doi.org/10.59249/EARX2427
46. Meng X et al (2021) Short term associations of ambient nitrogen dioxide with daily total, cardiovascular, and respiratory mortality: multilocation analysis in 398 cities. BMJ 372:n534. https://doi.org/10.1136/bmj.n534
47. World Health Organization (2021) WHO air quality guidelines. Particulate matter (PM2.5, PM10), ozone, nitrogen dioxide, sulfur dioxide and carbon monoxide. World Health Organization, Geneva. chrome-extensiohttps://iris.who.int/bitstream/handle/10665/345329/9789240034228-eng.pdf
48. Calderón-Garcidueñas L et al (2002) Air pollution and brain damage. Toxicol Pathol 30(3):373–389. https://doi.org/10.1080/01926230252929954
49. Hahad O et al (2020) Ambient air pollution increases the risk of cerebrovascular and neuropsychiatric disorders through induction of inflammation and oxidative stress. Int J Mol Sci 21(12):1–24. https://doi.org/10.3390/IJMS21124306
50. Jia Z et al (2018) Exposure to ambient air particles increases the risk of mental disorder: findings from a natural experiment in Beijing. Int J Environ Res Public Health 15(1):160. https://doi.org/10.3390/IJERPH15010160
51. Thomson EM, Filiatreault A, Guénette J (2019) Stress hormones as potential mediators of air pollutant effects on the brain: rapid induction of glucocorticoid-responsive genes. Environ Res 178:108717. https://doi.org/10.1016/J.ENVRES.2019.108717
52. Ehsanifar M et al (2021) Hippocampal inflammation and oxidative stress following exposure to diesel exhaust nanoparticles in male and female mice. Neurochem Int 145:104989. https://doi.org/10.1016/J.NEUINT.2021.104989
53. Salvi A, Liu H, Salim S (2019) Involvement of oxidative stress and mitochondrial mechanisms in air pollution-related neurobiological impairments. Neurobiol Stress 12:100205. https://doi.org/10.1016/J.YNSTR.2019.100205
54. Zundel CG et al (2022) Air pollution, depressive and anxiety disorders, and brain effects: a systematic review. Neurotoxicology 93:272–300. https://doi.org/10.1016/J.NEURO.2022.10.011
55. Herting MM et al (2019) Outdoor air pollution and brain structure and function from across childhood to young adulthood: a methodological review of brain MRI studies. Front Public Health 7:332. https://doi.org/10.3389/FPUBH.2019.00332
56. Lubczyńska MJ et al (2020) Exposure to air pollution during pregnancy and childhood, and white matter microstructure in preadolescents. Environ Health Perspect 128(2):27005. https://doi.org/10.1289/EHP4709

57. Borroni E et al (2022) Air pollution exposure and depression: a comprehensive updated systematic review and meta-analysis. Environm Pollut 292(Pt A):118245. https://doi.org/10.1016/J.ENVPOL.2021.118245
58. Braithwaite I et al (2019) Air pollution (particulate matter) exposure and associations with depression, anxiety, bipolar, psychosis and suicide risk: a systematic review and meta-analysis. Environ Health Perspect 127(12):126002. https://doi.org/10.1289/EHP4595
59. Cao T et al (2023) The relationship between air pollution and depression and anxiety disorders—a systematic evaluation and meta-analysis of a cohort-based study. Int J Soc Psychiatry 70:241. https://doi.org/10.1177/00207640231197941
60. Generaal E et al (2019) Not urbanization level but socioeconomic, physical and social neighbourhood characteristics are associated with presence and severity of depressive and anxiety disorders. Psychol Med 49(1):149–161. https://doi.org/10.1017/s0033291718000612
61. Trushna T et al (2020) Effects of ambient air pollution on psychological stress and anxiety disorder: a systematic review and meta-analysis of epidemiological evidence. Rev Environ Health 36(4):501–521. https://doi.org/10.1515/REVEH-2020-0125
62. Antonsen S et al (2020) Exposure to air pollution during childhood and risk of developing schizophrenia: a national cohort study. Lancet Planet Health 4(2):e64–e73. https://doi.org/10.1016/S2542-5196(20)30004-8
63. Attademo L et al (2017) Environmental pollution and risk of psychotic disorders: a review of the science to date. Schizophr Res 181:55–59. https://doi.org/10.1016/J.SCHRES.2016.10.003
64. Khan A et al (2019) Environmental pollution is associated with increased risk of psychiatric disorders in the US and Denmark. PLoS Biol 17(8):e3000353. https://doi.org/10.1371/JOURNAL.PBIO.3000353
65. Li D et al (2023b) Long-term exposure to ambient air pollution, genetic susceptibility, and the incidence of bipolar disorder: a prospective cohort study. Psychiatry Res 327:115396. https://doi.org/10.1016/J.PSYCHRES.2023.115396
66. Hwang IY et al (2022) Association of short-term particulate matter exposure with suicide death among major depressive disorder patients: a time-stratified case-crossover analysis. Sci Rep 12(1):8471. https://doi.org/10.1038/S41598-022-12421-Z
67. Davoudi M et al (2021) Association of suicide with short-term exposure to air pollution at different lag times: a systematic review and meta-analysis. Sci Total Environ 771:144882. https://doi.org/10.1016/J.SCITOTENV.2020.144882
68. Papadogeorgou G et al (2019) Low levels of air pollution and health: effect estimates, methodological challenges, and future directions. Curr Environ Health Rep 6(3):105–115. https://doi.org/10.1007/S40572-019-00235-7
69. Aguglia A et al (2021) Meteorological variables and suicidal behavior: air pollution and apparent temperature are associated with high-lethality suicide attempts and male gender. Front Psych 12:653390. https://doi.org/10.3389/FPSYT.2021.653390
70. Bhui K et al (2023) Air quality and mental health: evidence, challenges and future directions. BJPsych Open 9(4):e120. https://doi.org/10.1192/BJO.2023.507
71. Karnauskas KB, Miller SL, Schapiro AC (2020) Fossil fuel combustion is driving indoor CO2 toward levels harmful to human cognition. GeoHealth 4(5):e2019GH000237. https://doi.org/10.1029/2019GH000237
72. Park J et al (2023) Association of long-term exposure to air pollution with chronic sleep deprivation in South Korea: a community-level longitudinal study, 2008-2018. Environ Res 228:115812. https://doi.org/10.1016/J.ENVRES.2023.115812
73. Wallace DA et al (2023) Is exposure to chemical pollutants associated with sleep outcomes? A systematic review. Sleep Med Rev 70:101805. https://doi.org/10.1016/J.SMRV.2023.101805
74. Bernardini F et al (2019) Air pollutants and daily number of admissions to psychiatric emergency services: evidence for detrimental mental health effects of ozone. Epidemiol Psychiatr Sci 29:e66. https://doi.org/10.1017/S2045796019000623
75. Liu JJ et al (2019) Ambient fine particulate matter is associated with increased emergency ambulance dispatches for psychiatric emergencies. Environ Res 177:108611. https://doi.org/10.1016/J.ENVRES.2019.108611
76. Liang Z et al (2019) The association between short-term ambient air pollution and daily outpatient visits for schizophrenia: a hospital-based study. Environ Pollut 244:102–108. https://doi.org/10.1016/J.ENVPOL.2018.09.142
77. Bernardini F et al (2020) Air pollutants and daily hospital admissions for psychiatric care: a review. Psychiatr Serv 71(12):1270–1276. https://doi.org/10.1176/appi.ps.201800565
78. Duan J et al (2018) Is the serious ambient air pollution associated with increased admissions for schizophrenia? Sci Total Environ 644:14–19. https://doi.org/10.1016/J.SCITOTENV.2018.06.218
79. Qiu X et al (2022) Associations of short-term exposure to air pollution and increased ambient temperature with psychiatric hospital admissions in older adults in the USA: a case-crossover study. Lancet Planet Health 6(4):e331–e341. https://doi.org/10.1016/S2542-5196(22)00017-1
80. Tao J et al (2023) Impacts of PM2.5 before and after COVID-19 outbreak on emergency mental disorders: a population-based quasi-experimental and case-crossover study. Environ Pollut 334:122175. https://doi.org/10.1016/J.ENVPOL.2023.122175
81. Wei Q et al (2022) Oxidative stress-mediated particulate matter affects the risk of relapse in schizophrenia patients: air purification intervention-based panel

study. Environ Pollut 292(Pt B):118348. https://doi.org/10.1016/J.ENVPOL.2021.118348
82. Wang L et al (2023) Ecological correlation between short term exposure to particulate matter and hospitalization for mental disorders in Shijiazhuang, China. Sci Rep 13(1):11412. https://doi.org/10.1038/S41598-023-37279-7
83. Landrigan PJ et al (2019) Pollution and children's health. Sci Total Environ 650(Pt 2):2389–2394. https://doi.org/10.1016/J.SCITOTENV.2018.09.375
84. Theron LC et al (2022) A systematic review of the mental health risks and resilience among pollution-exposed adolescents. J Psychiatr Res 146:55–66. https://doi.org/10.1016/J.JPSYCHIRES.2021.12.012
85. Danese A, Baldwin JR (2017) Hidden wounds? Inflammatory links between childhood trauma and psychopathology. Annu Rev Psychol 68:517–544. https://doi.org/10.1146/ANNUREV-PSYCH-010416-044208
86. Copeland WE et al (2015) Adult functional outcomes of common childhood psychiatric problems: a prospective, longitudinal study. JAMA Psychiatry 72(9):892–899. https://doi.org/10.1001/JAMAPSYCHIATRY.2015.0730
87. Ruiz-Sobremazas D et al (2023) Uncovering the link between air pollution and neurodevelopmental alterations during pregnancy and early life exposure: a systematic review. Neurosci Biobehav Rev 152:105314. https://doi.org/10.1016/J.NEUBIOREV.2023.105314
88. Saez M et al (2018) The association between exposure to environmental factors and the occurrence of attention-deficit/hyperactivity disorder (ADHD). A population-based retrospective cohort study. Environ Res 166:205–214. https://doi.org/10.1016/J.ENVRES.2018.05.009
89. Volk HE et al (2013) Traffic-related air pollution, particulate matter, and autism. JAMA Psychiatry 70(1):71–77. https://doi.org/10.1001/JAMAPSYCHIATRY.2013.266
90. Xie H et al (2023) Affective disorder and brain alterations in children and adolescents exposed to outdoor air pollution. J Affect Disord 331:413–424. https://doi.org/10.1016/J.JAD.2023.03.082
91. Liu S et al (2021) Long-term exposure to ambient air pollution and road traffic noise and asthma incidence in adults: the Danish Nurse cohort. Environ Int 152:106464. https://doi.org/10.1016/j.envint.2021.106464
92. Luan Y et al (2021) High-frequency noise-induced hearing loss disrupts functional connectivity in non-auditory areas with cognitive disturbances. Neurosci Bull 37:720. https://doi.org/10.1007/s12264-021-00663-2
93. Münzel T et al (2014) Cardiovascular effects of environmental noise exposure. Eur Heart J 35:829. https://doi.org/10.1093/eurheartj/ehu030
94. European Commision (2017) 2nd report from the Commission to the European Parliament and the Council on the implementation of the Environmental Noise Directive in accordance with Article 11 of the Directive. http://eur-lex.europa.eu. Accessed 22 Jan 2022
95. European Environment Agency (2020) Environmental noise in Europe. https://www.eea.europa.eu/publications/environmental-noise-in-europe. Accessed 11 Jan 2022
96. World Health Organization Regional Office for Europe (2011) Burden of disease from environmental noise. Copenaghen, Denmark. https://www.euro.who.int/__data/assets/pdf_file/0008/136466/e94888.pdf. Accessed 31 Jan 2022
97. European Environment Agency (2018) Environmental indicator report. www.eea.europa.eu. Accessed 20 Jan 2021
98. Basner M et al (2014) Auditory and non-auditory effects of noise on health. Lancet 383:1325–1332. https://doi.org/10.1016/S0140-6736(13)61613-X
99. Clark C, Crumpler C, Notley H (2020) Evidence for environmental noise effects on health for the United Kingdom policy context: a systematic review of the effects of environmental noise on mental health, wellbeing, quality of life, cancer, dementia, birth, reproductive outcomes, and cognition. Int J Environ Res Public Health 17(2):393. https://doi.org/10.3390/ijerph17020393
100. Tortorella A et al (2022) New determinants of mental health: the role of noise pollution. A narrative review. Int Rev Psychiatry 34(7–8):783–796. https://doi.org/10.1080/09540261.2022.2095200
101. Hunter JC, Hayden KM (2018) The association of sleep with neighborhood physical and social environment. Public Health 162:126–134. https://doi.org/10.1016/j.puhe.2018.05.003
102. Guski R, Schreckenberg D, Schuemer R (2017) WHO environmental noise guidelines for the European region: a systematic review on environmental noise and annoyance. Int J Environ Res Public Health 14:1539. https://doi.org/10.3390/ijerph14121539
103. Hahad O et al (2019) Environmental noise-induced effects on stress hormones, oxidative stress, and vascular dysfunction: key factors in the relationship between cerebrocardiovascular and psychological disorders. Oxid Med Cell Longev 2019:4623109. https://doi.org/10.1155/2019/4623109
104. Alyan E et al (2021) Frontal electroencephalogram alpha asymmetry during mental stress related to workplace noise. Sensors (Basel) 21(6):1–12. https://doi.org/10.3390/S21061968
105. Herzog J et al (2019) Acute exposure to nocturnal train noise induces endothelial dysfunction and pro-thromboinflammatory changes of the plasma proteome in healthy subjects. Basic Res Cardiol 114(6):46. https://doi.org/10.1007/S00395-019-0753-Y

106. Schmidt FP et al (2013) Effect of nighttime aircraft noise exposure on endothelial function and stress hormone release in healthy adults. Eur Heart J 34(45):3508. https://doi.org/10.1093/EURHEARTJ/EHT269
107. Schmidt FP et al (2021) The impact of aircraft noise on vascular and cardiac function in relation to noise event number: a randomized trial. Cardiovasc Res 117(5):1382–1390. https://doi.org/10.1093/CVR/CVAA204
108. Hahad O et al (2018) Annoyance to different noise sources is associated with atrial fibrillation in the Gutenberg Health Study. Int J Cardiol 264:79–84. https://doi.org/10.1016/J.IJCARD.2018.03.126
109. Hahad O et al (2021) Midregional pro atrial natriuretic peptide: a novel important biomarker for noise annoyance-induced cardiovascular morbidity and mortality? Clin Res Cardiol 110(1):29–39. https://doi.org/10.1007/S00392-020-01645-6
110. Eze IC et al (2020) Incidence of depression in relation to transportation noise exposure and noise annoyance in the SAPALDIA study. Environ Int 144:106014. https://doi.org/10.1016/j.envint.2020.106014
111. Seidler A et al (2017) Association between aircraft, road and railway traffic noise and depression in a large case-control study based on secondary data. Environ Res 152:263–271. https://doi.org/10.1016/j.envres.2016.10.017
112. Hao G et al (2021) Associations of PM2.5 and road traffic noise with mental health: evidence from UK Biobank. Environ Res 207:112221. https://doi.org/10.1016/J.ENVRES.2021.112221
113. Monazzan Esmaielpour MR et al (2021) Investigating the effect of noise exposure on mental disorders and the work ability index among industrial workers. Noise Vibr Worldw 53:3. https://doi.org/10.1177/09574565211052690
114. Díaz J et al (2020) Short-term effects of traffic noise on suicides and emergency hospital admissions due to anxiety and depression in Madrid (Spain). Sci Total Environ 710:136315. https://doi.org/10.1016/j.scitotenv.2019.136315
115. Alimohammadi I et al (2018) Effect of chronic noise exposure on aggressive behavior of automotive industry workers. Int J Occup Environ Med 9(4):170–175. https://doi.org/10.15171/ijoem.2018.1375
116. Tregellas JR et al (2009) Increased hippocampal, thalamic, and prefrontal hemodynamic response to an urban noise stimulus in schizophrenia. Am J Psychiatry 166(3):354–360. https://doi.org/10.1176/appi.ajp.2008.08030411
117. Evandt J et al (2017) A population-based study on nighttime road traffic noise and insomnia. Sleep 40(2). https://doi.org/10.1093/sleep/zsw055
118. Erfurth A (2021) Schlaf und serotonin. Psychopraxis Neuropraxis 24(6):318–319. https://doi.org/10.1007/S00739-021-00768-3
119. Klompmaker JO et al (2019) Associations of combined exposures to surrounding green, air pollution and traffic noise on mental health. Environ Int 129:525–537. https://doi.org/10.1016/j.envint.2019.05.040
120. Okokon EO et al (2018) Traffic noise, noise annoyance and psychotropic medication use. Environ Int 119:287–294. https://doi.org/10.1016/j.envint.2018.06.034
121. Poulsen AH et al (2019) Impact of long-term exposure to wind turbine noise on redemption of sleep medication and antidepressants: a nationwide cohort study. Environ Health Perspect 127(3):37005. https://doi.org/10.1289/EHP3909
122. Chen Y, Jones C, Dunse N (2021) Coronavirus disease 2019 (COVID-19) and psychological distress in China: does neighbourhood matter? Sci Total Environ 759:144203. https://doi.org/10.1016/j.scitotenv.2020.144203
123. Ma J et al (2018) A multilevel analysis of perceived noise pollution, geographic contexts and mental health in Beijing. Int J Environ Res Public Health 15(7):1479. https://doi.org/10.3390/ijerph15071479
124. Shiue I (2015) Neighborhood epidemiological monitoring and adult mental health: European Quality of Life Survey, 2007–2012. Environ Sci Pollut Res 22(8):6095–6103. https://doi.org/10.1007/s11356-014-3818-3
125. Cerletti P et al (2020) The independent association of source-specific transportation noise exposure, noise annoyance and noise sensitivity with health-related quality of life. Environ Int 143:105960. https://doi.org/10.1016/j.envint.2020.105960
126. Dzhambov AM, Lercher P (2019) Road traffic noise exposure and depression/anxiety: an updated systematic review and meta-analysis. Int J Environ Res Public Health 16(21):4134. https://doi.org/10.3390/ijerph16214134
127. Hammersen F, Niemann H, Hoebel J (2016) Environmental noise annoyance and mental health in adults: findings from the cross-sectional German health update (GEDA) study 2012. Int J Environ Res Public Health 13(10):954. https://doi.org/10.3390/ijerph13100954
128. Jensen HAR, Rasmussen B, Ekholm O (2018) Neighbour and traffic noise annoyance: a nationwide study of associated mental health and perceived stress. Eur J Pub Health 28(6):1050–1055. https://doi.org/10.1093/eurpub/cky091
129. Oiamo TH, Luginaah IN, Baxter J (2015) Cumulative effects of noise and odour annoyances on environmental and health related quality of life. Soc Sci Med 146:191–203. https://doi.org/10.1016/j.socscimed.2015.10.043
130. Dzhambov A et al (2017) Residential road traffic noise and general mental health in youth: the role of noise annoyance, neighborhood restorative quality, physical activity, and social cohesion as potential mediators. Environ Int 109:1–9. https://doi.org/10.1016/j.envint.2017.09.009
131. Golmohammadi R et al (2021) Role of individual and personality traits in occupational

noise-induced psychological effects. Appl Acoust 173:107699. https://doi.org/10.1016/J.APACOUST.2020.107699
132. Kou L, Kwan MP, Chai Y (2021) Living with urban sounds: understanding the effects of human mobilities on individual sound exposure and psychological health. Geoforum 126:13–25. https://doi.org/10.1016/J.GEOFORUM.2021.07.011
133. Baudin C et al (2018) Aircraft noise and psychological ill-health: the results of a cross-sectional study in France. Int J Environ Res Public Health 15(8):1642. https://doi.org/10.3390/ijerph15081642
134. Nazneen S, Raza A, Khan S (2020) Assessment of noise pollution and associated subjective health complaints and psychological symptoms: analysis through structure equation model. Environ Sci Pollut Res 27(17):21570–21580. https://doi.org/10.1007/s11356-020-08655-x
135. Stansfeld S et al (2021) Road traffic noise, noise sensitivity, noise annoyance, psychological and physical health and mortality. Environ Health 20(1):32. https://doi.org/10.1186/s12940-021-00720-3
136. Weyde KV et al (2017) Nocturnal road traffic noise exposure and children's sleep duration and sleep problems. Int J Environ Res Public Health 14(5):491. https://doi.org/10.3390/ijerph14050491
137. Dreger S et al (2015) Environmental noise and incident mental health problems: a prospective cohort study among school children in Germany. Environ Res 143(Pt A):49–54. https://doi.org/10.1016/j.envres.2015.08.003
138. Hjortebjerg D et al (2016) Exposure to road traffic noise and behavioral problems in 7-year-old children: a cohort study. Environ Health Perspect 124(2):228–234. https://doi.org/10.1289/ehp.1409430
139. Carpenter JS, Robillard R, Hickie IB (2015) Variations in the sleep-wake cycle from childhood to adulthood: chronobiological perspectives. Chronophysiol Ther 5:37–49. https://doi.org/10.2147/CPT.S41765
140. Paksarian D et al (2020) Association of Outdoor Artificial Light at night with mental disorders and sleep patterns among US adolescents. JAMA Psychiatry 77(12):1266–1275. https://doi.org/10.1001/JAMAPSYCHIATRY.2020.1935
141. Phillips AJK et al (2019) High sensitivity and interindividual variability in the response of the human circadian system to evening light. Proc Natl Acad Sci U S A 116(24):12019–12024. https://doi.org/10.1073/PNAS.1901824116
142. Dzhambov AM et al (2018) Pathways linking residential noise and air pollution to mental ill-health in young adults. Environ Res 166:458–465. https://doi.org/10.1016/j.envres.2018.06.031
143. Falchi F et al (2016) The new world atlas of artificial night sky brightness. Sci Adv 2(6):e1600377. https://doi.org/10.1126/SCIADV.1600377
144. Tähkämö L, Partonen T, Pesonen AK (2019) Systematic review of light exposure impact on human circadian rhythm. Chronobiol Int 36(2):151–170. https://doi.org/10.1080/07420528.2018.1527773
145. Cleary-Gaffney M, Espey B, Coogan AN (2022) Association of perceptions of artificial light-at-night, light-emitting device usage and environmental noise appraisal with psychological distress, sleep quality and chronotype: a cross sectional study. Heliyon 8(11):e11284. https://doi.org/10.1016/J.HELIYON.2022.E11284
146. Dominoni DM, Borniger JC, Nelson RJ (2016) Light at night, clocks and health: from humans to wild organisms. Biol Lett 12(2):20160015. https://doi.org/10.1098/RSBL.2016.0015
147. Repova K et al (2022) Melatonin as a potential approach to anxiety treatment. Int J Mol Sci 23(24):16187. https://doi.org/10.3390/IJMS232416187
148. Lin LZ et al (2022) Outdoor light at night, overweight, and obesity in school-aged children and adolescents. Environ Pollut 305:119306. https://doi.org/10.1016/J.ENVPOL.2022.119306
149. Argentiero A, Cerqueti R, Maggi M (2021) Outdoor light pollution and COVID-19: the Italian case. Environ Impact Assess Rev 90:106602. https://doi.org/10.1016/J.EIAR.2021.106602
150. Coogan AN et al (2020) Perceptions of light pollution and its impacts: results of an Irish citizen science survey. Int J Environ Res Public Health 17(15):1–7. https://doi.org/10.3390/IJERPH17155628
151. Lahiri A et al (2020) Effect of light pollution on self-reported sleep quality and its components: comparative assessment among healthy adult populations in a rural and an urban area of West Bengal, India. Indian J Public Health 64(3):229–235. https://doi.org/10.4103/IJPH.IJPH_265_20
152. Wang LB et al (2022) Association between exposure to outdoor artificial light at night and sleep disorders among children in China. JAMA Netw Open 5(5):E2213247. https://doi.org/10.1001/JAMANETWORKOPEN.2022.13247
153. Min JY, Min KB (2018) Outdoor artificial nighttime light and use of hypnotic medications in older adults: a population-based cohort study. J Clin Sleep Med 14(11):1903–1910. https://doi.org/10.5664/JCSM.7490
154. Obayashi K et al (2022) Associations between indoor light pollution and unhealthy outcomes in 2,947 adults: cross-sectional analysis in the HEIJO-KYO cohort. Environ Res 215(Pt 2):114350. https://doi.org/10.1016/J.ENVRES.2022.114350
155. Cho JR et al (2013) Let there be no light: the effect of bedside light on sleep quality and background electroencephalographic rhythms. Sleep Med 14(12):1422–1425. https://doi.org/10.1016/J.SLEEP.2013.09.007
156. Helbich M, Browning MHEM, Huss A (2020) Outdoor light at night, air pollution and depressive symptoms: a cross-sectional study in The Netherlands. Sci Total Environ 744:140914. https://doi.org/10.1016/J.SCITOTENV.2020.140914

157. Esaki Y et al (2020) Association between light exposure at night and manic symptoms in bipolar disorder: cross-sectional analysis of the APPLE cohort. Chronobiol Int 37(6):887–896. https://doi.org/10.1080/07420528.2020.1746799
158. Esaki Y et al (2022) Effect of nighttime bedroom light exposure on mood episode relapses in bipolar disorder. Acta Psychiatr Scand 146(1):64–73. https://doi.org/10.1111/ACPS.13422
159. Carta M, Preti A, Akiskal H (2018) Coping with the new era: noise and light pollution, hyperactivity and steroid hormones. Towards an evolutionary view of bipolar disorders. Clin Pract Epidemiol Ment Health 14(1):33–36. https://doi.org/10.2174/1745017901814010033
160. Kim KH et al (2015) A study on the risk perception of light pollution and the process of social amplification of risk in Korea. Environ Sci Pollut Res Int 22(10):7612–7621. https://doi.org/10.1007/S11356-015-4107-5

Social and Cultural Determinants of Suicide

16

Giuseppe Sarli, Lorenzo Polidori, and Maurizio Pompili

Abstract

Suicide is a complex phenomenon deeply rooted in the sociocultural background, influenced by several aspects of society, with some of those playing a crucial role in determining suicide risk. It is not easy to drag out univocal results when dealing with social and cultural determinants of suicide; on the other hand, it is more fruitful to analyze the tight bond between them and suicide risk. In 1897, Émile Durkheim was the first to theorize the impact of society on suicide, especially regarding anomie, the disruption of society's balance, and the upheaval of its values.

Education, marital status, and job position are dimensions of the individual's sphere. Each of those influences suicide risk in different ways, leaning on specific dynamics between the individual and the society. The same can be said about social class belongingness; in this specific context, social and economic factors are combined in influencing individuals' suicide risk.

Focusing on minorities, they represent vulnerable subjects in society; studying the phenomenon of suicide in these subpopulations is a not to be missed opportunity. The Interpersonal Theory of Suicide (ITS) proposed by Joiner represents a theoretical framework explaining the role of lack of social integration and the belief of being a burden for significant others. The constantly growing phenomenon of migration highlighted the need to studying society's impact on migrants' suicide risk. The same complex, multifactorial and bidirectional bond connects society with sexual minorities and suicide risk among them.

Keywords

Suicide · Suicide prevention · Social psychiatry · Interpersonal Theory of Suicide · Minorities

Despite the huge effort made to prevent suicide, it still represents a leading cause of death, ranking among the first ten causes of death in the world. Data from the Centers for Disease Control and Prevention showed that suicide is responsible for over 47,000 deaths in the United States in 2021 [1], which means that almost 130 people die by

G. Sarli · L. Polidori
Psychiatry Residency Training Program, Faculty of Medicine and Psychology, Sapienza University of Rome, Rome, Italy
e-mail: giuseppe.sarli@uniroma1.it; lorenzo.polidori@uniroma1.it

M. Pompili (✉)
Department of Neurosciences, Mental Health and Sensory Organs, Suicide Prevention Center, Sant'Andrea Hospital, Sapienza University of Rome, Rome, Italy
e-mail: maurizio.pompili@uniroma1.it

A. Fiorillo, S. De Giorgi (eds.), *Social Determinants of Mental Health*, Sustainable Development Goals Series, https://doi.org/10.1007/978-3-031-70165-8_16

suicide every day in America. Furthermore, nearly 12 million adults seriously thought about suicide, 3.5 million planned a suicide attempt, and 1.4 million attempted suicide in 2019. Moreover, suicide rates increased by 30% from 1999 to 2018 in the United States [2]. Suicide is an incredibly intricate and multifactorial phenomenon with a two-way bond with society. Suicide has huge distressing effects on families, communities, and societies; on the other side, important social stressors can determine suicide. The Office of Disease Prevention and Health Promotion defines the social determinants of health as "conditions in the environment in which people are born, live, learn, work, play, worship, and age that affect a wide range of health, functioning, and quality-of-life outcomes and risks" [3]. Research findings based on young adult samples have provided empirical evidence about the social determinants of factors (low socioeconomic status, unequal distribution of resources, disadvantaged neighborhood) and subsequent inequalities in suicide rates.

Some sociocultural theoretical frameworks have been proposed to describe the complexity of the suicidal phenomenon from a sociological point of view. In this sense, social isolation is for many authors a strong and reliable predictor of suicidal ideation, attempts, along with lethal behaviors. These suicidal behaviors result associated with various facets of social isolation that can be due to various causes, such as losing spouse through divorce or death, living in a disaggregated family, living alone, having scarce social supports or networks, and being restricted in a single person cell [4].

A classical social theory is the social integration theory, derived from the pioneeristic works of Durkheim and other late nineteenth-century social scientists. Social integration indicates the quality and quantity of ties binding an individual to the wider society, their community, and their significant others [5]. The Durkheim work from 1897 suggests that social integration can be both insufficient and excessive. Either way, the result is an increase in the suicide rate. When there is excessive social integration, individual interests are dominated by group interest, leading to what Durkheim called the altruistic from of suicide. Otherwise, lack of integration leads to the egoistic form of suicide [6]. Moving from social integration theory, suicide rates are elevated among groups with low domestic integration [5].

Another widely employed social theory is the Interpersonal Theory of Suicide (ITS) proposed by Joiner [7]. This theoretical framework proposes that a lack of social integration and the belief of being a burden for significant others can lead to suicide. The ITS offers to consider three fundamental constructs: thwarted belongingness, perceived burdensomeness, and the acquired capability for suicide [4]. Thwarted belongingness refers to social isolation or the lack of social connectedness. This last one concept represents a human psychological need, that if unmeet can lead to suicidal ideation. The term perceived burdensomeness refers to the belief of being a burden for significant others. This perception could be developed after family conflict, job loss, and physical illness, and contribute to suicidal ideation. Last, moving from ITS, to switching from suicidal ideation to proper suicidal attempts, an acquired capability for suicide is needed. This term refers to the condition characterized by reduced death fear and increased pain tolerance. Repeated exposure to fearful experiences and painful experiences can produce a development of suicide capability [4]. The ITS had been widely applied to minorities, such as migrants, sexual and gender minorities, and neurodiverse individuals [8–11].

16.1 Socioeconomic Factors and Suicide Risk

16.1.1 Marital Status

Many researchers have investigated the relationship between marital status and suicide risk. The first to point this out was Durkheim in 1897, who noticed a lower suicide risk among married individuals when compared with unmarried ones [6]. He postulated that the reason for such evidence is that marriage relates with emotional support, social integration, and stability, while not having a stable partner promotes social isolation that increases suicide risk [6]. The conclusions of research on this topic are similar and univocal. Being married means lower mortality risk in general [12–14] and, when talking about suicide, it stands for decreased risk when compared to widowhood, separation, divorce, and never being married [15–21]. The increased suicide risk in these subpopulations is two to ten times higher, even after controlling for socioeconomic variables [22, 23]. The role of being married as a protective factor has an important gender difference, it is remarkably strong among men, while women display weaker and sometimes uncertain correlation [15–17, 19, 21, 24]. In the same study carried out in Italy, widowed men showed a 13 times higher suicide risk, while women had a 1.7 higher risk [24]. A possible explanation for this strong great difference between men and women could be found in women's relationships within and outside the family. They are usually more integrated with relatives, friends, and community members. This may mean stronger social support and reduced risk of isolation, a well-known risk factor for suicide. This dynamic is probably more representative among older women than among younger ones. The latter have lifestyles that are more and more similar to men's. Perhaps due to this generational gap, marital status has a reduced impact on older women [24]. The increased suicide risk among divorced women may be due to the greater financial difficulties and ostracism in being competitive in the work market, especially among older women [25].

The cultural background is a strong pabulum deeply related to marital status. In Italy, as in the other Roman Catholic countries, we can find a visceral cultural and religious norm of "starting a family." This may be seen as a protective factor as suggested by the very low-risk profile in these countries [24] where marriage and children are significant and where (especially in Italy) divorce is still unusual [24].

Having children is another crucial aspect in determining suicide risk. Several studies showed that parenting reduces suicide risk among women, while results are not univocal for men [18, 19, 26–28].

Having one or more children implements social integration into the marriage itself and may increase social cohesiveness in the relationships between partners. Theoretically, this can overestimate the effect of being married. On the other side, the parenting bond is a strong social and emotional tie that is lasting, even after the end of a marriage; it can be considered a protective factor against suicide among those unmarried [27].

16.1.2 Education

A rich body of research investigated the relationship between education and morbidity and/or mortality, showing the importance of education in shaping health status, health-related behaviors, and psychosocial factors. These studies highlighted not only differences in the prevalence of risk behaviors such as tobacco and alcohol use but also differential returns to risk factors, proving there may be important differences in access and ability to benefit from health care and medical assistance [29, 30]. The impact of education on mental health is well documented in literature [30–32]. Back in the years, in 1880, Enrico Morselli, examining the phenomenon of suicide across Europe, noticed that higher levels of education were associated with a higher risk of suicide; moreover, he found gender differences, with males at higher risk than women. However, Durkheim in his theory postulated that lower education might increase suicide risk [6].

Higher education levels have been found protective against suicide; more specifically, men and women aged >25 displayed the lowest rates of suicide, while those with high school degree showed the highest. Men with such degrees had twice the risk of dying by suicide than those with college degrees. Furthermore, interpersonal problems and substance abuse were more common among subjects with a lower education level [30]. An interesting result was found in Finland: good performances at school had a protective role against suicide while, in a group of psychotic patients, high premorbid education achievements were related to higher suicide risk [33]. Other studies found a negative association between education level and suicide risk with a less consistent pattern among women [22, 34]. Some works showed a non-linear correlation between suicide risk and education attainment [35, 36] or even no correlation at all [37]. Conversely, among the Italian population, a significant correlation was found between higher levels of education and completed suicide [32].

Finding an explanation of education as a protective factor is easier. As stated above, having higher levels of education means easier access to the healthcare system, a higher probability of having employment and being better integrated in society. Discussing the positive association between education level and suicide risk is harder. Education may be a synonym of high expectation in certain domains, such as a person's career achievement, higher income, life quality, and satisfaction or certain psychological needs. Facing failures may play a central role in individual perceptions toward suicide. For those with education attainment, high achievements, or expected to do well in life, any setbacks or failures may trigger strong and powerful psychological reactions[32].

16.1.3 Work's Influence on Suicide

Work represents a central element of human life since it is the column of its subsistence; furthermore, it is not only related to workers' and their families' needs, but it can be seen as the engine and the pivot of world's economy. Work itself is a market with countless position in a huge range of sectors that vary between societies and over time. Every employment requires experience, expertise, and/or education background. A worker position in the market tends to be stable over time, even if this paradigm is strictly related to society. There are some categories of people not performing paid work: unemployed (persons willing to work but unable to find position), disabled (persons judged incapable of working), students (persons full-time committed to study, ideally in preparation to enter the work market), and the retired (persons who have worked). Thus, most of any population is somehow connected to a work market.

Each position in the work market determines, in broad terms, what kind of physical environment the employee will spend their time in and the amount and type of stress their body will be exposed to. The same can be said about the mental environment and the psychological pressure. Furthermore, different work situations offer various possibilities for stress relief, such as independent decision-making (Karasek and Theorell 1990). Beyond the mental stimuli coming from the work itself, we also must consider the social work environment made of persons close to oneself in terms of location, activities, and social status. This can be seen as the second most important social environment in a working individual's life besides home. Job position is a strong social marker, often used as an indicator of one's position in the society. It is also a major determinant of one's life chances through the economic, sociopsychological, and physical conditions it implies. Work is one of the greatest ties between a society's member and the society itself since it is a crucial factor in defining one's belonging to a certain social class.

The health of each member of the society is strongly related to their employment [38] and mental health is no exception. Suicide behavior is known to be partly socially affected, then it seems obvious that different job positions have different influences on this phenomenon.

Data regarding the kind of occupation are controversial and far from being univocal. A meta-analysis of 34 studies showed that elementary professions have a higher risk of suicide when compared with the general population. In contrast, workers with higher levels of skills and professionals had the lowest risk of suicide [39]. Stack and colleagues analyzed data from 1990 regarding 21 States in United States, founding higher risk of suicide among dentists, physicians, artists, and carpenters, while elementary school teachers, postal workers, and clerks showed a significantly lower risk [40]. Kposowa studied industrial occupational groups in the United States in 10 years [41]. He found that people working in the mining industry showed the highest relative risk of suicide compared to finance, insurance, and real estate employees (4.39 times higher). A higher risk was found among construction, business, and repair service. In Denmark, high suicide rates were found among medical doctors, nurses, plant and machine operators, drivers, mobile drivers, and mobile plant operators. Architects, engineers, and technicians proved to be at the lowest risk [42, 43].

There are several hypotheses behind different suicide rates between different occupations. Some jobs present very stressful episodes regularly base or have permanent difficult situation such as dealing with specific subpopulation regularly or have permanent difficult situations such as dealing with specific subpopulations regularly or having permanent difficult situations such as dealing with certain subpopulations or depending on customers. In some cases, occupational groups might face economic difficulties that can be either temporary or permanent. For example, farmers can be afflicted by different kinds of economic crises related to the market or agriculture itself [44].

Some occupations have direct knowledge of the means of suicide and sometimes also a privileged access to them. Medical doctors and healthcare professionals probably have the highest level of expertise in this context [42, 43, 45–47]. The suicide risk of American physicians has been calculated to be more than 2 (2.45) times higher than the average of the working-age population, when controlling for demographic variables. A gender difference has been highlighted when discussing easy access to suicide-related methods: women showed a significantly higher risk [48]. Military employees [49, 50], policemen [51], and even the large agricultural populations of many developing countries [52–55] are also thus endangered. However, studies on military or police suicides do not always show higher rates among these groups [56–58]. Agricultural workers can be considered the numerically largest subpopulation at risk of suicide if we consider the easy and direct access to toxic and chemical substances adopted in agriculture that can also be employed for committing suicide.

Another important element regarding the "occupational" risk of committing suicide is related to the nature of the occupation itself. Some character and personality traits make a person prone to occupy a certain job position. In the same way, some works might be done more frequently by people at higher risk of suicide. It's been hypothesized that people with depressive traits can more often be found among psychiatrists. Furthermore, some difficult life paths more often lead to jobs that are not chosen freely but imposed by necessity which might determine a higher suicide risk. The high rates observed among unskilled workers may be partly due to such processes. Furthermore, different occupational groups are composed differently in terms of sex, age, ethnic group, marital state, etc. Here, the occupational suicide risk reflects the one related to the demographic group.

There is also a theory speculating that some jobs expose workers to circumstances that can somehow be related to suicide. As better explained later when we talk about Durkheim's classical theory, people in commercial professions might be more exposed to suicide risk. At the same time, those whose occupation does not fit with their role might suffer from status incompatibility ("role strain") as explained by Gibbs and Martin [59].

Another crucial aspect insisting in one's everyday life is the work environment. While occupation and social class belongingness are the same, the work environment is changeable, depending on working conditions, society conditions, and adoption of new technologies. Work environment is thought to play an active role in determining causation of suicide, even more than class and occupation, since it affects the individual's life more directly and every day. Its effect relates to the permanent features of the occupation, while the workload and the social side of the environment are mainly related to the place of work. Those situation with few to no possibilities to grow on the professional side are associated with a more than double the risk of suicide among men, while the same increase of the risk among women can be observed in hectic and monotonous jobs. An increased suicide risk can be highlighted among nurses, especially when the stress load at the workplace is combined with a high domestic stress [60]. Also, knowing that their occupation leads to exposition to dangerous substances can be seen as a stress, as shown during the Chernobyl nuclear accident [61]. Heavy workloads and long working hours can deeply affect mental health and company rebuilding process or corporate merger [62]. The hierarchical structure of an organization may be a source of conflict that can result in bullying and, finally, lead to suicide [63].

The work environment might potentially have a negative effect even on the employee's family; a relationship between father's adverse work condition and suicide among their children has been proven [64].

The absence of a stable job can affect mental health too. Unemployment can be considered as a risk factor when talking about suicide. It may increase the impact of stressful life events; it may indirectly cause suicide by increasing the risk factors that have an important role in determining suicide (e.g., mental illness, medical issues, and financial difficulties); or it may be a non-causal association because of cooccurring factors that predict both unemployment and suicide [65]. Researchers controlling for social factors variables found an approximately two times higher suicide risk among the unemployed [37]; the possible explanations may lie in the health selection or residual confounding. Health selection means that poor health (both mental and physical) precedes and predicts both unemployment and death causing an association between unemployment and suicide. A British study proved this theory, showing that long-standing illness can dramatically reduce the probability of staying employed and finding occupation [66]. According to this, a weaker association of unemployment with poor health would be expected in societies with high unemployment rates, since a larger proportion of the society is unemployed (not only those with poor health). However, findings in this context are mixed. In the United Kingdom, a similarly strong association of unemployment with all causes of mortality (including suicide) was found in times of both high and low unemployment [67].

On the other hand, Finnish researchers found a lower relative risk of suicide for the unemployed compared with employed during a period of high unemployment rates [68]. Other than health selection, socioeconomic, or other variables might be the reason for the association of unemployment with suicide. Being unemployed showed a two to three times higher risk of suicide compared to being employed. This risk is attributable to confounding by mental illness (and all the socioeconomic features related to it) [65].

Some researchers speculated about a "paradoxal" theory, according to which lower suicide rates among the unemployed should be expected in areas with high unemployment since unemployment might represent "normality" in these societies. However, the scientific evidence proved the opposite [69, 70].

16.1.4 The Role of Social Class on Suicide

Many researchers have studied the relationship between social class and suicide. Especially among men, those with low income or education show higher rates of suicide than those with higher income or education level; more specifically, those employed in manual work have higher rates than those in non-manual work; even lower-ranking office clerks often display higher suicide rates than those from the higher echelons [19, 71–74]. The differences in suicide rates between the lowest and highest classes are typically two- or threefold.

A longitudinal study in Scotland [75] found that people from lower classes living in the less served areas had a ten times higher risk of suicide. Another study run in Finland between 1991 and 2000 proved a 10% difference in life expectancy due to suicide mortality between manual workers and non-manual workers from upper classes[76].

In Japan, miners aged 20–64 were found to show a five times higher standardized all-cause mortality then managers in 1985 [77]. This means that five miners' suicides produced the same proportional measure of "suicide risk" as one managerial suicide.

On the other hand, Stack [40] found in the United States that the significantly higher risks for suicide among manual workers became no longer significant when they controlled for demographic differences between occupational groups. This result underlines the importance of other co-occurring factors, such as divorce. Being divorced/not having a stable partner is known to increase suicide risk, especially among men [78]. Men from lower classes display a higher risk of divorce because of other social positions and all its disadvantages. Then, it is difficult to understand whether suicide risk, in this scenario, is more affected by either the social position or the marital status. Controlling for other variables can sometimes unveil the potential role and implication of other factors and reconsider those of others [42, 43]. The scenario is more controversial for the female population. Some studies showed results more or less similar to those among the male population [72, 79, 80], while others highlighted a higher risk for suicide among women in higher classes [81], and others found either inconsistent relations [22, 82], or none at all [73]. These non-unidirectional findings may reflect the evolving role of women in modern society; furthermore, women's role in the sociocultural environment is less defined by work and income than men. However, there are still elements such as social exclusion, stigma, and negative experiences that are more often related to belonging to lower classes that, alongside unhealthy lifestyles, can contribute to an increase the risk of suicide [75].

It is important to underline how social class relates to suicide not only considering the economic and social status but it must be seen in relation to its cultural aspects and context.

In the late nineteenth century, Emile Durkheim was a pioneer in considering the impact of socioeconomic factors on suicide risk [6, 83]. He spotlighted the correlations between suicide and measures of social integration and regulation, defined as society's moral and normative demands individuals [84]. Durkheim speculated that equality in income and wealth is a protective factor against suicide. He theorized that income inequality undermines social integration and leads to social instability. On the other side, Durkheim also hypothesized that poverty may have a protective role against suicide since wealth could lead people to believe they are dependent only on themselves, which may strengthen feelings of loneliness and social disintegration. Durkheim's theories and literature documenting the impact of economic factors on health [85, 86] have driven the growth of substantial research on the relationship between suicidal behavior and economic conditions, especially in high-income countries. Alongside inequalities, economic shocks, either boom or recession, have their influence on suicide [60]. The 2006–2008 global crisis has been proved to increase suicide rates and an even higher rate can be recorded in the poorest classes of society left behind during the recovery process or hit harder from the crisis [87, 88].

Furthermore, these rates tend to remain high among economically vulnerable subjects even after the economic recovery since this subpopulation might take more time to align with the upper social classes [89]. However, it is important to clarify that a wide range of sociocultural, geographic, and demographic variables can influence the bond between social class belongingness, poverty, and suicide. Sometimes, studies focused on specific sub-population can highlight associations that are not significant at the national or international level. After the last global financial crisis, people from rural areas in Portugal showed higher vulnerability to suicide, while nothing was found in the general population [90].

We can also find socioeconomic elements playing a protective role against suicide. During the most recent recession, in the Mediterranean area, the crisis's impact on individuals has been mitigated by the strong family network that represents a pillar in these societies. In Nordic societies, the social welfare safety net had the same role in contrasting suicide after the economic instability led by the fall of Soviet Union [91].

16.1.5 Prevention Strategies

Regarding the occupational context, three strategies can be employed to reduce suicide risk: (a) reduction in unemployment policies, (b) control of the access to occupation-related mean of suicide, and (c) improving access for mental problems at the workplace [92–94].

There are no univocal thoughts about the actual role of unemployment policies in preventing suicide [95, 96]. There is an important research body supporting the efficacy of employment policies in reducing suicide risk and their inclusion in prevention strategies. Especially during economic crisis, these measures might be crucial in preventing suicide, primarily among younger subjects [97]. Conversely, no relation has been proven between suicide decline among young people and the adoption of unemployment reduction policies in an Australian study [98]. As stated above, each result must be seen in the society in which it was carried out. Similar results suggested that among those admitted to the psychiatric care, suicidality was less common in the unemployed group compared to the employed group; this may be due to work-related stressors that can increase suicide risk, primarily for those with an existing vulnerability [99].

Focusing on the access to suicide methods, there is a common believe that its control is both easy to reach and effective [100].

The workplace must be seen as a not to be missed occasion to prevent suicide, since a huge amount of people can be reached through it. However, there is a difficulty related to relative rarity of suicides, stigma, and the motivation of employers to commit to it [101]. The effectiveness of such strategy can be deduced by the positive experience carried out in the US Air Force, where suicide-prevention programs led to the impressive result of a reduction of a 33% of suicides in a 5-years period [102]. Also, supportive strategies for the early detection of depression can be incredibly useful, as well as general mental health promotion campaigns for occupational risk to reduce stress on the workplace and make it precious occasion to promote mental well-being [103].

16.2 Minorities

16.2.1 Migrants, Refugees, Asylum Seekers, Indigenous People, and Ethnic Minorities

Migration is the process by which single individual or a mass of individuals move from one country, region, or place of residence to another, with the expectation of settling down in the new location temporarily or permanently [104]. Purposes of migration are represented by the will to advance one's opportunity or life quality, escape from an oppressive political context, or finding a place where specific cultural needs are more adequately met [105]. Often, this process involves a shift in the cultural setting [106]. Not only the reasons for but also the duration of the migratory process represent sources of extraordinary stress for the migrants and for their families [106]. The migration process differs from one individual to another, and not every migrant goes through the same experiences during this transition. Nevertheless, the migration process and both pre- and post-migrations phases seem to represent causes of intense psychological distress, which can contribute to the development of mental health problems and suicidal behaviors [107, 108]. Several studies highlight how social connection and belonging are key components for mental health and how they can prevent suicidal behaviors [109]. In this sense, connection with and support by a broader community, such as religious communities, along with family networks, are protective factors against suicidal behaviors; on the contrary, isolation and lack of connection and support represent risk factors [110].

Indeed, distance from family of origin and worries for family back home increase suicidal risk [111]. Overall, several factors can contribute to suicidal risk in migrants, such as ethnic discrimination in the host country, acculturation stress, traditional religious and cultural norms (including beliefs about mental illness and suicide), traumatic experiences along with torture before and during the migration process, language and health services barriers, and shame linked to mental illness [112]. Specific considerations are needed for refugees and asylum seekers, which often have been exposed to extremely traumatic experiences such as war, repression, and physical trauma (including torture). These experiences can further increase risk of mental problems and suicide [113].

The migratory phenomenon can be further subdivided in three stages. *Pre-migration*, the first phase, is characterized by the decision to leave and the planning of the process. During this stage, factors that can predispose the individual to developing mental disorders are represented by personality structure, a history of adverse childhood experiences, forced migration, and persecution. Proper *migration*, the second stage, is the effective relocation process from the native country to the host country. Cultural bereavement is the central factor for developing psychiatric disorder in this stage. The third phase is the *post-migration* stage. In this phase, migrants have reached their migratory destination, trying to establish in the new country. Challenges of post-migration stage are "culture shock," the failing of the migration process, and the quality of acceptance from the host country [104, 114]. In all three phases, there could be a worsening in mental health, along with the development of several mental disorders such as depressive disorders, anxiety disorders, post-traumatic stress disorder (PTSD), somatization disorders, and suicide [114–118].

Newcomer migrants often find brand new and extremely different relationships and social networks, which can produce significant distress and cultural shock. Acculturation stress and lack of social support can increase suicidal risk in new migrants [119]. The term acculturation refers to the process occurring during the post-migration period, where migrants from a different cultural context begin to acquire the cultural features of the host country, including values and behaviors [105]. Acculturation occurs at both individual and societal levels. Moreover, the terms *psychological acculturation* and *adaptation* describe psychological consequences and outcomes resulting from the individual experience of acculturation. Two factors influence and define the acculturation process: *cultural maintenance*, contact, *and participation.* Different forms of acculturation are described from the combination of these two factors. Different forms of acculturation are described from the combination of these two factors *separation*, *assimilation*, *marginalization*, and *integration* [120]. Outcomes of the acculturation process and responses to acculturation stress can impact the mental health of migrants and suicidal behaviors [121, 122]. In fact, acculturation stress and lack of support among migrants have been demonstrated that can increase suicidal risk [119, 123]. This is particularly true for individuals migrating from collectivistic societies to individualistic societies, who may face some challenges in adapting to the new cultural context [104]. Moreover, refugees and asylum seekers, who are often forced to migrate, appear to be less acculturated and experience intense alienation, with a significant increase in suicidal ideation rates [119].

Talking about the proper suicidal dimension in the migrants' population, a recent systematic review highlights how migrants and ethnic minorities are at increased suicide risk when confronted with general population [113]. Literature on the theme is heterogenous, with some studies indicating higher suicide risk in migrants versus natives, and other sustaining the contrary. This variance in between the studies reinforces the diversity among different groups of migrants [105]. Concerning ethnic minorities, it seems to be a higher suicide risk in these individuals concerning the native. Another recent meta-analysis has estimated the rate for suicidal ideation, plan, and attempts, with pooled rates of 16%, 6%, and 4%, respectively. The suicidal dimension was more represented in women, and there was a tenfold difference between refugees and migrants for concerns suicidal behaviors [124]. Worldwide, there are some common patterns concerning suicidal behaviors, with women experiencing more suicidal ideation and attempts following the so-called "*gender paradox in suicide*" [125]. This is particularly true for migrant females, who show higher rates of suicidal behaviors when confronted with native women, mostly among young female who moved from sociocentric to individualistic social contexts

[126, 127]. Several reasons can explain differences in suicidal risk between migrant male and females, such as reasons for migrating, economic disadvantage, cultural conflicts, and pressure deriving from observing familial expectations [105, 128]. Some differences appear also among first, second generations, and native, with first-generation migrants offering to consider lower suicide rates when confronted with the other two groups, in line with "*healthy migrant effect*" [105]. Again, when talking about young migrants, literature appears to be heterogenous [129]. Last, a pre-eminent role in the definition of the suicidal patterns rates in migrants is played by the influence of the cultural and social norms of the country of origin [130]. Overall, suicidal rates for migrant individuals tend to converge with the ones of the natives over time [5].

Literature about suicidal risk in indigenous people is rare, with some difficulties in identifying an internationally accepted definition of indigenous. Given this, it is fundamental to underline how suicide prevention interventions in indigenous should consider the challenge in promoting mental health in societies with heterogenous values, languages, and ethno-cultural backgrounds [131]. These same considerations are also valid when assessing suicidal risk in migrants, refugees, and asylum seekers, as well as other ethnic minorities, with integration consisting in the most favorable strategy of response to acculturation stress in terms of mental health benefits [132].

16.2.2 Sexual and Gender Minorities

In recent years, there has been a growing interest in understanding and assessing mental health in sexual and gender minorities, particularly in suicidal behaviors. Although Western world's social and political landscapes show some substantial improvement, there remain significant individual and religious discrimination in other place [133]. Given this, several important changes should be considered, such as the legalization of homosexual relationships and same-sex marriage, same-sex marriage, and gender recognition. These social and cultural developments do underline greater acceptance of gender and sexual minorities, with a significant rise of youths self-identifying as non-binary, transgender, or fluid [134, 135].

It is fundamental to offer proper definitions when assessing mental health and suicidal dimension in sexual and gender minorities. Talking about sex, we do refer to anatomical sex assigned to children at birth. This definition moves from sexual characteristics, such as chromosomes, sexual hormones, gonads, and genitals. Furthermore, intersexual individuals show sexual characteristics at birth non-fitting typical female or male presentations. The term gender is addressed as the role constructed, mediated, and regulated in and by the social context, referring to activities and behaviors typically associated with male or female sex. Moving from this, the term transgender and trans are used to define individuals whose gender is not in line with birth-assigned sex. Nowadays, transgender can be considered as an umbrella term including other identities such as gender non-conforming, gender non-binary, gender variant, and gender fluid, indicating representations not aligning with culturally defined experiences of cis genderism. Last, sexuality involves sexual and emotional attraction to others [136]. Again, the contemporary context offers several different and complex categorizations of sexuality, such as heterosexuality, homosexuality, pansexuality, and asexuality.

The broader term LGBTQ+ is an acronym indicating a community in which different sexual orientations and gender identity experiences are resumed, going from gay, lesbian, and bisexual for what concerns sexual orientation to transgender, intersexual, questioning, gender fluid, non-binary, questioning, and two-spirits for gender identification [137, 138].

Intersectional frameworks are frequently used to assess mental health in gender and sexual minorities, considering various other status such as age, religion, ethnicity, and ability/disability [133].

Although these conditions are no longer considered pathological [139], many studies worldwide underline how sexual and gender minorities show worse outcomes in mental health. Several studies demonstrated that gay, lesbian, and bisexual individuals have a higher risk for mental disorders when confronted with heterosexual peers. In fact, in environments characterized by antihomosexual hostility, LGB youths are prone to internalize a sense of shame, resulting in internalized homophobia [140]. Internalizing homophobia can lead to long-term mental health challenges, including suicidal behaviors. The most represented diagnoses among sexual minorities are depression, anxiety disorders, substance use disorders, and suicidal behavior [141, 142]. Specifically, bisexual and homosexual men are three times more likely to develop psychological distress and suffer panic attacks than heterosexual men [138]. Moreover, there are some intergroup differences, with bisexual individuals offering to consider higher rates of depression and suicidality when confronted with lesbians and gays [142]. This seems particularly true for bisexual women and males who have sex with male (MSM) bisexual [143]. These same considerations remain valid for gender minorities, with several lines of evidence indicating a higher prevalence of psychiatric disorders in transgender individuals, confronted with both cisgender individuals and general populations [144]. Talking about transgender individuals, these individuals show a higher prevalence of several conditions, such as depression, anxiety disorders, self-harm and suicidal behaviors, substance use disorder, eating disorders, trauma and stress-related disorders, personality disorders, and neurodevelopmental disorders with autism spectrum disorder above all [144–147]. Same data are available for gender non-conforming individuals, in particular the youths, for which higher prevalence rates for depression, anxiety disorders, substance use disorders, trauma and stress-related disorders, and non-suicidal self-injuries and suicide have been described [148, 149]. Proper gender dysphoria diagnosis offers to consider specific comorbidity: among Axis I disorders the more frequent are mood and anxiety disorders, along with substance use disorders [148–150].

Regarding the suicidal dimension, increased self-harm and suicidal risk has been highlighted for both sexual and gender minority individuals [151]. For sexual minorities, many studies suggest that non-heterosexual individuals, both adults and youths, have a significantly higher lifetime prevalence of suicidal ideation and attempts along with life-threatening behaviors in comparison with heterosexual individuals [152, 153]. Among LGBTQ+ youths with experiences of self-harm and suicide, victimization and mental health difficulties were highly prevalent [154]. Bisexual individuals show a higher risk of suicide, followed by gay/lesbian individuals [143, 152].

Transgender individuals offer to consider augmented self-harm and suicidal risk when confronted with cisgender peer and the general population [144, 155]. Also, the wider group of gender non-conforming individuals is more prone to suffer from bullying and stigmatization, which may lead to a higher prevalence of suicidal ideation and attempts [149]. Overall, suicidal ideation seems higher among male-to-female (MTF), then female-to-male (FTM), and lowest among gender non-conforming individuals. Conversely, suicidal attempts occur mostly among FTM, then MTF, and last in gender non-conforming [155]. Moreover, some evidence suggests that there could be a reduction in suicide risk following gender-affirming treatment. However, literature on the theme is heterogeneous and some authors afford that some level of suicidal risk remains after these treatments [156]. Another recent cohort study highlights how transgender individuals have higher mortality rates when confronted with cisgender persons, particularly for death due to external causes, but also for what concerns suicide [156].

Some conceptual frameworks have been proposed to try to theoretically assess the augmented suicidal risk in sexual and gender minorities. Among these, the Minority Stress Model suggests how discrimination experiences and homo/trans-phobia can negatively affects the mental health of sexual and gender minorities, putting them at increased risk for suicide [157, 158]. This model defines three different sources of distress associated with suicide risk: *internalized homo/trans-phobia*, *experiences of discrimination and violence*, and *stigma*, followed by expectations of rejection and discrimination. Throughout this model several psychiatric conditions have been associated with sexual and gender minorities, such as depression, substance use disorder, and suicide and self-harm [157, 159–163].

In conclusion, although stigmatization, systemic discrimination, rejection, isolation, and violence can produce resilience among sexual and gender minorities, literature underlines how these experiences represent unique risk factors for LGBTQ+ individuals, leading to mental disorders such as depression, anxiety, and substance abuse disorder, along with suicidal thoughts and behaviors. It is crucial to understand that these experiences shape some recurring themes across the life course of these individuals, who struggle to overcome guilt, shame, stigma, and internalized minority stress and to try to come out and take pride in their sexual and gender identity [133]. Moving from this, tailored suicide prevention programs for sexual and gender minorities should focus on decreasing barriers for accessing mental health services, ensure a safer society for sexual and genders minorities, empower community-based and community-driven interventions, and increase the knowledge on the suicidal phenomenon, on the stigma, and on the increased suicide risk in sexual and gender minorities [164].

16.2.3 Prevention Strategies

Regarding suicide prevention among migrants and ethnic minorities, some authors propose strategies deeply rooted in community-based interventions that combine Brief Intervention and Contact (BIC) and Safety Planning volunteers-delivered [165].

Focusing on sexual and gender minorities, tailored suicide prevention programs should aim to decrease barriers for accessing mental health services, ensure a safer society for these special subpopulations, empower community-based and community-driven interventions, and increase the knowledge on the suicidal phenomenon, on the stigma, and on the well documented increased suicidal risk among these individuals [164].

References

1. Curtin SC, Garnett MF, Ahmad FB (2022) Provisional numbers and rates of suicide by month and demographic characteristics: United States, 2021. https://doi.org/10.15620/CDC:120830
2. Hedegaard H, Curtin SC, Warner M (2020) Increase in suicide mortality in the United States, 1999-2018. NCHS Data Brief:1–8
3. Social Determinants of Health - Healthy People 2030 | health.gov (n.d.) www.document. https://health.gov/healthypeople/priority-areas/social-determinants-health. Accessed 9 Mar 2023
4. Van Orden KA, Witte TK, Cukrowicz KC, Braithwaite SR, Selby EA, Joiner TE (2010) The interpersonal theory of suicide. Psychol Rev 117:575–600. https://doi.org/10.1037/A0018697
5. Kposowa AJ, McElvain JP, Breault KD (2008) Immigration and suicide: the role of marital status, duration of residence, and social integration. Arch Suicide Res 12:82–92. https://doi.org/10.1080/13811110701801044
6. Durkheim E (1988) Le suicide: étude de sociologie
7. Joiner TE (2005) Why people die by suicide. Harvard University Press, Cambridge, pp 1–288
8. Chang CJ, Dorrell KD, Feinstein BA, Depp CA, Ehret BC, Selby EA (2023) Testing the interpersonal theory of suicide in a sample of sexual minority young adults: attention to within-group differences. Suicide Life Threat Behav 53:415–425. https://doi.org/10.1111/SLTB.12952
9. Dow D, Morgan L, Hooker JL, Michaels MS, Joiner TE, Woods J, Wetherby AM (2021) Anxiety, depression, and the interpersonal theory of suicide in a community sample of adults with autism spectrum disorder. Arch Suicide Res 25:297–314. https://doi.org/10.1080/13811118.2019.1678537
10. Kene P, Brabeck KM, Kelly C, DiCicco B (2016) Suicidality among immigrants: application of the interpersonal-psychological theory. Death Stud 40:373–382. https://doi.org/10.1080/07481187.2016.1155675
11. Triece PA, Oddo LE, Hill RM, Pettit JW, Meinzer MC (2020) Investigation of the interpersonal theory of suicide in the context of attention-deficit/hyperactivity disorder symptomatology and suicide ideation. Suicide Life Threat Behav 50:1198–1204. https://doi.org/10.1111/SLTB.12683
12. Kravdal Ø, Grundy E, Keenan K (2018) The increasing mortality advantage of the married: the role played by education. Demogr Res 38:471–512. https://doi.org/10.4054/DEMRES.2018.38.20

13. Lillard LA, Panis CWA (1996) Marital status and mortality: the role of health. Demography 33:313–327. https://doi.org/10.2307/2061764/METRICS
14. Murray JE (2000) Marital protection and marital selection: evidence from a historical-prospective sample of American men. Demography 37:511–521. https://doi.org/10.1353/DEM.2000.0010
15. Denney JT, Rogers RG, Krueger PM, Wadsworth T (2009) Adult suicide mortality in the United States: marital status, family size, socioeconomic status, and differences by sex. Soc Sci Q 90:1167. https://doi.org/10.1111/J.1540-6237.2009.00652.X
16. Kposowa AJ (2000) Marital status and suicide in the National Longitudinal Mortality Study. J Epidemiol Community Health 54:254. https://doi.org/10.1136/JECH.54.4.254
17. Luoma JB, Pearson JL (2002) Suicide and marital status in the United States, 1991–1996: is widowhood a risk factor? Am J Public Health 92:1518. https://doi.org/10.2105/AJPH.92.9.1518
18. Lusyne P, Page H (2008a) The impact of children on a parent's risk of suicide following death of a spouse, Belgium 1991-96. Popul Stud (NY) 62:55–67. https://doi.org/10.1080/00324720701788566
19. Qin P, Agerbo E, Mortensen PB (2003) Suicide risk in relation to socioeconomic, demographic, psychiatric, and familial factors: a national register-based study of all suicides in Denmark, 1981-1997. Am J Psychiatry 160:765–772. https://doi.org/10.1176/APPI.AJP.160.4.765
20. Smith JC, Mercy JA, Conn JM (1988) Marital status and the risk of suicide. Am J Public Health 78:78. https://doi.org/10.2105/AJPH.78.1.78
21. Wyder M, Ward P, De Leo D (2009) Separation as a suicide risk factor. J Affect Disord 116:208–213. https://doi.org/10.1016/J.JAD.2008.11.007
22. Lorant V, Kunst AE, Huisman M, Costa G, Mackenbach J (2005a) Socio-economic inequalities in suicide: a European comparative study. Br J Psychiatry 187:49–54. https://doi.org/10.1192/BJP.187.1.49
23. Yip PSF, Thorburn J (2004) Marital status and the risk of suicide: experience from England and Wales, 1982-1996. Psychol Rep 94:401–407. https://doi.org/10.2466/PR0.94.2.401-407
24. Masocco M, Pompili M, Vichi M, Vanacore N, Lester D, Tatarelli R (2008) Suicide and marital status in Italy. Psychiatry Q 79:275–285. https://doi.org/10.1007/S11126-008-9072-4
25. Næss EO, Mehlum L, Qin P (2021) Marital status and suicide risk: temporal effect of marital breakdown and contextual difference by socioeconomic status. SSM Popul Health 15:100853. https://doi.org/10.1016/J.SSMPH.2021.100853
26. Andrés AR, Collings S, Qin P (2010) Sex-specific impact of socio-economic factors on suicide risk: a population-based case-control study in Denmark. Eur J Pub Health 20:265–270. https://doi.org/10.1093/EURPUB/CKP183
27. Øien-Ødegaard C, Hauge LJ, Reneflot A (2021) Marital status, educational attainment, and suicide risk: a Norwegian register-based population study. Popul Health Metrics 19:1–11. https://doi.org/10.1186/S12963-021-00263-2/FIGURES/2
28. Qin P, Agerbo E, Westergard-Nielsen N, Eriksson T, Mortensen PB (2000) Gender differences in risk factors for suicide in Denmark. Br J Psychiatry 177:546–550. https://doi.org/10.1192/BJP.177.6.546
29. Lleras-Muney A (2005) The relationship between education and adult mortality in the United States. Rev Econ Stud 72:189–221. https://doi.org/10.1111/0034-6527.00329
30. Phillips JA, Hempstead K (2017) Differences in U.S. suicide rates by educational attainment, 2000–2014. Am J Prev Med 53:e123–e130. https://doi.org/10.1016/j.amepre.2017.04.010
31. Dalgard OS, Mykletun A, Rognerud M, Johansen R, Zahl PH (2007) Education, sense of mastery and mental health: results from a nation wide health monitoring study in Norway. BMC Psychiatry 7:1–9. https://doi.org/10.1186/1471-244X-7-20/TABLES/5
32. Pompili M, Vichi M, Qin P, Innamorati M, De Leo D, Girardi P (2013) Does the level of education influence completed suicide? A nationwide register study. J Affect Disord 147:437–440. https://doi.org/10.1016/J.JAD.2012.08.046
33. Alaräisänen A, Miettunen J, Lauronen E, Räsänen P, Isohanni M (2006) Good school performance is a risk factor of suicide in psychoses: a 35-year follow up of the northern Finland 1966 birth cohort. Acta Psychiatr Scand 114:357–362. https://doi.org/10.1111/J.1600-0447.2006.00800.X
34. Kposowa AJ (2001) Unemployment and suicide: a cohort analysis of social factors predicting suicide in the US National Longitudinal Mortality Study. Psychol Med 31:127–138. https://doi.org/10.1017/S0033291799002925
35. Shah A, Bhandarkar R (2009) The relationship between general population suicide rates and educational attainment: a cross-national study. Suicide Life Threat Behav 39:463–470. https://doi.org/10.1521/SULI.2009.39.5.463
36. Shah A, Chatterjee S (2008) Is there a relationship between elderly suicide rates and educational attainment? A cross-national study. Aging Ment Health 12:795–799. https://doi.org/10.1080/13607860802427986
37. Lewis G, Sloggett A (1998) Suicide, deprivation, and unemployment: record linkage study. BMJ 317:1283–1286. https://doi.org/10.1136/BMJ.317.7168.1283
38. Marmot M, Allen JJ (2014) Social determinants of health equity. Am J Public Health 104:S517. https://doi.org/10.2105/AJPH.2014.302200
39. Milner A, Spittal MJ, Pirkis J, LaMontagne AD (2013) Suicide by occupation: systematic review and meta-analysis. Br J Psychiatry 203:409–416. https://doi.org/10.1192/BJP.BP.113.128405

40. Stack S (2001) Occupation and suicide. Soc Sci Q 82:384–396. https://doi.org/10.1111/0038-4941.00030
41. Kposowa AJ (1999) Suicide mortality in the United States: differentials by industrial and occupational groups. Am J Ind Med 36:645–652. https://doi.org/10.1002/(SICI)1097-0274(199912)36:6
42. Agerbo E, Gunnell D, Bonde JP, Bo Mortensen P, Nordentoft M (2007a) Suicide and occupation: the impact of socio-economic, demographic and psychiatric differences. Psychol Med 37:1131–1140. https://doi.org/10.1017/S0033291707000487
43. Agerbo E, Sterne JAC, Gunnell DJ (2007b) Combining individual and ecological data to determine compositional and contextual socioeconomic risk factors for suicide. Soc Sci Med 64:451–461. https://doi.org/10.1016/J.SOCSCIMED.2006.08.043
44. Labovitz S, Hagedorn R (1971) An analysis of suicide rates among occupational categories. Sociol Inq 41:67–72. https://doi.org/10.1111/J.1475-682X.1971.TB01201.X
45. Hawton K, Clements A, Simkin S, Malmberg A (2000) Doctors who kill themselves: a study of the methods used for suicide. QJM 93:351–357. https://doi.org/10.1093/QJMED/93.6.351
46. Hawton K, Malmberg A, Simkin S (2004) Suicide in doctors: a psychological autopsy study. J Psychosom Res 57:1–4. https://doi.org/10.1016/S0022-3999(03)00372-6
47. Stark C, Hopkins P, Gibbs D, Rapson T, Belbin A, Hay A (2004) Trends in suicide in Scotland 1981-1999: age, method and geography. BMC Public Health 4:49. https://doi.org/10.1186/1471-2458-4-49
48. Milner A, Witt K, Maheen H, LaMontagne AD (2017) Access to means of suicide, occupation and the risk of suicide: a national study over 12 years of coronial data. BMC Psychiatry 17:1–7. https://doi.org/10.1186/S12888-017-1288-0/TABLES/5
49. Desjeux G, Labarère J, Galoisy-Guibal L, Ecochard R (2004) Suicide in the French armed forces. Eur J Epidemiol 19:823–829. https://doi.org/10.1023/B:EJEP.0000040527.59987.B2
50. Mahon MJ, Tobin JP, Cusack DA, Kelleher C, Malone KM (2005) Suicide among regular-duty military personnel: a retrospective case-control study of occupation-specific risk factors for workplace suicide. Am J Psychiatry 162:1688–1696. https://doi.org/10.1176/APPI.AJP.162.9.1688
51. Schmidtke A, Fricke S, Lester D (1999) Suicide among German federal and state police officers. Psychol Rep 84:157–166. https://doi.org/10.2466/PR0.1999.84.1.157
52. Coloma C, Hoffman JS, Crosby A (2006) Suicide among Guaraní Kaiowá and Nandeva youth in Mato Grosso do Sul, Brazil. Arch Suicide Res 10:191–207. https://doi.org/10.1080/13811110600662505
53. Khan MM (2002) Suicide on the Indian subcontinent. Crisis 23:104–107. https://doi.org/10.1027/0227-5910.23.3.104
54. Nwosu SO, Odesanmi WO (2001) Pattern of suicides in Ile-Ife, Nigeria. West Afr J Med 20:259–262
55. Recena MCP, Pires DX, Caldas ED (2006) Acute poisoning with pesticides in the state of Mato Grosso do Sul, Brazil. Sci Total Environ 357:88–95. https://doi.org/10.1016/J.SCITOTENV.2005.04.029
56. Hem E, Haldorsen T, Aasland OG, Tyssen R, Vaglum P, Ekeberg Ø (2005) Suicide rates according to education with a particular focus on physicians in Norway 1960-2000. Psychol Med 35:873–880. https://doi.org/10.1017/S0033291704003344
57. Loo R (2003) A meta-analysis of police suicide rates: findings and issues. Suicide Life Threat Behav 33:313–325. https://doi.org/10.1521/SULI.33.3.313.23209
58. Stack S, Kelley T (1994) Police suicide: an analysis. Am J Police 13(4):73–90
59. Gibbs J, Martin W (1964) Status integration and suicide. University of Oregon Press, Eugene
60. Wasserman D (2020) Oxford textbook of suicidology and suicide prevention. Oxford University Press, Oxford
61. Rahu K, Rahu M, Tekkel M, Bromet E (2006) Suicide risk among Chernobyl cleanup workers in Estonia still increased: an updated cohort study. Ann Epidemiol 16:917–919. https://doi.org/10.1016/J.ANNEPIDEM.2006.07.006
62. Westerlund H, Ferrie J, Hagberg J, Jeding K, Oxenstierna G, Theorell T (2004) Workplace expansion, long-term sickness absence, and hospital admission. Lancet 363:1193–1197. https://doi.org/10.1016/S0140-6736(04)15949-7
63. Nielsen MB, Nielsen GH, Notelaers G, Einarsen S (2015) Workplace bullying and suicidal ideation: a 3-wave longitudinal Norwegian study. Am J Public Health 105:e23–e28. https://doi.org/10.2105/AJPH.2015.302855
64. Aleck O, Stefania M, James T, James D, Ruth H, Lisa C, Amber L, Clyde H (2006) The impact of fathers' physical and psychosocial work conditions on attempted and completed suicide among their children. BMC Public Health 6:1–9. https://doi.org/10.1186/1471-2458-6-77/COMMENTS
65. Blakely TA, Collings SCD, Atkinson J (2003b) Unemployment and suicide. Evidence for a causal association? J Epidemiol Community Health 57:594–600. https://doi.org/10.1136/JECH.57.8.594
66. Bartley M, Owen C (1996) Relation between socioeconomic status, employment, and health during economic change, 1973-93. BMJ 313:445–449. https://doi.org/10.1136/BMJ.313.7055.445
67. Jones D, Goldblatt P, Fox AJ (1987) Unemployment and mortality: comparison of the 1971 and 1981 longitudinal study census samples. Br Med J (Clin Res Ed) 294:86. https://doi.org/10.1136/BMJ.294.6564.86
68. Martikainen PT, Valkonen T (1996) Excess mortality of unemployed men and women during a period of rapidly increasing unemployment.

Lancet 348:909–912. https://doi.org/10.1016/S0140-6736(96)03291-6
69. Åhs AMH, Westerling R (2006) Mortality in relation to employment status during different levels of unemployment. Scand J Public Health 34:159–167. https://doi.org/10.1080/14034940510032374
70. Martikainen P, Mäki N, Blomgren J (2004) The effects of area and individual social characteristics on suicide risk: a multilevel study of relative contribution and effect modification. Eur J Popul 20:323–350. https://doi.org/10.1007/S10680-004-3807-1/METRICS
71. D'Souza AJ, Blakely TA, Woodward A (2008) The effect of eradicating poverty on childhood unintentional injury mortality in New Zealand: a cohort study with counterfactual modelling. J Epidemiol Community Health 62:899–904. https://doi.org/10.1136/jech.2007.068072
72. Kim MD, Hong SC, Lee SY, Kwak YS, Lee CI, Hwang SW, Shin TK, Lee SM, Shin JN (2006) Suicide risk in relation to social class: a national register-based study of adult suicides in Korea, 1999-2001. Int J Soc Psychiatry 52:138–151. https://doi.org/10.1177/0020764006061254
73. Kwan YK, Ip WC, Kwan P (2005) Gender differences in suicide risk by socio-demographic factors in Hong Kong. Death Stud 29:645–663. https://doi.org/10.1080/07481180591004543
74. Stack S (2000) Suicide: a 15-year review of the sociological literature part I: cultural and economic factors. Suicide Life Threat Behav 30:145–162. https://doi.org/10.1111/J.1943-278X.2000.TB01073.X
75. Platt S (2016) Inequalities and suicidal behavior. In: The international handbook of suicide prevention: second edition. Wiley, New York, pp 258–283. https://doi.org/10.1002/9781118903223.CH15
76. Mäki NE, Martikainen PT (2007) Socioeconomic differences in suicide mortality by sex in Finland in 1971-2000: a register-based study of trends, levels, and life expectancy differences. Scand J Public Health 35:387–395. https://doi.org/10.1080/14034940701219618
77. Fujioka M, Mori H, Yoshinaga K, Kaneko J (2002) Comparison of occupational mortality between the Nordic countries and Japan, with analysis by age group in Japan, using micro-data and the statistical pattern analysis (SPA) method. Bull Labour Stat
78. Kyung-Sook W, SangSoo S, Sangjin S, Young-Jeon S (2018) Marital status integration and suicide: a meta-analysis and meta-regression. Soc Sci Med 197:116–126. https://doi.org/10.1016/J.SOCSCIMED.2017.11.053
79. Pensola TH, Martikainen P (2003) Effect of living conditions in the parental home and youth paths on the social class differences in mortality among women. Scand J Public Health 31:428–438. https://doi.org/10.1080/14034950310003980
80. Steenland K, Halperin W, Hu S, Walker JT (2003) Deaths due to injuries among employed adults: the effects of socioeconomic class. Epidemiology 14:74–79. https://doi.org/10.1097/00001648-200301000-00017
81. Kelly S, Charlton J, Jenkins R (1995) Suicide deaths in England and Wales, 1982-92: the contribution of occupation and geography. Popul Trends:16–25
82. Blakely T, Atkinson J, O'Dea D (2003a) No association of income inequality with adult mortality within New Zealand: a multi-level study of 1.4 million 25–64 year olds. J Epidemiol Community Health 57:279–284. https://doi.org/10.1136/JECH.57.4.279
83. Taylor S (1982) Durkheim and the study of suicide. Springer, Berlin. https://doi.org/10.1007/978-1-349-16792-0
84. Bearman PS (1991) The social structure of suicide. Sociol Forum 6:501–524. https://doi.org/10.1007/BF01114474/METRICS
85. Lund C, Breen A, Flisher AJ, Kakuma R, Corrigall J, Joska JA, Swartz L, Patel V (2010) Poverty and common mental disorders in low and middle income countries: a systematic review. Soc Sci Med 71:517–528. https://doi.org/10.1016/J.SOCSCIMED.2010.04.027
86. Wilkinson RG, Pickett KE (2006) Income inequality and population health: a review and explanation of the evidence. Soc Sci Med 62:1768–1784. https://doi.org/10.1016/J.SOCSCIMED.2005.08.036
87. Hong J, Knapp M, Mcguire A (2011) Income-related inequalities in the prevalence of depression and suicidal behaviour: a 10-year trend following economic crisis. World Psychiatry 10:40. https://doi.org/10.1002/J.2051-5545.2011.TB00012.X
88. Milner A, Morrell S, LaMontagne AD (2014) Economically inactive, unemployed and employed suicides in Australia by age and sex over a 10-year period: what was the impact of the 2007 economic recession? Int J Epidemiol 43:1500–1507. https://doi.org/10.1093/IJE/DYU148
89. Chan CH, Caine ED, You S, Fu KW, Chang SS, Yip PSF (2014) Suicide rates among working-age adults in South Korea before and after the 2008 economic crisis. J Epidemiol Community Health 1978(68):246–252. https://doi.org/10.1136/JECH-2013-202759
90. Santana P, Costa C, Cardoso G, Loureiro A, Ferrão J (2015) Suicide in Portugal: spatial determinants in a context of economic crisis. Health Place 35:85–94. https://doi.org/10.1016/j.healthplace.2015.07.001
91. Wahlbeck K, McDaid D (2012) Actions to alleviate the mental health impact of the economic crisis. World Psychiatry 11:139–145. https://doi.org/10.1002/J.2051-5545.2012.TB00114.X
92. Singh B, Jenkins R (2000) Suicide prevention strategies—an international perspective. Int Rev Psychiatry 12:7–14. https://doi.org/10.1080/09540260074058

93. Taylor SJ, Kingdom D, Jenkins R (1997) How are nations trying to prevent suicide? An analysis of national suicide prevention strategies. Acta Psychiatr Scand 95:457–463. https://doi.org/10.1111/J.1600-0447.1997.TB10132.X
94. Wasserman D (2004) Evaluating suicide prevention: various approaches needed. World Psychiatry 3:153
95. Goldney RD (2005) Suicide prevention: a pragmatic review of recent studies. Crisis 26:128–140. https://doi.org/10.1027/0227-5910.26.3.128
96. Makinen IH (1999) Effect on suicide rate of having reduced unemployment is uncertain. BMJ 318:941. https://doi.org/10.1136/bmj.318.7188.941
97. De Leo D, Evans R (2004) International suicide rates and prevention strategies 1. Hogrefe & Huber Publishers, Cambridge
98. Morrell S, Page AN, Taylor RJ (2007) The decline in Australian young male suicide. Soc Sci Med 64:747–754. https://doi.org/10.1016/J.SOCSCIMED.2006.09.027
99. Agerbo E (2005) Effect of psychiatric illness and labour market status on suicide: a healthy worker effect? J Epidemiol Community Health 59:598. https://doi.org/10.1136/JECH.2004.025288
100. Gunnell D, Frankel S (1994) Prevention of suicide: aspirations and evidence. BMJ 308:1227. https://doi.org/10.1136/BMJ.308.6938.1227
101. Lewis G, Hawton K, Jones P (1997) Strategies for preventing suicide. Br J Psychiatry 171:351–354. https://doi.org/10.1192/BJP.171.4.351
102. Knox KL, Litts DA, Talcott GW, Feig JC, Caine ED (2003) Risk of suicide and related adverse outcomes after exposure to a suicide prevention programme in the US Air Force: cohort study. BMJ 327:1376–1378. https://doi.org/10.1136/BMJ.327.7428.1376
103. Platt S, Hawton K (2002) Suicidal behaviour and the labour market. In: International handbook of suicide and attempted suicide. Wiley-Blackwell, Hoboken
104. Bhugra D, Gupta S, Bhui K, Craig T, Dogra N, Ingleby JD, Kirkbride J, Moussaoui D, Nazroo J, Qureshi A, Stompe T, Tribe R (2011) WPA guidance on mental health and mental health care in migrants. World Psychiatry 10:2. https://doi.org/10.1002/J.2051-5545.2011.TB00002.X
105. Montgomery A, Bhugra D (2021) Suicide among migrants. In: Oxford textbook of suicidology and suicide prevention. Oxford Academic, Oxford, pp 233–240. https://doi.org/10.1093/MED/9780198834441.003.0028
106. Bhugra D, Jones P (2001) Migration and mental illness. Adv Psychiatr Treat 7:216–222. https://doi.org/10.1192/APT.7.3.216
107. Carta MG, Bernal M, Hardoy MC, Haro-Abad JM, Kovess V, Brugha T, Lehtinen V, Angermeyer MC, Xavier M, Kittel F, Fryers T, Aongusa BN, Stefansson CG, Poulsen HD, Pull C, Abad JMH, Katschnig H, Madianos MG, Dalgard OS, Bijl R, Rutz W, Henderson JH, Lafortune G, Mateos R, Bebbington P, Caldas de Almeida JM, Dahl A, Joukaama M, Mavrey V, Morosini P, Nettelbladt P, Ormel J, Rouillon F, Walsh D, Wancata J, Weyerer S, Demyttenaere K, McColl K, Capuano F, Gagnon J, Hill T, Morgan Z, Taub N, Smith J (2005) Migration and mental health in Europe (the state of the mental health in Europe working group: Appendix 1). Clin Pract Epidemiol Ment Health 1:13. https://doi.org/10.1186/1745-0179-1-13
108. Cho YB, Haslam N (2010) Suicidal ideation and distress among immigrant adolescents: the role of acculturation, life stress, and social support. J Youth Adolesc 39:370–379. https://doi.org/10.1007/S10964-009-9415-Y
109. Aran N, Card KG, Lee K, Hogg RS (2023) Patterns of suicide and suicidal ideation in relation to social isolation and loneliness in newcomer populations: a review. J Immigr Minor Health 25:415–426. https://doi.org/10.1007/S10903-022-01422-9
110. Lai DWL, Li L, Daoust GD (2017) Factors influencing suicide behaviours in immigrant and ethnocultural minority groups: a systematic review. J Immigr Minor Health 19:755–768. https://doi.org/10.1007/S10903-016-0490-3
111. Hagaman AK, Sivilli TI, Ao T, Blanton C, Ellis H, Lopes Cardozo B, Shetty S (2016) An investigation into suicides among Bhutanese refugees resettled in the United States between 2008 and 2011. J Immigr Minor Health 18:819–827. https://doi.org/10.1007/S10903-015-0326-6
112. Berardelli I, Tarsitani L, Sarubbi S, Pinucci I, Rogante E, Cifrodelli M, Erbuto D, Lester D, Innamorati M, Pompili M (2023) Suicide risk and suicide risk factors among immigrants in Italy: a bi-center matched sample study. Int J Soc Psychiatry 69:111–116. https://doi.org/10.1177/00207640211072425
113. Forte A, Trobia F, Gualtieri F, Lamis DA, Cardamone G, Giallonardo V, Fiorillo A, Girardi P, Pompili M (2018) Suicide risk among immigrants and ethnic minorities: a literature overview. Int J Environ Res Public Health 15:1438. https://doi.org/10.3390/IJERPH15071438
114. Mesa-Vieira C, Haas AD, Buitrago-Garcia D, Roa-Diaz ZM, Minder B, Gamba M, Salvador D, Gomez D, Lewis M, Gonzalez-Jaramillo WC, Pahud de Mortanges A, Buttia C, Muka T, Trujillo N, Franco OH (2022) Mental health of migrants with pre-migration exposure to armed conflict: a systematic review and meta-analysis. Lancet Public Health 7:e469–e481. https://doi.org/10.1016/S2468-2667(22)00061-5
115. Aragona M, Pucci D, Carrer S, Catino E, Tomaselli A, Colosimo F, Lafuente M, Mazzetti M, Maisano B, Geraci S (2011) The role of post-migration living difficulties on somatization among first-generation immigrants visited in a primary care service. Ann Ist Super Sanita 47:207–213. https://doi.org/10.4415/ANN_11_02_13
116. Hynie M (2018) The social determinants of refugee mental health in the post-migration context: a criti-

cal review. Can J Psychiatr 63:297–303. https://doi.org/10.1177/0706743717746666
117. Miller KE, Rasmussen A (2017) The mental health of civilians displaced by armed conflict: an ecological model of refugee distress. Epidemiol Psychiatr Sci 26:129–138. https://doi.org/10.1017/S2045796016000172
118. Perreira KM, Ornelas I (2013) Painful passages: traumatic experiences and post-traumatic stress among immigrant Latino adolescents and their primary caregivers. Int Migr Rev 47:976–1005. https://doi.org/10.1111/IMRE.12050
119. Ratkowska KA, De Leo D (2013) Suicide in immigrants: an overview. Open J Med Psychol 2:124–133. https://doi.org/10.4236/ojmp.2013.23019
120. Berry JW (1997) Immigration, acculturation, and adaptation. Appl Psychol 46:5–34. https://doi.org/10.1111/J.1464-0597.1997.TB01087.X
121. Choy B, Arunachalam K, Gupta S, Taylor M, Lee A (2020) Systematic review: acculturation strategies and their impact on the mental health of migrant populations. Public Health Pract (Oxf) 2:100069. https://doi.org/10.1016/J.PUHIP.2020.100069
122. Gupta A, Leong F, Valentine JC, Canada DD (2013) A meta-analytic study: the relationship between acculturation and depression among Asian Americans. Am J Orthopsychiatry 83:372–385. https://doi.org/10.1111/AJOP.12018
123. Hovey JD, King CA (1996) Acculturative stress, depression, and suicidal ideation among immigrant and second-generation Latino adolescents. J Am Acad Child Adolesc Psychiatry 35:1183–1192. https://doi.org/10.1097/00004583-199609000-00016
124. Amiri S (2022) Prevalence of suicide in immigrants/refugees: a systematic review and meta-analysis. Arch Suicide Res 26:370–405. https://doi.org/10.1080/13811118.2020.1802379
125. Canetto SS, Sakinofsky I (1998) The gender paradox in suicide. Suicide Life Threat Behav 28:1–23. https://doi.org/10.1111/J.1943-278X.1998.TB00622.X
126. Bhugra D, Baldwin DS, Desai M, Jacob KS (1999a) Attempted suicide in west London, II. Inter-group comparisons. Psychol Med 29:1131–1139. https://doi.org/10.1017/S0033291799008922
127. Bhugra D, Desai M, Baldwin DS (1999b) Attempted suicide in west London, I. Rates across ethnic communities. Psychol Med 29:1125–1130. https://doi.org/10.1017/S0033291799008910
128. Spallek J, Reeske A, Norredam M, Nielsen SS, Lehnhardt J, Razum O (2015) Suicide among immigrants in Europe—a systematic literature review. Eur J Pub Health 25:63–71. https://doi.org/10.1093/EURPUB/CKU121
129. Basu A, Boland A, Witt K, Robinson J (2022) Suicidal behaviour, including ideation and self-harm, in young migrants: a systematic review. Int J Environ Res Public Health 19:8329. https://doi.org/10.3390/IJERPH19148329/S1
130. Ide N, Kõlves K, Cassaniti M, De Leo D (2012) Suicide of first-generation immigrants in Australia, 1974-2006. Soc Psychiatry Psychiatr Epidemiol 47:1917–1927. https://doi.org/10.1007/S00127-012-0499-4
131. Hughes J, Durkee T, Hadlaczky G (2021) Suicide and attempted suicide among indigenous people. In: Oxford textbook of suicidology and suicide prevention. Oxford Academic, Oxford, pp 241–248. https://doi.org/10.1093/MED/9780198834441.003.0029
132. Yoon E, Chang CT, Kim S, Clawson A, Cleary SE, Hansen M, Bruner JP, Chan TK, Gomes AM (2013) A meta-analysis of acculturation/enculturation and mental health. J Couns Psychol 60:15–30. https://doi.org/10.1037/A0030652
133. Keeley H, Súilleabháin FÓ, Leane M (2021) Sexual and gender minority populations and suicidal behaviours. In: Oxford textbook of suicidology and suicide prevention. Oxford Academic, Oxford, pp 353–360. https://doi.org/10.1093/MED/9780198834441.003.0042
134. Cohen-Kettenis PT, Pfäfflin F (2010) The DSM diagnostic criteria for gender identity disorder in adolescents and adults. Arch Sex Behav 39:499–513. https://doi.org/10.1007/S10508-009-9562-Y
135. Zucker KJ, Seto MC (2015) Gender dysphoria and paraphilic sexual disorders. In: Rutter's child and adolescent psychiatry: sixth edition. Wiley, New York, pp 983–998. https://doi.org/10.1002/9781118381953.CH69
136. Yarns BC, Abrams JM, Meeks TW, Sewell DD (2016) The mental health of older LGBT adults. Curr Psychiatry Rep 18:60. https://doi.org/10.1007/S11920-016-0697-Y
137. Tinney J, Dow B, Maude P, Purchase R, Whyte C, Barrett C (2015) Mental health issues and discrimination among older LGBTI people. Int Psychogeriatr 27:1411–1416. https://doi.org/10.1017/S1041610214002671
138. Yıldız E (2018) Suicide in sexual minority populations: a systematic review of evidence-based studies. Arch Psychiatr Nurs 32:650–659. https://doi.org/10.1016/J.APNU.2018.03.003
139. American Psychiatric Association (2013) Diagnostic and statistical manual of mental disorders. American Psychiatric Association, Virginia. https://doi.org/10.1176/APPI.BOOKS.9780890425596
140. Rivers I (2004) Recollections of bullying at school and their long-term implications for lesbians, gay men, and bisexuals. Crisis 25:169–175. https://doi.org/10.1027/0227-5910.25.4.169
141. Lewis NM (2009) Mental health in sexual minorities: recent indicators, trends, and their relationships to place in North America and Europe. Health Place 15:1029–1045. https://doi.org/10.1016/J.HEALTHPLACE.2009.05.003
142. Wittgens C, Fischer MM, Buspavanich P, Theobald S, Schweizer K, Trautmann S (2022) Mental health in people with minority sexual orientations: a meta-analysis of population-based studies. Acta Psychiatr

Scand 145:357–372. https://doi.org/10.1111/ACPS.13405
143. Pompili M, Lester D, Forte A, Seretti ME, Erbuto D, Lamis DA, Amore M, Girardi P (2014) Bisexuality and suicide: a systematic review of the current literature. J Sex Med 11:1903–1913. https://doi.org/10.1111/JSM.12581
144. Pinna F, Paribello P, Somaini G, Corona A, Ventriglio A, Corrias C, Frau I, Murgia R, El Kacemi S, Galeazzi GM, Mirandola M, Amaddeo F, Crapanzano A, Converti M, Piras P, Suprani F, Manchia M, Fiorillo A, Carpiniello B (2022) Mental health in transgender individuals: a systematic review. Int Rev Psychiatry 34:292–359. https://doi.org/10.1080/09540261.2022.2093629
145. Polidori et al. (2023) Risk of suicide attempt with gender diversity and neurodiversity. https://doi.org/10.1016/j.psychres.2023.115632
146. Thrower E, Bretherton I, Pang KC, Zajac JD, Cheung AS (2020) Prevalence of autism spectrum disorder and attention-deficit hyperactivity disorder amongst individuals with gender dysphoria: a systematic review. J Autism Dev Disord 50:695–706. https://doi.org/10.1007/S10803-019-04298-1
147. Warrier V, Greenberg DM, Weir E, Buckingham C, Smith P, Lai MC, Allison C, Baron-Cohen S (2020) Elevated rates of autism, other neurodevelopmental and psychiatric diagnoses, and autistic traits in transgender and gender-diverse individuals. Nat Commun 11:3959. https://doi.org/10.1038/S41467-020-17794-1
148. Lin Y, Xie H, Huang Z, Zhang Q, Wilson A, Hou J, Zhao X, Wang Y, Pan B, Liu Y, Han M, Chen R (2021) The mental health of transgender and gender non-conforming people in China: a systematic review. Lancet Public Health 6:e954–e969. https://doi.org/10.1016/S2468-2667(21)00236-X
149. Surace T, Fusar-Poli L, Vozza L, Cavone V, Arcidiacono C, Mammano R, Basile L, Rodolico A, Bisicchia P, Caponnetto P, Signorelli MS, Aguglia E (2021) Lifetime prevalence of suicidal ideation and suicidal behaviors in gender non-conforming youths: a meta-analysis. Eur Child Adolesc Psychiatry 30:1147–1161. https://doi.org/10.1007/S00787-020-01508-5
150. de Freitas LD, Léda-Rêgo G, Bezerra-Filho S, Miranda-Scippa Â (2020) Psychiatric disorders in individuals diagnosed with gender dysphoria: a systematic review. Psychiatry Clin Neurosci 74:99–104. https://doi.org/10.1111/PCN.12947
151. Marchi M, Arcolin E, Fiore G, Travascio A, Uberti D, Amaddeo F, Converti M, Fiorillo A, Mirandola M, Pinna F, Ventriglio A, Galeazzi GM (2022) Self-harm and suicidality among LGBTIQ people: a systematic review and meta-analysis. Int Rev Psychiatry 34:240–256. https://doi.org/10.1080/09540261.2022.2053070
152. Di Giacomo E, Krausz M, Colmegna F, Aspesi F, Clerici M (2018) Estimating the risk of attempted suicide among sexual minority youths: a systematic review and meta-analysis. JAMA Pediatr 172:1145–1152. https://doi.org/10.1001/JAMAPEDIATRICS.2018.2731
153. Hottes TS, Bogaert L, Rhodes AE, Brennan DJ, Gesink D (2016) Lifetime prevalence of suicide attempts among sexual minority adults by study sampling strategies: a systematic review and meta-analysis. Am J Public Health 106:e1–e12. https://doi.org/10.2105/AJPH.2016.303088
154. Williams AJ, Jones C, Arcelus J, Townsend E, Lazaridou A, Michail M (2021) A systematic review and meta-analysis of victimisation and mental health prevalence among LGBTQ+ young people with experiences of self-harm and suicide. PLoS One 16:e0245268. https://doi.org/10.1371/JOURNAL.PONE.0245268
155. Adams N, Hitomi M, Moody C (2017) Varied reports of adult transgender suicidality: synthesizing and describing the peer-reviewed and gray literature. Transgend Health 2:60. https://doi.org/10.1089/TRGH.2016.0036
156. Jackson D (2023) Suicide-related outcomes following gender-affirming treatment: a review. Cureus 15:e36425. https://doi.org/10.7759/CUREUS.36425
157. Hatzenbuehler ML, Nolen-Hoeksema S, Erickson SJ (2008) Minority stress predictors of HIV risk behavior, substance use, and depressive symptoms: results from a prospective study of bereaved gay men. Health Psychol 27:455–462. https://doi.org/10.1037/0278-6133.27.4.455
158. Meyer IH (2003) Prejudice, social stress, and mental health in lesbian, gay, and bisexual populations: conceptual issues and research evidence. Psychol Bull 129:674. https://doi.org/10.1037/0033-2909.129.5.674
159. De Lange J, Baams L, Van Bergen DD, Bos HMW, Bosker RJ (2022) Minority stress and suicidal ideation and suicide attempts among LGBT adolescents and young adults: a meta-analysis. LGBT Health 9:222–237. https://doi.org/10.1089/LGBT.2021.0106
160. Goldbach JT, Tanner-Smith EE, Bagwell M, Dunlap S (2014) Minority stress and substance use in sexual minority adolescents: a meta-analysis. Prev Sci 15:350–363. https://doi.org/10.1007/S11121-013-0393-7
161. Pellicane MJ, Ciesla JA (2022) Associations between minority stress, depression, and suicidal ideation and attempts in transgender and gender diverse (TGD) individuals: systematic review and meta-analysis. Clin Psychol Rev 91:102113. https://doi.org/10.1016/J.CPR.2021.102113
162. Testa RJ, Michaels MS, Bliss W, Rogers ML, Balsam KF, Joiner T (2017) Suicidal ideation in transgender people: gender minority stress and interpersonal theory factors. J Abnorm Psychol 126:125–136. https://doi.org/10.1037/ABN0000234

163. Thoma BC, Eckstrand KL, Montano GT, Rezeppa TL, Marshal MP (2021) Gender nonconformity and minority stress among lesbian, gay, and bisexual individuals: a meta-analytic review. Perspect Psychol Sci 16:1165–1183. https://doi.org/10.1177/1745691620968766
164. Ferlatte O, Salway T, Oliffe JL, Saewyc EM, Holmes C, Schick L, Purdie A, Damstrom-Albach DD, Mantler ERG, Ho D, Knight R (2020) It is time to mobilize suicide prevention for sexual and gender minorities in Canada. Can J Public Health 111:737–742. https://doi.org/10.17269/S41997-020-00316-3
165. Haroz EE, Decker E, Lee C (2018) Evidence for suicide prevention and response programs with refugees: a systematic review and recommendations. A report prepared by: Evidence for suicide prevention and response programs with refugees: a systematic review and recommendations. United Nations High Commissioner for Refugees, Geneva, p 2

17 Trauma and Mental Health: Individual and Collective Traumas

Claudia Carmassi, Sara Fantasia, Virginia Pedrinelli, Silvia Mammarella, Laura Giusti, and Rita Roncone

Abstract

This chapter briefly reports the history of the term “trauma” and the evolution in the years of the nosography of post-traumatic stress disorder (PTSD). We will describe the main trauma-related disorders in the current nosography, including the complex PTSD (cPTSD), recently introduced in the International Classification of Diseases, 11th revision (ICD-11). Psychopharmacological treatments and psychological interventions for the management of PTSD will be reported. As individual trauma, Prolonged Grief Disorder (PGD) will be described, whose diagnostic criteria have been only recently introduced by the American Psychiatric Association in the Diagnostic and Statistical Manual of Mental Disorders-5th Edition Text Revision (DSM-5-TR). Concerning collective traumas, the most recent natural disasters occurred in our country are briefly reported, with more details for the L’Aquila 2009 earthquake. The social impact of the latter and the long-lasting consequences confirm the broader scientific literature concerning the reciprocal influence of the social environment on mental health and well-being.

Keywords

Trauma · Post-traumatic stress disorder · Complex post-traumatic stress disorder · Prolonged grief disorder · Natural disasters · Earthquake · Post-traumatic stress disorder management · Resilience · Post-traumatic growth · Social dimensions of disasters

17.1 Introduction

The term trauma comes from the Greek τραύμα and means trauma wound, alteration of trōma; related to the Greek titrōskein = wound, tetrainein = puncture [1], is generally used to describe two conditions [2]:

C. Carmassi (✉) · S. Fantasia · V. Pedrinelli
Department of Clinical and Experimental Medicine, University of Pisa, Pisa, Italy
e-mail: claudia.carmassi@unipi.it

S. Mammarella · L. Giusti · R. Roncone
Department of Life, Health and Environmental Sciences, University of L’Aquila, L’Aquila, Italy
e-mail: silvia.mammarella@univaq.it; laura.giusti@univaq.it; rita.roncone@univaq.it

A. Fiorillo, S. De Giorgi (eds.), *Social Determinants of Mental Health*, Sustainable Development Goals Series, https://doi.org/10.1007/978-3-031-70165-8_17

- Physical trauma: a tissue injury caused by an external physical, biological, or radiological agent.
- Psychological trauma: a state of mental or behavioral disturbance resulting from severe mental or emotional stress.

In the context of mental health, trauma is an experience that occurs during a highly emotionally charged event and may be followed by the onset of psychiatric symptoms [2].

Recognition of psychological trauma as part of the human condition is not recent: indeed, references to the psychological consequences of war can be found as far back as the ancient Greeks (e.g., in Homer's Iliad). In the seventeenth century, Samuel Pepys noted the occurrence of sleep disturbances and intrusive thoughts in response to the "Great Fire" in London in 1666 [3]. However, discussions about the concept of trauma and its consequences have persisted throughout more recent years, with different terms being used to define them. In particular, the "Railway Spine" and "Shell Shock" should be cited, among many others. The former was used in the late 1800s to refer to disturbances in uninjured passengers following a railroad accident. It was originally attributed to an underlying neurological physical injury from the accident, specifically chronic or subacute inflammation of the spinal meninges. However, Page drew attention to the similarity between "railroad spine" and traumatic hysteria, suggesting that they were forms of the same phenomenon and highlighting the psychological effects of the fear of being involved in a railroad accident [4].

The term "Railway Spine" was replaced by the term "Shell Shock" with the outbreak of the World War I. It referred to anxiety, fatigue, and sleep disorders that occurred in the World War I soldiers and which were initially attributed to physical brain damage as a result of exposure to bomb blasts [3]. However, since many affected soldiers had not been close to the explosions, the term "War Neurosis" was introduced [5].

A shift from the conceptualization of trauma as a neurological injury to a psychological–psychoanalytic theorization of traumatic neurosis is due to the development of Freudian and post-Freudian theories [4].

As for the official nosography, the American Psychiatric Association [6] included "Gross Stress Reaction" in the first Diagnostic and Statistical Manual of Mental Disorders (DSM-I) of the 1952. This diagnosis, however, assumed that reactions to the trauma would disappear within 6 months of the event. This diagnosis was dropped by the DSM-II [7] which, in contrast, included the "adjustment reaction to adult life," limiting to three examples of trauma: unwanted pregnancy with suicidal ideation, fear related to military combat, and Ganser syndrome (characterized by incorrect answers to questions) in prisoners facing a death sentence [5]. The diagnosis of post-traumatic stress disorder (PTSD), whose definition was based on studies of Vietnam War veterans and Holocaust survivors, was introduced in the DSM-III in 1980 only [8].

The definitions of PTSD and trauma-related disorders have undergone an important evolution up to the most recent editions of the DSM and International Classification of Diseases (ICD). One of the most relevant changes that occurred in the DSM-5 was the introduction of a specific chapter for stress- and trauma-related disorders [9], including PTSD, which was removed from the Anxiety Disorders Chapter. Consistently, the definition of a "traumatic event" also changed significantly. The Criterion A of the DSM-5-TR [10] defines a traumatic event as follow: "*The person was exposed to: death, threatened death, actual or threatened serious injury, or actual or threatened sexual violence, in the following way(s): direct exposure, witnessing the trauma, learning that a relative or close friend was exposed to a trauma, indirect exposure to aversive details of the trauma, usually in the course of professional duties (e.g., first responders, medics).*"

Although the evidence that traumas most associated with PTSD are combat exposure among men and rape and sexual molestation among women [11], epidemiological surveys aimed at estimating the incidence and prevalence of PTSD have highlighted the impact of methodological, trauma-related factors on the rates of the disorder. In its original definition [8], PTSD referred to the exposure to a very limited number of traumatic events, including combat or war exposure, rape and sexual trauma, and human-made or natural disasters [12, 13]. Gradually, however, traumatic events have been expanded to include a broader range of experiences, all of which involve actual or threatened death, serious injury, or sexual violence in some way. Currently, the DSM also includes life-threatening illnesses, or debilitating medical conditions limited to sudden medical emergencies or catastrophes, highlighting the need for the event to be sudden and severely dangerous, with major attention on the urgency and abruptness of the perceived threat [14]. Despite the official nosography, the debate continues.

17.2 Post-traumatic Stress Disorder (PTSD) and Main Trauma-Related Disorders

Post-Traumatic Stress Disorder (PTSD) is a psychopathological condition resulting from the direct or indirect experience of a traumatic event involving actual or threatened death, serious injury, or sexual violence [10]. This disorder is characterized by chronic course, poor response to pharmacotherapy, and significant impairment in occupational, social and family roles, leading to a poor quality of life and increased risk of suicide [15–19].

According to the DSM 5-TR, PTSD has a lifetime prevalence of 6.1–8.3% [10]. Trauma most commonly associated with PTSD are war exposure among men and rape and sexual assault among women [11]. However, epidemiologic studies aimed at estimating the incidence and prevalence of PTSD following exposure to a traumatic event come to very different conclusions, even when the same types of traumatic events are considered.

Several individual, social, and event-related risk factors influence the risk of developing PTSD and the presentation of the disorder following a traumatic event. Pre-injury, injury-related, and post-injury risk factors can be identified for mental health problems. Consistent risk factors include female gender, a history of mental health problems or trauma, the type of injury, and the degree of pain reported [20]. In addition, PTSD rates are higher in certain occupational groups, such as veterans and people working at high risk of traumatic exposure (e.g., police, firefighters, emergency medical personnel) [10].

According to the DSM-5-TR, a diagnosis of PTSD requires significant exposure to a traumatic event (Criterion A) that caused the onset of symptoms belonging to four clusters: intrusive symptoms (Criterion B); persistent avoidance of stimuli associated with the traumatic event (Criterion C), negative alterations in cognition or mood related to the trauma (Criterion D), and a marked change in arousal and reactivity (Criterion E). These symptoms must persist for more than 1 month (Criterion F) and significantly impair the person's ability to function in one or more areas (Criterion G).

The temporal criterion (criterion F) is helpful for the differential diagnosis with Acute Stress Disorder (ASD), which is also included in the DSM-5-TR. ASD occurs within 30 days after a severe traumatic event and is characterized by heterogeneous symptoms ranging from intrusive symptoms to hypervigilance and dissociative reactions, and is considered one of the main precursors of PTSD [21, 22]. However, a diagnosis of ASD does not define all individuals who will develop PTSD [21]. In fact, post-traumatic symptoms may be delayed for months or years before the criteria for PTSD are met, defining a PTSD subtype with delayed expression.

The DSM 5-TR also distinguishes the dissociative subtype based on the presence of persistent dissociative symptoms, such as depersonalization or derealization. Subjects with the dissociative subtype often have a history of multiple traumas, childhood trauma, and higher suicide rate [23–25].

One of the most debated issues in the field of PTSD is the achievement of threshold criteria in terms of number of symptoms to fulfill the diagnosis. In fact, restrictive criteria exclude a high number of individuals who present psychiatric symptoms following a traumatic event. Thus, partial, subthreshold, or subsyndromal PTSDs have been proposed. The term "subsyndromal PTSD" refers to those syndromes in which the threshold for symptom criteria is not met, but at least one symptom of each criterion is present; whereas "partial PTSD" refers to a clinical condition in which the symptoms of a given criterion are absent [26]. Although these subtypes are highly prevalent, they are not included (yet) in the official nosography.

More recently, dimensional approaches to PTSD have been proposed, such as the trauma and loss spectrum, with its related assessment instrument (trauma and loss self report, TALS-SR) [27–30]. The TALS-SR, in fact, is based on a multidimensional approach to post-traumatic stress disorder that includes a range of threatening or frightening experiences, as well as a variety of potentially significant losses, to which an individual can be exposed to; furthermore, it explores the spectrum of peritraumatic reactions and post-traumatic symptoms that may derive from either trauma or losses, targeting soft signs and subthreshold conditions, as well as temperamental and personality traits that may represent risk factors for the development of the disorder. A significant burden of post-traumatic spectrum on subjects' mental health in the aftermath of individual or mass trauma has been demonstrated, not only in the general population but also in other mental disorders, particularly bipolar disorders [31].

The 11th revision of the International Classification of Diseases (ICD-11) of the World Health Organization [32] introduced the complex PTSD (cPTSD) in this chapter of stress-related disorders, which includes clusters of PTSD symptoms (ICD-11 defines three and not four symptom clusters) associated with self-organization disorder (DSO). DSO is defined by the three symptom clusters of affective dysregulation, negative self-concept, and relationship disorders. Although the type of trauma is not used for the differential diagnosis, PTSD and cPTSD are typically distinguished by the nature of the triggering events: cPTSD is more commonly associated with interpersonal and early childhood trauma, while PTSD is more commonly associated with non-interpersonal and adult trauma [33].

To summarize, the subjective experience of trauma and the resulting symptoms vary considerably in space and time, leading to clinical symptoms that are attributable to trauma but may or may not be labeled as PTSD [34].

17.3 An Individual Trauma: The Specific Case of the "Loss of a Close One" and the Prolonged Grief Disorder

Grief is a physiological reaction to the death of a loved one that is associated with pain and adjustment difficulties, but which in its natural course involves a progressive, albeit slow, recovery through four phases: the attainment of full awareness of the loss and its consequences; the development of alternative ways of relating to the deceased; the redefinition of personal goals and projects [35]; and the transition to integrated grief that lasts throughout life and evolves (e.g., there may be episodes of heightened longing or sadness triggered by anniversaries, celebratory life events or other losses that usually subside within a short period) [36]. This process can deviate from its natural course, leading to various psychopathological pictures.

One of the first studies on the manifestations of physiological and pathological grief was that of Freud in his publication on mourning and melancholia in 1917, in which he introduced the concept of grief [37]. Currently, *grief* is defined as a person's emotional response to a loss; *mourning* is the outward expression of grief (i.e., the cultural and religious customs surrounding death); *bereavement* is the time of mourning and grieving after a loss; *anticipatory grief* is the reaction to an expected loss, as in the case of family members of people with a terminal illness; and *disenfranchised grief* occurs when people suffer a loss that is not or cannot be openly acknowledged, publicly mourned or socially supported, such as the loss of a patient in healthcare workers or parents with perinatal loss [38].

Several studies have focused on the psychopathological manifestations following the loss of a loved one, leading to the definition of a specific clinical picture of pathological grief, namely Prolonged Grief Disorder (PGD), which has been recognized for the first time in the DSM-5-TR. Consistently, there is evidence of the relationship between grief and other mental disorders, particularly major depression and PTSD [37, 39] .

PGD is a maladaptive grief reaction lasting at least 12 months (6 months in children and adolescents) after the death of a person with whom the grieving person had a close relationship (criterion A) [10]. The temporal criterion distinguishes physiological pain from maladaptive reactions. However, the duration of adaptive grief can vary individually and across cultures.

The prevalence of PGD is still unknown since the diagnostic criteria have been introduced only recently. However, previous studies conducted according to the diagnostic criteria for complicated grief found a prevalence after a significant bereavement of 6.7% and of 3.7% in the general sample. Risk factors for PGD include female gender, low income, advanced age (>61 years), the loss of a child or spouse, or cancer as the cause of death [40].

The grief reaction triggered by the loss can have characteristics that overlap with those of a depressive episode. However, despite common elements (i.e., sadness, hypnotic disturbances, difficulties in concentrating, thoughts of death), some differences allow a differential diagnosis. In grief reaction, feelings of emptiness and loss predominate, with a dysphoric mood associated with thoughts or memories of the deceased that, therefore, occur in waves and may be accompanied by positive emotions. Self-esteem is maintained or, if self-deprecating thoughts are present, they are usually perceived as failings towards the deceased (e.g., not visiting often enough, not telling the deceased how much he or she was loved) [10, 41]. Finally, thoughts of death focus on the possibility of being reunited with the deceased. In contrast, in a major depressive episode, depressed mood is persistent, not associated with specific thoughts or worries, with a limited ability to experience joy and positive emotions. Self-deprecation and thoughts of death are associated with a desire to end one's life because of a sense of uselessness, a perception of oneself as unworthy of life, or an inability to cope with the pain of depression [10, 41]. Finally, it is important to emphasize that loss can trigger not only a grief reaction but also the development of major depression or the exacerbation of an existing episode.

People may also experience loss through the violent or accidental death of a loved one, an event that falls under criterion A of PTSD according to the DSM 5-TR (i.e., a death that is categorized as a traumatic event). In this case, both PGD and PTSD may occur, which also overlap in some elements, such as a sense of shock, intrusive images, avoidance of stimuli related to the death, feelings of alienation from others, insomnia, and difficulties in concentrating. However, the symptomatic core of PGD is represented by yearning and desire, whereas the main symptom in PTSD is fear of a threat. Indeed, in PTSD, there are elements such as hypervigilance to threats, the excessive response to fear, and nightmares, which are generally not present in PGD, where sadness is more prominent. In addition, the content of the intrusive thoughts is different: in PTSD, they relate to the traumatic event and trigger reactions of fear and horror, whereas in persistent grief, they relate to the deceased person and can also be comforting [10, 41, 42].

17.4 Collective Traumas: Natural Disasters in Italy

Considering the vast field of interest in trauma, in the following paragraphs we will focus on collective trauma from natural disasters that have affected our country recently and which have allowed us to study the main consequences on the mental health of the population. Due to the high number of Italian scientific works related to L'Aquila earthquakes and the fact that two authors have personally lived that experience

(R.R., L.G.), more space will be given to the natural catastrophe that struck L'Aquila in 2009.

17.4.1 The L'Aquila Earthquake in April 2009

At 3.32 a.m. on April 6, 2009, central Italy was struck by a 6.3 magnitude earthquake. The earthquake caused severe damage to the thirteenth-century town of L'Aquila, considering the high vulnerability level of its historic buildings—mainly concentrated in the city center. The earthquake also caused significant damage to several medieval hill villages in the surrounding areas, killing 309 residents, injuring over 1600, and leaving approximately 70,000 people homeless. Approximately 44,000 people found accommodations in tented camps close to their residences, and an additional 20,000 people were housed in hotels on the Abruzzo Adriatic Sea coast. Others sought shelter with friends and relatives throughout Italy. The earthquake also caused severe damage to St. Salvatore General Hospital in L'Aquila, where the psychiatric inpatient unit and outpatient services were located. They were moved into tents (Fig. 17.1). During the 6 months post-earthquake, several aftershocks occurred (22 shocks with a local magnitude of 4.0 or higher) [43].

Several studies have been carried out on the consequences of this seismic event, more than those published on similar events in Italy [44]. Indeed, mental health was intensively studied in the L'Aquila earthquake, while its effects on mortality, cardiovascular outcomes, and health systems were less frequently evaluated [45].

Immediately after the L'Aquila earthquake, in the first 4 weeks, the incidence rate of acute stress disorder (ASD) in help-seekers at the tent of the General Hospital Psychiatric Unit at San Salvatore Hospital, only partially functioning, was 4.9% for full ASD, and 39.3% for partial ASD [46]. The strongest predictor of traumatic stress reactions was having been trapped/injured under rubble during the earthquake. At the same time, the adoption of an "acceptance" coping style seemed to reduce the likelihood of developing ASD.

Positive symptoms increased significantly from the pre- to post-earthquake assessment in first-episode schizophrenia subjects, and they scored significantly worse in cognitive functions assessment within 3 months after the earthquake. In contrast, symptom severity and cognitive performances did not change in subjects affected by chronic schizophrenia [47]. Incidence of post-traumatic stress disorder (PTSD) was between 12% and 37.5% in different samples of the population [28, 48].

Having been diagnosed as affected by partial ASD was not the strongest predictor of PTSD [49]. At 6-month follow-up, the most relevant predictor of PTSD for individuals seeking treatment at the General Hospital Psychiatric Unit within the first month following the L'Aquila

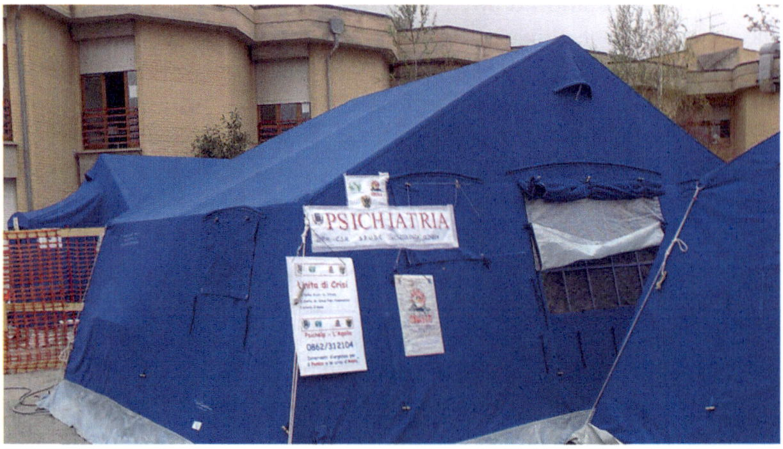

Fig. 17.1 The location of the outpatient service of the S. Salvatore Hospital, L'Aquila. (Photo R.R.)

earthquake was the persistent fear of aftershocks, followed by working memory impairment (backward digit span), suggesting an essential role of neurocognitive variables in PTSD [49]. Ten months after the earthquake, gender, age, and epicenter proximity were reported as relevant risk factors for PTSD [29, 48, 50].

Six months after the earthquake, an increase in psychotropic prescriptions was found [51], with a 37% increase in new prescriptions for antidepressants and a 129% increase in antipsychotic prescriptions associated with older age and female gender. Compared to the previous utilization of mental health services (2008), informatic system data showed a significant decrease in their utilization in the period 2009–2010 [52], mainly because 12 months after the earthquake, only 25% of the population was able to return to their home and mostly were displaced in hotels of the nearby towns.

An extensive mental health survey conducted between March and December 2010 on a total of 1078 young subjects found a marked increase in substance abuse [53]. Around 30% of the sample had a psychiatric morbidity. Use of alcohol, tobacco, and cannabis increased both in subjects affected by psychiatric disorders and in healthy young people. Among psychiatric cases, none reported a reduced use of these substances following the disaster. However, the study also showed a positive aspect [53]; in fact, 119 healthy young people (15.5%) reported a reduced use of cannabis after the earthquake and a significant improvement in well-being compared to those with increased assumptions. Those who reduced the use of cannabis reported more intimate relationships, a changed sense of priorities, a greater appreciation of life, and a greater sense of personal strength.

Real-world variables related to population distress and the naturalistic recovery from natural disasters were studied [43]. Many residents had found their way to recover through "writing, telling the story," by analogy with narrative medicine, thus estimating the positive effect of "emotional disclosure" on health. Residents produced many materials (books, web blogs, videos), with the implementation of a database of memories. L'Aquila residents have developed a more positive attitude towards Facebook and other social media. Their engagement with social media became integrated into their daily lives to cope with the loss of previous social relationships, to get information about recreational opportunities, or to get organized for public events despite the displacement [43].

A daily connection to the Facebook social network for more than 1 h per day for at least 2 years was studied in 2013 in a population-based cross-sectional study carried out to determine if continued use of online social networks correlated with depression, PTSD, and adverse quality of life (QOL) outcomes in an adult population previously exposed to L'Aquila earthquake [54]. Social network use among adults 25–54 years old positively impacted mental health outcomes following a disaster, helping to maintain, if not improve, quality of life regarding social relationships and psychological distress [54].

The increased utilization of social media platforms was reported also immediately after the 2010–2011 Canterbury earthquakes in New Zealand. To promote well-being messages, the Facebook page "All Right?" was an effective tool in the broader public health toolkit post-disaster. The platform also brought survivors closer by making individuals feel part of a broader social network [55].

Years later, a Facebook page in Italy, "Emergenza Sordi," was created to disseminate information online to deaf people immediately after the Amatrice 2016 August earthquake, with a page including a video with subtitles, Italian sign language, and service numbers. Facebook page obtained unexpectedly several accesses and satisfaction from deaf adults and families with deaf children, as well as hearing family relatives and caregivers [56].

17.4.2 The Long-Lasting Impact of Natural Disasters

Collective traumas, such as earthquakes, have long-lasting consequences. In L'Aquila, 21 months after the earthquake, suicidal behaviors were more frequent in young PTSD earthquake survivors compared to subthreshold PTSD and healthy controls [57]. Interestingly, a role of spiritual coping was detected as a protective factor for suicidality [58]. The relationship between lifetime mood symptoms and PTSD was investigated in the same sample, highlighting a relationship between lifetime depressive and manic symptoms and PTSD, with a particular impact of the latter on the number of traumatic exposures and maladaptive behaviors [59].

One of the first studies showing the negative impact of a natural catastrophic event on mental health was a general practitioner study carried out in 1987–1997 in three areas of the province of Naples: Pozzuoli, a town exposed to significant seismic events in September–October 1983 (shocks ranging from 2 to 6 on the Mercalli scale), Monteruscello, a village built to accommodate the victims of the earthquake, and Monte di Procida, a town selected as a control since it is situated near Pozzuoli and not significantly affected by the earthquake [60]. The prevalence of psychiatric disorders in the subjects exposed to seismic events of Pozzuoli and Monteruscello was greater than in the control population of Monte di Procida, with an increased relative risk of mental disorders of more than four times in subjects reporting more social problems exposed to the seismic event. The psychopathological impact seemed to be partially mediated by the social issues caused by the event [60].

The population of Pozzuoli was also included in studies concerning the "Irpinia" earthquake, a major earthquake (6.9, Richter Scale) that struck Southern Italy on November 23, 1980. More than 3000 deaths and 8000 injuries and 280,000 homeless were reported. Men working at the Olivetti Factory in Napoli with damage from this earthquake had higher levels of psychological distress 7 years after the earthquake compared to men who did not report damages. A third of these men reported PTSD symptoms. Additionally, participants residing in Pozzuoli, exposed to the 1980 earthquake and experiencing the continuous swarm of Bradyseism (the gradual upward or downward shifting of the land) between 1983 and 1984, reported higher levels of distress 4 years later if they experienced financial loss and/or were evacuated [61]. Increased distress was reported by permanently relocated men, while those who were evacuated, but returned to their original homes, reported distress levels comparable to their non-evacuated co-workers. Additionally, among evacuated men, only those whose relocation placed them at an increased distance from family and/or friends reported distress levels higher than the non-evacuated, resulting in disrupted social networks [62, 63].

In May 1998, Southern Italy, particularly the Campania region, was again affected by another natural disaster, the Sarno landslide. In a few hours, 14 landslides came down from Mount Saro and hit the inhabited areas of Sarno. Most material damage and human losses were recorded in the village of Episcopio. Many buildings were destroyed or damaged, and 137 people were killed [64]. The psychosocial consequences of a natural disaster identified high levels of psychiatric morbidity in the population of Sarno 12 months after the 1998 landslide, showing that more than 25% of the population met the criteria for PTSD. Around 60% were identified as "probable cases," suggesting that the psychosocial impact of the event is not time-limited [64].

A lower rate (14.5%) of subjects affected by PTSD was observed 6 months after the 2002 earthquake in Molise (a rural region of Italy) [65]. On October 31 and November 1, 2002, two earthquakes struck the sparsely populated region of Molise in Southern Italy. The first one measured 5.4 on the Richter scale and triggered a sequence of minor earthquakes lasting for several days. In the events, 30 people died, 27 of whom were children trapped in an elementary school, and up to 40% of buildings became temporarily or permanently uninhabitable. Notably, national and international media at the time reported the death of the school children, promoting an intense emotional response to that tragic event.

On August 24, 2016, an earthquake measuring 6.2 on the moment magnitude scale hit Central Italy, destroying the city of Amatrice and the nearby villages. The earthquake affected the whole Central Italy, involving 140 municipalities. The event was followed by several aftershocks, the strongest of which recorded a magnitude 5.3 just an hour after the main shock. The earthquake caused 299 victims, 388 injuries, and around 41,000 displaced people. Three years after the earthquake of Amatrice, the health status of the 51 survivors extricated from the rubble was investigated, taking into account the type of sedation administered during the extrication phase [66]. More than 90% were treated for PTSD, depression and anxiety. At the time of the study, concerning analyses on quality of life, only 10 survivors out of 51 perceived their health status as good; the others reported psychological disorders. Early sedation with ketamine directly in the disaster setting seemed to promote prophylaxis and reduce the risk of developing trauma-related disorders (TRDs) in the buried victims [66].

If most studies confirm the long-term impact of natural disasters on mental health, Priebe et al. study [59] does not align with such findings. On September 4, 1997, the region Marche in Central Italy was struck by an earthquake with a strength of 4.5 on the Richter scale, which was followed by stronger quakes with a strength of 5.5 and 5.8 on September 26 and a large number of minor quakes during the following 6 months. In Camerino, a small town in the Marche region close to the epicenter of the main earthquake, various buildings, including the main church, collapsed, and parts of the city were destroyed. Nobody died in Camerino, but 11 people died in the neighboring region of Umbria. Eight years later, the earthquake had a negative impact on the mental health of the affected population. Possible reasons included the relatively weak nature of the earthquake, strong community support that helped to overcome mental distress, the long period (8 years) between the occurrence of the earthquake and the study, and the capacity of people to maintain or restore mental health after a natural disaster in the long term [67]. Another earthquake occurred in Camerino in 2016; the impact of the second exposure in the same cohort showed that 16.9% of the sample had reached the PTSD threshold, compared to the 0.5% in 2005 [68]. Therefore, the positive long-term response after one earthquake does not represent a protective factor in experiencing positive outcomes after another exposure [68].

17.4.3 The Add-On Impact of Collective Traumas

Economic crises and the coronavirus disease 2019 (COVID-19) pandemic seemed to have an add-on effect of prior collective trauma. The adverse effects of the economic crisis seemed to add to the long-term consequences on survivors' psychological well-being, as in the province of Modena, in Northern Italy, which was struck by the earthquake in 2012. In fact, the Great Recession, which caused tangible costs worldwide in terms of cuts in employment and income, showed a more substantial effect in areas struck by the earthquake than in the rest of Italy [69].

During the COVID-19 pandemic, the role of prior traumas, which seem to increase reactivity to and potential harm of new traumas [70], was confirmed by a recent study conducted in L'Aquila in 2021 on depression in women balancing "work–life" responsibilities and caregiving. The likelihood of manifesting moderate depression was approximately four times higher in women who were exposed to the 2009 L'Aquila earthquake and reported it as a highly traumatic collective experience [71]. This variable increased its predictive power by more than double when women reported severe depression, highlighting a vulnerability to life-event stressors 12 years later [71].

17.5 Management of PTSD

The correct management of PTSD begins with the correct recognition of symptoms and the correct definition and sharing (with the subject and caregivers) of treatment goals (see Table 17.1).

According to shared international guidelines [72], trauma-focused psychotherapy that includes exposure, in particular trauma-focused cognitive behavioral therapy (CBT) and eye movement desensitization and reprocessing (EMDR), is rec-

Table 17.1 Management of PTSD

PTSD recognition	Assessing the clinical picture of persons in primary and secondary care Screening of people involved in a major disaster, refugees and asylum seekers
Definition and sharing of treatment goals	Safety of the person and others by assessing suicidality and self- or other-harmful ideation Symptom reduction, relapse prevention, and recovery Management of comorbidities
Prevention of PTSD	Trauma-focused CBT for those who have acute stress disorder or clinically significant symptoms of PTSD and have been exposed to one or more traumatic events within the last month NO drug treatment, especially no benzodiazepines
Treatment of PTSD	Trauma-focused CBT or EMDR Selective serotonin reuptake inhibitors (SSRI), such as sertraline, or venlafaxine Antipsychotics, such as risperidone, in addition to psychological therapies, if the disabling symptoms and behaviors do not respond to other drugs or psychological treatment

ommended for the prevention and treatment of PTSD. Conversely, pharmacotherapy is not recommended for the prevention of PTSD, but for the treatment of subjects who prefer pharmacotherapy (the therapeutic decision should always be shared with the affected person) or in whom the intensity of post-traumatic stress symptoms or the presence of comorbidities interferes with the skills required to carry out correctly the psychotherapeutic process (e.g., subjects with depression and resulting motivational and cognitive deficits).

Pharmacological treatments can be effective for both the main symptoms of PTSD and comorbidities. First-choice drugs are selective serotonin reuptake inhibitors (SSRIs), particularly sertraline, because of their greater efficacy compared with placebo, their tolerability, and the greater robustness of the evidence regarding the number and size of studies supporting their efficacy compared with those of other pharmacological categories [72, 73]. In line with the National Institute for Health and Care Excellence (NICE) guidelines, venlafaxine can be used as an alternative [72].

Symptoms that do not respond well to serotonin and norepinephrine reuptake inhibitors (SNRIs) and SSRIs, including sleep pattern disorders, may require polypharmacy. In subjects who do not respond to therapy or who exhibit prevalent psychotic symptoms, second-generation antipsychotics should be considered, either as monotherapy or in combination with SSRIs, with risperidone and quetiapine being the most studied [74].

An important clarification concerns the use of benzodiazepines, particularly in the immediate post-traumatic phase, which has been widely discussed in the past and is not currently recommended in both prevention and treatment of PTSD because of the lack of scientific evidence for their efficacy in this disorder and because they reduce the effectiveness of exposure psychotherapies. Moreover, drugs with addictive properties should be avoided given the high comorbidity with addictive disorders in these subjects [72, 73, 75].

Studies on other types of interventions, e.g., ketamine or 3,4-methylenedioxymethamphetamine (MDMA) in combination with psychotherapy, are still limited, although promising [76, 77].

17.6 Psychological Treatment for Collective Traumas

A critical task is to distinguish trauma survivors who will suffer transient stress reactions from those who will experience stress reactions that will develop into a more persistent mental disorder [78] and will need support.

EMDR and CBT are recommended for the treatment of PTSD [79, 80], although not often adequately implemented in clinical practice [81].

Referring to the natural disaster reported above, EMDR is included among the early psychological interventions, defined as treatment initiating within 3 months after the traumatic event to prevent or treat post-traumatic stress disorder, ongoing distress, or acute stress disorder.

In the Emilia Romagna earthquake, an early EMDR intervention was implemented in a large sample of individuals exposed to the disaster [82]. The study evaluated the effects of EMDR administered in the acute phase, while the shocks were still occurring, with severe aftershocks that went on for many months, preventing people from feeling safe at home or indoors. Results suggest that EMDR is a viable treatment option in response to a disaster and in reducing psychological distress, representing an acceptable strategy for acutely traumatized individuals [82].

Starting from the experience of treating survivors of the L'Aquila earthquake [83], a manualized CBT trauma intervention was developed for a "delayed" treatment [84].

American researchers have paid great attention to the development of specific treatments that help people to overcome the consequences of severe trauma, such as that following the terroristic attack on the Twin Towers in New York on September 11, 2001, in which almost 3000 people died [85], and following natural severe disasters, such as those caused by the hurricanes in Florida in 2004.

Hamblen et al. (2006) developed a specific cognitive behavioral treatment for the survivors of Hurricane Katrina in 2005 [86] and for those who survived the Hurricane Sandy in New York in 2012 [87]. The treatment, as part of a larger mental health trauma response, was designed to be implemented no sooner than 60 days post-trauma. This treatment is for individuals who show more than normal transient stress and who require more than traditional crisis counseling because of persistent post-traumatic symptoms that negatively affect their quality of life. The approach is transdiagnostic and multi-symptomatic.

Table 17.2 Sessions, content, and goals of the trauma-focused CBT in the Italian Manual [73]

Sessions	Content	Goals
1	Psychoeducation: Common reactions • Fear and anxiety • Anger • Sadness and depression • Guilt and shame Symptoms of depression Symptoms of anxiety Alcohol and substance use Sleep Diet Physical health Functioning (relationship, work, finances) Grief/bereavement Symptoms of post-traumatic stress disorder	To learn what the users experienced during the disaster and establish treatment goals To understand the users' symptoms and educate them about common post-disaster reactions To develop a case conceptualization of how the disaster currently impacts the person and to make the person feel that you have a handle on their problems and how to help them
2	Breathing retraining The importance of pleasant activities Pleasant activities list Scheduling pleasant activities Coping strategies Homeworks	To teach the person a strategy to control physical tension and anxiety through breathing so that they can apply it themselves Review the activities that the person finds pleasant and find ways to increase both pleasure and the number of activities to engage in
3	Understanding cognitive restructuring Guide to thoughts and feelings Upsetting situations log Homeworks	To have users understand the connection between their thoughts and feelings To have users understand that certain feelings are related to specific thoughts
4	Problematic thinking styles 5 steps of cognitive restructuring, CR The action plan Homeworks	To teach users to identify problematic thinking styles that they may be using To teach users the 5 steps of cognitive restructuring

(continued)

Table 17.2 (continued)

Sessions	Content	Goals
5	Problem-solving Homework	To teach clients the 6 steps of structured problem-solving
6–12	Practicing CR Identify trauma-related thoughts When the 5 steps aren't working Homeworks	To identify a problematic trauma-related thought, to challenge the thought, and to either come up with a new, more balanced thought or an action plan (problem-solving) for how to handle the upsetting situation in the future
13	Progress review and review of treatment Aftercare plan Conclude treatment	To review the three components of the treatment and remind users of the skills they have learned to cope with upsetting thoughts Plan the "after treatment" "Say goodbye" in a healthy way and, if necessary, refer the user to another specialist

The Italian CBT-trauma is a manualized, 13-session intervention that primarily focuses on identifying and challenging maladaptive trauma-related beliefs [84]. The intervention includes four main components: psychoeducation, breathing retraining, behavioral activation, and cognitive restructuring. Users receive a workbook and complete assignments to reinforce the skills they have learned in session [88]. Sessions, contents, and the main goals for every session are described in Table 17.2.

Starting from March 2011, at the end of the training carried out in L'Aquila conducted by Jennifer Gottlieb, the L'Aquila psychiatry group applied CBT focused on psychological suffering following natural disasters and significant traumas in around a hundred users showing persistent post-traumatic symptoms following the 2009 L'Aquila earthquake. Good improvements were observed at clinical level, with symptom reduction and restoring of functioning. Most users were also treated with psychopharmacological therapy (80% with antidepressants). This CBT trauma intervention is now routinely used by mental health professionals, with good clinical results.

17.7 Resilience and Post-traumatic Growth

As we have seen, traumatic events have many negative physical and psychological consequences. However, psychopathological symptoms do not necessarily develop after exposure to adversity, trauma, or other significant sources of stress, as the individual and the community can adapt to those events. Therefore, the concepts of resilience and post-traumatic growth (PTG) have recently been introduced into the psychological and psychiatric fields.

The term "resilience" traditionally defines the ability of a material to return to its original shape or position after being bent, compressed, or stretched, and has been used in the human sciences to refer to the ability of an individual to return to the level of functioning before the adverse event [89, 90]. Most of the available scientific literature conceptualizes it as an outcome, i.e., the absence of symptoms or the maintenance of a state of mental health after a trauma, with attention focused on the stress response systems. Alternative models based on the neurobiology of affiliation have been recently proposed, incorporating oxytocin, the affiliative brain, and biobehavioral synchrony as key elements. This model has emphasized the three tenets defining resilience: plasticity, sociality, and meaning [91].

The term post-traumatic growth (PTG) refers to the psychological changes resulting from a traumatic event, such as achieving a higher level of functioning compared to before the trauma [92, 93]. While the concept of PTG does not deny the adverse effects of trauma, it recognizes the possibility of growth that can occur along with pain and suffering [83, 92, 94]. PTG areas include appreciation for life, relationships with others, new possibilities, personal strength, and spiritual change [93]. It is interesting to note that even if female gender is a risk factor for developing PTSD, women tend to report more significant benefits than men. However, the data on the mechanisms underlying post-traumatic growth are still incomplete and often come from studies with significant methodological limitations. Thus, it is impossible to identify with certainty the factors contributing to positive outcomes following trauma [95, 96].

Overall, available data point to the multifactorial nature of resilience and post-traumatic growth. Being empowerable, resilience, and post-traumatic growth are potential targets for new intervention and prevention strategies for individuals and communities [97].

17.8 Beyond Individual Resilience: The Social Impact of Disaster and Resilience in the Community of L'Aquila

Disasters impact individuals and groups [98] and always have a severe social impact on the multiple dimensions of local community well-being.

Several studies have investigated the social consequences, not just the psychological ones caused by the L'Aquila earthquake, that caused a massive displacement of the population. The government constructed 19 new towns composed of two-and three-storey apartment buildings with pendulum base isolation, the project C.A.S.E (Complessi Antisismici Sostenibili ed. Ecocompatibili), and 24 villages of smaller prefabs, M.A.P. (Moduli Abitativi Provvisori) without base isolation [99]. They were located in isolated places, in conservation lands or farmland, far from the core city of L'Aquila (Fig. 17.2). The delivery of the C.A.S.E. units started on September 29, 2009, with about 500 apartments and continued at a pace of approximately 300 apartments a week until March 2010. The C.A.S.E. units cost more than 20 times compared

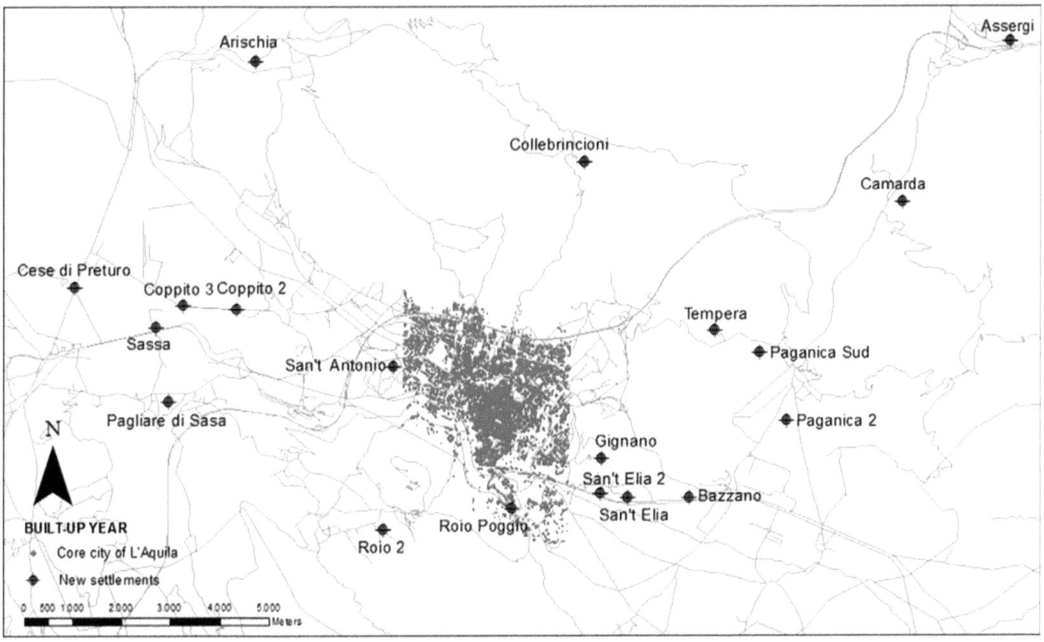

Fig. 17.2 Location of new settlements, inner city and old town in L'Aquila. Servizio per L'informazione Territoriale e la Telematica—Ufficio Sistema Informativo Geografico—Regione Abruzzo. MICRODIS Project—Commission's Sixth Framework Programme

to a basic prefabricated dwelling [100]. This quick and expensive housing solution involved problems such as lack of essential services, urban facilities (churches, schools, pharmacies, post offices, supermarkets, social centers, sports centers, and so on), limited public transportation (low and not reliable frequencies), social fragmentation, and functional living [99]. The social and logistic issues of new housing had a profound effect on the population as a whole, but mainly on older people, who were less self-sufficient in terms of mobility and were deprived of friendships, social gatherings, and places of worship, isolated and unable to re-establish their everyday lives or their contacts with friends [101]. Three years after the earthquake, older people living in the new towns and temporary housing of L'Aquila had a worse perception of their quality of life than those who owned or rented a house. Furthermore, immediately after the earthquake, a 26.9% increase in the number of hospitalizations due to cardiovascular diseases was found in older adults [102].

Spatial connectivity was identified as a recovery process indicator after the earthquake, integrating variables such as distance, travel time, and quality of public transportation service: the distance between the new settlements and the inner city strongly influenced the preference to either stay or move and the discomfort of their residents [99]. The analysis of the relationship between urban facilities, collaboration networks, and lack of spatial resilience in the recovery process in L'Aquila demonstrated a strong relationship where the preference to search for another housing site decreased with the increasing number of urban facilities in the settlement and increased with travel distance to the urban core of L'Aquila. The allocation of facilities to supply essential services seemed to neglect other community needs during recovery, reducing the community's resilience [103]. Indeed, the concept of "urban" depends not so much on the quantity of housing but more on the presence and quality of services.

Fragmentation and dispersion of inhabitants were (and still are) the main characteristics of the new socio-spatial configuration in the post-disaster period in L'Aquila [104]. In fact, resettling greatly impacts people and communities. The magnitude of its social impact typically dominates the life of the people and their community for many years [105].

In 2013, using the methodology of Participatory-Participating Research Action (PPRA), a widespread discomfort among the inhabitants of L'Aquila shaped by a negative rating on life conditions and context was found [106]: adults provided poor quality evaluations about the present and difficulties in figure out their future. For young people, even though the spatial projection into the present appeared more objective, the projection into the future turned out to be more pessimistic than adults. Finally, the discomfort was shaped by a deterioration in coexistence and a high perception of insecurity, especially among those living in the new residential earthquake-proofing complex CASE [106]. The author expressed her concern about the quality of the relationship between inhabitant and territory and the consequences on the population's comfort in the present and the future since they may influence individual behaviors (such as fear, loneliness, and alcohol abuse), as well as collective behaviors, (such as vandalism of public goods and spaces).

David Alexander, Professor at the Institute for Risk and Disaster Reduction at University College London, formerly Chief Senior Scientist at the Global Risk Forum in Davos, Switzerland (2011–2012), was very critical and equally lucid about the long-medium-term recovery processes after L'Aquila earthquake [107]. He discussed the first questionable policy decision in the L'Aquila case, where no measures were implemented to protect livelihoods and foster employment. Following the L'Aquila earthquake 2009, some 16,000 jobs were lost in the L'Aquila province, which were not recouped in the following 2 years [108]. Economic and employment difficulties were the common denominator of both PTSD (4.1%) and major depression (5.8%) [109]. Individuals with economic difficulties were nearly twice as likely to develop PTSD symptoms (odds ratio [OR] = 2.3) compared to individuals without economic difficulties, and they were more than three times more likely to develop MD (OR = 3.5).

As for the Val Belice earthquake in Western Sicily, Alexander foresaw economic stagnation, stalled reconstruction, alienation of the local population, fiscal deprivation, and corruption, which tend to perpetuate rather than reducing vulnerability to disasters. He argued that in the Belice and L'Aquila cases, the central government virtually suppressed local governance or direct democratic participation in recovery decision-making with its stop-start paternalism [107].

Sharing the vision of poor management of the disaster recovery process, Imperiale and Vanclay adopted the term "disaster capitalism" [110]. Their critiques focused on the actions of the Government of Italy and the Department of Civil Protection, paying little attention to the role of local authorities, hindering local communities from learning, transforming, and building resilience, and then facilitating corruption.

The disaster recovery should include local communities and initiatives in decision-making, consistent with the affected places' spatial, socioeconomic, and cultural complexity. Indeed, the obstacles to local community participation, because of the city's spatial fragmentation and the lack of common facilities for inhabitants to meet, were barriers to develop collaborative networks necessary to build resilience.

The increase in the use of internet technologies by local citizens who utilized platforms such as Facebook, Twitter, YouTube, and blogs represented an attempt to reconstruct the offline local public spaces of communication damaged or destroyed by the quake [111, 112]. A year after the tragedy, on April 11, 2010, to protest against the Italian state due to the problem of the debris that continued to be unremoved from the histori-

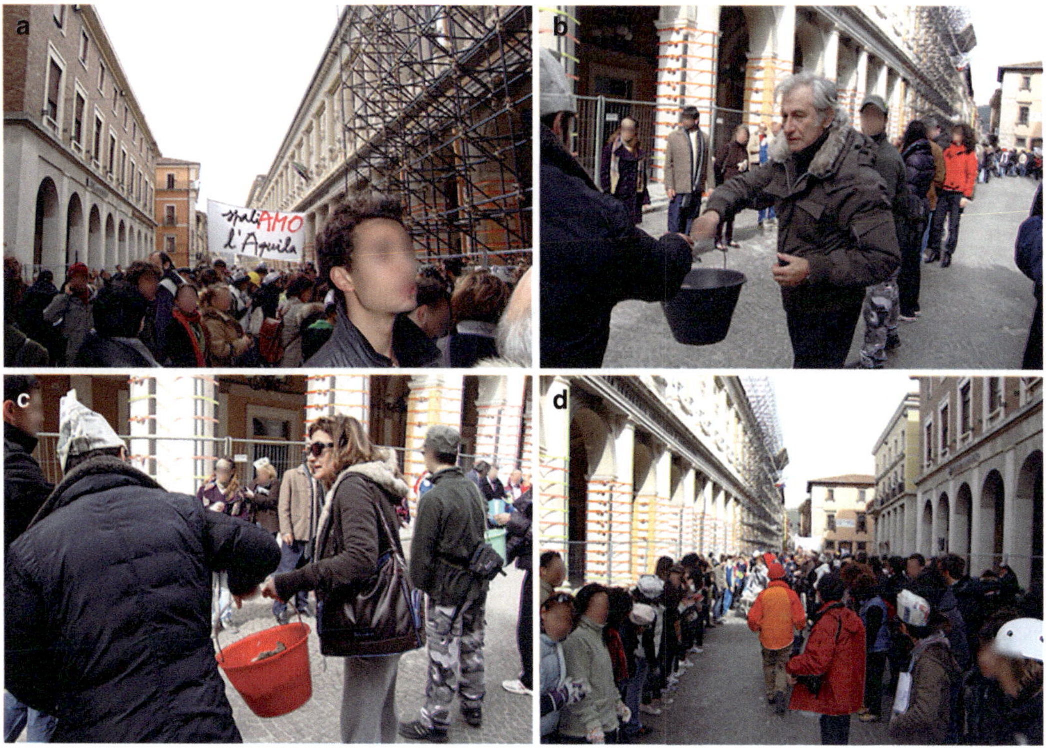

Fig. 17.3 Participation in the protest of the people of the wheelbarrows, L'Aquila, April 11, 2010. (Photo R.R.). (**b**) Prof. Massimo Casacchia, Full Professor of Psychiatry, Uiversity of L'Aquila (Italy) and Director of the Psychiatric Ward (actually Professor Emeritus of Psychiatry), actively participates in the protest with a bucket of debris in the human chain of citizens, as does R.R. with the red bucktet (**c**)

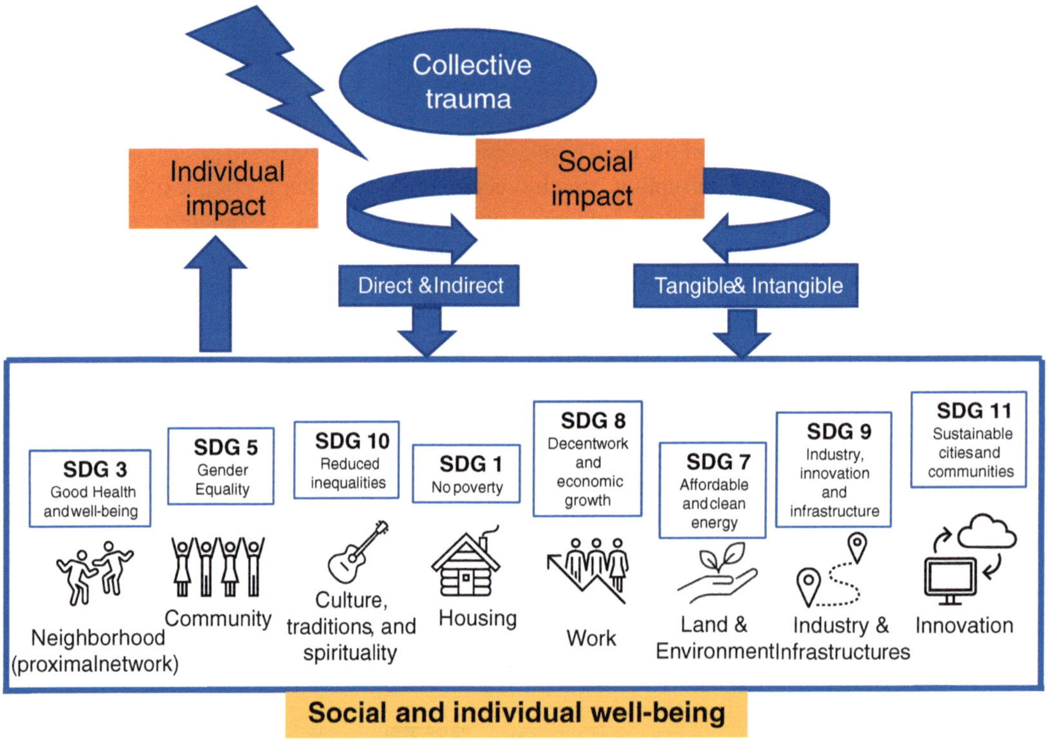

Fig. 17.4 The social impacts of disasters (collective traumas). (Modified by Imperiale and Vanclay [110, 114]; Smyth and Vanclay [115])

cal city center, some citizens decided to flee into the streets with their wheelbarrows and autonomously remove the rubble. They built a human chain, passing buckets from hand to hand, claiming to be an active part of the reconstruction (Fig. 17.3). These people aim to involve citizenship in the decisional processes regarding L'Aquila reconstruction, in contrast to the government's bottom-up strategies.

Despite this attempt, if it seems, therefore, difficult to talk about disaster resilience (DR), as a shared and dynamic process integrating the capacities of individuals and communities, for the L'Aquila 2009 earthquake, still the contribution of Forino reported emergent groups (EGs), as a potential resource for DR [113]. EGs were defined as "private citizens who work together in pursuit of collective goals relevant to actual or potential disasters but whose organization has not yet become institutionalized." He analyzed the EG's ideas and initiatives in reconstructing the city, suggesting that integrating these contributions into institutional strategies would have more successfully targeted the needs of local communities during reconstruction [113].

The long-lasting social and economic consequences of the earthquake affecting the community, with more than 10,000 people still living in temporary housing, and slow rebuilding [114] and the COVID-19 pandemic have led to a situation where, for L'Aquila residents, life in the town has never truly "returned to normal" [63]. Anyway, in L'Aquila, since April 5, 2010, every year at night, a long torchlight residents' procession winds through the city to remember the victims of the seismic event in a collective survival identity ritual and to promote hope in the future.

Inspired by the Social Framework for Projects [115] and the social disaster impact described by Imperiale and Vanclay [114], we propose a model to describe the social impact of disasters and the main affected areas (Fig. 17.4) based on the Sustainable Development Goals (SDGs) of the 2030 Agenda, which include a set of 17 SDGs related to ending poverty, fighting inequality and injustice, and tackling climate change [116]. As depicted in Fig. 17.3, all the areas similarly contribute to social and individual well-being after a collective trauma, and every distinction between these two dimensions sounds artificial, unifying the concept of biopsychosocial well-being as a whole.

17.9 Conclusions

This chapter is not intended to exhaust the broad issues related to individual and collective traumas. Indeed, traumas have assumed an ever-increasing importance, with particular reference to studies on their impact on life trajectories. Exposure to severe stressors and subsequent traumas can accumulate and affect individuals' epigenetic, psychosocial, physiological, and behavioral attributes and social conditions in which families, communities, and social groups live and work [117]. Likewise, social and economic inequities may contribute to poor mental health outcomes. The task of psychiatrists is to work for the early detection of traumas and conduct integrated interventions to contain psychopathology and mitigate social hazards.

References

1. Kolaitis G, Olff M (2017) Psychotraumatology in Greece. Eur J Psychotraumatol 8(Suppl 4):135175
2. Heber A, Testa V, Groll D, Ritchie K, Tam-Seto L, Mulligan A et al (2023) Glossary of terms: a shared understanding of the common terms used to describe psychological trauma, version 3.0. Health Promot Chronic Dis Prev Can 43(10–11):S1–S999
3. Kock WJ, Douglas KS, Nicholls TL, O'Neill ML (2005) Psychological injuries: forensic assessment, treatment, and law. Oxford University Press, Oxford
4. Harrington R (1996) The "railway spine" diagnosis and Victorian responses to PTSD. J Psychosom Res 40(1):11–14
5. Friedman JM (2013/2024) History of PTSD in veterans: Civil War to DSM-5. https://www.ptsd.va.gov/understand/what/history_ptsd.asp#:~:text=In%201952%2C%20the%20American%20Psychiatric,such%20as%20disaster%20or%20combat
6. American Psychiatric Association (1952) Diagnostic and statistical manual of mental disorders. American Psychiatric Association, Washington, DC
7. American Psychiatric Association (1968) Diagnostic and statistical manual of mental disorders, DMS-II, 2nd edn. American Psychiatric Association, Washington, DC
8. American Psychiatric Association (1980) Diagnostic and statistical manual of mental disorders, DSM-III, 3rd edn. American Psychiatric Association, Washington, DC
9. American Psychiatric Association (2013) Diagnostic and statistical manual of mental disorders, DSM-5, 5th edn. American Psychiatric Association, Washington, DC
10. American Psychiatric Association (2022) Diagnostic and statistical manual of mental disorders, DSM-5-TR, 5th edn. Text revision. American Psychiatric Association, Washington, DC
11. Kessler RC, Sonnega A, Bromet E, Hughes M, Nelson CB (1995) Posttraumatic stress disorder in the National Comorbidity Survey. Arch Gen Psychiatry 52(12):1048–1060
12. Magruder KM, Goldberg J, Forsberg CW, Friedman MJ, Litz BT, Vaccarino V et al (2016) Long-term trajectories of PTSD in Vietnam-era veterans: the course and consequences of PTSD in twins. J Trauma Stress 29(1):5–16
13. Mgoqi-Mbalo N, Zhang M, Ntuli S (2017) Risk factors for PTSD and depression in female survivors of rape. Psychol Trauma 9(3):301–308
14. Friedman MJ, Resick PA, Bryant RA, Brewin CR (2011) Considering PTSD for DSM-5. Depress Anxiety 28(9):750–769
15. Schnurr PP, Lunney CA (2016) Symptom benchmarks of improved quality of life in PTSD. Depress Anxiety 33(3):247–255
16. Glassman LH, Mackintosh MA, Talkovsky A, Wells SY, Walter KH, Wickramasinghe I et al (2019) Quality of life following treatment for PTSD: comparison of videoconferencing and in-person modalities. J Telemed Telecare 25(2):123–127
17. Bosch J, Mackintosh MA, Wells SY, Wickramasinghe I, Glassman LH, Morland LA (2020) PTSD treatment response and quality of life in women with childhood trauma histories. Psychol Trauma 12(1):55–63
18. Chou PH, Ito M, Horikoshi M (2020) Associations between PTSD symptoms and suicide risk: a comparison of 4-factor and 7-factor models. J Psychiatr Res 129:47–52
19. Holliday R, Hoffmire CA, Martin WB, Hoff RA, Monteith LL (2021) Associations between justice involvement and PTSD and depressive symptoms, suicidal ideation, and suicide attempt among post-9/11 veterans. Psychol Trauma 13(7):730–739
20. Sareen J, Erickson J, Medved MI, Asmundson GJ, Enns MW, Stein M et al (2013) Risk factors for post-injury mental health problems. Depress Anxiety 30(4):321–327

21. Fiorillo A, Sampogna G, Giallonardo V, Del Vecchio V, Luciano M, Albert U, Carmassi C, Carrà G, Cirulli F, Dell'Osso B, Nanni MG, Pompili M, Sani G, Tortorella A, Volpe U (2020) Effects of the lockdown on the mental health of the general population during the COVID-19 pandemic in Italy: Results from the COMET collaborative network. Eur Psychiatry 28;63(1):e87. https://doi.org/10.1192/j.eurpsy.2020.89.
22. Zhonghu Z (2015) A systematic review of the relationship between ASD and PTSD. J Int Psychiatry
23. Terr LC (1991) Childhood traumas: an outline and overview. Am J Psychiatry 148(1):10–20
24. Stein DJ, Koenen KC, Friedman MJ, Hill E, McLaughlin KA, Petukhova M et al (2013) Dissociation in posttraumatic stress disorder: evidence from the world mental health surveys. Biol Psychiatry 73(4):302–312
25. Foote B, Smolin Y, Neft DI, Lipschitz D (2008) Dissociative disorders and suicidality in psychiatric outpatients. J Nerv Ment Dis 196(1):29–36
26. Mylle J, Maes M (2004) Partial posttraumatic stress disorder revisited. J Affect Disord 78(1):37–48
27. Dell'Osso L, Carmassi C, Rucci P, Conversano C, Shear MK, Calugi S, Maser JD, Endicott J, Fagiolini A, Cassano GB (2009) A multidimensional spectrum approach to post-traumatic stress disorder: comparison between the structured clinical interview for trauma and loss spectrum (SCI-TALS) and the self-report instrument (TALS-SR). Compr Psychiatry 50(5):485–490
28. Dell'Osso L, Carmassi C, Massimetti G, Conversano C, Daneluzzo E, Riccardi I et al (2011) Impact of traumatic loss on post-traumatic spectrum symptoms in high school students after the L'Aquila 2009 earthquake in Italy. J Affect Disord 134(1–3):59–64
29. Carmassi C, Akiskal HS, Yong SS, Stratta P, Calderani E, Massimetti E, Akiskal KK, Rossi A, Dell'Osso L (2013) Post-traumatic stress disorder in DSM-5: estimates of prevalence and criteria comparison versus DSM-IV-TR in a non-clinical sample of earthquake survivors. J Affect Disord 151(3):843–848
30. Carmassi C, Akiskal HS, Bessonov D, Massimetti G, Calderani E, Stratta P, Rossi A, Dell'Osso L (2014) Gender differences in DSM-5 versus DSM-IV-TR PTSD prevalence and criteria comparison among 512 survivors to the L'Aquila earthquake. J Affect Disord 160:55–61
31. Carmassi C, Bertelloni CA, Cordone A, Cappelli A, Massimetti E, Dell'Oste V, Dell'Osso L (2020) Exploring mood symptoms overlap in PTSD diagnosis: ICD-11 and DSM-5 criteria compared in a sample of subjects with bipolar disorder. J Affect Disord 276:205–211
32. WHO (2019/2021) International classification of diseases, eleventh revision (ICD-11). WHO, Geneva
33. Rossi R, Socci V, Pacitti F, Carmassi C, Rossi A, Di Lorenzo G et al (2022) The Italian version of the international trauma questionnaire: symptom and network structure of post-traumatic stress disorder and complex post-traumatic stress disorder in a sample of late adolescents exposed to a natural disaster. Front Psych 13:859877
34. Stein DJ, Seedat S, Iversen A, Wessely S (2007) Post-traumatic stress disorder: medicine and politics. Lancet 369(9556):139–144
35. Carmassi C, Conversano C, Pinori M, Bertelloni CA, Dalle Luche R, Gesi C, et al (2016) [Complicated grief in DSM-5 era]. Riv Psichiatr 51(6):231–237
36. Zisook S, Iglewicz A, Avanzino J, Maglione J, Glorioso D, Zetumer S et al (2014) Bereavement: course, consequences, and care. Curr Psychiatry Rep 16(10):482
37. Carmassi C, Bertelloni CA, Dell'Osso L (2018) Grief reactions in diagnostic classifications of mental disorders. In: Bui E (ed) Clinical handbook of bereavement and grief reactions. Humana Press, Boston, pp 301–332
38. Mughal S, Azhar Y, Mahon MM, Siddiqui WJ (2023) Grief reaction and prolonged grief disorder. StatPearls Publishing, Treasure Island
39. Dell'Osso L, Carmassi C, Musetti L, Socci C, Shear MK, Conversano C, Maremmani I, Perugi G (2012). Lifetime mood symptoms and adult separation anxiety in patients with complicated grief and/or post-traumatic stress disorder: a preliminary report. Psychiatry Res 15;198(3):436–40
40. Kersting A, Brahler E, Glaesmer H, Wagner B (2011) Prevalence of complicated grief in a representative population-based sample. J Affect Disord 131(1–3):339–343
41. Shear MK, Simon N, Wall M, Zisook S, Neimeyer R, Duan N et al (2011) Complicated grief and related bereavement issues for DSM-5. Depress Anxiety 28(2):103–117
42. Lichtenthal WG, Cruess DG, Prigerson HG (2004) A case for establishing complicated grief as a distinct mental disorder in DSM-V. Clin Psychol Rev 24(6):637–662
43. Casacchia M, Pollice R, Roncone R (2012) The narrative epidemiology of L'Aquila 2009 earthquake. Epidemiol Psychiatr Sci 21(1):13–21
44. Stratta P, Rossetti MC, di Michele V, Rossi A (2016) Effects on health of the L'Aquila (Central Italy) 2009 earthquake. Epidemiol Prev 40(2 Suppl 1):22–31
45. Ripoll Gallardo A, Alesina M, Pacelli B, Serrone D, Iacutone G, Faggiano F et al (2016) [Medium- and long-term health effects of the L'Aquila earthquake (Central Italy, 2009) and of other earthquakes in high-income countries: a systematic review]. Epidemiol Prev 40(2 Suppl 1):14–21
46. Casacchia M, Bianchini V, Mazza M, Pollice R, Roncone R (2013) Acute stress reactions and associated factors in the help-seekers after the L'Aquila earthquake. Psychopathology 46(2):120–130

47. Pollice R, Bianchini V, di Mauro S, Mazza M, Verni L, Roncone R et al (2012) Cognitive function and clinical symptoms in first-episode psychosis and chronic schizophrenia before and after the 2009 L'Aquila earthquake. Early Interv Psychiatry 6(2):153–158
48. Dell'Osso L, Carmassi C, Massimetti G, Daneluzzo E, Di Tommaso S, Rossi A (2011) Full and partial PTSD among young adult survivors 10 months after the L'Aquila 2009 earthquake: gender differences. J Affect Disord 131(1–3):79–83
49. Roncone R, Giusti L, Mazza M, Bianchini V, Ussorio D, Pollice R et al (2013) Persistent fear of aftershocks, impairment of working memory, and acute stress disorder predict post-traumatic stress disorder: 6-month follow-up of help seekers following the L'Aquila earthquake. Springerplus 2(1):636
50. Dell'Osso L, Carmassi C, Massimetti G, Stratta P, Riccardi I, Capanna C, Akiskal KK, Akiskal HS, Rossi A (2013) Age, gender and epicenter proximity effects on post-traumatic stress symptoms in L'Aquila 2009 earthquake survivors. J Affect Disord 146(2):174–180
51. Rossi A, Maggio R, Riccardi I, Allegrini F, Stratta P (2011) A quantitative analysis of antidepressant and antipsychotic prescriptions following an earthquake in Italy. J Trauma Stress 24(1):129–132
52. Stratta P, de Cataldo S, Bonanni RL, Rossi A (2015) Community mental health service utilization after the L'Aquila earthquake. Community Ment Health J 51(4):504–508
53. Pollice R, Bianchini V, Roncone R, Casacchia M (2011) Marked increase in substance use among young people after L'Aquila earthquake. Eur Child Adolesc Psychiatry 20(8):429–430
54. Masedu F, Mazza M, Di Giovanni C, Calvarese A, Tiberti S, Sconci V et al (2014) Facebook, quality of life, and mental health outcomes in post-disaster urban environments: the L'Aquila earthquake experience. Front Public Health 2:286
55. Calder K, D'Aeth L, Turner S, Begg A, Veer E, Scott J et al (2020) Evaluation of the all right? Campaign's Facebook intervention post-disaster in Canterbury, New Zealand. Health Promot Int 35(1):111–122
56. Rotondi L, Zuddas M, Marsella P, Rosati P (2019) A Facebook page created soon after the Amatrice earthquake for deaf adults and children, families, and caregivers provides an easy communication tool and social satisfaction in maxi-emergencies. Prehosp Disaster Med 34(2):137–141
57. Carmassi C, Bertelloni CA, Dell'Oste V, Luperini C, Marazziti D, Rossi R et al (2021) PTSD and suicidal behaviors amongst L'Aquila 2009 earthquake young survivors. Front Public Health 9:590753
58. Stratta P, Capanna C, Riccardi I, Carmassi C, Piccinni A, Dell'Osso L, Rossi A (2012) Suicidal intention and negative spiritual coping one year after the earthquake of L'Aquila (Italy). J Affect Disord 136(3):1227–1231
59. Dell'Osso L, Stratta P, Conversano C, Massimetti E, Akiskal KK, Akiskal HS et al (2014) Lifetime mania is related to post-traumatic stress symptoms in high school students exposed to the 2009 L'Aquila earthquake. Compr Psychiatry 55(2):357–362
60. Maj M, Starace F, Crepet P, Lobrace S, Veltro F, De Marco F et al (1989) Prevalence of psychiatric disorders among subjects exposed to a natural disaster. Acta Psychiatr Scand 79(6):544–549
61. Bland SH, O'Leary ES, Farinaro E, Jossa F, Trevisan M (1996) Long-term psychological effects of natural disasters. Psychosom Med 58(1):18–24
62. Bland SH, O'Leary ES, Farinaro E, Jossa F, Krogh V, Violanti JM et al (1997) Social network disturbances and psychological distress following earthquake evacuation. J Nerv Ment Dis 185(3):188–194
63. Bland SH, Valoroso L, Stranges S, Strazzullo P, Farinaro E, Trevisan M (2005) Long-term follow-up of psychological distress following earthquake experiences among working Italian males: a cross-sectional analysis. J Nerv Ment Dis 193(6):420–423
64. Catapano F, Malafronte R, Lepre F, Cozzolino P, Arnone R, Lorenzo E et al (2001) Psychological consequences of the 1998 landslide in Sarno, Italy: a community study. Acta Psychiatr Scand 104(6):438–442
65. Priebe S, Grappasonni I, Mari M, Dewey M, Petrelli F, Costa A (2009) Posttraumatic stress disorder six months after an earthquake: findings from a community sample in a rural region in Italy. Soc Psychiatry Psychiatr Epidemiol 44(5):393–397
66. Petrucci E, Cofini V, Pizzi B, Sollecchia G, Cascella M, Stefano N et al (2023) Health status perception and psychological sequelae in buried victims: an observational study on survivors of the earthquake in Amatrice (Italy), three years later. Prehosp Disaster Med 38(2):193–198
67. Priebe S, Marchi F, Bini L, Flego M, Costa A, Galeazzi G (2011) Mental disorders, psychological symptoms and quality of life 8 years after an earthquake: findings from a community sample in Italy. Soc Psychiatry Psychiatr Epidemiol 46(7):615–621
68. Altamore F, Grappasonni I, Laxhman N, Scuri S, Petrelli F, Grifantini G et al (2020) Psychological symptoms and quality of life after repeated exposure to earthquake: a cohort study in Italy. PLoS One 15(5):e0233172
69. Starace F, Mungai F, Sarti E, Addabbo T (2016) Being hit twice: the psychological consequences of the economic crisis and an earthquake. Int J Soc Psychiatry 62(4):345–349
70. Pazderka H, Shalaby R, Eboreime E, Mao W, Obuobi-Donkor G, Agyapong B et al (2022) Isolation, economic precarity, and previous mental health issues as predictors of PTSD status in females living in Fort McMurray during COVID-19. Front Psych 13:837713
71. Giusti L, Mammarella S, Del Vecchio S, Salza A, Casacchia M, Roncone R (2023) Deepening depres-

sion in women balancing work-life responsibilities and caregiving during the COVID-19 pandemic: findings from gender-specific face-to-face street interviews conducted in Italy. Behav Sci (Basel) 13(11):892
72. The National Institute for Health and Care Excellence (2018) Post-traumatic stress disorder guideline. https://www.nice.org.uk/guidance/ng116/resources/posttraumatic-stress-disorder-pdf-66141601777861
73. Williams T, Phillips NJ, Stein DJ, Ipser JC (2022) Pharmacotherapy for post traumatic stress disorder (PTSD). Cochrane Database Syst Rev 3(3):CD002795
74. Compean E, Hamner M (2019) Posttraumatic stress disorder with secondary psychotic features (PTSD-SP): diagnostic and treatment challenges. Prog Neuro-Psychopharmacol Biol Psychiatry 88:265–275
75. Jessell L, Stanhope V, Manuel JI, Mateu-Gelabert P (2020) Factors associated with benzodiazepine prescribing in community mental health settings. J Subst Abus Treat 109:56–60
76. Yavi M, Lee H, Henter ID, Park LT, Zarate CA Jr (2022) Ketamine treatment for depression: a review. Discov Ment Health 2(1):9
77. Latimer D, Stocker MD, Sayers K, Green J, Kaye AM, Abd-Elsayed A, Cornett EM, Kaye AD, Varrassi G, Viswanath O, Urits I (2021) MDMA to treat PTSD in adults. Psychopharmacol Bull 51(3):125–149
78. Bryant RA (2011) Acute stress disorder as a predictor of posttraumatic stress disorder: a systematic review. J Clin Psychiatry 72(2):233–239
79. International Society for Traumatic Stress Studies (2018) Posttraumatic stress disorder prevention and treatment guidelines: methodology and recommendations. http://www.istss.org/getattachment/Treating-Trauma/New-ISTSS-Prevention-and-Treatment-Guidelines/ISTSS_PreventionTreatmentGuidelines_FNL-March-19-2019.pdf.aspx
80. Watkins LE, Sprang KR, Rothbaum BO (2018) Treating PTSD: a review of evidence-based psychotherapy interventions. Front Behav Neurosci 12:258
81. Neill EL, Zarling A, Weems CF (2023) Therapist use of cognitive behavior therapy and eye movement desensitization and reprocessing components for the treatment of posttraumatic stress disorder in practice settings. Front Psychol 14:1158344
82. Saltini A, Rebecchi D, Callerame C, Fernandez I, Bergonzini E, Starace F (2018) Early eye movement desensitisation and reprocessing (EMDR) intervention in a disaster mental health care context. Psychol Health Med 23(3):285–294
83. Bianchini V, Roncone R, Giusti L, Casacchia M, Cifone MG, Pollice R (2015) PTSD growth and substance abuse among a college student community: coping strategies after 2009 L'Aquila earthquake. Clin Pract Epidemiol Ment Health 11:140–143
84. Hamblen JL, Roncone R, Giusti L, Casacchia M (2018) La sofferenza psicologica da disastri naturali e traumi importanti. Trattamento cognitivo-comportamentale. Manuale per gli operatori. Il Pensiero Scientifico Editore, Roma
85. Silver RC, Holman EA, McIntosh DN, Poulin M, Gil-Rivas V (2002) Nationwide longitudinal study of psychological responses to September 11. JAMA 288(10):1235–1244
86. Hamblen JL, Norris FH, Pietruszkiewicz S, Gibson LE, Naturale A, Louis C (2009) Cognitive behavioral therapy for postdisaster distress: a community based treatment program for survivors of Hurricane Katrina. Admin Pol Ment Health 36(3):206–214
87. Hamblen JL, Norris FH, Symon KA, Bow TE (2017) Cognitive behavioral therapy for postdisaster distress: a promising transdiagnostic approach to treating disaster survivors. Psychol Trauma 9(Suppl 1):130–136
88. Hamblen JL, Roncone R, Giusti L, Casacchia M (2018) La sofferenza psicologica da disastri naturali e traumi importanti. Trattamento cognitivo-comportamentale. Quaderno di lavoro per l'utente
89. Cathomas F, Murrough JW, Nestler EJ, Han MH, Russo SJ (2019) Neurobiology of resilience: interface between mind and body. Biol Psychiatry 86(6):410–420
90. Babić R, Babić M, Rastović P, Ćurlin M, Šimić J, Mandić K, Pavlović K (2020) Resilience in health and illness. Psychiatr Danub 32(Suppl 2):226–232
91. Feldman R (2020) What is resilience: an affiliative neuroscience approach. World Psychiatry 19(2):132–150
92. Senol-Durak E, Di Tella M, Romeo A (2023) Editorial: post-traumatic growth. Front Psychol 14:1227892
93. Magne H, Jaafari N, Voyer M (2021) [Post-traumatic growth: some conceptual considerations]. Encéphale 47(2):143–150
94. Bianchini V, Giusti L, Salza A, Cofini V, Cifone MG, Casacchia M et al (2017) Moderate depression promotes posttraumatic growth (Ptg): a young population survey 2 years after the 2009 L'Aquila earthquake. Clin Pract Epidemiol Ment Health 13:10–19
95. Carmassi C, Stratta P, Massimetti G, Bertelloni CA, Conversano C, Cremone IM, Miccoli M, Baggiani A, Rossi A, Dell'Osso L (2014) New DSM-5 maladaptive symptoms in PTSD: gender differences and correlations with mood spectrum symptoms in a sample of high school students following survival of an earthquake. Ann Gen Psychiatry 13:28.
96. Jayawickreme E, Infurna FJ, Alajak K, Blackie LER, Chopik WJ, Chung JM et al (2021) Posttraumatic growth as positive personality change: challenges, opportunities, and recommendations. J Pers 89(1):145–165

97. Berkes F, Ross H (2013) Community resilience: toward an integrated approach. Soc Nat Resour 26(1):5–20
98. Tierney KJ (2007) Businesses and disasters: vulnerability, impacts, and recovery. In: Rodríguez H, Quarantelli EL, Dynes RR (eds) Handbook of disaster research. Springer, New York, pp 275–296
99. Contreras D, Blaschke T, Kienberger S, Zeil P (2013) Spatial connectivity as a recovery process indicator: the L'Aquila earthquake. Technol Forecast Soc Chang 80(9):1782–1803
100. Calvi, Michele G (2009) Reconstruction between temporary and definitive: the CASE project. Progettazione Sismica 3:221–250
101. Giuliani AR, Mattei A, Santilli F, Clori G, Scatigna M, Fabiani L (2014) Well-being and perceived quality of life in elderly people displaced after the earthquake in L'Aquila, Italy. J Community Health 39(3):531–537
102. Sofia S, Melone A, Manzoli L, De Ciantis P, Varrato E, Di Filippo R et al (2012) Cardiovascular and cerebrovascular events pre- and post-earthquake of 6 April 2009: the Abruzzo's experience. Am J Hypertens 25(5):556–560
103. Contreras D, Blaschke T, Hodgson ME (2017) Lack of spatial resilience in a recovery process: case L'Aquila, Italy. In: Technological forecasting and social change, vol 121. Elsevier, Amsterdam, pp 76–88
104. Castellani S, Palma F, Calandra LM (2016) [The new territorial configuration of L'Aquila (Central Italy) after the 2009 earthquake and places and behaviours changes of everyday life]. Epidemiol Prev 40(2 Suppl 1):82–92
105. Vanclay F (2017) Project-induced displacement and resettlement: from impoverishment risks to an opportunity for development? Impact Assess Proj Apprais 35(1):3–21
106. Calandra LM (2016) [Between perception and reality: towards an assessment of socio-territorial discomfort in L'Aquila (Central Italy) after the earthquake]. Epidemiol Prev 40(2 Suppl 1):72–81
107. Alexander D (2013) An evaluation of medium-term recovery processes after the 6 April 2009 earthquake in L'Aquila, Central Italy. Environ Hazards 12(1):60–73
108. SVIMEZ (2009) Rapporto 2009 sull'Economia del Mezzogiorno. Il Mulino Editore, Bologna
109. Gigantesco A, Mirante N, Granchelli C, Diodati G, Cofini V, Mancini C et al (2013) Psychopathological chronic sequelae of the 2009 earthquake in L'Aquila, Italy. J Affect Disord 148(2–3):265–271
110. Imperiale AJ, Vanclay F (2021) The mechanism of disaster capitalism and the failure to build community resilience: learning from the 2009 earthquake in L'Aquila, Italy. Disasters 45(3):555–576
111. Farinosi M, Treré E (2010) Inside the "People of the Wheelbarrows": participation between online and offline dimension in the postquake social movement. J Community Inform 6(3)
112. Farinosi M, Treré E (2011) Between the square and the net: civic engagement and participation in a post-earthquake movement. SSRN Electron J
113. Forino G (2014) Disaster recovery: narrating the resilience process in the reconstruction of L'Aquila (Italy). Geografisk Tidsskrift-Danish J Geogr 115(1):1–13
114. Imperiale AJ, Vanclay F (2021) Conceptualizing community resilience and the social dimensions of risk to overcome barriers to disaster risk reduction and sustainable development. Sustain Dev 29(5):891–905
115. Smyth E, Vanclay F (2017) The Social Framework for Projects: a conceptual but practical model to assist in assessing, planning and managing the social impacts of projects. Impact Assess Proj Apprais 35(1):65–80
116. United Nations (2015) Sustainable development goals. https://sustainabledevelopment.un.org
117. Allen J, Balfour R, Bell R, Marmot M (2014) Social determinants of mental health. Int Rev Psychiatry 26(4):392–407

Urbanization and Mental Health 18

Mauro Percudani, Matteo Porcellana,
Ilaria Di Bernardo, and Carla Morganti

Abstract

Almost 55% of today's population live in cities and this rate is expected to increase in the next decades. Urbanization is a direct consequence of globalization as well as industrialization, social migration, and economic and political transitions.

Urbanization affects mental health through social, economic, and environmental factors. It has been shown that common mental syndromes are highly prevalent in the cities, even if many data are frequently controversial.

Social disparities, social insecurity, pollution, and lack of contact with nature are some of recognized factors affecting urban mental health.

We begin by exploring the neurobiological processes mediating the impact of urbanization on mental health.

Subsequently, we delve into the link among urbanicity and risk of psychosis, depressive disorders, suicide, and addiction disorders.

Furthermore, we explore patterns of care for psychiatric patients living in big cities.

This chapter underscores the critical importance of considering mental health in the context of increasing urbanization.

Sustainable urbanization is key to successful development. Well-managed urbanization, informed by an understanding of population trends over the long run, can help to maximize the benefits of agglomeration while minimizing environmental degradation and other potential adverse impacts of growing number of city dwellers. Health, social, and economic professionals should form partnerships for operational preventive and service solutions.

Adequate policies to adapt to that process should be advocated and pursued. Urban mental health may be improved by designing cities to provide residents with regular access to green spaces, opportunities for physical activities, facilitated social interactions, and fostered feelings of safety.

Keywords

Urbanization · Neurourbanism · Psychosis
Depressive disorders · Addiction disorders
Patterns of care

M. Percudani (✉)
Departments of Mental Health and Addiction Services, Niguarda Hospital, Milan, Italy

Dipartimento di Salute Mentale e delle Dipendenze, ASST GOM "Niguarda", Milan, Italy
e-mail: mauro.percudani@ospedaleniguarda.it

M. Porcellana · I. Di Bernardo · C. Morganti
Departments of Mental Health and Addiction Services, Niguarda Hospital, Milan, Italy
e-mail: matteo.porcellana@ospedaleniguarda.it; ilaria.dibernardo@ospedaleniguarda.it; carla.morganti@ospedaleniguarda.it

A. Fiorillo, S. De Giorgi (eds.), *Social Determinants of Mental Health*, Sustainable Development Goals Series, https://doi.org/10.1007/978-3-031-70165-8_18

18.1 Introduction

Today, almost 55% of the population live in cities and this rate is expected to increase in the next decades. Urbanization is a direct consequence of globalization as well as of industrialization, social migration, economic turmoil, and political transitions [1]. Global megatrends, including climate change and urbanization, are shaping, and changing rapidly the way we live. These changes have had and will continue to have an effect on our health and well-being [2].

Megacities are intended when the population is over ten million, like Mexico City, Sao Paulo, and Mumbai, where we observe a rapid and massive growth and expansion. There are problems with urban sprawl or conurbation, emerging favelas, and other complex social phenomena. But the effect of urbanization on health can be observed also in smaller European cities, such as London, Paris, Milan, and Rome.

In many megacities and in mid-size cities, urbanization is associated with the following risk factors: increased population density, socioeconomic disparities (e.g., poverty, social isolation), environmental pollution (e.g., heavy metals, traffic pollution, noise exposure), lack of natural spaces, and social stressors (such as high social demands, social instability, perceived insecurity, inequalities).

Globalization increases the move of people both within country and across countries. Migration is a global reality of our time. There are two types of migration: internal (rural to urban) migration and international migration, mostly from disadvantaged countries to more developed economies. Both processes may flow from premigration triggers and decisions to the migration itself to the postmigration adaptation.

International migrants may be pushed out of their origin-homes not only by poverty, but also because of violent conflicts, unsafe life, oppression, and discrimination. Their migration journey may be arduous and dangerous. Upon arrival at destination, they might confront hostile, unwelcoming, and entrenched residents. They need to adapt to a different language and culture. The cultural adaptation is easier for younger people and may be leveraged to accelerate and enhance assimilation. Some mental health problems, including depression and posttraumatic stress disorder (PTSD), are often the result of the journey. Thus, urbanization may produce several health-related physical and mental health problems.

Urbanization affects mental health through social, economic, and environmental factors. It has been shown that common mental disorders are highly prevalent in the cities, even if data are still controversial. Social disparities, social insecurity, pollution, and lack of contact with nature are some of recognized factors affecting urban mental health [3].

Cities can expose vulnerable people to socio-economic disparities and discrimination, but also to a sensory input overload. At the contrary, nature and natural landscapes may reduce stress with an effect on the autonomic nervous system [4]. Living in or growing up in urban environments is associated with an increased prevalence of mental disorders [5]. Findings are most robust for urban residence at birth and during childhood, suggesting an important impact of urban factors on the developing organism [6], with higher rates of autism spectrum disorders (incidence rate ratios (IRRs) birth: 2.28; childhood: 2.85) in those born or grown up in big cities [7].

Epidemiological findings suggest that the risk of urbanicity is increased in those with a genetic liability for mental health conditions, as in the case of psychosis [8, 9]. Many studies have shown that urban living is associated with a higher perception of insecurity and personal risk of violence both in the general population and in people with schizophrenia (SZ). Insecurity, violence, trauma, and a degraded neighborhood reduce social support/interaction and affect well-being and mental health. Social interactions and support may be also reduced by social stigma and discrimination.

The process of urbanization may be associated with adaptational stress. Even though urban life may provide opportunities and positive impacts on many people, it may cause a chronic stressful situation on others [10]. Living in a city can offer benefits, such as health centers of excellence, culture opportunities, and other facilities, but it has also been observed that physical and mental health problems can be more frequent in those living in towns. Stress is a reaction to some perceived threats as well as to some urban factors: time pressure, unhealthy lifestyles, convenient diet, pollution, vehicles traffic, violence and crime, job insecurity, little social support, difficulty in social connections, and high distances.

In correlation with data above, urban lifestyle is also associated with higher metabolic, cardiovascular, and cancer risks, which lead to poorer mental health. In fact, comorbidities are higher in urban settings and common mental disorders are more likely to be associated with diabetes, stroke, hypertension, respiratory disorders, alcoholism, substance abuse, and chronic infections (e.g., HIV) [11].

Cultural forms and cultural norms heavily influence mental health and urbanicity. Youth culture gangs, games, entertainment, and access to substances and alcohol significantly influence the mental health of young people. At the same time, those at higher risk of developing mental disorders might be drawn toward living in urban or deprived areas as for a selective migration [12, 13].

All these observations pinpoint that the interaction between urbanicity and polygenic risk score in the transmission of mental disorders should be better understood. Using this approach for other environmental exposures, the EU-GEI study suggests that both early-life adversities and cannabis use interact with molecular genetic risk state in the development of psychosis [14].

Several studies show a huge variation on the risk of different disorders, including time of exposure (e.g., developmental vs. current) and geographic region. Thus, there is the need for systematic research to assess periods of risk in conjunction with multiple individual (e.g., polygenic risk) and contextual factors (e.g., specific risk of urban living) [15].

A large-population study in adolescents showed that those who perceived higher levels of threat in their neighborhood were more likely to have psychotic experiences [16]. These results remain true also after adjusting for variables such as levels of crime, individual disorder, and neighborhood- and family-level socioeconomic status, suggesting that the subjective perception of the urban environment is an important target for research and intervention.

Initial evidence links urbanicity to changes in neural activation and structure [15]. For example, a low childhood socioeconomic status has been associated with a range of brain structural and functional changes [17, 18], with the strongest effects in the most disadvantaged children [19].

Initial neuroimaging studies suggest possible neurobiological pathways that mediate urbanicity effects on cognitive functioning and mental health. Future studies need to systematically investigate multiple mechanisms that could underlie the urban effect on the brain (e.g., exposure to toxic or noise pollution, and social stressors) [15].

On the contrary, there is convincing evidence for positive effects of the short-term experience of nature on well-being and cognition, which may occur through largely unconscious processes affecting attention and the activity of the autonomous nervous system [20]. Environmental epigenetics suggest that urban characteristics (e.g., exposure to pollution or social density) biochemically influence the phenotypical development and might help to understand delayed temporality and intergenerational urban effects [21].

In summary, urban lifestyle can affect mental health according to a number of evidence. Litman [22] proposed a list of factors/mechanisms associated with mental health in the urban settings: social stress, substance abuse, social isolation and loneliness, noise and pollution, crime and insecurity, crowding and reduced privacy, economic stress, poor physical activity, transport conditions, and inadequate access to nature.

Studies on urbanity and self-reported happiness [23, 24] indicate that self-reported happiness (or life satisfaction) tends to increase with: financial situation (incomes relative to living costs and peers' incomes), family status (being in a stable family), work status (having a secure and satisfying job), health (being healthy and physically active), community connections and close friends (also called community cohesion or social capital), social inclusiveness (being a visible minority reduces happiness), personal freedom and security (having civil rights and feeling safe), positive attitudes, and beliefs in a higher power.

Sustainable urbanization is key to successful development. Well-managed urbanization, informed by an understanding of population trends, can help to maximize the benefits of agglomeration while minimizing environmental degradation and other potential adverse impacts of city dwellers. Health, social, and economic professionals should form partnerships for operational preventive and service solutions [25].

Adequate policies to adapt to that process should be advocated and pursued. Negligent management of urbanization may result in a ticking bomb of eventual social unrest concerning food, housing, jobs, transportation, and other daily needs [25]. Urban mental health may be improved by designing cities providing residents with regular access to green spaces, opportunities for physical activities, facilitated social interactions, and fostered safety.

18.2 Urbanization and Neuroscience

The effects of urbanization on psychiatric disorders have deep roots in the biological bases of neural systems involved in mood regulation, emotions, and behaviors. The urban environment can interact with neurobiological systems influencing susceptibility to and onset of various psychiatric disorders. Neuroscientific research contributes to explore the neurobiological processes mediating the impact of urbanization on mental health. In this regard, some authors identified a new academic discipline, named *Neurourbanism*, that aims to investigate the consequences of urban living on mental health, and on the brain in general [26].

18.2.1 Neurotransmitters, Stress Response Systems, and Mood Dysregulation

Psychiatric disorders, such as depression, bipolar disorder, and psychosis, are associated with imbalances in neurotransmitters in the nervous system. Serotonin, dopamine, and norepinephrine, for instance, play a crucial role in mood and emotion regulation. The urban environment can influence these systems through chronic stress. Exposure to air pollution and social isolation contribute to mood dysregulation and susceptibility to psychiatric disorders [3, 5, 27, 28]. Urbanization introduces a range of stressors that can disrupt the regulation of catecholaminergic systems and neuronal circuits involved in stress response [15, 29].

Chronic stress, often a hallmark of urban living, has been linked to changes in neurochemical systems [29]. Urbanization can exacerbate chronic stress, activating the stress response system; the constant demands and pressures of city life can lead to an overactive hypothalamic-pituitary-adrenal (HPA) axis, resulting in elevated cortisol levels [29–31]. Prolonged exposure to elevated cortisol levels can influence brain structure and function. Cortisol can impact the hippocampus, a brain area critical for memory and emotion regulation [15]. Changes in the hippocampus have been associated with mood disorders and cognitive impairments, contributing to symptoms of anxiety, depression, and other psychiatric disorders. The stress-induced hormonal shift can influence serotonin receptors, impacting on mood regulation and increasing susceptibility to mood disorders [32]. Additionally, exposure to air pollutants commonly found in urban environments has been associated with altered dopamine signaling, potentially affecting reward pathways and contributing to conditions like bipolar disorder [33]. These findings underscore the connection between urbanization, chronic stress, and psychiatric vulnerability [15].

18.2.2 Immune System and Inflammation

The connection between systemic inflammation and psychiatric disorders is an emerging area of interest. Air pollution and stress associated with urbanization can trigger widespread multisystemic inflammatory responses, which can influence neuronal function through communication between the immune system and the brain.

Chronic inflammation can damage brain cells and affect neurotransmitter function, increasing the risk of several psychiatric manifestations, such as mood and anxiety disorders [34].

Indeed, the immune system's role extends beyond physical protection; it also communicates with the brain, shaping mood and behaviors. Urban environments, rife with pollution and psychological stressors, can stimulate inflammatory responses in the body. This inflammation triggers the release of cytokines that can cross the blood-brain barrier and impact brain function. Elevated cytokine levels have been found recently in both depression and anxiety [34, 35].

18.2.3 Neural Plasticity and Adaptation

The neural system is characterized by plasticity, the ability to adapt to new stimuli and to reorganize neural network in response to new experiences and environments. However, urbanization's rapid pace and sensory overload can improve this adaptability to its limits. Social isolation, sensory overstimulation, and exposure to stressors can influence neural plasticity in ways that predispose to the onset of psychiatric disorders. Overall, the urban environment triggers the brain with stimuli, challenging its ability to filter and process information effectively. As a result, neural circuits responsible for emotion regulation and cognitive control may become strained [3].

In this regard the *Mirror Neuron Theory* (mirror neuron system is a pathway of specialized neuronal cells that "mirrors" the behaviors of other subjects) has defined brain areas involved in reaction to external behaviors, including the perigenual anterior caudal cortex (PACC), the premotor cortex, and the right dorsolateral prefrontal cortex (RDLPFC). *PACC* is connected to limbic and frontal brain areas and is involved in emotional regulation, cognitive processing, and contingency learning. RDLPFC located in the frontal lobes governs executive functions encompassing cognitive flexibility, manipulation of spatial representation in the working memory, and decision-making process. According to the Mirror Neuron Theory, PACC may play an important role in the process of anxiety response about social and urban context requirements, while RDLPFC may be involved in the manipulation of spatial representation and urban environment, that seems to be characterized by a greater visual complexity than rural contexts [36].

Furthermore, a hyperactivation of amygdale (a pivotal component of the limbic system that orchestrates emotional processing, particularly fear appraisal and threat recognition) has been found in people living in urban environments. Sustained urban stress could lead to amygdale hyperactivity and be related to the selection of stimuli with a relevant salience that may be increased in urban settings. This sort of *over-identification*, related to an increased attribution of self-involvement in urban settings, characterizes several psychiatric conditions, such as anxiety and psychotic disorders [15].

A recent study on 156,075 subjects [37] showed the relationship between typical urban contexts and specific patterns of affective, anxiety, and emotional instability symptoms. The study found three environmental profiles of urban living that may influence specific psychiatric conditions, mediated by distinct neurobiological substrates (Table 18.1).

In conclusion, the biological bases of psychiatric disorders related to urbanization develop through an intricate interplay of interaction between environmental factors and neural processes. Understanding how the urban environment can influence brain biology paves the way for targeted prevention and treatment. Designing cities that consider neural and psychological impacts can contribute to reduce the burden of psychiatric disorders associated with urbanization.

Table 18.1 Distinct urban environmental profiles, correlated psychiatric symptoms and neurobiological substrates [37]

Urban environmental profiles	Symptoms groups	Brain regions volume reduction	Genetic pathways
High degrees of deprivation and air pollution; lesser extent traffic; short distance to infrastructural facilities; lack of green spaces	Affective symptoms: – Unenthusiasm – Tiredness – Loneliness	Reward processing (13 brain regions): – Ventral striatum – Cerebellar Crus I and II – Amygdala – Superior frontal gyrus	Stress response (22 genes): – CRHR1 – MAPT – ARL17B
Green spaces; long distance to waste; energy facilities; presence of lakes-river-sea	Anxiety symptoms: – Anxious – Tense – Nervous	Emotional regulation (11 brain regions): – Inferior frontal regions – Amygdala – Cerebellar regions (Crus I, lobule VIII)	Serotonin metabolism (11 genes): – EXD3 – TRIM – NOLC1
Density of land use and infrastructure	Emotional instability symptoms: – Highly strung – Feeling miserable – Mood swings	Emotion response (13 brain regions): – Frontal pole – Amygdala – Precentral gyrus – Insular cortex – Cerebellum	Cerebellar development (6 genes): – ITF74 – TMPO – LFHC

18.3 Urbanicity and Risk of Psychosis

Urbanicity encapsulates the transformation of rural landscapes into bustling metropolises. This transformation brings the exploration of its impact on mental health. The intricate relationship between urbanicity and risk of psychosis has been investigated by many authors, giving an insight into how the cityscape might shape the vulnerability to this complex mental disorder.

Urbanicity is a multifaceted concept including various dimensions of urban development. From the densely populated neighborhoods to the towering skyscrapers, cities beckon with promises of opportunity and excitement. However, the urban landscape also carries its shadows, as it molds the experience of daily life and influences the mental wellbeing of its inhabitants. Noise pollution, congestion, and social isolation are stressors that influence mental health.

The dynamics of urban living foster a unique social landscape. While cities offer unparalleled diversity, they can also cultivate a sense of disconnection. The fast pace of life can leave individuals feeling socially fragmented, leading to a potential erosion of social support networks. This isolation, combined with the challenges of city life, might contribute to the vulnerability to psychosis.

Schizophrenia (SZ) is a severe mental disorder that typically emerges in late adolescence and persists throughout adult life, affecting about 1% of the population. The direct and indirect costs of SZ-related disorders amount to 93.9 billion euros. High levels of disease-related incapacity to work, early retirement, and high hospitalization rates lead to a high disease burden. Genetically, SZ is highly heritable, with heritability estimated at 80%, and monozygotic twin concordance at 45%. In addition to genetics, exposure to different environmental factors at different stages during development contributes to the risk of developing schizophrenia that is the result of the interaction between these two risk factors, rather than being the result of their independent effect [38].

As already reported in the beginning of 1990s by Faris and Dunahm [39], risk of psychosis is higher in people living in big cities. In the following decades, a consistent number of large studies confirmed the higher prevalence of psychosis in urban settings in the United Kingdom, Germany, the United States, and in North Europe, but not in Spain and Italy [3].

The higher prevalence of schizophrenia-spectrum disorders in urban settings has been explained by several hypotheses, including the social drift hypothesis, the gene–environment interaction, the exposure to environmental factors, and the lower detection in rural areas. In particular, the social drift hypothesis is based on the evidence that individuals with SZ deal with a progressive social and economic deterioration and move to more deprived areas, whereas families at risk for SZ are more likely to move to urban areas. In a systematic review on the risk of psychosis according to urbanicity [40], the majority of investigators define urbanicity by degrees of population density, either as population per square kilometer or, most commonly, as number of inhabitants within a defined location. In most studies, urbanicity is associated with an approximately twofold increased risk of psychosis, though associations indicating a fourfold risk increase have been reported in early-onset cases. Only two reports found no significant differences in rates of psychosis according to urbanicity.

Another recent study suggests that urban living might be linked to an increased risk of psychosis, particularly when urban exposure occurs in pre-adolescence [41]. However, the mechanisms underlying this association are unclear. Saxena and Dodell-Feder [41] utilized 1-year follow-up data from a large nationwide study of pre-adolescents in the United States (n = 7979) and found that factors related to increased number of psychotic-like experiences were: annual average particulate matter (PM), with a diameter of 2.5 μm or less (PM2.5); proximity to roads; census-level home at-risk for exposure to lead paint; census-level poverty, and census-level income disparity. These same urban-related exposures were also related to the persistence of psychosis after 1 year.

Psychosocial stressors are a hallmark of urban living. Adverse childhood experiences, discrimination, and urban violence can serve as chronic stressors that impact on mental health. The accumulation of stress over time might lead to vulnerability to psychosis. As individuals strive to navigate the urban environment, the wear and tear of these stressors could potentially alter brain function and contribute to the development of mental disorders.

The urban environment extends beyond the psychological realm and can influence biological processes. Air pollution and exposure to toxins might contribute to inflammation in the brain, potentially impacting neural pathways related to psychosis. Genetic predisposition and gene–environment interactions might also play a role in the heightened vulnerability to psychosis in urban environments.

Since more than three decades, schizophrenia (SZ) has been regarded as a neurodevelopmental disorder [42] in which genetic and environmental risk factors influence connectivity in neuronal circuits during vulnerable developmental periods. These risk factors induce disturbance of macro- and micro-connectivity in brain regions involving the prefrontal, temporal, and parietal cortices and the hippocampus. On the molecular and cellular levels, a disturbed synaptic plasticity, loss of oligodendrocytes, and impaired myelination have been shown in brain regions of SZ patients. However, the association between urbanicity and psychosis is heterogeneous and driven by multiple risk and protective factors that act differently in different ethnic groups and countries.

Fett et al. [43] highlight the need for global, multidisciplinary investigations that incorporate epidemiology, neuroscience, experimental psychology, sociology, and urban planning, an approach that was recently presented as "neurourbanism." This research needs to pinpoint risk (e.g., pollution, disease exposure, unemployment, social fragmentation, or migration) and protective urban factors (e.g., resources, political freedom, and low social control) and their interactions. Sensitive periods of maximum risk (e.g., urban birth, upbringing, and current urbanicity) should be systematically investigated, while considering effects of cumulative urban exposure [43].

To mitigate the potential impact of urbanicity on the risk of psychosis, a multifaceted approach is required. Community support programs, early intervention services, and accessible mental health care can contribute to reduce the burden of psychosis in urban areas. Urban planning should prioritize green spaces and environments that foster community connections. The integration of mental health considerations into urban policies can pave the way for a more mentally supportive urban landscape.

In summary, urban environment holds both allure and challenges, with its potential impact on mental health becoming increasingly evident. Understanding this relationship is crucial not only for individuals' wellbeing, but also for urban planning and public health policies. As societies continue their urban journey, the imperative to create cities that nurture mental health becomes vital. By addressing the multifaceted factors contributing to psychosis risk in urban environments, communities can forge a path toward a better mental health for all.

18.4 Urbanization and Depressive Disorders

Although recently the focus of researchers and clinicians is on the link between urbanicity and schizophrenia, the most prevalent mental disorders linked to urbanicity are depression and anxiety [37].

Urbanization stands as a hallmark of human progress, reshaping landscapes and lives as populations flock to cities in pursuit of opportunity and advancement. However, this march toward urban living has cast a spotlight on a growing concern: the toll it takes on mental wellbeing. In the midst of skyscrapers and bustling streets, a quieter struggle unfolds—that of depressive disorders.

Different factors intertwine urbanization and depression. The allure of urban living is undeniable, offering a cornucopia of experiences, careers, and connections. Cities are magnets for innovation and cultural exchange, fostering an environment conducive to personal and professional growth. Paradoxically, the rapid urban expansion comes with a psychological cost. The "urban paradox" suggests that the same dynamics that make cities attractive—competition, diversity, and dynamism—can also breed mental health problems. The pressure to keep pace in an ever-moving environment can fuel stress, anxiety, and ultimately contribute to depressive disorders.

Within the tapestry of urban life, certain threads stand out as contributors to the fabric of depressive disorders. The sprawling concrete landscapes that attract dreamers also isolate them. Social isolation becomes a shadow, as city dwellers navigate crowds while feeling disconnected. The perpetual buzz of traffic and construction, the ever-present hum of noise pollution, infiltrates minds, chipping away at tranquility. The very air they breathe, tainted by pollutants, can cast a pall over mental wellbeing. These factors, often intensified by the urban experience, increase susceptibility to depressive disorders.

In the heart of the city, a cacophony of interactions unfolds—brief glances shared on subways, hurried conversations in coffee shops, fleeting connections in the digital realm. Yet, among this vibrant mosaic, a silent struggle with loneliness and social disconnectedness persists. The urban lifestyle can foster superficial relationships and paradoxical isolation. Social media and technology, meant to connect, can amplify feelings of inadequacy as individuals curate a facade of success. This constant comparison can lead to a distorted self-perception, further entangling the link between urban living and depressive disorders.

Biological findings are crucial for understanding urban mental health problems. Using functional MRI (magnetic resonance imaging) in three independent studies, Lederbogen et al. [44] have shown that city living is associated with increased amygdala activity, whereas urban upbringing affects the perigenual anterior cingulate cortex, a key region regulating amygdala activity, negative affect, and stress.

A study conducted by Luciano et al. [45] represents one of the first attempts to explore the role of perceived insecurity on the outcome of patients with mood or anxiety disorders. Their main finding is a common sense of perceived insecurity among the sample, which can be due to recent changes in modern society (e.g., terroristic attacks, mass-murders, and natural disasters, but also to changes in family structure and reduced social cohesion, which have lost their buffering effect). Another factor that contributed to increase this insecurity is the loss of a structured and rigorous society, where ties and rules were clear and well defined. This loss has generated a "liquid society," characterized by lack of social cohesion and remoteness among people [46]. The second most important finding is the presence of higher levels of perceived insecurity in persons living in big cities, probably due to the rapid expansion of urban agglomerations, which has been chaotic and dysregulated. Neighborhood social cohesion influences mental health at population level, with increased risk to develop depression and anxiety disorders in neighborhoods with a lower social cohesion, independently by the individual characteristics.

A systematic review [47] has shown that house and built environment with poor house quality, lack of green areas, noise, and air pollution were more clearly related to depressive disorders than the population density, aesthetics, and walkability of living environment and availability of services.

Wang et al. [48] investigated the relationship between urbanization and depressive symptoms in China, focusing on the influence of neighborhood social capital, given its potential protective effect on mental health. Inconsistently with other studies, they found that depression was less prevalent in urban areas and explained this difference by the healthy migration hypothesis, that is, healthy and optimistic rural people are most likely to migrate to more urbanized areas, leaving behind those at risk of depression. Another possible explanation is that residents living in less urbanized areas generally have less knowledge about depression and fewer resources to cope with it than those in more urbanized areas.

Purtle et al. [49] conducted a systematic review and meta-analysis about urban–rural differences in older adult depression, suggesting that converging trends of urbanization and aging could increase the global burden of depression. However, there is a difference across contexts: in developed countries, the odds of depression are significantly higher in urban than rural residents, whereas this association is not true in developing countries.

Xu et al. [37] found that affective symptoms were positively correlated with environmental factors, including a profile of social deprivations, air and sound pollution, measure of street network accessibility (street radial and centrality), traffic, and density of urban infrastructures (factories, retail, office, and community). The same group was negatively correlated with distance to urban facilities and green space proximity (percentage of domestic gardens, natural environment, and green space). Finally, authors described how the environment might affect the brain and mental health, by reducing regional brain volumes and influencing genes involved in pertinent biological pathways.

In summary, as the world continues its urban march, the imperative to address mental health in cities becomes more pressing. The relationship between urbanization and depressive disorders calls for a holistic approach that includes urban planning, mental health awareness, and community support.

18.5 Urbanization and Suicide

Suicide mortality is recognized as a severe public health issue worldwide [50], being one of the leading causes of global deaths affecting millions of families, communities, and individuals every year. About 700,000 suicide cases occur each year, and even more attempted suicides. The suicide phenomenon is complex and multidimensional, with the involvement of compositional and contextual factors.

Significant geographic variations in suicide mortality trends between and within countries, as well as between urban and rural areas have been reported by several epidemiological studies, although the association between suicide and urban areas is not universally accepted. Urban lifestyle has been historically associated with higher rates of suicidality [51]. Urban living is synonymous with dynamism, diversity, and innovation but, although stimulating, it also increases the levels of stressors on individuals. The pressure to succeed, to maintain social appearance, and to keep up with the frenetic pace of city life can all take a toll. These psychological stressors can amplify feelings of hopelessness, contributing to the troubling rise of suicide rates in urban areas. Moreover, the anonymity offered by city life can obscure individuals' struggles, making it easier for those suffering to go unnoticed. The same factors that attract individuals can also increase vulnerability to mental health challenges and, ultimately, to suicide. Urban environments, though densely populated, can foster feelings of social disconnection and alienation that contribute to increase suicidal thoughts and behaviors.

On the contrary, more recent evidence has shown a declining trend in suicidality in urban settings and an increase in rural areas in many countries including Europe, the United States, New Zealand, China, Canada, and Australia. Suicidality in rural areas can be due social isolation, easier access to lethal means, aging, socioeconomic decline, stigmatization toward people with mental health problems, poor availability of mental health services, lower social support, and climate challenges. Despite popular clichés about anonymous city-dwelling cited above, rural living also leads to social isolation, resulting in less intimate face-to-face contacts with family and friends, which, in turn, increases suicidal risk [52].

In a longitudinal study on adolescents and young adults aged 10–24 years, Fontanella et al. [52] examined rural and urban differences in youth suicide mortality in the United States over time and stratified by sex. From January 1, 1996, to December 31, 2010, a total of 66,595 young people died by suicide; rates of suicide were approximately double in rural areas than in urban areas for both sexes. Male suicide rates significantly declined in urban areas but remained relatively stable in rural areas; in females, suicide rates significantly increased in the most urban and rural areas. Rates of suicide by firearm and hanging/suffocation are disproportionately higher in rural areas compared with urban ones.

Helbich et al. [53], examining the effect of 14 different urbanicity indicators on urban–rural suicide associations in Germany, found a higher suicide risk in those living in rural areas compared to those living in urban areas. Reccord et al. [54] carried out an observational study of all suicide deaths ($N = 972$) among Newfoundland and Labrador (urban and rural regions of Canada) residents between 1997 and 2016. Compared to suicides committed by people living in urban contexts, those living in rural areas who died by suicide were younger, less likely to have had prior suicide attempts or a psychiatric disorder, more likely to use firearms or hanging, and had a higher mean blood alcohol content at the time of death. Also, Casant and Helbich [50] in their review of 24 papers found higher suicide rates in rural areas in most ecological and cross-sectional studies. Although rural suicide rates among males exceeded those among males in urban areas, there is no urban–rural difference in female suicides. Suicide methods also vary between urban and rural areas; firearms and poisoning by pesticides are more frequently used in rural areas.

Access to mental health care can be challenging in both urban and rural areas. Stigma and lack of awareness can stop individuals from seeking help. The spread of mental health services does not always translate into accessibility for all residents. In many countries, there are discrepancies in the availability of mental health resources and efforts to bridge this gap should be made through initiatives like community clinics, helplines, and online support platforms.

To address the issue of elevated suicide rates, a multipronged approach is needed. Public awareness campaigns can shatter stigma and encourage open conversations about mental health. Mental health education in schools and workplaces equips individuals with tools to recognize and address signs of mental distress.

Efforts to offer social support at the local level could reduce the suicide risk in rural and urban residents; designing spaces that promote social interaction and community cohesion may also help in reducing the suicide risk in rural areas compared to urban ones.

18.6 Urbanization and Addiction Disorders

With the rapid growth of cities, a parallel rise in various social and health issues, including addiction disorders, has been observed. Urban environments can increase accessibility to substances; moreover, social interactions and various forms of entertainment represent potential catalysts for addiction disorders. High levels of stress, boredom, and fast-paced lifestyles can contribute to feelings of isolation and the desire to seek relief through substances or addictive behaviors such as gambling disorder or other types of pathological Internet use (PIU; e.g., Internet gaming, compulsive online sexual behaviors/cyberpornography, Internet-related buying or shopping disorder, Internet-related gambling disorder, cyberbullying, cyberchondria, and social media/network forum use) [55]. As cities continue to grow, the prevalence of addiction disorders can become a pressing concern.

The complex interaction between urbanization and addiction disorders can be due to several factors, such as:

- *Socioeconomic disparities and vulnerability*: Urbanization can exacerbate socioeconomic disparities, which can impact susceptibility to addiction disorders. Marginalized communities may face limited access to education, health care, and employment opportunities, leading to increased stress and a higher likelihood of addictive behaviors as maladaptive coping strategies [56].
- *The role of urban design*: Rates of addiction are significantly influenced by the layout and design of urban spaces. Walkability, access to green spaces, and community facilities can enhance mental wellbeing and serve as protective factors against addiction. Conversely, deprived neighborhoods might foster isolation contributing to substance abuse [56].
- *Neurobiological mechanisms*: Urbanization's effects on neural processes interact with the intricate neurobiology of substance use disorder (SUD). Urban environment can influence the release of stress-related neurotransmitters, such as corticotropin-releasing factor (CRF), thereby modulating the reward pathways implicated in substance-seeking behaviors. Moreover, the mesocorticolimbic dopamine system, which is integral to reward processing, can be sensitized or dysregulated by the stressors inherent to urban living, potentially shaping the development and persistence of SUD (for a more detailed description of the neurobiological mechanisms, please refer to the previous section "Urbanization and Neuroscience") [3, 8, 56].
- *Digital urbanism and behavioral addictions*: The digital age has brought a new dimension of urbanization, the so-called digital urbanism. Constant connectivity and virtual interactions have given rise to behavioral addictions, such as Internet gaming disorder or online gambling disorder. While the majority of subjects take advantage from a positive use of Internet, some can develop Problematic Internet Use. This "umbrella term" encompasses a wide range of repetitive disabling behaviors characterized by compulsivity and addiction (See Box 18.1). As people navigate the virtual cityscape, these addictive behaviors can present unique challenges for clinicians, researchers, and policymakers [55].

Box 18.1 Internet Addiction Disorder (IAD) and Pathological Internet Use (PUI)

In 1995, Internet Addiction Disorder was first identified by Ivan Goldberg as a loss of control in use of the Internet resulting in functional impairment. In 1996, Kimberly Young conducted an empirical investigation on the phenomenon and described a list of symptoms drawn from the characteristics of pathological gambling.

Despite the term internet addiction disorder (IAD) remains widely used nowadays to indicate internet-related psychopathology, the term pathological internet use (PIU) is preferable. Indeed, just a few of the clinical manifestations of PIU exhibit similarities with established behavioral addictions (i.e., gambling disorder, social media addiction, and gaming disorder). Other subtypes of PIU, such as digital searching for medical information (cyberchondria) or digital hoarding, may be more similar to obsessive-compulsive related disorders. Moreover, other forms of PIU, such as internet social-media/forum use, appear more related to social anxiety and demonstrate the phenomenon of "FOMO," fear of missing out, from online activities and relationships. Finally, some forms of online shopping, cyberbullying, and cyberpornography present clinical features that are characteristic of impulse control disorders and/or sexual disorders [55, 63].

18.6.1 Urbanization and Substance Use Disorders

As urbanization continues its global improvement, the concomitant rise in substance use disorder (SUD) presents a multifaceted challenge to public health. The intricate interplay between urbanization and SUD requires a comprehensive exploration of the sociocultural, neurobiological, and environmental factors that contribute to the increase of substance abuse in urban environments.

The urban environment, with its accelerated pace, competitive demands, and noise pollution, poses an unprecedented array of stressors on residents. Such stressors can foster psychological distress and maladaptation, potentially making individuals more susceptible to substance use as a coping strategy [57, 58].

The increased availability of substances in urban contexts is influenced by several factors, such as growing economies, international trade, reduced prices, and access to the Internet [56]. Internet and the "dark web" created alternative uncontrollable routes of drug distribution, thus inducing sellers to move to a more convenient and globalized distribution system that involves mainly novel psychoactive substances and prescription drugs [56]. A national investigation of Saudi Arabian students showed a strong association between use of illicit drugs and heavy use of Internet [59]. Several recent studies [59–61] have investigated the differences in the use of new psychoactive substances between rural and urban areas, reporting conflicting findings. In fact, there were found no differences between urban and rural contexts in the use of novel psychoactive substances in a sample of Italian adolescents [59], while use of new psychoactive substances was higher in the non-metropolitan county of Norfolk than in urban areas in a sample of UK students [60].

Furthermore, the increased consumption of substances in specific urban contexts (i.e., Latin American countries) could be due to changes in pattern of family relationships, such as breakdown of traditional family structure due to transnational urban migration of parents without their children [56]. Overall, urbanization dramatically reconfigures social networks, influencing the dynamics of social support and normative behaviors. The anonymity afforded by urban environments can facilitate peer influence and the propagation of substance use norms. Homelessness can also influence substance abuse in big cities [56]. A recent investigation conducted in New York showed higher rates of past year drug use, alcohol misuse, and lifetime opioid overdose in homeless patients accessing emergency departments [62]. Conversely, urban settings may offer opportunities for implementing targeted intervention strategies, leveraging the expanded reach of social services and community programs. Prevention and treatment services tailored to emerging mental health needs due to global urbanization are needed.

18.6.2 Urbanization and Pathological Internet Use

The dynamic mechanisms through which urban environment may foster excessive Internet use, leading to pathological Internet use (PIU), are complicated and not yet fully elucidated [63].

Urbanization facilitates the creation of a digital ecosystem that perpetuates connectivity. In urban environments, Internet represents an essential tool for working, communicating, and leisure activities. Moreover, the stressful urban lifestyle may foster individuals to find relaxation in the immersive world of Internet. This behavior is further reinforced by the continuous connectivity made possible by smartphones and high-speed Internet services, establishing the basis for a problematic use of Internet. Urbanization's influence on psychological vulnerabilities contributes to the allure of Internet addiction. The anonymity and depersonalization afforded by urban environments can foster a sense of dissociation, prompting individuals to seek validation and interaction through online platforms. The instant gratification provided by social media interactions with the dopamine-driven loops inherent in digital engagement can create a vicious cycle in individuals predisposed to impulsive behaviors or in those grappling feelings of loneliness and isolation [55].

The urban environment contains triggers that amplify PIU; the proliferation of Wi-Fi hotspots, digital displays, and pervasive advertising ensure that the allure of the online realm remains constantly present. Additionally, urban areas provide fertile grounds for the development and indulgence in immersive digital experiences, such as virtual reality and online gaming, further increasing the risk of PIU in urban areas.

A comprehensive response to PIU within urban contexts requires a multifaceted approach. Public awareness campaigns, targeted educational programs, and school-based interventions can foster digital literacy and promote responsible online behavior. Developing spaces that encourage in-person interactions, such as community centers and green spaces, can also be extremely useful to reduce Internet use in big cities. Collaborative initiatives involving mental health professionals, educators, policymakers, and urban planners can shape a holistic framework for mitigating PIU impact within the context of urbanization [63].

Recently, Ko et al. conducted a review on the association between urbanization and Internet addiction disorder (IAD) [63]. Despite several studies on the prevalence of IAD in urban contexts have been carried out, relatively a few studies have explored differences in IAD between rural and urban contexts. In the review by Ko et al. [63], nine studies [64–72] found a positive association between urbanization and IAD, three studies [73–75] found a negative association, and five studies [76–80] showed no association. Although the results were not completely conclusive, more than half of the studies identified a positive association between IAD and urbanization. The authors concluded that green open spaces and sport facilities should be implemented in urban areas in order to promote and facilitate physical activities and social interaction.

In summary, the relationship between urbanization and PIU reflects the intricate intersection of technological advances and evolving behavioral patterns. The complex challenges posed by PIU within urbanization require innovative and interdisciplinary strategies that transcend traditional boundaries, emphasizing the importance of collaborative efforts in mitigating its impact and fostering a harmonious coexistence between urbanization and digital connectivity.

18.7 Patterns of Psychiatric Care for Patients Living in Big Cities

The urban landscape is a dynamic and intricate tapestry of human interactions, culture, and bustling activities. In the heart of these cities, individuals with psychiatric disorders have to challenge not only their mental health problems, but also the complexities of urban life. As urbanization continues to grow, understanding the unique needs and barriers faced by these individuals is crucial for shaping effective and compassionate care strategies.

In big cities, the availability of mental health services can vary dramatically from one neighborhood to another; while some areas might boast a plethora of clinics and specialists, others might face a scarcity of resources, leaving individuals underserved. For instance, downtown districts might have bustling private practices, while marginalized communities struggle to access even the most basic care. The disparity in access is further compounded by issues such as long waiting lists, insurance limitations, and out-of-pocket costs. Initiatives to bridge this gap include the establishment of community mental health centers strategically located in underserved areas and the implementation of mobile clinics to provide care directly to those in need.

The urban environment, with its mix of cultures and diversity, presents a unique challenge in dealing with mental health stigma. While cities offer the potential for openness and acceptance, the flip side is the increased visibility of individuals seeking psychiatric care. Help-seeking can be either facilitated or hampered by culturally rooted attitudes toward mental health. Communities including people with different backgrounds might have differing views on mental health and treatment of mental disorders, leading to reduced utilization of care services. Overcoming stigma requires culturally sensitive approaches that consider these nuances and actively engage community leaders and policymakers.

One key strategy for addressing inequalities in mental health care is to ensure integration of mental health services with primary care. Mental health care must be a crucial component of primary care serving overall population [81]. Homelessness is an unfortunate reality in many urban centers, and its relationship with mental health is well known. Homeless individuals often suffer from psychiatric conditions, with the urban environment intensifying their problems. Almost in all countries poor people have a higher risk of developing mental disorders, so poverty is considered both a determinant and a consequence of poor mental health [82]. In response, innovative programs recognizing the need for a holistic approach have emerged, providing not only psychiatric treatment but also housing solutions. By offering safe and stable living environments, these programs break the cycle of homelessness and psychiatric distress.

Another issue in urban areas is the large spread of substances through the Internet. The so-called dotcom generation, composed by urban young people accessing the Internet daily, can easily find information as well as buy illicit drugs on the web with a large variety of offers and a few limitations. Young adults often migrate from rural to urban areas for studying or working and they may be exposed to social stress leading to addictive behaviors [60, 83].

On the other hand, the digital age has generated new possibilities for delivery of mental health care in urban areas. Telepsychiatry platforms offer remote access to care and are particularly useful in big cities, where traffic and distance can be significant barriers to treatment. However, the digital divide remains a challenge, as not all individuals have access to the necessary technology or Internet connectivity. Initiatives to address this divide include community centers with Internet access and partnership with telecommunication companies to provide affordable options for underserved populations.

Several community-driven support systems have blossomed among the crowded streets in big cities. Peer support groups, often led by individuals who have faced similar mental health problems, offer a unique avenue for sharing experiences and improving coping strategies. The collaboration between local organizations, non-governmental agencies, and mental health providers has resulted in safe spaces and resources for those seeking support.

The landscape of urban mental health is shaped by local policies and advocacy strategies. Positive changes in care accessibility have often been driven by advocacy groups that highlight the importance of mental health and push for policy reform. Collaborative efforts between mental health professionals, governmental agencies, and advocacy organizations have resulted in initiatives that focus on improving mental health care infrastructure, increasing funding for mental health services, and promoting mental health awareness campaigns in urban environments.

In Italy, the 1978 reform of psychiatric services initiated the closure of psychiatric hospitals encouraging the development of a widespread and complex network of community mental health facilities [84]. The Italian community model was implemented earlier than in the rest of the world and relevant efforts were made to move away from the institutional model and to implement the community model of mental health care. Psychiatric care of the population of a catchment area is ensured by the Department of Mental Health and Addiction Services, which provide a network of community services, including outreach teams, hospital wards, and day-care and residential facilities. Data about service provision are regularly collected by the mental health information system.

This organizational model is centered on multidisciplinary teams led by consultant psychiatrists and including clinical psychiatrists, psychologists, nurses, social workers, occupational therapists, rehabilitation counsellors, and auxiliary staff. Each Department should provide the full range of psychiatric care, from acute emergency treatment to long-term rehabilitation.

The concept of integration is based on packages of care that can be defined as a cluster of services provided to an individual based on carefully constructed components. Patients' care can be provided in four possible different settings: Community Mental Health Centers, Day-Care Facilities, General Hospital Psychiatric Units, and Community Residential Facilities. Lora et al. [85] highlighted that currently community care is more focused on the delivery of biological treatments than on psychosocial-oriented care. The only sustainable way to close the psychosocial gap is to empower nurses, rehabilitation therapists, and social workers as providers of psychosocial interventions through a wide and structural process of task shifting. Moreover, newly taken-in-care cases receive less intensive and continuous care than the more chronic ones. In Italy, as in other countries, the implementation of Early Intervention Services using structured clinical pathways for young patients is incomplete and addressing this gap in care must be prioritized.

Another model of treatment based on personalized care is the Personal Health Budget (PHB). According to the long-term plan of the UK National Health Service (NHS), personalized care is one of five major practical changes needed to ensure a service fit for the future. This implies that people will get more control over their health and more personalized care when they need it.

The person with a PHB (or their representative) should: (1) be central in developing their personalized care and support plan and agree who is involved in; (2) be able to agree upon the outcomes they want to achieve; (3) get the money needed for health care and support; (4) have enough money to meet the health and well-being needs; and (5) be able to use the money to meet their outcomes in ways and at times that make sense to them.

In conclusion, as cities continue to evolve, the future of mental health care holds promises and challenges. Integrating mental health care into primary care settings is a potential solution for increasing access and reducing stigma. Continued investment in education and awareness campaigns will play a pivotal role in reshaping public perceptions and reducing the stigma surrounding mental health. Furthermore, the ongoing advancement of technology offers opportunities for more efficient care delivery, although efforts must be made to ensure equitable access for all residents.

References

1. Bhugra D, Ventriglio A, Castaldelli-Maia JM et al (2019) Urban mental health. Oxford University Press, Oxford
2. Pasanen TP, Kajosaari A (2023) Special issue: place, space, and mental health. Int J Environ Res Public Health 20:5055. https://doi.org/10.3390/ijerph20065055
3. Ventriglio A, Torales J, Castaldelli-Maia JM, De Berardis D, Bhugra D (2021) Urbanization and emerging mental health issues. CNS Spectr 26(1):43–50. https://doi.org/10.1017/S1092852920001236. Epub 2020 Apr 6. PMID: 32248860
4. Ulrich RS, Simons RF, Losito BD, Fiorito E, Miles MA, Zelson M (1991) Stress recovery during exposure to natural and urban environments. J Environ Psychol 11:201–230
5. Peen J, Schoevers RA, Beekman AT, Dekker J (2010) The current status of urban-rural differences in psychiatric disorders. Acta Psychiatr Scand 121:84–93
6. Toulopoulou T, Picchioni M, Mortensen PB, Petersen L (2017) IQ, the urban environment, and their impact on future schizophrenia risk in men. Schizophr Bull 43:1056–1063
7. Lauritsen MB, Astrup A, Pedersen CB, Obel C, Schendel DE, Schieve L et al (2014) Urbanicity and

autism spectrum disorders. J Autism Dev Disord 44:394–404
8. Krabbendam L, Van Os J (2005) Schizophrenia and urbanicity: a major environmental influence—conditional on genetic risk. Schizophr Bull 31:795–799
9. van Os J, Kenis G, Rutten BP (2010) The environment and schizophrenia. Nature 468:203
10. Halbreich U (2021) Stress: a global multidimensional common denominator. Br J Psychiatry Adv 27:142–144
11. Kessler RCP, Chiu WTA, Demler OM et al (2005) Prevalence, severity, and comorbidity of 12-month DSMIV disorders in the National Comorbidity Survey Replication. Arch Gen Psychiatr 62:617–627
12. Colodro-Conde L, Couvy-Duchesne B, Whitfield JB, Streit F, Gordon S, Kemper KE, De Zeeuw EL (2018) Association between population density and genetic risk for schizophrenia. JAMA Psychiatry 75:901–910
13. Sariaslan A, Fazel S, D'Onofrio BM, Langstrom N, Larsson H, Bergen SE et al (2016) Schizophrenia and subsequent neighborhood deprivation: revisiting the social drift hypothesis using population, twin and molecular genetic data. Transl Psychiatry 6:e796
14. Guloksuz S, Pries LK, Delespaul P, Kenis G, Luykx JJ, Lin BD, van Os J (2019) Examining the independent and joint effects of molecular genetic liability and environmental exposures in schizophrenia: results from the EUGEI study. World Psychiatry 18:173–182
15. Lidia K, van Vugt M, Conus P, Söderström O, Empson LA, van Os J, Fett A-KJ (2021) Understanding urbanicity: how interdisciplinary methods help to unravel the effects of the city on mental health. Psychol Med 51:1099–1110. https://doi.org/10.1017/S0033291720000355
16. Newbury J, Arseneault L, Caspi A, Moffitt TE, Odgers CL, Fisher HL (2018) Cumulative effects of neighborhood social adversity and personal crime victimization on adolescent psychotic experiences. Schizophr Bull 44:348–358
17. Farah MJ (2017) The neuroscience of socioeconomic status: correlates, causes, and consequences. Neuron 96:56–71
18. McDermott CL, Seidlitz J, Nadig A, Liu S, Clasen LS, Blumenthal JD et al (2019) Longitudinally mapping childhood socioeconomic status associations with cortical and subcortical morphology. J Neurosci 39:1365
19. Noble KG, Houston SM, Brito NH, Bartsch H, Kan E, Kuperman JM et al (2015) Family income, parental education and brain structure in children and adolescents. Nat Neurosci 18:773
20. Berto R (2014) The role of nature in coping with psycho-physiological stress: a literature review on restorativeness. Behav Sci 4:394–409
21. Guthman J, Mansfield B (2012) The implications of environmental epigenetics: a new direction for geographic inquiry on health, space, and nature-society relations. Prog Hum Geogr 37:486–504
22. Todd L (2017) Urban sanity: understanding urban mental health impacts and how to create saner, happier cities. Victoria Transport Policy Institute, Victoria. www.vtpi.org/urban-sanity.pdf
23. Ballas D (2013) What makes a 'happy city'? Cities 32(1):S39–S50. https://doi.org/10.1016/j.cities.2013.04.009
24. Helliwell JF, Layard R, Sacks JD, De Neve JE, Atkin LB, Wang S (2022) World happiness report 2022. Sustainable Development Solutions Network, New York
25. Halbreich U (2023) Impact of urbanization on mental health and well being. Curr Opin Psychiatry 36(3):200–205
26. United Nations Department of Economic and Social Affairs—UN-DESA world urbanization prospects (2018) (Early 2022 update revision). Accessed 9 Dec 2022
27. Freeman H (1984) Mental health and the environment, 1st edn. Churchill Livingstone, London
28. Dohrenwend BP, Dohrenwend BS (1974) Psychiatric disorders in urban settings. In: Caplan G (ed) American handbook of psychiatry. Basic Books, New York, pp 424–447
29. Steinheuser V, Ackermann K, Schonfeld P, Schwabe L (2014) Stress and the city: impact of urban upbringing on the (re)activity of the hypothalamus-pituitary-adrenal axis. Psychosom Med 76:678–685
30. Selten J-P, Cantor-Graae E (2005) Social defeat: risk factor for schizophrenia? Br J Psychiatry 187:101–102
31. Selten J-P, van der Ven E, Rutten BP, Cantor-Graae E (2013) The social defeat hypothesis of schizophrenia: an update. Schizophr Bull 39:1180–1186
32. Yang, Zhao Y, Wang Y, Liu L, Zhang X, Li B, Cuia R (2015) The effects of psychological stress on depression. Curr Neuropharmacol 13:494–504
33. Berghorst LH, Kumar P, Greve DN, Deckersbach T, Ongur D, Dutra SJ, Pizzagalli DA (2016) Stress and reward processing in bipolar disorder: a functional magnetic resonance imaging study. Bipolar Disord 18(7):602–611. https://doi.org/10.1111/bdi.12444. Epub 2016 Nov 10. PMID: 27870507; PMCID: PMC5234857
34. Zunszain PA, Hepgul N, Pariante CM (2013) Inflammation and depression. Curr Top Behav Neurosci 14:135–151. https://doi.org/10.1007/7854_2012_211. PMID: 22553073
35. Peirce JM, Alviña K (2019) The role of inflammation and the gut microbiome in depression and anxiety. J Neurosci Res 97(10):1223–1241. https://doi.org/10.1002/jnr.24476. Epub 2019 May 29
36. Rizzolatti G, Craighero L (2004) The mirror neuron system. Ann Rev Neurosci 27(169–192):96
37. Xu J, Liu N, Polemiti E, Garcia-Mondragon L, Tang J, Liu X, Lett T, Yu L, Nöthen MM, Feng J, Yu C, Marquand A, Schumann G, The environMENTAL Consortium (2023) Effects of urban living environments on mental health in adults. Nat Med 29(6):1456–1467. https://doi.org/10.1038/s41591-023-02365-w. Epub 2023 Jun 15. PMID: 37322117; PMCID: PMC10287556

38. Wahbeh MH, Avramopoulos D (2021) Gene-environment interactions in schizophrenia: a literature review. Genes (Basel) 12(12):1850. https://doi.org/10.3390/genes12121850. PMID: 34946799; PMCID: PMC8702084
39. Faris R, Dunahm H (1939) Mental disorders in urban areas. University of Chicago Press, Chicago
40. March D, Hatch SL, Morgan C, Kirkbride JB, Bresnahan M, Fearon P, Susser E (2008) Psychosis and place. Epidemiol Rev 30:84–100. https://doi.org/10.1093/epirev/mxn006. Epub 2008 Jul 30. PMID: 18669521
41. Saxena A, Dodell-Feder D (2022) Explaining the association between urbanicity and psychotic-like experiences in pre-adolescence: the indirect effect of urban exposures. Front Psych 11(13):831089. https://doi.org/10.3389/fpsyt.2022.831089. PMID: 35360125; PMCID: PMC8962621
42. Schmitt A, Falkai P, Papiol S (2023) Neurodevelopmental disturbances in schizophrenia: evidence from genetic and environmental factors. J Neural Transm (Vienna) 130(3):195–205. https://doi.org/10.1007/s00702-022-02567-5. Epub 2022 Nov 12. PMID: 36370183; PMCID: PMC9660136
43. Fett AJ, Lemmers-Jansen ILJ, Krabbendam L (2019) Psychosis and urbanicity: a review of the recent literature from epidemiology to neurourbanism. Curr Opin Psychiatry 32(3):232–241. https://doi.org/10.1097/YCO.0000000000000486. PMID: 30724751; PMCID: PMC6493678
44. Lederbogen F, Kirsch P, Haddad L, Streit F, Tost H, Schuch P, Wüst S, Pruessner JC, Rietschel M, Deuschle M, Meyer-Lindenberg A (2011) City living and urban upbringing affect neural social stress processing in humans. Nature 474(7352):498–501. https://doi.org/10.1038/nature10190. PMID: 21697947
45. Luciano M, De Rosa C, Del Vecchio V, Sampogna G, Sbordone D, Atti AR, Bardicchia F, Bertossi F, Calò S, Cava L, Ciafone M, De Fazio P, Di Iorio G, Fantini E, Ferrari S, Ginanneschi A, Gotelli S, Macina A, Mulè A, Papanti D, Pingani L, Pinna F, Piselli M, Signorelli MS, Tarricone I, Tarsitani L, Ventriglio A, Carrà G, Catapano F, Fiorillo A (2016) Perceived insecurity, mental health and urbanization: results from a multicentric study. Int J Soc Psychiatry 62(3):252–261. https://doi.org/10.1177/0020764016629694. Epub 2016 Feb 19. PMID: 26896027
46. Bauman Z (2005) Liquid life. Polity Press, Cambridge
47. Rautio N, Filatova S, Lehtiniemi H, Miettunen J (2018) Living environment and its relationship to depressive mood: a systematic review. Int J Soc Psychiatry 64(1):92–103. https://doi.org/10.1177/0020764017744582. Epub 2017 Dec 6. PMID: 29212385
48. Wang R, Xue D, Liu Y, Chen H, Qiu Y (2018) The relationship between urbanization and depression in China: the mediating role of neighborhood social capital. Int J Equity Health 17(1):105. https://doi.org/10.1186/s12939-018-0825-x. PMID: 30041631; PMCID: PMC6056990
49. Purtle J, Nelson KL, Yang Y, Langellier B, Stankov I, Diez Roux AV (2019) Urban-rural differences in older adult depression: a systematic review and meta-analysis of comparative studies. Am J Prev Med 56(4):603–613. https://doi.org/10.1016/j.amepre.2018.11.008. Epub 2019 Feb 16. PMID: 30777704
50. Casant J, Helbich M (2022) Inequalities of suicide mortality across urban and rural areas: a literature review. Int J Environ Res Public Health 19(5):2669. https://doi.org/10.3390/ijerph19052669. PMID: 35270369; PMCID: PMC8909802
51. Durkheim E (1897/1951) Suicide: a study in sociology. Routledge, London
52. Fontanella CA, Hiance-Steelesmith DL, Phillips GS, Bridge JA, Lester N, Sweeney HA, Campo JV (2015) Widening rural-urban disparities in youth suicides, United States, 1996-2010. JAMA Pediatr 169(5):466–473. https://doi.org/10.1001/jamapediatrics.2014.3561. PMID: 25751611; PMCID: PMC4551430
53. Helbich M, Blüml V, de Jong T, Plener PL, Kwan MP, Kapusta ND (2017) Urban-rural inequalities in suicide mortality: a comparison of urbanicity indicators. Int J Health Geogr 16(1):39. https://doi.org/10.1186/s12942-017-0112-x. PMID: 29084555; PMCID: PMC5663034
54. Reccord C, Power N, Hatfield K, Karaivanov Y, Mulay S, Wilson M, Pollock N (n.d.) Rural-urban differences in suicide mortality: an observational study in Newfoundland and Labrador, Canada: Différences de la Mortalité Par Suicide en Milieu Rural-Urbain: Une Étude
55. Fineberg N, Demetrovics Z, Stein D, Ioannidis K, Potenza M, Grünblatt E, Chamberlain S (2018) Manifesto for a European research network into problematic usage of the internet. Eur Neuropsychopharmacol 28(11):1232–1246
56. Morgan M (2019) Pathways between urbanization and harmful substance use. Curr Opin 32(3):218
57. Szabo CP (2018) Urbanization and mental health: a developing world perspective. Curr Opin Psychiatry 31:256
58. Turner S, Mota N, Bolton J et al (2018) Self-medication with alcohol or drugs for mood and anxiety disorders: a narrative review of the epidemiological literature. Depress Anxiety 35:851–860
59. AlSayyari A, AlBuhairan F (2018) Relationship of media exposure to substance use among adolescents in Saudi Arabia: results from a national study. Drug Alcohol Depend 191:174–180
60. Martinotti G, Lupi M, Carlucci L, Cinosi E, Santacroce R, Acciavatti T, Chillemi E, Bonifaci L, Janiri L, Di Giannantonio M (2015) Novel psychoactive substances: use and knowledge among adolescents and young adults in urban and rural areas. Hum Psychopharmacol 30(4):295–301. https://doi.org/10.1002/hup.2486. PMID: 26216566

61. Roderick E, Penney J, Murrells T et al (2018) Epidemiology of adolescent substance use in Norfolk schools. QJM 111:699–706
62. Doran KM, Rahai N, McCormack RP et al (2018) Substance use and homelessness among emergency department patients. Drug Alcohol Depend 188:328–333
63. Ko CH, Yen JY, Lin PC (2022) Association between urbanization and internet addiction. Curr Opin Psychiatry 35(3):219–225. https://doi.org/10.1097/YCO.0000000000000780. Epub 2022 Jan 25. PMID: 35081557
64. Cao H, Sun Y, Wan Y et al (2011) Problematic internet use in Chinese adolescents and its relation to psychosomatic symptoms and life satisfaction. BMC Public Health 11:802
65. Stavropoulos V, Alexandraki K, Motti-Stefanidi F (2013) Recognizing internet addiction: prevalence and relationship to academic achievement in adolescents enrolled in urban and rural Greek high schools. J Adolesc 36:565–576
66. Ying Ying C, Awaluddin SM, Kuang Kuay L, Siew Man C, Baharudin A, Miaw Yn L, Sahril N, Omar MA, Ahmad NA, Ibrahim N (2020) Association of internet addiction with adolescents' lifestyle: a national school-based survey. Int J Environ Res Public Health 18(1):168. https://doi.org/10.3390/ijerph18010168. PMID: 33383635; PMCID: PMC7801949
67. Park S, Jeon HJ, Son JW et al (2017) Correlates, comorbidities, and suicidal tendencies of problematic game use in a national wide sample of Korean adults. Int J Ment Health Syst 11:35
68. Yasuma N, Watanabe K, Nishi D et al (2019) Urbanization and internet addiction in a nationally representative sample of adult community residents in Japan: a cross-sectional, multilevel study. Psyachiatr Res 273:699–705
69. Yasuma N, Nishi D, Watanabe K et al (2021) Association between urban upbringing and compulsive internet use in Japan: a cross-sectional, multilevel study with retrospective recall. Int J Environ Res Public Health 18:9890
70. Li L, Xu DD, Chai JX et al (2018) Prevalence of internet addiction disorder in Chinese university students: a comprehensive meta-analysis of observational studies. J Behav Addict 7:610–623
71. Chen Y, Kang Y, Gong W et al (2016) Investigation on internet addiction disorder in adolescents in Anhui, People's Republic of China. Neuropsychiatr Dis Treat 12:2233–2236
72. Prakash S (2017) Internet addiction among junior doctors: a cross-sectional study. Indian J Psychol Med 39:422–425
73. Li Y, Zhang X, Lu F et al (2014) Internet addiction among elementary and middle school students in China: a nationally representative sample study. Cyberpsychol Behav Soc Netw 17:111–116
74. Yen CF, Ko CH, Yen JY et al (2009) Multidimensional discriminative factors for internet addiction among adolescents regarding gender and age. Psychiatry Clin Neurosci 63:357–364
75. Pawtowska B, Zygo M, Potembska E et al (2015) Prevalence of internet addiction and risk of developing addiction as exemplified by a group of polish adolescents from urban and rural areas. Ann Agric Environ Med 22:129–136
76. Tsiolka E, Bergiannaki ID, Margariti M et al (2017) Dysfunctional internet behaviour symptoms in association with personality traits. Psychiatriki 28:211–218
77. Nemati Z, Matlabi H (2017) Assessing behavioral patterns of internet addiction and drug abuse among high school students. Pyschol Res Behav Manag 10:39–45
78. Puharić Z, Stašević I, Ropac D, Petričević N, Jurišić I (2014) Istrazivanje čimbenika nastanka ovisnosti o internetu [A study investigating the factors of internet addiction]. Acta Med Croatica 68(4–5):361–373. Croatian. PMID: 26285469
79. Poli R, Agrimi E (2012) Internet addiction disorder: prevalence in an Italian student population. Nordic J Psychiatr 66:55–59
80. Hamza A, Sharma MK, Anand N et al (2019) Urban and rural pattern of internet use among youth and its association with mood state. J Family Med Prim Care 8:2602–2606
81. Ngui EM, Khasakhala L, Ndetei D, Roberts LW (2010) Mental disorders, health inequalities and ethics: a global perspective. Int Rev Psychiatry 22(3):235–244. https://doi.org/10.3109/09540261.2010.485273. PMID: 20528652; PMCID: PMC2935265
82. Murali V, Oyebode F (2004) Poverty, social inequality and mental health. Adv Psychiatr Treat 10:216–224
83. Schifano F, Leoni M, Martinotti G, Rawaf S, Rovetto F (2003) Importance of cyberspace for the assessment of the drug abuse market: preliminary results from the Psychonaut 2002 project. Cyberpsychol Behav 6(4):405–410. https://doi.org/10.1089/109493103322278790. PMID: 14511453
84. Lora A, Barbato A, Cerati G, Erlicher A, Percudani M (2012) The mental health system in Lombardy, Italy: access to services and patterns of care. Soc Psychiatry Psychiatr Epidemiol 47:447–454
85. Lora A, Monzio Compagnoni M, Allevi L, Barbato A, Carle F, D'avanzo B, Di Fiandra T, Ferrara L, Gaddini A, Leogrande M, Saponaro A, Scondotto S, Tozzi VD, Carbone S, Corrao G; 'QUADIM project' and 'Monitoring and assessing diagnostic-therapeutic paths (MAP)' working groups of the Italian Ministry of Health (2022) The quality of mental health care delivered to patients with schizophrenia and related disorders in the Italian mental health system. The QUADIM project: a multi-regional Italian investigation based on healthcare utilisation databases. Epidemiol Psychiatr Sci 31:e15. https://doi.org/10.1017/S2045796022000014. PMID: 35156603; PMCID: PMC8851066

19 The Impact of Job on Mental Health

Pasquale De Fazio, Renato de Filippis, Antonio Ventriglio, and Antonello Bellomo

Abstract

Both work and unemployment can serve as significant protective and/or risk factors for mental health in different ways. Indeed, employment provides individuals with a sense of purpose, structure, economic stability, and social interaction, contributing positively to their mental well-being. Conversely, unemployment can lead to financial stress, loss of self-esteem, and social isolation, all of which can exacerbate mental health issues. However, the connection between work, unemployment, and major psychiatric disorders is complex and varied. Prolonged unemployment can increase the risk of developing severe mental health illnesses, particularly in young adults. In addition, individuals facing unemployment are more vulnerable to suicidal ideation and behavior due to the emotional toll of job loss. Addressing these risks requires a holistic approach that encompasses not only employment support but also mental health services. Moreover, work holds also the potential to be a therapeutic and rehabilitative element within the framework of mental health care. Meaningful employment can provide a sense of accomplishment and purpose for individuals recovering from mental illness. Supported employment programs and inclusive workplaces can play a vital role in the recovery process, promoting social integration and improving self-esteem. Recognizing work as a therapeutic opportunity underscores the importance of a comprehensive approach to mental health care that includes vocational support alongside clinical treatment. This chapter aims to explore these implications of work and unemployment in mental health.

Keywords

Employment · Mental health · Job Empowerment · Workplace · Stigma

19.1 Introduction

Work—considered from an anthropological point of view—has moved from the category of duty to that of right and necessity in a relatively short time, representing the most relevant social element of affirmation and personal growth.

From a psychiatric point of view, work has taken on particular interest in recent years: in

P. De Fazio (✉) · R. de Filippis
Psychiatry Unit, Department of Health Sciences, University Magna Graecia of Catanzaro, Catanzaro, Italy
e-mail: defazio@unicz.it

A. Ventriglio · A. Bellomo
Department of Clinical and Experimental Medicine, University of Foggia, Foggia, Italy
e-mail: antonello.bellomo@unifg.it

A. Fiorillo, S. De Giorgi (eds.), *Social Determinants of Mental Health*, Sustainable Development Goals Series, https://doi.org/10.1007/978-3-031-70165-8_19

fact, its presence or lack seems capable of generating numerous mental health issues, including anxiety, depression, and increased suicidality risk. On the other hand, it has been shown that people suffering from a serious mental disorder, in most cases, have never worked or have rarely started working and those who work are strongly affected by the presence of stigma. It should also be considered that the COVID-19 pandemic has also played a role in modifying the classic paradigm of in-person work, quickly and ubiquitously spreading the option of teleworking, with economic and commuting advantages but making social interaction more difficult. Indeed, as telecommuting and mobile work arrangements continue to proliferate due to advancements in digitalization, these adaptable work models are rapidly extending to encompass various employee categories, thereby reshaping working conditions and the quality of jobs. On this regard, research demonstrated that occasional telecommuters enjoy the highest job quality, while highly mobile telecommuters experience the lowest job quality and struggle with work-life balance. Home-based telecommuters, particularly women, exhibit superior outcomes in terms of working time quality and intensity, albeit at the expense of reduced skills and autonomy, income, and career prospects [1].

Finally, with a view to the empowerment and recovery of patients with serious mental disorders, work becomes an important rehabilitation opportunity for people with mental disorders.

In this chapter, we will try to outline the role of work in mental health following these three guidelines: (1) mental health in the workplace; (2) work difficulties for people with mental disorders; (3) the role of work for patients with serious mental disorders.

19.2 Mental Health and the Workplace

According to the Organization for Economic Cooperation and Development [2], 5% of the working population in high-income countries suffer from serious mental health illnesses, and a further 15% have mental health issues of moderate severity.

The mental disorders most often found among workers include depression, anxiety disorders, sleep disorders, adjustment disorders, and other stress-related conditions, such as burnout [3]. These disorders would be related to poor working conditions, defined as "work stress factors."

Depressive disorder is a fairly common mental health problem in the workplace. It is associated with poor quality of life and work functioning, with a significant impact not only on the work management, but also on society in general. Workplace depressive disorders include mild and sub-clinical to severe forms, associated with greater levels of disability and an increased risk of relapse [4]. Anxiety disorders can also be linked to stressful factors in the workplace, with negative effects on work performance, relationships with colleagues and the quality of the work performed. The concepts of "workplace anxiety" and "workplace phobia" have recently been introduced; in particular, phobia seems to be the most serious form of anxiety, defined as a phobic reaction with symptoms of panic occurring when thinking of or approaching the workplace and highly correlated with absenteeism [5]. Work-related anxiety disorders must be distinguished from other phenomena with social impact, such as workplace bullying (mobbing) and burnout syndrome.

Mobbing is defined as the set of negative behaviors conducted against an employee frequently and for a prolonged period of time by colleagues or supervisors [6]; it is a working condition rather than a real mental disorder. Burnout is a syndrome linked to chronic stress in the workplace and is characterized by emotional exhaustion with loss of energy, depersonalization or cynicism, emotional detachment in the workplace, reduced professional effectiveness and productivity. The effects of burnout on mental health include insomnia, depressive symptoms, increased use of psychotropic drugs and antidepressants, and increased likelihood of hospitalization for mental disorders. Burnout is also highly linked to suicidal ideation and suicidal attempts in diverse occupations [7].

19.3 Work as a Risk Factor for Mental Disorders: The Psychosocial Model

Over the last 30 years, the complex relationship between psychological well-being and the work environment has been explained through various psychosocial models [3]. In particular, it has been documented that well-being at work is influenced by various factors, relating both to the workplace and to the characteristics of the workers and to the individual's living environment. Individual vulnerability factors include cognitive abilities, coping strategies, social support, and temperament factors. A particularly relevant risk factor is the negative affectivity, with a prevalence of negative emotions such as pessimism and anger.

In addition, also the precarious employment is associated with an adverse effect on mental health, supported by moderate-quality evidence in a recent systematic review, although high-quality prospective studies remain limited as well as studies stratifying gender differences [8–10].

Other factors that increase the risk of developing mental disorders in the workplace include high job demands, low decision-making freedom, poor support at work, imbalance between effort and rewards, job insecurity, atypical work, conflicts in the workplace, and stress related to the role within the organization [3]. These models will be briefly exposed in the following paragraphs.

19.3.1 The Job Demand-Control-Support Model (JDCS)

According to the demand-control-support model of work, work activities with high performance required (increased workload and little time available), when associated with poor decision-making freedom, may lead to high-tension situations that induce greater risk of developing mental disorders. The model was subsequently complemented by workplace social support, which could play a moderating role [11].

19.3.2 The Effort-Reward Imbalance Model (ERI)

The effort-reward imbalance model is based on the experience of the balance between the efforts made at work and the rewards received by the worker. According to this model, the most stressful working conditions are those in which the knowledge obtained in the workplace does not correspond to the effort expended. In particular, the lack of reciprocity between the worker's high effort and low reward generates negative emotions in the worker, with long-term negative effects on mental health. Greater susceptibility to these stress responses can be found in people with a coping style characterized by rigidity, excessive emotional involvement, and the desire for hypercontrol [12].

19.3.3 The Organizational Justice Model

The organizational justice model refers to the correct application of rules and social norms within companies. This model refers to the appropriateness in the distribution of resources and benefits (distributive justice), in the allocation of resources (procedural justice), in the treatment received from the authority, and in the level of information sharing (relational justice). It has been recently demonstrated that this model leads to high levels of job satisfaction [13].

19.3.4 Job Insecurity and Organizational Changes

Organizational changes, such as downsizing, relocation, mergers, and increased workload, are increasingly frequent in companies. An inverse relationship has been observed between organizational changes and mental health, although this association tends to lose significance in prospective studies, suggesting an important role of adaptation over time to organizational changes. Frequent changes in work organization, as well as economic difficulties, can lead the worker to a perception of poor job security which, in turn, increases the risk of mental disorders, burnout syndrome, and depression.

19.3.5 Job Insecurity and Atypical Working Hours

Available evidence suggests that temporary employees have greater psychological morbidity than permanent employees. Several studies have demonstrated the association between atypical working hours and an increase in depressive and anxious symptoms. In particular, the risk would increase when 40 h per week or 8 h per day are exceeded [14]. However, a recent meta-analysis highlighted only a slight increase in risk for depressive disorders, with a stronger association for females [15]. Sleep disorders, on the contrary, are strongly correlated to increased workloads, with a greater risk of sleep disorders and burnout syndrome in shift workers [16].

19.3.6 Workplace Conflicts and Mobbing

The impact of workplace conflicts on mental health is limited, while mobbing causes an increase in depressive, anxiety, and stress-related symptoms [17]. Furthermore, mobbing also increases the risk of suicidal ideation, although this association is not supported by adequate evidence [18]. The financial and psychological consequences of bullying are considerable, resulting in increased absenteeism, staff turnover, lower work commitment, and low job satisfaction [17].

19.3.7 Role-Stress

The impact of role-stress on mental health has been assessed in terms of role-ambiguity (when an employee lacks information about his or her role and responsibilities) and role-conflict (when there are two or more opposing expectations with respect to the employee's role). Schmidt et al. [19] documented that both conflict and role-ambiguity are related to an increase in depressive symptoms.

19.3.8 The Integrated Model

The risk factors and models of interaction between workplace stress and mental health overlap and it is not appropriate to consider the various models in isolation. Recently, Harvey et al. [3] proposed an integrated model that identifies three clusters of risk factors in the workplace: (1) disequilibrium in the workplace (excessive work demands, low decision-making freedom, poor social support); (2) uncertainty at work (low decision-making freedom, low procedural justice, frequent organizational changes, job insecurity, temporary employment status); (3) lack of value and respect internally of the work environment (low procedural justice, low relational justice, temporary employment status, poor social support).

19.4 Unemployment and Mental Disorders

The presence of a mental disorder or psychological distress has often been considered a risk factor for unemployment, since individuals who suffer from psychological distress have a greater tendency to leave or not find a job. On the other hand, unemployment is a condition that independently has a significant negative impact on physical and mental health. Indeed, a study investigating the link between the extent of unemployment experienced during the severe Swedish recession of 1992–1996 and subsequent mortality over a 6-year period, revealed that the risk of mortality rises with the duration of unemployment, with different patterns observed for men and women. The underlying causes of death demonstrate varying associations with the duration of unemployment, highlighting the complex interplay between unemployment and mortality outcomes [20].

Reasons why unemployment worsens mental health include: changes in living standards, income insecurity, stigma and loss of self-esteem, and loss of social contacts. In particular, unemployment can be associated with a loss of status within the social network, family and community in general, with consequent loss of self-esteem. Individuals who have been unemployed for many years have a double risk of developing depressive and anxiety disorders compared to employed workers or compared to those who have only been unemployed for a short period. Numerous studies conducted after the 2008 European economic crisis have documented that unemployed people are more likely to develop depressive symptoms, to be more stressed and to perceive a lower well-being and quality of life compared to individuals with a job [21].

Furthermore, the impact of unemployment on mental health varies by age and being unemployed at a young age also has an impact in adulthood, regardless of other experiences of job loss [22]. Some factors specific to youth, such as the uncertainty linked to the transition to adulthood and changes in social relationships, can contribute to the development of a depressive condition in young, unemployed adults. Unemployment among young people correlates with a reduction in both physical and mental health levels as well as an increase in the consumption of alcohol, drugs, and cigarettes. Finally, unemployment represents a risk factor for suicidality, with a greater risk in the first 5 years after job loss [23]. The association between unemployment and the risk of suicide is due to the interaction of numerous factors, such as increased risk of developing a depressive disorder, economic difficulties, reduction in the possibility of accessing healthcare, interruption of treatments in progress.

For instance, during the economic crisis, an upsurge in suicidal tendencies was observed in Europe, particularly in Greece. These reports garnered significant media attention and became a topic of discussion among political parties [24, 25]. Existing literature indicates that deep economic crises are associated with a rise in suicides, but a clear cause-and-effect relationship remains elusive. The prevailing consensus, both in scientific literature and the media, is that the economic crisis poses a more or less universal risk to the entire population, affecting virtually anyone. However, recent studies challenge this notion by revealing that suicide rates increased several months before unemployment rates did. Moreover, when focusing on Greece, where the economic crisis has been more severe and prolonged, the examination of age and gender-specific suicide rates does not align with a simple "male gender" and "unemployment" interaction.

Considering these factors, along with the observation that even prosperous countries with low unemployment rates like Germany and Norway have experienced a rise in suicides, another possible explanation emerges [24]. It suggests that changes in the socioeconomic landscape, particularly in employment conditions, have placed excessive strain on vulnerable populations, such as individuals with mental health issues, leading to increased suicide rates. The issue at hand is that much of the existing literature treats the economic crisis and austerity measures as generic risk factors affecting the entire population, leading to broad, one-size-fits-all recommendations. Unfortunately, individuals at risk of suicide are not recognized as such; instead, they are often treated as ordinary, healthy individuals who respond to generic adverse events with suicidal behavior [24].

In the recent recession, rising unemployment had a greater impact on suicide rates in countries with less developed protection measures (Eastern and Southern Europe). In contrast, the increase in the number of unemployed in Scandinavia, a country with the highest level of worker protection, did not have particularly clear consequences on the risk of suicide. Furthermore, the impact of economic recession on mental health is dependent on the country's national income. In high-income countries, the effect of unemployment on mental health is less marked, as workers have greater availability of unemployment benefits, debt reduction programs, and social assistance [26]. In Southern Italy, unemployment has a negative impact not only on the possibility of developing a mental disorder, but also on the perception of health [27]. Barriers to employment for people with mental disorders are summarized in Table 19.1.

Table 19.1 Barriers to employment for people with mental disorders

Stigma
Discrimination
Lack of policies
Fear of losing one's rights
Work environment intolerant to changes in employee productivity
Concerns about rising health care and insurance costs

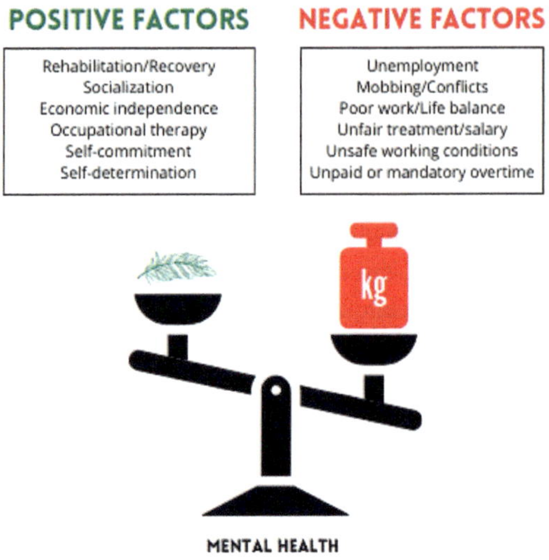

Fig. 19.1 The relationship between job and mental health: positive and negative factors

19.4.1 Prevention Interventions

The growing costs of mental disorders related to work stress and their impact on individual and social functioning require the development of effective prevention strategies. Although guidelines are available in various countries around the world to address work disability induced by mental disorders or stress-related symptoms, these guidelines are difficult to find, poorly applicable and of poor quality [28].

Interventions aimed at solving mental health problems in the workplace have been developed by various areas of expertise, including occupational doctors, psychiatrists, psychologists, hygienists, and workers responsible for workplace safety. The consequence is the difficulty of adopting truly integrated preventive approaches, as there is often a tendency to focus only on one area of intervention. For an intervention to be preventive, it is necessary to modify and minimize the associated risk factors at work, promote positive and protective factors within the workplace, and manage disorders, regardless of the cause (Fig. 19.1).

19.5 Work as a Rehabilitative Opportunity for Patients with Mental Disorders

The majority of patients with serious mental disorders do not have a job [29] and only 30–40% of patients manage to find a job and keep it over time.

Workers with mental disorders often are unable to perform adequate work due to problems with concentration, attention, and planning. Nonetheless, the majority of patients with mental disorders want to find work, although the search for stable work is made difficult by numerous factors, among which stigma plays a predominant role. In fact, patients with mental health problems are often forced to be fired or resign by their employers when they become aware of psychiatric problems. For this reason, many patients do not declare in the workplace that they are suffering from mental health disorders for fear of being discriminated against, creating a daily internal state of tension for fear of being discovered. When the pathology becomes known, problems of discrimination arise, since it is a common belief that patients suffering from mental disorders are not able to work. In fact, the general population believes that giving a job to a person with mental disorders is an act of charity that is inconsistent with the needs of the workplace [30] (Table 19.1). Furthermore, fewer than four out of ten employers are willing to hire people with serious mental disorders, especially given the costs resulting from absenteeism, reduced productivity during employment, coverage of absent staff and early retirement.

Another obstacle for the employment of patients with serious mental disorders is due to the changing world of work, which increasingly requires greater social skills and communication skills, which are often lacking in this group of people.

Although patients with mental disorders have enormous difficulties in functioning at work, the role of work in the recovery process is now widely documented. In fact, participation in work can have positive effects on long-term personal and social functioning, the reduction of symptoms and relapse rates. Having a job can make individuals feel more appreciated, foster a sense of belonging and acceptance, and actively contribute to social development [31].

One of the objectives of the recovery process is to promote, maintain, and build one's identity, also through work. In fact, the income deriving from work allows patients to achieve financial self-sufficiency, to be independent from their family and to improve their quality of life. Employment also provides non-financial benefits, in terms of defining the self and improving levels of self-esteem, which allows one to improve social interactions and develop adaptive coping strategies.

Another fundamental element in promoting job placement is the recognition of individual strengths. The Individual Placement and Support (IPS) model is based on individualized support that aims to strengthen the person's skills, resources, and support during the different phases that characterize the encounter with the world of work.

Numerous mental disorders, particularly chronic and severe conditions like those within the schizophrenia-spectrum, are incapacitating conditions that profoundly affect the social and cognitive functioning of individuals, including their ability to engage in work activities. Consequently, individuals grappling with these conditions often exhibit a specific vulnerability in terms of their socioeconomic circumstances, necessitating targeted social safety nets and rehabilitation measures, which may encompass disability benefits or assistance with job placement. Individuals afflicted by psychoses were found to be more prone to unemployment, reported greater levels of occupational impairment, and received more incentives and rehabilitation interventions. These results underscore the disabling nature of schizophrenia-spectrum disorders and emphasize the crucial need for psychosocial support and interventions within a framework that prioritizes recovery-oriented treatment [32].

The IPS model, born in Great Britain, stands out for being a personalized approach to the user's work needs starting from their own preferences with support in finding a job within the competitive job market. The main characteristics of the IPS model are summarized in Table 19.2. This model is currently the standard for the rehabilitation of unemployed adults with serious mental disorders. The probability of finding competitive employment for individuals treated with IPS is approximately double compared to patients receiving other rehabilitation interventions [33].

Other interventions aimed at employing people with mental health problems include the clubhouse model. The clubhouses are based on the principles of empowerment, i.e., the achievement of self-awareness and control over one's choices, decisions, and actions, both in the context of personal relationships and in that of social life, and recovery.

These principles are implemented through co-management (members and staff manage the clubhouse together), peer help (mutual and structured support among members), and non-medicalized (medical and psychotherapeutic interventions are performed by professionals independent of the staff). Clubhouses offer a range of activities and support, including social and recreational events and help with accessing education, employment, and housing. However, few studies exist on the effectiveness of clubhouses, and existing studies suggest only moderate or low levels of evidence regarding their effectiveness [34].

Table 19.2 Operational characteristics of Individual Placement and Support (IPS)

Individual placement and support (IPS)	Patient choice
	Individualized job search
	Extended pre-placement
	Integration with and within the treatment group
	Involvement of specialist figures

Although available data indicates that 60% of people with serious mental health problems can succeed in their jobs when using employment support services, a recent survey estimated that only 2% of them receive interventions for job placement. Rehabilitative interventions have continued to spread across states and countries, but only a few regions have made IPS available to a large portion of eligible people with psychiatric disabilities [33]. The main obstacles to the widespread implementation of these interventions for job placement appear to be the scarcity of financial resources and the lack of attention toward people who are indigent and stigmatized by mental illness. Other obstacles in implementing these models include organizational and systematization difficulties, barriers related to specialized employment skills and personal aptitudes.

Work can significantly improve the quality of life and income of people with psychiatric disabilities; consequently, the clinical course of the disease can also improve, reducing the costs of healthcare treatment over time and promoting social inclusion processes.

The next critical step in clinical practice is to ensure global access to high-quality job placement services. Therefore, future efforts should focus on workplace accommodations, greater investment in evidence-based return-to-work programs, and efforts to popularize early intervention programs [35].

19.6 Conclusion

The significance of employment within mental health care cannot be overstated. Unemployment exacerbates mental health issues, while gaining employment can enhance mental well-being, even for individuals grappling with severe mental illnesses [36]. In this chapter, we advocated for a fresh approach to mental health treatment that prioritizes employment. Supported employment, an evidence-backed intervention, holds the potential to assist the majority of individuals with mental health disabilities in achieving success in competitive, integrated workplaces. Distinguishing itself from many other mental health treatments, employment fosters self-reliance and yields other valuable outcomes, including increased self-confidence, the respect of peers, personal income, and community integration. It not only proves effective as a short-term intervention but also stands out as one of the few approaches that reduces reliance on the mental health system over time.

Authors' Contributions All authors have actively contributed to the chapter and approved it in its current form.

References

1. Rodríguez-Modroño P, López-Igual P (2021) Job quality and work-life balance of teleworkers. Int J Environ Res Public Health 18(6):3239. https://doi.org/10.3390/ijerph18063239. PMID: 33800995; PMCID: PMC8003956
2. Organization for Economic Cooperation and Development (OECD) (2023) Statistics news releases. https://www.oecd.org/sdd/statisticsnewsreleases.htm
3. Harvey SB, Modini M, Joyce S et al (2017) Can work make you mentally ill? A systematic meta-review of work-related risk factors for common mental health problems. Occup Environ Med 74:301–310
4. Greenberg PE, Fournier AA, Sisitsky T et al (2015) The economic burden of adults with major depressive disorder in the United States (2005 and 2010). J Clin Psychiatry 76:155–162
5. Muschalla B, Linden M (2009) Workplace phobia—a first explorative study on its relation to established anxiety disorders, sick leave, and work-directed treatment. Psychol Health Med 14(5):591–605. https://doi.org/10.1080/13548500903207398
6. Einarsen S, Hoel H, Zapf D (2010) The concept of bullying and harassment at work in the work place developments in theory, research, and practice. CRC Press, New York, pp 3–39
7. Oh DJ, Shin YC, Oh KS, Shin DW, Jeon SW, Cho SJ (2023) Examining the links between burnout and suicidal ideation in diverse occupations. Front Public Health 11:1243920. Published 2023 Sep 7. https://doi.org/10.3389/fpubh.2023.1243920
8. Rönnblad T, Grönholm E, Jonsson J, Koranyi I, Orellana C, Kreshpaj B, Chen L, Stockfelt L, Bodin T (2019) Precarious employment and mental health: a systematic review and meta-analysis of longitudinal studies. Scand J Work Environ Health 45(5):429–443. https://doi.org/10.5271/sjweh.3797. Epub 2019 Jan 25. PMID: 31165899
9. Utzet M, Valero E, Mosquera I, Martin U (2020) Employment precariousness and mental health, understanding a complex reality: a systematic review. Int J Occup Med Environ Health 33(5):569–598. https://doi.org/10.13075/ijomeh.1896.01553. Epub 2020 Sep 17. PMID: 32940256

10. Valero E, Martin U, Bacigalupe A, Utzet M (2021) The impact of precarious jobs on mental health: a gender-sensitive literature review. Int Arch Occup Environ Health 94(4):577–589. https://doi.org/10.1007/s00420-020-01605-7. Epub 2020 Nov 24. PMID: 33236281
11. Portoghese I, Galletta M, Leiter MP, Finco G, d'Aloja E, Campagna M (2020) Job demand-control-support latent profiles and their relationships with interpersonal stressors, job burnout, and intrinsic work motivation. Int J Environ Res Public Health 17(24):9430. https://doi.org/10.3390/ijerph17249430. PMID: 33339208; PMCID: PMC7765581
12. van Vegchel N, de Jonge J, Bosma H, Schaufeli W (2005) Reviewing the effort-reward imbalance model: drawing up the balance of 45 empirical studies. Soc Sci Med 60(5):1117–1131. https://doi.org/10.1016/j.socscimed.2004.06.043
13. Ekingen E (2023) The effect of organizational justice on job performance and the mediating role of job satisfaction: a study on nurses. Hosp Top 101(2):103–112. https://doi.org/10.1080/00185868.2021.1969874
14. Bannai A, Tamakoshi A (2014) The association between long working hours and health: a systematic review of epidemiological evidence. Scand J Work Environ Health 40:5–18
15. Watanabe K, Imamura K, Kawakami N (2016) Working hours and the onset of depressive disorder: a systematic review and metaanalysis. Occup Environ Med 73:877–884
16. Cheng WJ, Cheng Y (2017) Night shift and rotating shift in association with sleep problems, burnout and minor mental disorder in male and female employees. Occup Environ Med 74:483–488
17. Verkuil B, Atasayi S, Molendijk ML (2015) Workplace bullying and mental health: a meta-analysis on cross-sectional and longitudinal data. PLoS One 10:e0135225
18. Leach LS, Poyser C, Butterworth P (2017) Workplace bullying and the association with suicidal ideation/thoughts and behaviour: a systematic review. Occup Environ Med 74:72–79
19. Schmidt S et al (2014) Uncertainty in the workplace: examining role ambiguity and role conflict, and their link to depression—a meta-analysis. Eur J Work Organ Psychol 23:91–106
20. Garcy AM, Vågerö D (2012) The length of unemployment predicts mortality, differently in men and women, and by cause of death: a six year mortality follow-up of the Swedish 1992-1996 recession. Soc Sci Med 74(12):1911–1920. https://doi.org/10.1016/j.socscimed.2012.01.034. Epub 2012 Mar 13. PMID: 22465382
21. Pelzer B, Schaffrath S, Vernaleken I (2014) Coping with unemployment: the impact of unemployment on mental health, personality, and social interaction skills. Work 48:289–295
22. Fergusson DM, McLeod GF, Horwood LJ (2014) Unemployment and psychosocial outcomes to age 30: a fixed-effects regression analysis. Aust N Z J Psychiatry 48:735–742
23. Milner A, Page A, LaMontagne AD (2013) Long-term unemployment and suicide: a systematic review and meta-analysis. PLoS One 8:e51333
24. Fountoulakis KN (2017) Employment insecurity, mental health and suicide. Psychiatriki 28(3):259–264. https://doi.org/10.22365/jpsych.2017.283.259. PMID: 29072190
25. Jónsdóttir U, Þórðardóttir EB, Aspelund T, Jónmundsson Þ, Einarsdóttir K (2020) The effect of the 2008 recession on well-being and employment status of people with and without mental health problems. Eur J Pub Health 30(4):761–766. https://doi.org/10.1093/eurpub/ckz192. PMID: 31800030
26. Antti U (2010) Economic crisis and mental health. Curr Opin Psychiatry 23:127–130
27. De Fazio P, Cerminara G, Calabrò G et al (2015) Unemployment, perceived health status and coping: a study in southern Italy. Work 53:219–224
28. Joosen MC, Brouwers EP, van Beurden KM et al (2015) An international comparison of occupational health guidelines for the management of mental disorders and stress-related psychological symptoms. Occup Environ Med 72:313–322
29. Nobel JH (2000) A legacy of failure: the inability of the federal-state vocational rehabilitation system to serve people with serious mental illness. National Alliance for the Mentally Illness, Arlington
30. Long PW (2005) Mental illness and work, 1995-2005. Canadian Psychiatric Association, Ottawa
31. Brown W, Kandirikirira N (2007) Engagement. In: Recovering mental health in Scotland. Report on narrative investigation of mental health recovery. Scottish Recovery Network, Glasgow
32. Ventriglio A, Latorre M, Calabretta MA, Cuomo A, Di Gioia I, Ducci G, Ghio L, Mallozzi A, Politi P, Suma D, Tarricone I, Valentini Gravinese G, Vita A, Essimh Working Group, Bellomo A (2023) Employment and social security/insurance among patients affected by mental disorders in Italy: a descriptive multicenter study. Int J Soc Psychiatry 69(7):1736–1748. https://doi.org/10.1177/00207640231174358. PMID: 37178011
33. Metcalfe JD, Drake R, Bond G (2018) Economic, labor, and regulatory moderators of the effect of individual placement and support among people with severe mental illness: a systematic review and meta-analysis. Schizophr Bull 44:22–31
34. Battin C, Bouvet C, Hatala C (2016) A systematic review of the effectiveness of the clubhouse model. Psychiatr Rehabil J 39:305–312
35. Frank RG, Glied SAM, Shields M (2021) Jobs for people with mental health conditions: trends and prospects. Psychiatr Serv 72(2):143–147. https://doi.org/10.1176/appi.ps.202000243. Epub 2020 Sep 23. PMID: 32966178; PMCID: PMC7869603
36. Drake RE, Wallach MA (2020) Employment is a critical mental health intervention. Epidemiol Psychiatr Sci 29:e178. https://doi.org/10.1017/S2045796020000906. PMID: 33148366; PMCID: PMC7681163

Sport and Mental Health

20

Francesca Cirulli, Chiara Ciacchella, and Barbara Collacchi

Abstract

People with mental disorder experience an increased risk of physical diseases due to the high rate of physical comorbidities, which leads to an overall reduced life expectancy compared to the general population. There is a great potential for physical activity and sport to overcome, at least partially, health inequality experienced by individuals with mental disorders. Indeed, an active lifestyle has been shown to bring important benefits to the general population as well as to individuals at risk or experiencing mental disorder. There is now sufficient scientific evidence to include this type of activity in psychoeducational interventions as it also has the potential for fostering social relationships, increasing resilience and combating stigma. While more basic research and specific clinical trials are needed to assess the potential (positive) interaction of physical activity with pharmacological and psychotherapeutic treatments, the current evidence and the guidelines issued by important scientific societies, such as the European Psychiatric Association (EPA), call for acting now to incorporate physical activity programmes as a new standard of care for mental disorders.

Keywords

Sport · Physical activity · Resilience · Mental health · Psychiatry

Mental disorders represent a significant portion of the global burden of disease and a major cause of disability worldwide [1, 2]. People with severe mental disorders are characterised by a reduced life expectancy compared to the general population, largely due to cardiovascular and metabolic disorders and by high comorbidity with respiratory and osteoarticular disorders as a result of unhealthy lifestyles (e.g. smoking, sedentary behaviours and reduced physical activity) [3–5]. Severe mental disorders are also accompanied by cognitive decline, social withdrawal and the impoverishment of emotional relationships, all elements that represent an important risk factor for health; in fact, social isolation and the resulting sense of loneliness are relevant determinants of mortality [6–9] and affect the incidence and prognosis of cardiometabolic diseases and other physical disorders [10].

Despite the proven effectiveness of pharmacological and psychotherapeutic therapies (alone or in combination) for the management of psychiatric

F. Cirulli (✉) · C. Ciacchella · B. Collacchi
Center for Behavioral Sciences and Mental Health, Istituto Superiore di Sanità, Rome, Italy
e-mail: francesca.cirulli@iss.it; chiara.ciacchella@uniroma1.it; barbara.collacchi@iss.it

A. Fiorillo, S. De Giorgi (eds.), *Social Determinants of Mental Health*, Sustainable Development Goals Series, https://doi.org/10.1007/978-3-031-70165-8_20

symptoms, these approaches have limited effects on physical health [11]. By contrast, pharmacotherapies, especially antipsychotics, have documented adverse effects on cardiometabolic health [12, 13]. It has now become clear that a multidimensional and multidisciplinary approach, which takes into consideration the person's global health and well-being, including active participation in physical activity and social life, is necessary for a more effective rehabilitation and social integration. Greater knowledge on the specific effects of physical activity and sports can help health practitioners, therapists, psychologists and psychiatrists to increase the quality of life and the general health of individuals with mental disorder.

20.1 Benefits of Physical Activity for the Overall Health of the General Population

According to World Health Organization (WHO) definitions, physical exercise is *any body movement made by skeletal muscles which requires waste of energy*, while 'sport training' is characterised by planning, organisation, temporal repetitiveness and a final or intermediate aim to improve, or maintain, one or many physical well-being factors. Regular physical activity contributes to improving muscular and cardiorespiratory fitness, preserving bone and functional health and maintaining a healthy body weight. Therefore, physical activity is known to play a key role in reducing the risk of developing cardiovascular and metabolic diseases [14]. Exercise could be useful in improving cognitive function [15–18], strengthening social and interpersonal skills, as well as preventing (or delaying the onset of) mental issues and neurodegenerative conditions in children and adults by promoting neuronal plasticity, attenuating anxiety and stress and improving sleep quality [19].

As such, physical activity could be an important adjunctive therapy for the treatment of psychopathologies and neurodegenerative diseases, as well as an important coping strategy for dealing with problems in daily life and for reducing stress and negative emotions [20].

It is also acknowledged that physical activity positively affects the physiological processes involved in the stress response. Stress-related processes are central to many mental disorders and can influence physical pathologies (e.g. cardiovascular diseases) [21] through a direct link between psychological processes and biological systems (neuroendocrine, autonomic and immune) [22].

An active line of research is currently exploring the neurobiological pathways that are engaged by lifestyle factors and how they can impact mental health. Adaptations to external circumstances can trigger a sophisticated communication process between the nervous, endocrine and immune systems. Among the many effectors involved in adaptation, neurotrophins produced by the brain (mainly brain-derived neurotrophic factor, BDNF) stand out as the most important biomarkers linking physical activity with brain health [23]. Neurotrophins increase as a consequence of exercise, promoting neuronal cell survival, differentiation, migration, dendritic arborisation and synaptic plasticity. By contrast, they are reduced following stress and in cases of psychiatric disorders, such as major depression. An increase in the expression of BDNF, as a result of physical exercise, could act positively on the structure and function of the hippocampus [24], a fundamental area of the central nervous system that is specifically affected by stress and is involved in the pathophysiology of mental disorders, including major depression. Other important targets of physical activity are inflammatory processes and the overall activity of the immune system, which is a phenotypic core of many physical and psychiatric disorders. In fact, exercise is able to strengthen the immune system, stimulating the active exchange of immune cells from the circulation to the tissues, promoting anti-inflammatory and anti-oxidant effects and delaying the onset of immunosenescence [25]. During exercise other organs, in addition to the skeletal muscle, can stimulate the release of systemic factors (myokines, irisin, BDNF, cytokines, adipokines) with important effects on both the body and the brain. These substances, upon reaching the central nervous system, could act in synergy with local factors stimulating the development of new nerve cells or increasing the number of synaptic connections, with positive effects on memory, learning, emotional and cognitive abilities, preventing or counteracting the physiopathology underlying many psychiatric disorders [23]. Indeed, physical activity has been shown to lead to important mood changes [26–28]. High levels of aerobic exercise have a protective effect against the development of depressive symptoms and major depression [29]. It is important to underline that, to produce significant effects on depressive symptoms, exercise must be of sufficient duration and intensity [30].

Further studies are still necessary to define the mechanisms underlying these effects and to better investigate the role of physical activity in mediating the association between stress, metabolic disorders and mood disorders [31].

20.2 Benefits of Physical Activity for People with Mental Disorders

A recent meta-review of Firth and colleagues has tried to establish the current evidence on the relationship between key modifiable health behaviours such as lifestyles (e.g. physical activity, diet, smoking and sleep) and the incidence of major mental disorders (e.g. depression, anxiety, stress-related disorders, attention-deficit/hyperactivity disorder [ADHD], bipolar disorder and schizophrenia) [32]. As an example, poor sleep has been found to increase the risk of suicidal behaviour in people suffering from mental disorder [33]. Unhealthy meals, smoking, insufficient exercise and sleep dysregulation have also been shown to contribute to the development of stress, inflammation and dysmetabolic conditions, which in turn have a main impact on mental health [34].

The main principles of lifestyle interventions for mental disease could be summarised as using behaviour change techniques, involving staff specifically trained and facilitating peer support to improve adherence to the interventions [32]. There is now a growing body of evidence indicating that, among lifestyle interventions, physical activity has a major protecting role for mental disorders and may provide effective complementary treatment for some of them. Physical activity has the potential to bring various benefits to people with serious mental disorders who experience numerous comorbidities related to their condition and lifestyle. Exercise therapy could be a valuable option in mental health care, both in terms of the psychological and physical health of those suffering from various psychological disorders. To date, there is considerable evidence to support the use of exercise-based interventions in the treatment of major depression and schizophrenia [35]. A prospective study recently demonstrated that physical activity has comparable effects to antidepressants in reducing depressive symptoms [28]. More specifically, the use of moderate-intensity aerobic exercise at a frequency of 2–3 times per week (a total of 150 min per week) can reduce depressive symptoms and improve cardiorespiratory fitness in individuals with major depression, as well as improve disease-related symptoms, cognitive functioning and quality of life in individuals suffering from schizophrenia [36–38]. In addition to improving mood and psychotic symptoms, exercise can also mitigate other comorbid conditions such as fatigue, pain and sleep disturbances [39]. Evidence on beneficial effects in people with bipolar disorder is still scarce and more research is needed for this specific disease [35]. Further research is necessary to establish whether the use of physical activity in the early stages of the disease can have long-term protective effects. Furthermore, there is still little information on the long-term outcomes effect of these interventions and whether they ultimately are able to improve the overall lifestyle of the person [4, 5].

Structured physical activity can be effectively integrated in therapeutic–rehabilitative programmes with the aim of counteracting some of the more important psychopathological symptoms, together with pharmacological and more cognitive-based therapies [40]. In psychosis, time, space and relationships are among the basic dimensions of existence most altered; in addition, it must be considered that there are important cognitive deficits relating to attention, memory, motor speed, while executive functions are impaired. Motor activity represents an important tool to act on all these domains at the same time, leading to the acquisition of a new self-awareness and an increase in self-esteem, which in turn can act as a stimulus to reduce the social withdrawal typical of psychosis. Together with increased body knowledge, a new awareness of space is progressively achieved. Action and movement aimed at technical sporting gestures are produced, that can positively affect the management of anxiety, fear, aggression and self-distrust. In the structured space of sporting activities, the individual can better adhere to reality and experience the concrete possibility of approaching the emotional world in a positive way, something that is always very limited, e.g. in psychotic patients. At a cognitive level, motor activity stimulates attention (looking after oneself with respect to others, following the coach's instructions), memory (remembering the rules of the game) as well as problem solving in order to develop 'technical' strategies that can be applied to sport practice. Executive functions are heavily involved, and as the motor activity becomes more complex and specialised—requiring quicker times in the implementation of the technical gesture—the resulting responses will also be processed more quickly.

In addition to positively influencing both the physical and psychological spheres, physical activity can contribute to improving social functioning and promoting social inclusion [41, 42], a very important aspect for people with mental disabilities, often subject to stigma and social isolation [43, 44]. Indeed, the rehabilitation context involving physical activity is often group-based and can allow observing and experiencing a series of experiential dynamics, becoming a tool for aggregation and relational experiences. Knowledge on these dynamics, however, is still limited and further studies are needed to evaluate the benefit of sport and physical activity for social functioning in individuals with severe mental disorders [45–49].

20.3 Implementation of Physical Activity-Based Interventions in Mental Health

The Ottawa Charter defines health promotion as *the process of enabling people to increase control over and improve their health. To reach a state of complete physical, mental and social well-being, an individual or group must be able to identify and to realize aspirations, to satisfy needs, and to change or cope with the environment.* Health is seen as a resource for everyday life and there are five main strategies for health promotion (e.g. build health public policy, create a supportive environment for health, strengthen community action for health, develop personal skills and re-orient health services). The WHO Guidelines on physical activity and sedentary behaviour provide evidence-based public health recommendations for children, adolescents, adults and older adults on the amount of physical activity (frequency, intensity and duration) required to offer significant health benefits and mitigate health risks [50].

As underlined throughout this chapter, to date there is a great amount of scientific evidence supporting the implementation of interventions based on physical activity in the field of mental health [4, 5, 51]. However, it is also necessary to take into account that there are currently several barriers that prevent involving people with serious mental disorders in these interventions. Among the most noticeable are: the side effects of pharmacological therapies, complications due to overweight and/or a suboptimal physical fitness, depressive symptoms, social isolation, unhealthy lifestyle, motivational factors and lack of resources and professional support [4, 5, 52–54].

Physical activity and exercise have been included in the National Institute for Health and Care Excellence (NICE) [55] and American Psychiatric Association (APA) [56] guidelines for the treatment and management of patients with major depression and in Lancet Psychiatry Commission recommendations for protecting the physical health of people with mental disorders [57]. Specific recommendations have also been drawn up by the European Psychiatric Association (EPA) and the International Organization of Physical Therapists in Mental Health (IOPTMH) for the development of interventions based on physical activity for people with serious mental disorders such as major depression, schizophrenia and bipolar disorder [35].

Both the *US Physical Activity Guidelines for Americans* and the *UK Chief Medical Officers' Physical Activity Guidelines* recommend attaining at least 150 min of moderate-to-vigorous physical activity per week for reducing the risk of depression (including postnatal depression). To preserve both overall mental health and cognitive functioning, both Canada's and Australia's *24-Hour Movement Guidelines* have adopted a 'whole day time-use' paradigm for young people, recommending that each day should include at least 60 min of moderate-to-vigorous exercise, several hours of light physical activity, no more than 2 h of sedentary leisure activities, and 8–11 h of uninterrupted sleep. The UK Royal College of Psychiatrist's position statement on public mental health also describes how the clustering of health-risk behaviours (which include smoking, lack of exercise and unhealthy eating) increases lifetime risk of mental disorder.

The European Psychiatric Association (EPA)'s guidelines on physical activity in people with mental disorder underline that there is sufficient evidence to recommend structured exercise training as an effective first-line treatment option for moderate depression and as an adjunctive intervention for improving symptomatic recovery in severe mental illness. Additionally, the Royal Australian and New Zealand College of Psychiatrists' clinical practice guidelines for mood disorders list exercise, smoking, diet and sleep as 'step zero' targets, to be addressed before implementation of pharmacotherapy and/or psychotherapy [32].

In 2023, WHO European Office for the Prevention and Control of Noncommunicable Diseases and members of the Sport Club for Health working group of the WHO European network for the promotion of Health-enhancing Physical Activity (HEPA Europe), under the leadership of the PROSCeSS research group, developed *The Health Promoting Sports Federation Implementation Guidance*. This document is designed to support those who run national sports federations (NSFs), including board members, management groups and employees, who are the individuals or groups responsible for developing strategic plans, directing and writing policies, promoting their sports and developing programmes and toolkits for sporting clubs and their members [58].

From all these documents, we have now an important platform of general rules useful for building rehabilitation programmes based on physical activity.

There is clear evidence indicating that, to be effective and motivating—observable in a reduction in dropouts—the intervention should be supervised by a qualified professional (professional sports coach) and be of sufficient intensity to obtain improvements in the physical sphere (e.g. in relation to cardiorespiratory fitness) [35]. Effective and safe programmes should, however, include the involvement of a multidisciplinary team, which also includes healthcare personnel, essential to take into consideration the person's psychosocial needs, the impact of the symptoms, the side effects of pharmacological therapies, previous experiences, preferences and motivations [59].

There is still limited information on the specific type of physical or sporting activity that can give the best results, or is the most suitable, for a specific psychopathology. As regards the frequency and duration of the intervention, the EPA recommends, for mild or moderate depression, an intervention to be carried out at least 2 or 3 times a week, at moderate intensity, for at least 40–45 min, under supervision of qualified sports technicians, with the aim of improving the symptoms of the pathology and physical fitness; in the case of schizophrenia, to improve symptoms, cognitive functions and quality of life, 150 min of vigorous aerobic exercise is recommended, performed weekly, always with adequate technical supervision.

Firth and colleagues, in their report on the Lancet Psychiatry Commission, tried to: (1) establish highly pertinent aspects of physical health-related morbidity and mortality that have transdiagnostic applications; (2) highlight the common modifiable factors that drive disparities in physical health; (3) present actions and initiatives for health policy and clinical services to address these issues; and (4) identify promising areas for future research that could identify novel solutions [57].

These authors describe how disparities could be reduced through evidence-based prescribing and better integration of physical and mental health care and how broader implementation of lifestyle interventions for mental disorder is required to reduce elevated cardiometabolic risk and attenuate medication side effects. More action from the governments is required to prevent discrimination and ensure equitable access to all aspects of health care for those with mental disorder. Overall, protecting the physical health of people with mental disorder should be considered an international priority for reducing the personal, social and economic burden of mental health conditions. For therapeutic effectiveness to be achieved, it is essential that a working methodology is established beforehand, in which the primary and secondary project objectives are clearly indicated. Specifically, it is essential to define the type and frequency of the activities (number of weekly sessions and duration of each session), technical contents and related purposes with respect to psychopathology, place where the activity takes place, whether individual or in a group (in this case number of participants), the expected results, and the multidisciplinary team involved [57].

The presence of a professional sports technician in the operational team can guarantee: the identification of the most suitable exercises in the various situations, adequate planning of their intensity and duration, and the study of a fitness programme that responds to the needs of the subjects and can be performed by them without encountering difficulties or frustrations. The problem of motivation and its support should be also highlighted. Psychiatric patients, particularly psychotic ones, tend to keep their lifestyles unchanged; any change can also cause experiences of anguish, interrupting a 'balance' that, however pathological, is still a form of defence against the disturbing external world. Therefore, the presence of a person 'external' to the medical–psychiatric field can be a strong stimulus towards change and a contact with an external world in which it is the sporting role that qualifies the person and no longer the pathology. Currently, sports professionals involved in this area are volunteers and not very numerous; their mental health skills are more the result of experience in the field than of adequate training courses [57].

Within the framework of the Erasmus + sport project (Sport Healing Rehabilitation, SPHERE) a set of training guidelines from a combination of current data and following a survey on the current practices of sport and physical activity for mental health in seven EU countries has been derived. These guidelines seek to best harness the psychological, physiological and social benefits of sport and physical activity to facilitate patient recovery in sport-based interventions (https://www.ecos-europe.com/sphere/wp-content/uploads/2020/12/2020_TheoreticalFramework.pdf). Furthermore, specific training programmes tailored towards professional sport coaches have been developed in order to improve their skills in engaging and involving patients with severe mental disorders in sport-based rehabilitation activities [60]. Overall, in the future, guidelines and training programmes are strongly needed to implement physical activity in psychiatric/sport settings, taking into account the needs and characteristics of non-conventional settings where professionals without a proper knowledge of psychiatric disorders are present, including sport professionals.

A growing body of research is now focused on digital phenotyping, mobile apps, Internet-based interventions (including Internet-based cognitive therapy and Internet-based self-help interventions) and virtual reality, as innovative tools for prevention and treatment [61]. Internet usage could have a tremendous potential to influence psychological well-being, both in prevention and treatment of mental disorder; however, emerging evidence suggests the need for clinician training and patient guidance for optimal benefit. Smith and colleagues, in their clinical review, have tried to summarise some recommendations across the broader area of digital mental health [62]. These innovative lines of research could be well applied to the field of sport and physical activity as they could be used to motivate and guide trainees even in the absence of a sport trainer. They could also be important tools to increase motivation and social interaction, also favouring adherence to the lifestyle programme.

In conclusion, despite a great deal of attention to the topic, to date there is still a strong need to develop replicable, accessible and motivating protocols for the widest possible spectrum of patients with serious mental disorders. The effectiveness of activities of different types, durations and intensities should be explored, as well as the role of different factors in motivating participation in physical activity [4, 5, 35, 59, 63–65]. Furthermore, future studies should include the potential side effects and risks (adverse events) of this type of activity for the population with mental disorders, as well as explore the economic sustainability [35].

20.4 Starting Early: Implementation of Physical Activity Programmes with Adolescents

Adolescence is a crucial period in an individual's life and the physical and psychological changes that occur at the onset of puberty mark the transition from childhood to adulthood [66]. The main challenges facing adolescents include reaching physical maturity, developing personal identity, seeking independence from the family environment and exploring new forms of intimate and social ties with the peer group [66]. Dealing with these challenges in a positive way protects the individual's health and well-being during and after this transition [66, 67]. For this reason, it is essential to support adolescents during their growth.

Nowadays, it is acknowledged that poor mental health is the leading cause of disability among adolescents and, according to a recent estimation, one in seven adolescents suffers from mental disorders (https://www.who.int/news-room/fact-sheets/detail/adolescent-mental-health). Prevalence rates of mental health issues increase especially from mid-adolescence (14–16 years) onwards and, when not properly treated, tend to persist into adulthood [68].

According to the WHO, depression and anxiety are the most common mental health issues among adolescents, severely affecting school attendance and performance. Moreover, social withdrawal resulting from these types of disorders fosters isolation and feelings of loneliness. It is important to note that suicide, which can be the extreme consequence of psychological burden, is the fourth leading cause of death in late adolescence (15–19 years). In addition, eating disorders (e.g. anorexia, bulimia and binge eating) and health-risk behaviours (e.g. smoking, substance use, perpetration of violence) begin during early adolescence and are dysfunctional strategies that adolescents adopt for coping with emotional difficulties [19].

A growing body of evidence suggests that physical activity-based programmes may be feasible interventions to prevent and mitigate psychological distress in adolescents [32, 69–74].

Research evidence indicates an inverse association between physical activity and depression, suggesting that adolescents who are involved in physical exercise programmes show fewer depressive symptoms [75]. Moreover, aerobic and resistance exercises, with moderate-to-vigorous intensity, can be used as an auxiliary treatment to improve depressive symptoms in youth [76–79]. A recent randomised controlled trial (RCT) study found that exercise intervention can significantly reduce symptoms of depression in hospitalised adolescents in psychiatric units [80]. It has been proposed that the recreational context that characterises physical exercise therapy brings a positive emotional response while reducing social withdrawal, lack of motivation and anhedonia [80, 81]. Importantly, administering the exercise programme at the initial phase of hospitalisation can promote the establishment of a working alliance between adolescent inpatients and mental health care providers [80].

Following the current scientific evidence, guidelines issued by the National Institute for Health and Care Excellence (NICE) of the UK indicate that an adolescent with depression should be encouraged to follow a supervised physical exercise programme [82]. Such a programme is structured over 10–12 weeks and includes up to 3 weekly sessions of moderate duration (45 min to 1 h) (NICE 2019).

In addition to exercise, participation in sports is also considered as a protective factor for depression in adolescence [71]. According to a recent study conducted on Italian adolescents, team-based sports moderate the association between bullying and depression [83]. Participation in sports can buffer against the negative effects of bullying by offering the opportunity to create a new positive social network [83]. In addition, the supportive atmosphere created among members of the same team helps to stem depressive tendencies such as rumination, inactivity and withdrawal [83]. Importantly, a 5-year longitudinal study has reported that young people performing sports from middle school onwards were less likely to have suicidal thoughts (including both thoughts and intentions) during high school compared to young sedentary people [84].

Despite the high prevalence rate of anxiety-related disorders among youths, the benefits of physical activity for adolescents are still poorly investigated. The current scientific literature appears promising as results show that anxiety symptoms are lower in adolescents who engage in daily physical exercises or participate in targeted physical activity interventions [85]. In particular, a recent meta-analytic study documented the effectiveness of mindfulness-based physical activity interventions (e.g. yoga) in reducing anxiety in clinical and non-clinical young populations [86]. This type of physical activity focuses on body movement, breathing and body awareness, which play a beneficial role in emotional regulation processes and anxiety management [86]. Coherently, a systematic review recommends participating in 30-min yoga sessions, at least 2–3 times a week for a total of 6–12 weeks, to significantly improve anxiety measures [87]. Although these indications are derived from the analysis of preliminary studies, they may be useful to consider when designing and implementing yoga-based programmes to improve anxiety symptoms in young people. It is also important to emphasise that participation in sporting activities reduces children's risk of developing anxiety symptoms in social situations [88]. This appears relevant from a preventive perspective since such activities, if encouraged during childhood, could also play a protective factor for adolescents.

The protective effect of physical activity and sports on risky behaviours has also been documented [89]. Involving a teenager in an active lifestyle can reduce the risk of alcohol consumption, reduced school attendance and increased delinquency [89]. In addition, high levels of physical exercise predict decreased rates of smoking (tobacco and marijuana) and use of illicit drugs during adolescence and early adulthood [90].

Several hypotheses have been proposed to explain the possible mechanisms underlying the beneficial effects of physical activity- and sport-based interventions for adolescents' mental health. The benefits of physical activity are certainly related to the physiological and neurobiological mechanisms underlying body movement [91]. However, this is not sufficient to fully understand the positive effect of physical activity interventions on mental health. Exercise and sports have a positive impact on self-esteem [76, 92, 93], which appears particularly relevant since the latter has a strong influence on the psychological state and health-compromising behaviours of adolescents [94]. Low levels of self-esteem, in fact, are associated with a wide range of mental health issues, such as depression, anxiety, eating problems, social isolation and suicidal ideation [94]. Furthermore, participating in physical activity programmes promotes autonomy and competence, which in turn have a positive impact on mental health [91]. Lastly, physical activity facilities, such as gyms or sports clubs, can become physically and emotionally safe environments to experience bonding and support, playing a key role in the social integration of adolescents, especially the most vulnerable ones [88], providing the opportunity to establish positive relationships with peers and adults in a stimulating environment that emphasises inclusion and a sense of belonging [71].

Ultimately, evidence of the importance of sport and physical activity for mental health promotion in adolescents is growing. Such knowledge should be used to promote the development of official guidelines for sport promotion to enable clinicians and sport professionals to plan tailored interventions focused on the specific needs of adolescents.

20.5 Conclusions

Physical activity brings important benefits both to the general population and to individuals at risk or experiencing mental disorders. Considering the average age of the European population, physical activity is also an important protective factor for active and healthy ageing; in fact, it offers benefits for musculoskeletal and cardiovascular health and counteracts age-related cognitive decline and the onset of chronic diseases and health disorders, including obesity and type 2 diabetes, as well as mental disorders such as major depression [95]. This type of activity should be included, more generally, in psychoeducational interventions that focus on the promotion of healthy lifestyles and social relationships, also with the aim of increasing resilience and coping strategies, combating stigma, as well as improving the overall participation of the person to community life, therefore increasing their autonomy [22, 51, 96, 97].

While there is a great potential for sport and physical activity in both prevention and care of mental disorder, a number of critical points still remain having to do with implementing current data and guidelines and promoting basic research to better understand the potential (positive) interaction of physical activity with pharmacological and psychotherapeutic treatments. This knowledge would be especially important as—most notably in the case of major depression—current pharmacological therapies are effective only in a portion of the population. As there is a potential for environmental conditions, including lifestyle, to overcome such therapeutic gap, clinical trials specifically addressing these aspects should be encouraged.

References

1. Rössler W, Joachim Salize H, Van Os J, Riecher-Rössler A (2005) Size of burden of schizophrenia and psychotic disorders. Eur Neuropsychopharmacol 15(4):399–409. https://doi.org/10.1016/J.EURONEURO.2005.04.009
2. Whiteford HA, Ferrari AJ, Degenhardt L, Feigin V, Vos T (2015) The global burden of mental, neurological and substance use disorders: an analysis from the Global Burden of Disease Study 2010. PLoS One 10(2):e0116820. https://doi.org/10.1371/JOURNAL.PONE.0116820
3. De Hert M, Dekker JM, Wood D, Kahl KG, Holt RIG, Möller HJ (2009) Cardiovascular disease and diabetes in people with severe mental illness position statement from the European Psychiatric Association (EPA), supported by the European Association for the Study of Diabetes (EASD) and the European Society of Cardiology (ESC). Eur Psychiatry 24(6):412–424. https://doi.org/10.1016/J.EURPSY.2009.01.005
4. Vancampfort D, Stubbs B, Sienaert P, Wyckaert S, De Hert M, Rosenbaum S, Probst M (2015a) What are the factors that influence physical activity participation in individuals with depression? A review of physical activity correlates from 59 studies. Psychiatria Danubina 27(3):210–224. https://www.researchgate.net/publication/282153728_What_are_the_factors_that_influence_physical_activity_participation_in_individuals_with_depression_A_review_of_physical_activity_correlates_from_59_studies
5. Vancampfort D, Stubbs B, Ward PB, Teasdale S, Rosenbaum S (2015b) Integrating physical activity as medicine in the care of people with severe mental illness. Aust N Z J Psychiatry 49(8):681–682. https://doi.org/10.1177/0004867415590831
6. Holt-Lunstad J, Smith TB, Layton JB (2010) Social relationships and mortality risk: a meta-analytic review. PLoS Med 7(7):e1000316. https://doi.org/10.1371/JOURNAL.PMED.1000316
7. House JS, Landis KR, Umberson D (1988) Social relationships and health. Science (NY) 241(4865):540–545. https://doi.org/10.1126/SCIENCE.3399889
8. Rico-Uribe LA, Caballero FF, Martín-María N, Cabello M, Ayuso-Mateos JL, Miret M (2018) Association of loneliness with all-cause mortality: a meta-analysis. PLoS One 13(1):e0190033. https://doi.org/10.1371/JOURNAL.PONE.0190033
9. Steptoe A, Shankar A, Demakakos P, Wardle J (2013) Social isolation, loneliness, and all-cause mortality in older men and women. Proc Natl Acad Sci U S A 110(15):5797–5801. https://doi.org/10.1073/PNAS.1219686110
10. Holt-Lunstad J (2018) Why social relationships are important for physical health: a systems approach to understanding and modifying risk and protection. Annu Rev Psychol 69:437–458. https://doi.org/10.1146/ANNUREV-PSYCH-122216-011902
11. Cella M, Preti A, Edwards C, Dow T, Wykes T (2017) Cognitive remediation for negative symptoms of schizophrenia: a network meta-analysis. Clin Psychol Rev 52:43–51. https://doi.org/10.1016/J.CPR.2016.11.009
12. Correll CU, Detraux J, De Lepeleire J, De Hert M (2015) Effects of antipsychotics, antidepressants and mood stabilizers on risk for physical diseases in people with schizophrenia, depression and bipolar disorder. World Psychiatry 14(2):119–136. https://doi.org/10.1002/WPS.20204

13. Weinmann S, Read J, Aderhold V (2009) Influence of antipsychotics on mortality in schizophrenia: systematic review. Schizophr Res 113(1):1–11. https://doi.org/10.1016/J.SCHRES.2009.05.018
14. Warburton DER, Bredin SSD (2017) Health benefits of physical activity: a systematic review of current systematic reviews. Curr Opin Cardiol 32(5):541–556. https://doi.org/10.1097/HCO.0000000000000437
15. Prakash RS, Voss MW, Erickson KI, Kramer AF (2015) Physical activity and cognitive vitality. Annu Rev Psychol 66:769–797. https://doi.org/10.1146/ANNUREV-PSYCH-010814-015249
16. Snowden M, Steinman L, Mochan K, Grodstein F, Prohaska TR, Thurman DJ, Brown DR, Laditka JN, Soares J, Zweiback DJ, Little D, Anderson LA (2011) Effect of exercise on cognitive performance in community-dwelling older adults: review of intervention trials and recommendations for public health practice and research. J Am Geriatr Soc 59(4):704–716. https://doi.org/10.1111/J.1532-5415.2011.03323.X
17. Stubbs B, Chen LJ, Chang CY, Sun WJ, Ku PW (2017) Accelerometer-assessed light physical activity is protective of future cognitive ability: a longitudinal study among community dwelling older adults. Exp Gerontol 91:104–109. https://doi.org/10.1016/J.EXGER.2017.03.003
18. Voelcker-Rehage C, Niemann C (2013) Structural and functional brain changes related to different types of physical activity across the life span. Neurosci Biobehav Rev 37(9 Pt B):2268–2295. https://doi.org/10.1016/J.NEUBIOREV.2013.01.028
19. WHO (2021) Physical activity fact sheet. World Health Organization, Washington, DC, pp 1–8
20. Caponnetto P, Casu M, Amato M, Cocuzza D, Galofaro V, La Morella A, Paladino S, Pulino K, Raia N, Recupero F, Resina C, Russo S, Terranova LM, Tiralongo J, Vella MC (2021) The effects of physical exercise on mental health: from cognitive improvements to risk of addiction. Int J Environ Res Public Health 18(24):13384. https://doi.org/10.3390/IJERPH182413384
21. Kivimäki M, Steptoe A (2018) Effects of stress on the development and progression of cardiovascular disease. Nat Rev Cardiol 15(4):215–229. https://doi.org/10.1038/NRCARDIO.2017.189
22. Steptoe A, Fancourt D (2019) Protecting physical health in people with mental illness. Lancet Psychiatry 6(11):889–890. https://doi.org/10.1016/S2215-0366(19)30393-1
23. Cooper C, Moon HY, Van Praag H (2018) On the run for hippocampal plasticity. Cold Spring Harb Perspect Med 8(4):a029736. https://doi.org/10.1101/CSHPERSPECT.A029736
24. Firth J, Stubbs B, Vancampfort D, Schuch F, Lagopoulos J, Rosenbaum S, Ward PB (2018) Effect of aerobic exercise on hippocampal volume in humans: a systematic review and meta-analysis. NeuroImage 166:230–238. https://doi.org/10.1016/J.NEUROIMAGE.2017.11.007
25. Nieman DC, Wentz LM (2019) The compelling link between physical activity and the body's defense system. J Sport Health Sci 8(3):201–217. https://doi.org/10.1016/J.JSHS.2018.09.009
26. Conn VS (2010) Anxiety outcomes after physical activity interventions: meta-analysis findings. Nurs Res 59(3):224–231. https://doi.org/10.1097/NNR.0B013E3181DBB2F8
27. Garcia-Falgueras A (2015) Psychological benefits of sports and physical activities. Br J Educ Soc Behav Sci 11(4):1–7. https://doi.org/10.9734/BJESBS/2015/21865
28. Verhoeven JE, Han LKM, Lever-van Milligen BA, Hu MX, Révész D, Hoogendoorn AW, Batelaan NM, van Schaik DJF, van Balkom AJLM, van Oppen P, Penninx BWJH (2023) Antidepressants or running therapy: comparing effects on mental and physical health in patients with depression and anxiety disorders. J Affect Disord 329:19–29. https://doi.org/10.1016/J.JAD.2023.02.064
29. Schuch FB, Vancampfort D, Firth J, Rosenbaum S, Ward PB, Silva ES, Hallgren M, De Leon AP, Dunn AL, Deslandes AC, Fleck MP, Carvalho AF, Stubbs B (2018) Physical activity and incident depression: a meta-analysis of prospective cohort studies. Am J Psychiatry 175(7):631–648. https://doi.org/10.1176/APPI.AJP.2018.17111194
30. Cooney GM, Dwan K, Greig CA, Lawlor DA, Rimer J, Waugh FR, McMurdo M, Mead GE (2013) Exercise for depression. Cochrane Database Syst Rev 2013(9):1203. https://doi.org/10.1002/14651858.CD004366.PUB6
31. Lincoln KD (2019) Social stress, obesity, and depression among women: clarifying the role of physical activity. Ethn Health 24(6):662–678. https://doi.org/10.1080/13557858.2017.1346190
32. Firth J, Solmi M, Wootton RE, Vancampfort D, Schuch FB, Hoare E, Gilbody S, Torous J, Teasdale SB, Jackson SE, Smith L, Eaton M, Jacka FN, Veronese N, Marx W, Ashdown-Franks G, Siskind D, Sarris J, Rosenbaum S et al (2020) A meta-review of "lifestyle psychiatry": the role of exercise, smoking, diet and sleep in the prevention and treatment of mental disorders. World Psychiatry 19(3):360–380. https://doi.org/10.1002/WPS.20773
33. Wang X, Cheng S, Xu H (2019) Systematic review and meta-analysis of the relationship between sleep disorders and suicidal behaviour in patients with depression. BMC Psychiatry 19(1):303. https://doi.org/10.1186/S12888-019-2302-5
34. Salvi V, Hajek T (2019) Editorial: Brain-metabolic crossroads in severe mental disorders-focus on metabolic syndrome. Front Psychiatry 10:492. https://doi.org/10.3389/FPSYT.2019.00492
35. Stubbs B, Vancampfort D, Hallgren M, Firth J, Veronese N, Solmi M, Brand S, Cordes J, Malchow B, Gerber M, Schmitt A, Correll CU, De Hert M, Gaughran F, Schneider F, Kinnafick F, Falkai P, Möller HJ, Kahl KG (2018) EPA guidance on physical activity as a treatment for severe mental illness:

a meta-review of the evidence and position statement from the European Psychiatric Association (EPA), supported by the International Organization of Physical Therapists in Mental Health (IOPTMH). Eur Psychiatry 54:124–144. https://doi.org/10.1016/J.EURPSY.2018.07.004
36. Firth J, Stubbs B, Rosenbaum S, Vancampfort D, Malchow B, Schuch F, Elliott R, Nuechterlein KH, Yung AR (2017) Aerobic exercise improves cognitive functioning in people with schizophrenia: a systematic review and meta-analysis. Schizophr Bull 43(3):546–556. https://doi.org/10.1093/SCHBUL/SBW115
37. Schuch FB, Vancampfort D, Richards J, Rosenbaum S, Ward PB, Stubbs B (2016) Exercise as a treatment for depression: a meta-analysis adjusting for publication bias. J Psychiatr Res 77:42–51. https://doi.org/10.1016/J.JPSYCHIRES.2016.02.023
38. Stubbs B, Rosenbaum S, Vancampfort D, Ward PB, Schuch FB (2016) Exercise improves cardiorespiratory fitness in people with depression: a meta-analysis of randomized control trials. J Affect Disord 190:249–253. https://doi.org/10.1016/J.JAD.2015.10.010
39. Hearing CM, Chang WC, Szuhany KL, Deckersbach T, Nierenberg AA, Sylvia LG (2016) Physical exercise for treatment of mood disorders: a critical review. Curr Behav Neurosci Rep 3(4):350–359. https://doi.org/10.1007/S40473-016-0089-Y
40. Harvey SB, Overland S, Hatch SL, Wessely S, Mykletun A, Hotopf M (2018) Exercise and the prevention of depression: results of the HUNT cohort study. Am J Psychiatry 175(1):28–36. https://doi.org/10.1176/APPI.AJP.2017.16111223
41. Bailey R (2005) Evaluating the relationship between physical education, sport and social inclusion. Educ Rev 57(1):71–90. https://doi.org/10.1080/0013191042000274196
42. Skinner J, Zakus DH, Cowell J (2008) Development through sport: building social capital in disadvantaged communities. Sport Manag Rev 11(3):253–275. https://doi.org/10.1016/S1441-3523(08)70112-8
43. Le Boutillier C, Croucher A (2010) Social inclusion and mental health. Br J Occup Ther 73(3):136–139. https://doi.org/10.4276/030802210X12682330090578
44. Linz SJ, Sturm BA (2013) The phenomenon of social isolation in the severely mentally ill. Perspect Psychiatr Care 49(4):243–254. https://doi.org/10.1111/PPC.12010
45. Carta MG, Maggiani F, Pilutzu L, Moro MF, Mura G, Sancassiani F, Vellante V, Migliaccio GM, Machado S, Nardi AE, Preti A (2014) Sailing can improve quality of life of people with severe mental disorders: results of a cross over randomized controlled trial. Clin Pract Epidemiol Ment Health 10(1):80–86. https://doi.org/10.2174/1745017901410010080
46. Manferdelli G, La Torre A, Codella R (2019) Outdoor physical activity bears multiple benefits to health and society. J Sports Med Phys Fitness 59(5):868–879. https://doi.org/10.23736/S0022-4707.18.08771-6
47. Perkins D (2010) Activation and social inclusion: challenges and possibilities. Aust J Soc Issues 45(2):267–287. https://doi.org/10.1002/J.1839-4655.2010.TB00178.X
48. Sancassiani F, Lorrai S, Cossu G, Cocco A, Trincas G, Floris F, Mellino G, Machado S, Nardi AE, Fabrici EP, Preti A, Carta MG (2017) The effects of "VelaMente?!" project on social functioning of people with severe psychosocial disabilities. Clin Pract Epidemiol Ment Health 13(1):220–232. https://doi.org/10.2174/1745017901713010220
49. Secker J, Hacking S, Kent L, Shenton J, Spandler H (2009) Development of a measure of social inclusion for arts and mental health project participants. J Ment Health 18(1):65–72. https://doi.org/10.1080/09638230701677803
50. WHO (2016) WHO guidelines on physical activity and sedentary behaviour. In: Handbook of youth sport. Routledge, London. https://www.who.int/publications/i/item/9789240015128
51. Sampogna G, Fiorillo A, Luciano M, Del Vecchio V, Steardo L, Pocai B, Barone M, Amore M, Pacitti F, Dell'Osso L, Di Lorenzo G, Maj M, Borriello G, De Rosa C, Giallonardo V, Malangone C, Savorani M, Longo L, Veneziani F et al (2018) A randomized controlled trial on the efficacy of a psychosocial behavioral intervention to improve the lifestyle of patients with severe mental disorders: study protocol. Front Psychiatry 9:235. https://doi.org/10.3389/FPSYT.2018.00235
52. Firth J, Rosenbaum S, Stubbs B, Gorczynski P, Yung AR, Vancampfort D (2016) Motivating factors and barriers towards exercise in severe mental illness: a systematic review and meta-analysis. Psychol Med 46(14):2869–2881. https://doi.org/10.1017/S0033291716001732
53. Vancampfort D, Correll CU, Probst M, Sienaert P, Wyckaert S, De Herdt A, Knapen J, De Wachter D, De Hert M (2013) A review of physical activity correlates in patients with bipolar disorder. J Affect Disord 145(3):285–291. https://doi.org/10.1016/J.JAD.2012.07.020
54. Vancampfort D, Knapen J, Probst M, Scheewe T, Remans S, De Hert M (2012) A systematic review of correlates of physical activity in patients with schizophrenia. Acta Psychiatr Scand 125(5):352–362. https://doi.org/10.1111/j.1600-0447.2011.01814.x
55. NICE (2010) Depression: The Treatment and Management of Depression in Adults (Updated Edition). Leicester (UK): British Psychological Society
56. APA (2010) Practice guideline for the treatment of patients with major depressive disorder (revision). Am J Psychiatry, 157(4 Suppl): 1–45
57. Firth J, Siddiqi N, Koyanagi A, Siskind D, Rosenbaum S, Galletly C, Allan S, Caneo C, Carney R, Carvalho AF, Chatterton ML, Correll CU, Curtis J, Gaughran F, Heald A, Hoare E, Jackson SE, Kisely S, Lovell

K et al (2019) The Lancet Psychiatry Commission: a blueprint for protecting physical health in people with mental illness. Lancet Psychiatry 6(8):675–712. https://doi.org/10.1016/S2215-0366(19)30132-4
58. WHO (2023) Inclusive, sustainable, welcoming national sports federations health promoting sports federation implementation guidance. WHO, Washington, DC
59. Carneiro L, Rosenbaum S, Mota MP, Schuch F, Ward PB, Vasconcelos-Raposo J (2017) Exercise as an essential therapeutic tool in mental health: closing the gap from research to practice, a Portuguese perspective. Acta Med Port 30(5):354–355. https://doi.org/10.20344/AMP.8436
60. Sampogna G, Borgi M, Collacchi B, Cirulli F, Cerino S, Rullo S, Di Vincenzo M, Luciano M, Di Tommaso V, Moliterni S, Bichi A, Garside J, Kivistö S, Iarion A, Fiorillo A (2022) Using sport-based interventions for people with severe mental disorders: results from the European EASMH study. Int Rev Psychiatry 34(7–8):837–847. https://doi.org/10.1080/09540261.2022.2106122
61. Linardon J, Cuijpers P, Carlbring P, Messer M, Fuller-Tyszkiewicz M (2019) The efficacy of app-supported smartphone interventions for mental health problems: a meta-analysis of randomized controlled trials. World Psychiatry 18(3):325–336. https://doi.org/10.1002/WPS.20673
62. Smith KA, Blease C, Faurholt-Jepsen M, Firth J, Van Daele T, Moreno C, Carlbring P, Ebner-Priemer UW, Koutsouleris N, Riper H, Mouchabac S, Torous J, Cipriani A (2023) Digital mental health: challenges and next steps. BMJ Ment Health 26(1):e300670. https://doi.org/10.1136/BMJMENT-2023-300670
63. Blumenthal JA, Sherwood A, Rogers SD, Babyak MA, Doraiswamy PM, Watkins L, Hoffman BM, O'Connell C, Johnson JJ, Patidar SM, Waugh R, Hinderliter A (2007) Understanding prognostic benefits of exercise and antidepressant therapy for persons with depression and heart disease: the UPBEAT study—rationale, design, and methodological issues. Clin Trials 4(5):548–559. https://doi.org/10.1177/1740774507083388
64. Farholm A, Sørensen M (2016) Motivation for physical activity and exercise in severe mental illness: a systematic review of intervention studies. Int J Ment Health Nurs 25(3):194–205. https://doi.org/10.1111/INM.12214
65. Stanton R, Reaburn P (2014) Exercise and the treatment of depression: a review of the exercise program variables. J Sci Med Sport 17(2):177–182. https://doi.org/10.1016/J.JSAMS.2013.03.010
66. Christie D, Viner R (2005) Adolescent development. BMJ 330(7486):301–304. https://doi.org/10.1136/BMJ.330.7486.301
67. Moghaddam H, Bahreini A, Ajilian Abbasi M, Fazli F, Saeidi M (2016) Adolescence health: the needs, problems and attention. Int J Pediatr 4(2):1423–1438. https://doi.org/10.22038/ijp.2016.6569
68. Guddal MH, Stensland SØ, Småstuen MC, Johnsen MB, Zwart JA, Storheim K (2019) Physical activity and sport participation among adolescents: associations with mental health in different age groups. Results from the Young-HUNT study: a cross-sectional survey. BMJ Open 9(9):e028555. https://doi.org/10.1136/BMJOPEN-2018-028555
69. Biddle SJH, Ciaccioni S, Thomas G, Vergeer I (2019) Physical activity and mental health in children and adolescents: an updated review of reviews and an analysis of causality. Psychol Sport Exerc 42:146–155. https://doi.org/10.1016/J.PSYCHSPORT.2018.08.011
70. Bjørnarå HB, Westergren T, Sejersted E, Torstveit MK, Hansen BH, Berntsen S, Bere E (2021) Does organized sports participation in childhood and adolescence positively influence health? A review of reviews. Prev Med Rep 23:101425. https://doi.org/10.1016/J.PMEDR.2021.101425
71. Boelens M, Smit MS, Raat H, Bramer WM, Jansen W (2021) Impact of organized activities on mental health in children and adolescents: an umbrella review. Prev Med Rep 25:101687. https://doi.org/10.1016/J.PMEDR.2021.101687
72. McCrary JM, Redding E, Altenmüller E (2021) Performing arts as a health resource? An umbrella review of the health impacts of music and dance participation. PLoS One 16(6):e0252956. https://doi.org/10.1371/JOURNAL.PONE.0252956
73. Pettitt RM, Brown EA, Delashmitt JC, Pizzo MN (2022) The management of anxiety and depression in pediatrics. Cureus 14(10):e30231. https://doi.org/10.7759/CUREUS.30231
74. Wang X, Cai ZD, Jiang WT, Fang YY, Sun WX, Wang X (2022) Systematic review and meta-analysis of the effects of exercise on depression in adolescents. Child Adolesc Psychiatry Ment Health 16(1):16. https://doi.org/10.1186/S13034-022-00453-2
75. Shen L, Gu X, Zhang T, Lee J (2022) Adolescents' physical activity and depressive symptoms: a psychosocial mechanism. Int J Environ Res Public Health 19(3):1276. https://doi.org/10.3390/IJERPH19031276
76. Ashdown-Franks G, Firth J, Carney R, Carvalho AF, Hallgren M, Koyanagi A, Rosenbaum S, Schuch FB, Smith L, Solmi M, Vancampfort D, Stubbs B (2020) Exercise as medicine for mental and substance use disorders: a meta-review of the benefits for neuropsychiatric and cognitive outcomes. Sports Med 50(1):151–170. https://doi.org/10.1007/S40279-019-01187-6
77. Bailey AP, Hetrick SE, Rosenbaum S, Purcell R, Parker AG (2018) Treating depression with physical activity in adolescents and young adults: a systematic review and meta-analysis of randomised controlled trials. Psychol Med 48(7):1068–1083. https://doi.org/10.1017/S0033291717002653
78. Hu MX, Turner D, Generaal E, Bos D, Ikram MK, Ikram MA, Cuijpers P, Penninx BWJH (2020) Exercise interventions for the prevention of depression: a systematic review of meta-analyses. BMC

Public Health 20(1):1255. https://doi.org/10.1186/S12889-020-09323-Y
79. Wegner M, Amatriain-Fernández S, Kaulitzky A, Murillo-Rodriguez E, Machado S, Budde H (2020) Systematic review of meta-analyses: exercise effects on depression in children and adolescents. Front Psych 11:81. https://doi.org/10.3389/FPSYT.2020.00081
80. Philippot A, Dubois V, Lambrechts K, Grogna D, Robert A, Jonckheer U, Chakib W, Beine A, Bleyenheuft Y, De Volder AG (2022) Impact of physical exercise on depression and anxiety in adolescent inpatients: a randomized controlled trial. J Affect Disord 301:145–153. https://doi.org/10.1016/J.JAD.2022.01.011
81. Carter T, Guo B, Turner D, Morres I, Khalil E, Brighton E, Armstrong M, Callaghan P (2015) Preferred intensity exercise for adolescents receiving treatment for depression: a pragmatic randomised controlled trial. BMC Psychiatry 15(1):247. https://doi.org/10.1186/S12888-015-0638-Z
82. Campisi SC, Krause KR, Chan BWC, Courtney DB, Bennett K, Korczak DJ, Szatmari P (2021) Eating, sleeping and moving recommendations in clinical practice guidelines for paediatric depression: umbrella review. BJPsych Open 7(6):e185. https://doi.org/10.1192/BJO.2021.1020
83. Holbrook HM, Voller F, Castellini G, Silvestri C, Ricca V, Cassioli E, Ivanova MY, Hudziak JJ (2020) Sport participation moderates association between bullying and depressive symptoms in Italian adolescents. J Affect Disord 271:33–38. https://doi.org/10.1016/J.JAD.2020.03.142
84. Taliaferro LA, Eisenberg ME, Johnson KE, Nelson TF, Neumark-Sztainer D (2011) Sport participation during adolescence and suicide ideation and attempts. Int J Adolesc Med Health 23(1):3–10. https://doi.org/10.1515/IJAMH.2011.002
85. Panza MJ, Graupensperger S, Agans JP, Doré I, Vella SA, Evans MB (2020) Adolescent sport participation and symptoms of anxiety and depression: a systematic review and meta-analysis. J Sport Exerc Psychol 42(3):201–218. https://doi.org/10.1123/JSEP.2019-0235
86. Carter T, Pascoe M, Bastounis A, Morres ID, Callaghan P, Parker AG (2021) The effect of physical activity on anxiety in children and young people: a systematic review and meta-analysis. J Affect Disord 285:10–21. https://doi.org/10.1016/J.JAD.2021.02.026
87. James-Palmer A, Anderson EZ, Zucker L, Kofman Y, Daneault J-F (2020) Yoga as an intervention for the reduction of symptoms of anxiety and depression in children and adolescents: a systematic review. Front Pediatr 8:78. https://doi.org/10.3389/FPED.2020.00078
88. Eime RM, Young JA, Harvey JT, Charity MJ, Payne WR (2013) A systematic review of the psychological and social benefits of participation in sport for children and adolescents: informing development of a conceptual model of health through sport. Int J Behav Nutr Phys Act 10:98. https://doi.org/10.1186/1479-5868-10-98
89. Nelson MC, Gordon-Larsen P (2006) Physical activity and sedentary behavior patterns are associated with selected adolescent health risk behaviors. Pediatrics 117(4):1281–1290. https://doi.org/10.1542/PEDS.2005-1692
90. Lynch WJ, Peterson AB, Sanchez V, Abel J, Smith MA (2013) Exercise as a novel treatment for drug addiction: a neurobiological and stage-dependent hypothesis. Neurosci Biobehav Rev 37(8):1622–1644. https://doi.org/10.1016/J.NEUBIOREV.2013.06.011
91. Doré I, Sylvester B, Sabiston C, Sylvestre MP, O'Loughlin J, Brunet J, Bélanger M (2020) Mechanisms underpinning the association between physical activity and mental health in adolescence: a 6-year study. Int J Behav Nutr Phys Act 17(1):9. https://doi.org/10.1186/S12966-020-0911-5
92. Dale LP, Vanderloo L, Moore S, Faulkner G (2019) Physical activity and depression, anxiety, and self-esteem in children and youth: an umbrella systematic review. Ment Health Phys Act 16:66–79. https://doi.org/10.1016/J.MHPA.2018.12.001
93. Das JK, Salam RA, Lassi ZS, Khan MN, Mahmood W, Patel V, Bhutta ZA (2016) Interventions for adolescent mental health: an overview of systematic reviews. J Adolesc Health 59(4S):754–762. https://doi.org/10.1016/J.JADOHEALTH.2016.06.020
94. Liu M, Wu L, Ming Q (2015) How does physical activity intervention improve self-esteem and self-concept in children and adolescents? Evidence from a meta-analysis. PLoS One 10(8):e0134804. https://doi.org/10.1371/JOURNAL.PONE.0134804
95. Zhao E, Tranovich MJ, Wright VJ (2014) The role of mobility as a protective factor of cognitive functioning in aging adults: a review. Sports Health 6(1):63–69. https://doi.org/10.1177/1941738113477832
96. Fenton L, White C, Gallant KA, Gilbert R, Hutchinson S, Hamilton-Hinch B, Lauckner H (2017) The benefits of recreation for the recovery and social inclusion of individuals with mental illness: an integrative review. Leis Sci 39(1):1–19. https://doi.org/10.1080/01490400.2015.1120168
97. Thompson Coon J, Boddy K, Stein K, Whear R, Barton J, Depledge MH (2011) Does participating in physical activity in outdoor natural environments have a greater effect on physical and mental wellbeing than physical activity indoors? A systematic review. Environ Sci Technol 45(5):1761–1772. https://doi.org/10.1021/ES102947T

Personal Recovery in People with Mental Disorders: The Achievement of a Meaningful Life

21

Luca Pellegrini and Umberto Albert

Abstract

The importance of personal recovery in mental health has grown in recent years: recovery is seen as a way to live a satisfying, hopeful, and contributing life despite limitations caused by mental illness. It involves various aspects such as self-management, personal productivity, and community engagement. The adoption of recovery perspectives by mental health services is a significant development in the field, focusing on the individual's agency and empowering them to take an active role in their recovery journey. Factors promoting personal recovery include personal agency, family support, structural, interpersonal, and intrapersonal factors. Exercise, nature, and socially interactive-based initiatives can improve mood and self-esteem; family psychoeducation can benefit family bonds and increase access to social and practical support, while digital technology can play a significant role in providing access to resources and enhancing treatment adherence. Relapse prevention in mental illness is crucial for maintaining stability: early intervention, medication adherence, and psychosocial interventions are key factors. On the other hand, stigma, lack of community support, lack of acceptance of one's self and limitations, and the presence of psychiatric symptoms can hinder recovery. Personal recovery in major depressive disorder (MDD) is an example of a recovery-oriented approach to mental disorders. Full functional recovery is a condition where patients can resume their usual activities, return to employment, and care for themselves. Personal recovery is the ultimate goal of treatment, involving accepting mental illness, discovering hope for the future, re-establishing a positive identity, developing meaning in life, taking control of one's life, and overcoming stigma.

Keywords

Personal recovery · Empowerment · Social support · Digital technology · Stigma · Major depressive disorder

L. Pellegrini
Department of Medicine, Surgery and Health Sciences, University of Trieste, Trieste, Italy

Department of Mental Health, UCO Clinica Psichiatrica, ASUGI, Trieste, Italy

School of Life and Medical Sciences, University of Hertfordshire, Hatfield, UK
e-mail: luca.pellegrini@units.it

U. Albert (✉)
Department of Medicine, Surgery and Health Sciences, University of Trieste, Trieste, Italy

Department of Mental Health, UCO Clinica Psichiatrica, ASUGI, Trieste, Italy
e-mail: ualbert@units.it

A. Fiorillo, S. De Giorgi (eds.), *Social Determinants of Mental Health*, Sustainable Development Goals Series, https://doi.org/10.1007/978-3-031-70165-8_21

21.1 Personal Recovery

In recent years, there has been a growing recognition of the importance of recovery in the field of mental health. Coinciding with a period of tightening budgets, a new hopeful theory of recovery from mental illness has gained prominence among mental health advocates. Its origins were largely in North America, and an early definition described how a person with mental illness can recover even though the illness is not "cured".

Recovery, in this context, is seen as a way of living a satisfying, hopeful, and contributing life even with the limitations caused by illness. The concept of recovery in mental illness goes beyond mere remission or symptomatic improvement; it is not just about the absence of symptoms, but about finding ways to live a fulfilling life despite the challenges posed by mental illness. It encompasses the achievement of a meaningful existence, one that is characterized by general functioning and a high quality of life; the process of recovery is not simply about finding stability, but rather about regaining a sense of hope and purpose in life [1].

Being a complex and multifaceted journey, recovery involves various aspects, such as self-management, personal productivity, and community engagement. The adoption of recovery perspectives by mental health service providers is a significant development in the field. This shift from a paternalistic, illness-oriented perspective to a collaborative, holistic, and autonomy-enhancing approach has the potential to transform the way mental health care is delivered and received. Recovery perspectives prioritize the individual's agency and empower them to take an active role in their own recovery journey; this shift also emphasizes the need for a holistic approach that takes into account the restoration of the sense of self.

The transition to a recovery-oriented mental health care system requires ongoing evaluation and monitoring to ensure its effectiveness and it is a multi-layered process, considering that recovery is a personal and individualized journey that each person with mental illness embarks upon, a dynamic and ongoing development, focusing on the individual's ability to live in fulfilled and satisfying way [2]. Recovery-focused collaborations are based on the belief that individuals with mental disorders can achieve their rewarding and pursed goals. These collaborations emphasize the importance of hope, healing, empowerment, and connection in the recovery course. Collaborative and autonomy-enhancing approaches in mental health care have the potential to transform the way services are delivered and received, and the Recovery Movement has gained significant traction in recent years as a way to address the challenges faced by individuals with severe mental illness [3].

21.2 Factors Promoting Personal Recovery

Factors promoting personal recovery in mental illness are manifold and involve various aspects of an individual's life (Table 21.1).

Several studies have explored these factors and shed light on the different elements that contribute to the recovery path. One important factor identified in the literature is *personal agency* or *self-determination*. Jaiswal et al. [4] found that personal agency was key to recovery from severe mental illness, as individuals who felt empow-

Table 21.1 Factors promoting personal recovery in people with mental disorders

Personal agency—self-determination	
Support provided by family members/community members	Emotional support Practical assistance Involvement in treatment decisions
Structural factors	Availability and accessibility of mental health services and resources
Interpersonal factors	Positive relationships with: healthcare providers, peers, other supportive individuals
Intrapersonal factors	Self-awareness Self-acceptance Development of coping strategies Self-compassion Hope

ered and in control of their own lives were more likely to experience positive outcomes. This sense of agency allows individuals to actively participate in their own recovery journey and make decisions that align with their goals and values.

Another significant factor is the *support provided by family members*. Chan et al. [5] and Chang and Chen [6] both highlight the positive impact of family support on personal recovery. Family support can manifest in various ways, such as emotional support, practical assistance, and involvement in treatment decisions. This support helps individuals feel understood, validated, and connected, which in turn promotes their recovery process.

In addition to personal agency and family support, Dell et al. [7] emphasize the importance of structural, interpersonal, and intrapersonal factors in promoting recovery. *Structural factors* refer to the availability and accessibility of mental health services and resources, while *interpersonal factors* involve positive relationships with healthcare providers, peers, and other supportive individuals. *Intrapersonal factors* encompass self-awareness, self-acceptance, and the development of coping strategies. These factors collectively contribute to creating an environment conducive to recovery. Furthermore, self-compassion has been identified as a mediating factor in the relationship between family support and recovery. Chan et al. [5] found that self-compassion played a significant role in the impact of family support on clinical and personal recovery. Self-compassion involves treating oneself with kindness, understanding, and acceptance, which can enhance an individual's ability to cope with challenges and setbacks during the recovery process.

The importance of *social networks*, including both family and community members, is also highlighted in the literature. Iseselo and Ambikile [8] found that patients' involvement in home activities, self-care management, and improved support systems were important factors in promoting recovery. Similarly, Chang and Chen [6] found that family social networks indirectly influenced personal recovery through the mediating effects of self-esteem and self-efficacy. These findings suggest that social connections and support systems play a crucial role in facilitating recovery.

Moreover, the concept of *hope* has been consistently identified as a factor promoting personal recovery. Several studies, including Jaiswal et al. [4] and Young et al. [9], have found that hope is positively associated with personal recovery. Hope provides individuals with a sense of optimism, motivation, and belief in the possibility of a better future, which can be instrumental in overcoming challenges and setbacks.

Other factors that have been identified in the literature include illness acceptance, adherence to treatment, environmental factors (such as a supportive environment and accessibility to mental health services), and the reduction of self-stigma [10–12]. These factors contribute to an individual's overall well-being and ability to navigate the recovery process.

Social support, in particular, has been found to enhance recovery outcomes, hope, and empowerment. In the absence of social support, individuals may experience feelings of frustration, apathy, and depression, which can hinder their recovery. Numerous studies have highlighted the positive impact of social support on mental health recovery and well-being [6, 7, 13–20]. Social support can be provided through various channels, including peer-to-peer support, community engagement, family support, and social networks. This synthesis explores the role of social support in promoting personal recovery in mental illness, drawing on relevant references. One study emphasizes the potential of peer-to-peer support and social media in the future of mental health care [17] and suggests that interventions delivered through social media platforms can be effective in reaching individuals with mental illness and providing them with social support. This finding highlights the importance of utilizing technology and online platforms to enhance social support networks for individuals with mental illness. Another study focuses on the experiences of individuals with severe mental illness using YouTube as a platform for peer support [18] and hints to the possibility that informal peers openly sharing their illness experiences on social media can support mental health recovery in individuals with severe mental illness. These results point out to the potential of social media platforms in facilitating social support and promoting personal recovery. Garverich and colleagues provide evidence of the positive associations between social support, community engagement, and mental health [14], emphasizing the importance of different types of social support in the recovery process among outpatient mental health service users. Effectiveness of exercise, nature, and socially interactive-based initiatives were found to improve mood and self-esteem in a clinical population [13]; this study suggests that combining exercise, nature, and social components in initiatives can play a key role in managing and supporting recovery from mental illness and highlights the potential of incorporating social interactions and nature-based activities in promoting personal recovery. Other authors [15] conducted a study examining the relationship between social support, activities, and recovery from serious mental illness and found that social network size and social support were correlated with recovery. In the study by Dell et al. [7], family psychoeducation is found to improve family bonds, increase access to social and practical support, and assist families in understanding how mental illness impacts their loved ones, underscoring the importance of family support and social connections in promoting personal recovery. Another research analyzes the relationships between insight, medication adherence, addiction, coping, and social support as determinants of clinical, functional, and personal recovery in patients with schizophrenia and other severe mental illnesses [19], underlining the interrelations between these concepts and their impact on recovery. Chang and Chen [6] investigated the relationship between family social networks, self-esteem, self-efficacy, and personal recovery among Chinese people with mental illness [6] and found that high perceived social support and larger social networks were related to high self-esteem among people with mental illness; their results highlight the positive impact of family social networks on personal recovery and emphasizes the role of social support in enhancing self-esteem. Roth and colleagues discussed the importance of perceived support for recovery and its relationship with the level of functioning among people with severe mental illness [20] and suggested that community-based services that embed recovery-oriented principles into care can support personal and social recovery, therefore pointing out the significance of community-based support services in promoting personal recovery. The role of peer support and supported employment services was investigated in another research [16] and found to reduce social isolation and optimizing recovery among individuals with mental illnesses on probation. Longmate et al. concluded by advocating that low levels of social support are associated with greater symptoms of mental illness.

Family is another pivotal factor that plays a crucial role in promoting personal recovery in mental illness. Research has shown that family caregivers of individuals with mental illness often experience significant stresses and burden [21]. These caregivers may also face challenges in accessing adequate support from mental health professionals [21]. Therefore, it is important for mental health nurses to provide psychosocial education and family interventions to help family caregivers cope with the stresses and stigmas associated with their relatives' mental illnesses [22]. Additionally, educating the public about mental health and illness through health promotion and education can contribute to better understanding and support for individuals with mental illness and their families [22].

Pets can also play a role in promoting recovery from serious mental illness. Research has shown that pet ownership can have positive effects on social, educational, and occupational functioning, as well as reducing loneliness [23]. This is particularly important as serious mental illnesses can often limit social networks and increase feelings of isolation [23]. Therefore, incorporating pet ownership into recovery plans may be beneficial for individuals with mental illness.

The recovery process for individuals with mental illness involves grieving the losses associated with their condition and adapting their social roles to a restructured sense of self [24]. This process is not limited to the individual with mental illness, but also extends to their family members [24]. Family members can experience their own recovery from the trauma of mental illness and play a supportive role in the recovery of their loved ones [25]. However, it is important to note that family members may also face challenges in their role, such as acting as stressors, displaying stigma, and lacking understanding [26]. Therefore, it is crucial for mental health professionals to provide support and interventions that address the needs of both individuals with mental illness and their families [26]. Family-focused practices have been identified as essential in supporting parents with mental illness in the context of their family [27]. The EASE framework (Engage, Assess, Support, Educate) provides a framework for clinicians to support parents with mental illness and strengthen their recovery within the context of their relationships [27]. Additionally, developing a recovery model specifically for parents in mental health and family services can help address the unique challenges faced by parents with mental illness who are caring for dependent children [28]. Attitudes towards disclosing a mental illness can also impact quality of life and recovery. Studies have shown a positive association between attitudes towards disclosing a mental illness, quality of life, and recovery [29]. This suggests that creating a supportive environment where individuals feel comfortable disclosing their mental illness can contribute to their overall well-being and recovery. Family support is associated with improved clinical and personal recovery outcomes, including symptom severity, social functioning, and work functioning [5]. Self-compassion has been identified as a potential mechanism underlying the impact of family support on recovery [5]. By fostering self-compassion, family support can contribute to the overall well-being and recovery of individuals with mental illness. However, high levels of family criticalness can have a negative impact on personal recovery, leading to low self-esteem and low levels of recovery. The impact of family support on recovery is not limited to mental health conditions. It also extends to physical health conditions, such as stroke recovery. Social support from family members can help stroke patients feel connected and motivated, leading to better recovery outcomes. Similarly, in the context of cognitive impairment, family support is crucial for resuming normal life and providing instrumental and supervisory care. Overall, a comprehensive and holistic approach that includes the involvement and support of family members is essential in promoting personal recovery in mental illness.

21.3 Technology, Internet, and Personal Recovery

Digital technology has the potential to play a significant role in promoting recovery from mental illness. It can provide individuals with mental illness access to resources and support, enhance treatment adherence, and improve overall mental health outcomes [30].

However, there are several factors that need to be considered to ensure the successful implementation and effectiveness of digital technology interventions for mental illness. One important consideration is the behavioral mechanisms underlying the management of mental health symptoms and the adoption of healthy behaviors. Naslund et al. emphasize the need to uncover specific behavioral mechanisms that effectively manage mental health symptoms, prevent relapse, and reinforce healthy behaviors [30, 31]. Understanding these mechanisms is crucial for developing digital interventions that target these behaviors and promote recovery. Another important aspect is the accessibility and usability of digital technology for individuals with mental illness. Tremain et al. [32] highlight the existence of a digital divide in mental health, where individuals with serious mental illnesses are excluded from receiving support through digital means due to a lack of access, skills, or confidence [31]. This exclusion needs to be addressed to ensure that digital technology interventions are accessible and beneficial for all individuals with mental illness. Furthermore, the therapeutic alliance between individuals with mental illness and digital mental health interventions is a crucial factor to consider. Tremain et al. [32] suggest that the therapeutic alliance, which is the collaborative relationship between the individual and the intervention, plays a significant role in the effectiveness of digital mental health interventions [31]. Building a strong therapeutic alliance in digital interventions can enhance engagement, adherence, and overall outcomes.

The use of mobile apps for mental health is a prevalent form of digital technology intervention. Torous et al. found that approximately 10% of psychiatric outpatients reported current usage of mental health apps [33]. However, it is important to note that the actual usage rates may vary depending on the clinic setting and patient population. Additionally, Lipschitz et al. highlight the importance of personalization in mental health apps, as insufficient personalization can limit their effectiveness [34]. Tailoring apps to individual needs and preferences can enhance engagement and improve outcomes. Digital technology interventions can also be particularly beneficial for specific populations, such as older adults and individuals with intellectual disabilities. Sheehan and Hassiotis emphasize the potential benefits of digital mental health interventions for individuals with intellectual disabilities, who often face barriers to fully embracing digital technology [35]. Similarly, Andrews et al. highlight the increasing uptake of digital technologies among older adults and the need to explore their attitudes toward using digital apps for maintaining good mental health [30].

In addition to individual-level interventions, digital technology can also support peer-to-peer support and social connections. Naslund et al. discuss the potential of social media platforms for individuals with mental illness to share their experiences and seek advice from others with similar conditions [17]. Peer support through digital platforms can provide valuable support and reduce feelings of isolation.

However, it is important to acknowledge the challenges and limitations of digital technology interventions for mental illness. The digital divide, as mentioned earlier, poses a significant barrier to access and utilization of digital interventions for individuals with mental illness. Additionally, concerns about privacy and security need to be addressed to ensure the ethical and responsible use of digital technology in mental health care [36].

Internet-based interventions have the potential to enhance mental health services and support self-management and recovery among individuals with mental illness [37]. These interventions can provide opportunities for individuals to connect with similar others online, challenge stigma, and increase consumer activation ([17], pp. 113–122). They have been shown to have positive effects on mental health outcomes, including decreasing depressive symptoms ([38], p. e10668). The internet can serve as a valuable source of information for individuals with mental illness, allowing them to access health information, seek support from peers, and gather coping strategies ([39], p. e15). It has become an influential source of information for people experiencing serious psychiatric conditions, such as schizophrenia spectrum disorders ([40], p. e1). In fact, a survey found that a large majority of individuals with serious mental illness have access to the internet via computers, smartphones, and tablets, which affords communication and socialization ([41], p. e12255). Internet-based interventions have been found to be effective for various mental health conditions, including depression ([42], pp. 8–15). They have the potential to bridge the gap in mental health services, particularly in low- and middle-income countries where access to traditional face-to-face interventions may be limited [43]. However, it is important to note that the usefulness of internet-based interventions may vary depending on the specific mental health condition. For example, they may be rated as more useful for sleep problems and anxiety, but less useful for psychiatric problems such as obsessive behaviors ([44], p. e15149; [45, 46]).

The concept of recovery is central to mental health services, and the internet can play a role in supporting recovery-oriented practice. Recovery-oriented interventions aim to help individuals with mental illness manage their illness and achieve personal recovery goals ([47], pp. 1344–1353). They focus on empowering individuals, promoting self-confidence, and enhancing personal control and self-reliance ([48], pp. 100–112). Internet-based interventions can provide resources and support for individuals on their recovery journey, helping them lead a satisfactory life despite the presence of debilitating symptoms [12]. It is worth noting that the implementation of internet-based interventions in routine mental health care can pose challenges. There is a need for further research to understand the barriers and facilitators to the use of internet interventions in mental health services ([49], pp. 261–270). In addition, the quality and effectiveness of internet interventions can vary, highlighting the importance of evidence-based practice and rigorous evaluation ([50], pp. 4–11).

The internet has, indeed, the potential to revolutionize mental health care and support recovery among individuals with mental illness. Internet-based interventions can provide opportunities for individuals to connect with peers, access information, and receive support. However, further research is needed to fully understand the impact and implementation of these interventions in mental health services.

21.4 Obstacles to Personal Recovery

Preventing relapse and recurrence in mental illness is a crucial aspect of treatment and recovery. It is important to address risk factors and implement strategies that can help individuals maintain stability and prevent the recurrence of symptoms. Several studies provide insights into effective approaches for relapse prevention in mental illness. One key factor in preventing relapse is early intervention and treatment. Wiersma et al. [51] emphasize the importance of timely mental health treatment in preventing further damage and deterioration. They suggest that an early warning and intervention strategy could prevent relapse and promote better outcomes. Similarly, Lewis et al. [52] highlight the need to improve the speed and quality of recovery and prevent future relapse in individuals with severe mental illness.

Medication adherence is another critical aspect of relapse prevention. Bidargaddi et al. [53] discuss the importance of early detection of *non-adherence to medication* in order to intervene and prevent relapse. They demonstrate how digitally automated non-adherence monitoring can be used to detect non-adherence and enable timely intervention. Psychosocial interventions and support systems also play a significant role in relapse prevention. Mudakavi and Rentala [54] emphasize that effective relapse prevention enables individuals to gain mastery over their symptoms and increase their sense of control over their lives. They point out to the importance of relapse prevention in improving the quality of life and enabling individuals to fully participate in work, leisure, and relationships. Family support and involvement can be a valuable resource in relapse prevention. Tlhowe et al. [55] suggest that utilizing the strengths of families can be a valuable approach in preventing relapse in mental health care. They highlight the need to explore the strengths of family members to help limit relapse in individuals with mental health conditions. Similarly, Muryani et al. [56] found that families play a crucial role in recognizing signs of relapse in family members with mental disorders. Psychoeducation and coping skills training are effective strategies for relapse prevention. Mueser et al. [57, 58] highlight that psychoeducation improves individuals' knowledge of mental illness, while coping skills training using cognitive-behavioral techniques helps individuals develop effective strategies to manage symptoms and prevent relapse. Furthermore, maintaining a supportive and therapeutic environment is essential for relapse prevention. Agenagnew and Kassaw [59] found that the support of families and effective social support can help limit relapse in individuals with mental illness. They pointed out to the need for an integrated approach that provides effective social support in relapse prevention.

Recovery from mental illness can be a complex and challenging process, as individuals face various obstacles along the way. These obstacles can hinder progress and make it difficult for individuals to achieve their recovery goals.

Several factors have been identified in the literature that contribute to these obstacles. One significant obstacle to recovery is the *stigma associated with mental illness*. Stigma can come from various sources, including mental health service providers ([60], pp. 526–531). Perceived provider stigma has been found to be associated with internalized stigma and disempowerment among mental health service users ([60], pp. 526–531). This stigma can lead to feelings of shame and self-criticism, which can hinder the recovery process and can also result in discrimination and social exclusion, limiting opportunities for individuals with mental illness [61]. Overcoming stigma and promoting acceptance of mental illness are crucial steps in the recovery process ([14], pp. 77–86).

Another obstacle to recovery is the *lack of support and understanding from the community*. The presence of a supportive environment and accessibility to mental health services have been identified as facilitators of recovery [11]. However, negative attitudes towards patients, inadequate human resources, and a lack of confidence in mental health professionals can hinder the recovery process ([62], pp. 200–210). It is essential to create a supportive and inclusive community that promotes recovery and provides individuals with the necessary resources and support to achieve their goals.

Acceptance of one's self and the limitations imposed by mental illness is another crucial factor in the recovery process ([63], pp. 44–51). Individuals need to search for meaning in their experience of mental illness and recovery, gain mastery over their experience and their lives, and reclaim their identity and self-worth ([63], pp. 44–51). This process of acceptance can be challenging, as individuals may struggle with *feelings of shame, guilt, and self-blame*. However, accepting one's self and the reality of living with a mental illness is a crucial step towards recovery.

The presence of psychiatric symptoms and the severity of mental illness can also pose obstacles to recovery. The experience of symptoms can impact an individual's ability to function in daily life and pursue their recovery goals ([64], pp. 540–547). It is essential for individuals to have access to evidence-based treatments and services that address their specific needs and support their recovery journey ([47], pp. 1344–1353).

Collaborative approaches to care, such as shared decision-making and person-centered care, have been shown to promote recovery-oriented practice and improve outcomes for individuals with mental illness ([65], pp. 783–788). Furthermore, the recovery process can be influenced by personal factors such as hope, illness acceptance, and adherence to treatment [11]. Hope plays a significant role in recovery, as it provides individuals with a sense of optimism and motivation to overcome challenges ([66], pp. 38–44). Illness acceptance involves acknowledging the limitations imposed by mental illness and finding ways to manage and cope with symptoms [11]. Adherence to treatment, including medication and therapy, is crucial for symptom management and overall well-being [11]. These personal factors can contribute to resilience and facilitate the recovery process. Creating a supportive and inclusive community, promoting acceptance and understanding, and providing evidence-based treatments and services are essential steps towards facilitating recovery in mental illness.

Isolation in recovery from mental illness is a complex and multifaceted issue that has significant implications for individuals' mental health and overall well-being. Several studies have explored the impact of isolation on mental health outcomes, particularly in the context of the COVID-19 pandemic. One study by Yang et al. [67] investigated the relationship between social isolation and mental health among college students during the high-risk period of COVID-19 transmission in Hubei, China. The study found that college students who received sufficient social support from online friends were able to avoid the negative effects of perceived social isolation on their mental health. On the other hand, an absence of sufficient social support from online friends exacerbated the negative effects of perceived social isolation on mental health. This suggests that social support plays a crucial role in mitigating the negative impact of isolation on mental health. Similarly, Xiong et al. [68] examined the impact of *social disconnectedness* on mental health problems during the COVID-19 pandemic in China. The study found that social disconnectedness indirectly led to mental health problems by increasing perceived isolation, the co-occurrence of social disconnectedness and perceived isolation had a significant impact on mental health outcomes. This highlights the importance of addressing both social disconnectedness and perceived isolation to promote mental well-being. In addition to the COVID-19 pandemic, social isolation has been identified as a significant factor affecting mental health in various populations. Cheng et al. [69] conducted a study on older adults in China and found that social isolation had a negative impact on mental health. The study also revealed that aging attitude played a significant mediating role between social isolation and mental health. This suggests that addressing social isolation alone may not be sufficient and that attitudes towards aging should also be considered in promoting mental well-being among older adults. Social isolation and loneliness have both been found to have negative impacts on mental health and Pai [70] discussed the physical and mental health consequences of social isolation and loneliness in the context of COVID-19. The study found that social isolation and loneliness were associated with negative outcomes, including anxiety, depression, and cognitive decline, emphasizing their detrimental effects on mental health and the need for interventions to address these issues.

Table 21.2 provides a summary of potential obstacles to personal recovery in people with mental disorders.

Table 21.2 Obstacles to personal recovery in people with mental disorders

Persistence and severity of psychiatric symptoms	Lack of access to evidence-based treatments and services
Relapses/recurrences	
Medication non-adherence	
Stigma associated with mental illness	Perceived provider stigma Internalized stigma
Lack of support and understanding from the community	Negative attitudes towards patients Inadequate human resources Lack of confidence in mental health professionals Perceived isolation/social disconnectedness
Feelings of shame, guilt, and self-blame	

21.5 Recovery in Depression as a "*New Paradigm*"

We will now focus the attention to personal recovery in major depressive disorder as an example of a recovery-oriented approach to mental disorders.

Recent investigations on the efficacy of antidepressants revealed that standard interventions were insufficient to achieve clinical recovery in many patients with major depressive disorder (MDD) [71]; hence, the emphasis on recovery from depression. Indeed, several clinical features associated with the naturalistic course of MDD, such as its chronicity, the associated high relapse rates, and the increasing probability of recurrences with each new episode [72–74], the frequent persistence and deleterious impact of residual symptoms [75–77], and the high comorbidity with physical illnesses, with long-term damaging effects on health and well-being greater than those associated with angina, arthritis, asthma, or diabetes [78–81], justify the recent interest in applying the concept of personal recovery to MDD. The lifetime prevalence of major depressive disorder is considerable (16.2%), and two-thirds of cases have an episodic recurrent course [82, 83]. More than 50% of MDD patients report unsatisfactory results from available interventions, with a high relapse rate 2 years after the disorder's onset [83–85]. Researchers and clinicians have been motivated by the magnitude of this public health issue to seek out improved treatments for this condition and to define more specific treatment objectives, such as response, remission, and recovery. In fact, these terms have evolved alongside the study of innovative therapeutic treatment strategies [86]. Response was defined as a 50% decrease from baseline in the total score on a standardized symptom scale (e.g., HAM-D, MADRS) and may be the most consistently defined term, widely used as the acute treatment objective. Remission is considered a more stringent definition of a positive endpoint and has been identified as the treatment objective for MDD since the late 1990s [87–89]. In clinical trials, remission is defined as a score reduction below a specific cutoff score on rating scales, and operationalized criteria have been proposed based on the specific rating scales used (e.g., HAM-D score 7; MADRS score 10). Unfortunately, only 30–40% of people with MDD achieve symptomatic remission after receiving an adequate course of antidepressants, and residual symptoms are often present. Cognitive dysfunctions (i.e., impairments in psychomotor speed, attention, verbal memory, executive functions) are among the most frequently encountered residual symptoms [90, 91], represent a substantial risk for relapse in depression [92], and are strongly related to impaired psychosocial functioning, some authors have proposed the term cognitive remission as a new primary treatment goal for MDD [93–95]. Continual functional impairment may have a negative impact on a patient's ability to return to daily life, delaying his or her functional recovery.

Full functional recovery is a condition in which the patient resumes his or her usual activities, returns to employment, and is able to care for himself or herself [80, 96]. Research demonstrates, in fact, that the prioritized therapeutic objective in MDD is the return to premorbid functioning, positive mental health, over the extinction of depressive symptomatology.

This historical shift from symptomatic remission to complete functional recovery as the treatment objective in clinical trials is mirrored by a similar trend in recent practice guidelines for mood disorders to identify more holistic objectives of mood disorder management. For instance, the CANMAT 2016 clinical guidelines for the management of adults with MDD state that the goals of acute treatment (8–12 weeks) are the remission of symptoms and the restoration of functioning, whereas the goals of the maintenance phase (6–24 months) are the return to full functioning and quality of life and the prevention of recurrence [97]. The more recent 2020 Royal Australian and New Zealand College of Psychiatrists clinical practice guidelines for mood disorders [98] explicitly recommend that "the aims of mood disorder treatment should go beyond symptom relief to include resilience and improve well-being"; this is especially recommended in the context of chronic and relapsing mood disorders, where an episode of care is also viewed as an opportunity to develop the patient's resilience against future episodes. Resilience is defined as the ability to adapt to and recoup from adversity; it is not merely the absence of vulnerability. Guidelines identify personal recovery as the ultimate aim of treatment, as the "process of adaptation to serious mental illness," and encourage clinicians to engage patients more actively [98]. The development of resilience "focuses on implementing new strategies, integrating new resources, and addressing weaknesses." The term personal recovery appears for the first time as the treatment objective for MDD.

Various definitions of personal recovery in severe mental disorder (SMD) have been proposed as well as a number of determinants of personal recovery. Nevertheless, all definitions of personal recovery include elements such as accepting mental illness, discovering hope for the future, re-establishing a positive identity, developing meaning in life, taking control of one's life through individual responsibility, spirituality, empowerment, overcoming stigma, and having supportive relationships [99]. Due to the complexity of the recovery concept, it is likely that a consensus definition of personal recovery has not yet been attained. The fact that there are at least five phases of recovery adds to the complexity [100]: (1) moratorium (i.e., denial, confusion, hopelessness, identity confusion, and self-protective withdrawal); (2) awareness (i.e., the initial appraisal that recovery is possible, with the possibility of a better life, including the development of the awareness of a possible self, other than that of being a patient with an SMD); (3) preparation, involves individuals initiating their journey towards recovery by acquiring knowledge about mental illness and the various services available to them. They actively engage in groups and establish connections with individuals who are at different stages of their own recovery process; (4) rebuilding, the most challenging stage of the recovery process. This entails a transformation towards a more positive identity, achieved through the reevaluation of previous values and the adoption of a new way of life. It involves assuming responsibility for the management of illness and taking control of one's own life. Additionally, it requires demonstrating perseverance by taking risks and enduring setbacks; (5) growth, another crucial aspect of the recovery process is, which refers to the acquisition of new skills for effectively managing symptoms and disabilities. Leamy et al. [101] provided one of the most exhaustive definitions of personal recovery; they developed a framework to comprehend the concept of personal recovery through a systematic review and narrative synthesis: the CHIME Framework. It consists of three interconnected superordinate categories of recovery, including recovery journey characteristics, recovery processes, and recovery stages. The acronym CHIME is derived from the framework's identified recovery process: Connectedness (i.e., peer and social group support, positive social relationships, support from others, and community membership); Hope and optimism (i.e., belief in the possibility of recovery, motivation to change, hope-inspiring relationships, positive thinking and valuing success, having ambitions and aspirations) are correlated with positive psychological outcomes; Identity (including identity dimensions, the capacity to reconstruct or redefine a positive sense of identity, and the ability to surmount stigma); Meaning in life (i.e., the meaning of mental illness experiences, spirituality, quality of life, meaningful life and social roles and objectives, the capacity to rehabilitate one's life); Empowerment (i.e., personal responsibility, control over one's life, a focus on one's strengths). Specifically, empowerment is a central concept of the World Health Organization's [102] vision for mental health promotion, and it is central to the concept of personal recovery. "No decision about me without me" is a user-led movement in the United Kingdom that sought to convert the English National Health Service into a recovery-oriented service system [103]. Empowerment refers to the capacity of individuals to become stronger and more self-assured, particularly in terms of regulating their own lives and asserting their rights. Empowerment helps to acquire autonomy and self-determination and to influence the decision-making process, thus influencing self-esteem and self-efficacy [104].

The process of personal recovery is characterized by three principal dimensions: inner experience, contribution from others, and participation in social activities [81]. The first category refers to patients' inner experiences of their illness, as well as their capacity to embrace themselves as individuals, as opposed to patients, and to see themselves as accountable for building an independent existence. In this context, recovery is the capacity to tolerate the impairment. Acceptance, which is not synonymous with giving up and submitting to symptoms, is the most difficult stage of the entire recovery process, but also the most important [105]. Hope, spirituality, empowerment, connection, purpose, self-identity, symptom management, and stigma are components of acceptance [106]. The second category refers to the support from relevant others, such as professionals, family members and other caregivers, acquaintances, and other patients, during the recovery process. Several therapeutic approaches, including cognitive remediation, psychoeducational interventions, and cognitive-behavioral approaches, have been demonstrated to be effective in facilitating the process of personal recovery, as part of professional support [107]. Independent of the therapeutic approach, a crucial element of professional support, which is strongly tied to the patient's rehabilitation, is the provision of a guide to the patient's symptoms and tools to help them surmount crises. Characteristics of mental health personnel associated with improved personal recovery are empathy and respect, active and attentive listening, and an interest in patients' concerns [108]. In recent years, the role of mental health professionals and the organization of mental health services have become central to the promotion of personal recovery. In fact, many nations have adopted mental health policies that emphasize recovery-oriented services and interventions [109, 110]. The recovery-oriented approaches provide a transformative conceptual framework for mental health practice, culture, and service delivery [110]. Multiple studies have demonstrated that spirituality is an important aspect of personal recovery, as religion can motivate and inspire patients to live their lives with greater acceptance [111, 112]. In addition, being a member of a faith community and having a religious affiliation are regarded as crucial components of a person's recovery [101]. Participation in social activities comprises the third element of personal recovery for patients. Patients can avoid seclusion and reduce detachment from reality by engaging in daily activity and maintaining contact with the outside world [111]. Having a stable job also helps maintain a sense of being able to contribute to society, feeling competent and valued by coworkers [108], while simultaneously reducing stigma and fostering a sense of independence from others. In addition, participation in recreational activities is a significant factor in the healing process. Participation in leisure activities allows individuals to be distracted from mental health issues, meet new people, and form social networks, thereby enhancing their social life [81]. Whitley and Drake [113] have proposed an integrated dimensional model of rehabilitation. It defines rehabilitation in terms of the following five dimensions: (1) clinical—reduction of symptoms; (2) existential—greater sense of hope, empowerment, and spiritual well-being; (3) functional—recovery of a meaningful role; (4) physical—promotion of physical health; and (5) social—consolidation of relationships with others and a sense of belonging in society. This framework provides an integrated approach with a focus on clinical and personal aspects of recovery (including a focus on physical health—and thus strategies implementing physical health) and may provide clinicians with a useful framework for identifying and promoting recovery-promoting strategies.

Recovery from MDD is still poorly understood. In fact, the majority of research on recovery has been conducted on patients with schizophrenia, other psychoses, and/or bipolar disorders. Patients with severe depression are underrepresented in consumer movements that have conceptualized the concept of personal recovery [71, 114]. Despite the fact that personal recovery is conceptualized as a process that can occur independently of patients' symptoms, a number of studies [115] have demonstrated that the type and severity of psychiatric symptoms can have varying effects on personal recovery. In actuality, the fundamental symptoms of schizophrenia, such as delusions and hallucinations, have a diminished impact on the patient's experience of recovery, whereas affective symptoms are viewed as a barrier to the recovery process of patients with schizophrenia [116]. In a sample of 105 patients with schizophrenia and bipolar disorder, the authors reported that personal recovery was predicted primarily by affective symptoms, while negative and positive symptoms were not associated with personal recovery. In addition, the severity of affective symptoms was more strongly associated with personal recovery in patients with non-psychotic disorders than in patients with schizophrenia.

Few studies have examined individual recovery from severe depression. The available evidence suggests that recovery from MDD is a complex, individualized, and multifaceted process. Several social, clinical, and contextual factors may be implicated in the recovery process [114], resulting in its complexity. Social support, measured as the extent of the social network, the subjective sensation of being supported by family or friends, the number of close relationships, and satisfaction with received support, is one of the most influential factors that can inhibit or promote the recovery process in MDD [117, 118]. According to Gladstone et al. [119], a significant proportion of individuals diagnosed with major depressive disorder (MDD) consider a lack of social support as a hindrance to their recovery process, with more than 50% expressing this sentiment. Interventions aimed at promoting the establishment and sustenance of supportive relationships may potentially serve as efficacious strategies for facilitating personal rehabilitation. However, the relationship between perceived poor social support and depression, leading to a delay in the recovery process, is complex: it is possible that the depressive state is associated with a negative perception of social support when this is not the case, but also that chronicity of depression or multiple recurrences of depression lead to the erosion of social support networks over time (a social scar of recurrent or chronic MDD). Consequently, it is crucial to thoroughly evaluate this aspect in the patient's actual existence. This also implies that clinicians should promptly recognize, diagnose, and treat MDD from its onset; an early personalized and optimized treatment is essential in terms of (a) pharmacologic compound or psychotherapeutic intervention, (b) appropriate dose (drug) or frequency (psychotherapeutic intervention), (c) right choice of the specific intervention according to the clinical subtype/predominant symptom dimension of MDD, and (d) quick adoption of alternative strategy. The duration of untreated illness and the absence of early change in depressive symptoms (e.g., 20% decrease in HAM-D score after 2 weeks) have been consistently associated with non-remission and/or relapses/recurrences, thereby impeding the personal recovery journey [120–122].

To promote recovery from depression, it is also essential to aggressively treat the complete spectrum of symptoms accompanying the episode, including residual symptoms and dysfunctions eventually caused by drug side effects (e.g., sexual dysfunctions). Integration of multiple treatment approaches (successively) may prove to be the most effective means of promoting individual recovery. Referring to the integrated model of recovery proposed by Whitley and Drake [113], these can be conceptualized as clinical recovery-promoting and personal recovery-contributing strategies. Other strategies that patients can implement with the help of healthcare providers include analyzing and changing dysfunctional beliefs (cognitive-behavioral treatments) and/or learning how to pay attention to mood changes (e.g., taking regular notes on mood changes) in order to recognize early signs of a relapse and implement appropriate strategies as soon as they become aware that their symptoms are intensifying [123]. Regarding contextual factors, it is crucial to note that patients and clinicians have varying perspectives on what comprises recovery from severe depression and what they deem essential for recovery from MDD [124–126]. In fact, the majority of physicians consider the reduction of the number and severity of depressive symptoms, as well as the improvement of patients' functioning, to be their primary treatment objectives, whereas patients are primarily concerned with the restoration of positive affect, such as having a meaningful life, being satisfied with personal relationships, and enhancing their concentration and personal strengths [127]. Moreover, across all phases of the disorder (acute, post-acute, and remission), perceptions of MDD symptoms and the associations between these symptoms and functioning differ significantly between patients and healthcare providers [128]. The findings of this latter study emphasize the need for enhanced patient-provider communication in order to establish appropriate treatment objectives. Different treatment outcome priorities between patients and clinicians can lead clinicians to systematically disregard all the components of personal recovery as an outcome to be attained, thereby decreasing the likelihood that patients will recover. An intriguing study found that discordance between what patients and physicians consider important in the definition of depression cure significantly affects clinical outcomes at 6 months: the subgroup with poor physician–patient agreement on expectations had a worse clinical outcome than the subgroup with excellent physician–patient agreement on expectations, with response rate differences between these groups ranging from 9% to 27% [127]. Again, the clinical complexity and heterogeneity of MDD in terms of predominant symptom dimensions, perceived different relevance of each symptom dimension according to patients' and healthcare providers' perspectives, subtype, chronicity, etc. emphasize the need for a personalized, individually tailored approach to the individual living with MDD [129].

Patients with MDD cite four main factors that can impede their recovery journey; the first is the lack of consensus on the nature of depression; having no personalized treatment, receiving insufficient information about proposed treatments, and a lack of discussion regarding medications (e.g., mechanisms of action, potential side effects, and time to response) are reported to be major impeding elements in the patient-clinician relationship. In this regard, practitioners may use psychoeducational consensus protocols to promote a stronger relationship and enhance shared decision making in MDD [130]. Other factors that patients with MDD perceive as having the potential to impede their rehabilitation are: (1) a precarious relationship with the clinician, including lack of trust in clinicians' abilities to treat depression, lack of continuity in treatment due to frequent changes in treating clinicians, inappropriate professional attitudes, and lack of professional guidance; (2) the unavailability of mental health care when needed, especially in emergency situations (long waiting lists, unavailability of treating clinician, and lack of care after symptom resolution are the most common causes); and (3) the stigma associated with seeking mental health care. Several approaches [131] have been proposed in recent years in an effort to facilitate recovery from depression. Self-management is one of the most promising approaches because it increases individualism, empowerment, and participation in social activities [123]. Self-management consists of both professional and user-driven strategies. Among the former have been proposed booklets, books, and e-health programs [132, 133]. Patients' perspectives on how they recovered from depression provide promising insights; an intriguing study [123] examined the strategies used by people recovering from depressive and anxiety disorders and classified them according to the model proposed by Whitley and Drake [113]; these strategies may be implemented in clinical practice to promote recovery. Self-management strategies used to promote clinical recovery include taking a proactive stance toward depression and its treatments (e.g., seeking information from mental health professionals about depressive symptoms and gaining insight into illness, taking your medication), managing daily symptoms (e.g., analyzing and changing your thoughts/emotions and behaviors), and remaining vigilant for signs and symptoms of potential relapses. Patients reported having a positive outlook, e.g., taking inspiration from someone who has previously recovered—well-known public figures with the same disorder, or people in support groups, having spiritual beliefs, using humor, developing a balanced sense of self (e.g., differentiating the illness from one's personality), and finding meaning (e.g. finding a project, a goal, a dream), among other strategies. Creating a routine (e.g., following a schedule, having and respecting regular rhythms—going to bed at a regular time) and proactively taking activities (e.g., engaging in pleasant activities and engaging in activities in which you can feel competent) were self-managed strategies that promoted functional recovery; again, the utility of this approach is that psychosocial interventions (led by healthcare providers but also led by peers) can be implemented in order to reduce relapse. Regaining and promoting physical health is another important aspect of rehabilitation; strategies that promote physical recovery include participating in sports, implementing good sleep hygiene, eating at regular times and well, and reducing consumption of alcohol, tobacco, and other substances. In this regard, it has to be borne in mind that physical health is compromised in mood disorders because of different contributors, some of them not modifiable such as genetic predisposition, other modifiable such as dysregulations in social rhythms, substance abuse, poor sleep hygiene, or side effects of medications. Individuals with the disorder and their healthcare providers can prevent physical complications and promote physical recovery. Last but not least, self-management strategies fostering social recovery reported by patients with depressive disorders included surrounding myself with people who make me feel better, avoiding negative people, and caring for others, such as family or friends [123].

21.6 Moving Forward

Despite the recent interest of the scientific community, much work remains to be done in order to define a clear and internationally recognized conceptualization of personal recovery and its dimensions for people living with severe depression. Too many questions remain unresolved, such as whether the process of personal recovery from depression is similar to or distinct from that of personal recovery from other severe mental disorders. The methodology employed in the various studies is extremely heterogeneous, and different instruments have been used to evaluate personal recovery, thereby obstructing comparisons across studies. In contrast to studies on the personal recovery of patients with schizophrenia or bipolar disorders, the lack of data makes it impossible to determine which aspects of recovery from severe depression should be prioritized. This information is necessary for clinicians to guide patients on their "journey to recovery." It is not a case that one of the most important factors slowing the process of recovery is the lack of professional support perceived by patients [83]. Patients with severe depression frequently view the clinician as an authority who makes treatment decisions on their behalf with little encouragement to attain autonomy, motivation, and self-management. Several authors have emphasized that the manner in which decisions are made during clinical encounters affects patients' recovery, and that the identification of treatment priorities should always be shared with patients, in accordance with the shared-decision making model, which is associated with better outcomes in terms of symptom reduction and improvement of psychosocial functioning, empowerment, and satisfaction with care received [104, 134]. Different perspectives have been reported between clinicians and patients regarding aspects of personal recovery for patients with severe depression; however, few studies ([124, 126, 127]; Baune et al. 2019) have explored the impact of these differences. Lastly, available studies on recovery from depression and other severe mental disorders demonstrate the need for a transition in psychiatric care delivery [135]. In actuality, there is a need to move away from a "treat-and-recover" approach, in which the provision of remedies with the goal of reengaging individuals in life is given priority [136].

For decades, mental health services have been organized around a clinical model of recovery, in which professionals diagnose and treat patients with the goal of reducing their symptoms, but do not consider the possibility of recovery from severe mental disorders beyond symptom reduction [137]. Numerous interventions, such as "Wellness Recovery Action Planning (WRAP)" [138], "Illness Management and Recovery Program (IMR)" [57, 58], and "REFOCUS" [139], are currently available to promote the personal recovery of users. Randomized controlled trials have demonstrated the efficacy of each of these approaches in promoting personal recovery in patients with severe mental disorders.

Authors' Contributions All authors have actively contributed to the chapter and approved it in its current form.

References

1. Escobedo-Aedo PJ et al (2022) Investigating the role of insight, decision-making and mentalizing in functional outcome in schizophrenia: a cross-sectional study. Behav Sci (Basel) 12:28. https://doi.org/10.3390/bs12020028
2. He S, Fang Y, Huang Z, Yu Y (2021) Validation of an 8-item recovery assessment scale (RAS-8) for people with schizophrenia in China. Health Qual Life Outcomes 19:119. https://doi.org/10.1186/s12955-021-01763-3
3. Parker RA (2012) A framework for funding culturally appropriate recovery for people affected by severe mental illness: a world view. https://doi.org/10.4038/sljpsyc.v2i2.4038
4. Jaiswal A, Carmichael K, Gupta S, Siemens T, Crowley P, Carlsson A, Brown N (2020) Essential elements that contribute to the recovery of persons with severe mental illness: a systematic scoping study. Front Psychiatry 11:586230. https://doi.org/10.3389/fpsyt.2020.586230
5. Chan K, Yip C, Tsui J (2023) Self-compassion mediates the impact of family support on clinical and personal recovery among people with mental illness. Mindfulness 14:720–731. https://doi.org/10.1007/s12671-023-02088-6
6. Chang C, Chen F (2022) Family social networks and personal recovery among Chinese people with mental illness in Hong Kong: the mediating effects of self-esteem and self-efficacy. Psychiatr Rehabil J 45:247–254. https://doi.org/10.1037/prj0000485
7. Dell N, Long C, Mancini M (2021) Models of mental health recovery: an overview of systematic reviews and qualitative meta-syntheses. Psychiatr Rehabil J 44:238–253. https://doi.org/10.1037/prj0000444
8. Iseselo M, Ambikile J (2020) Promoting recovery in mental illness: the perspectives of patients, caregivers, and community members in Dar Es Salaam, Tanzania. Psychiatry J 2020:3607414. https://doi.org/10.1155/2020/3607414
9. Young D, Ng P, Cheng D, Leung C (2018) A vocational recovery model for young people with mental illness: a pretest–posttest.

Res Soc Work Pract 29:495–505. https://doi.org/10.1177/1049731518757031
10. Connell M, King R, Crowe T (2011) Can employment positively affect the recovery of people with psychiatric disabilities? Psychiatr Rehabil J 35:59–63. https://doi.org/10.2975/35.1.2011.59.63
11. Kaewprom C, Curtis J, Deane F (2011) Factors involved in recovery from schizophrenia: a qualitative study of Thai mental health nurses. Nurs Health Sci 13:323. https://doi.org/10.1111/j.1442-2018.2011.00621.x
12. Xie H (2014) Voices of personal strengths and recovery: a qualitative study on people with serious mental illnesses with serious mental illnesses. https://doi.org/10.15405/epsbs.2014.05.4
13. Barton J, Griffin M, Pretty J (2011) Exercise-, nature- and socially interactive-based initiatives improve mood and self-esteem in the clinical population. Perspect Public Health 132:89–96. https://doi.org/10.1177/1757913910393862
14. Garverich S, Prener C, Guyer M, Lincoln A (2021) What matters: factors impacting the recovery process among outpatient mental health service users. Psychiatr Rehabil J 44:77–86. https://doi.org/10.1037/prj0000407
15. Hendryx M, Green C, Perrin N (2008) Social support, activities, and recovery from serious mental illness: stars study findings. J Behav Health Serv Res 36:320–329. https://doi.org/10.1007/s11414-008-9151-1
16. Longmate C, Lowder E, Givens A, Deinse T, Ghezzi M, Burgin S, Cuddeback G (2021) Social support among people with mental illnesses on probation. Psychiatr Rehabil J 44:70–76. https://doi.org/10.1037/prj0000428
17. Naslund J, Aschbrenner K, Marsch L, Bartels S (2016) The future of mental health care: peer-to-peer support and social media. Epidemiol Psychiatr Sci 25:113–122. https://doi.org/10.1017/s2045796015001067
18. Naslund J, Grande S, Aschbrenner K, Elwyn G (2014) Naturally occurring peer support through social media: the experiences of individuals with severe mental illness using YouTube. PLoS One 9:110171. https://doi.org/10.1371/journal.pone.0110171
19. Roosenschoon B, Kamperman A, Deen M, Weeghel J, Mulder C (2019) Determinants of clinical, functional and personal recovery for people with schizophrenia and other severe mental illnesses: a cross-sectional analysis. PLoS One 14:0222378. https://doi.org/10.1371/journal.pone.0222378
20. Roth C, Wensing M, Koetsenruijter J, Istvanovic A, Novotni A, Djurisic T, Shields-Zeeman L (2021) Perceived support for recovery and level of functioning among people with severe mental illness in Central and Eastern Europe: an observational study. Front Psych 12:732111. https://doi.org/10.3389/fpsyt.2021.732111
21. Reupert A, Maybery D, Cox M, Stokes E (2015) Place of family in recovery models for those with a mental illness. Int J Ment Health Nurs 24:495–506. https://doi.org/10.1111/inm.12146
22. Chang K, Horrocks S (2006) Lived experiences of family caregivers of mentally ill relatives. J Adv Nurs 53:435–443. https://doi.org/10.1111/j.1365-2648.2006.03732.x
23. Wisdom J, Saedi G, Green C (2009) Another breed of "service" animals: stars study findings about pet ownership and recovery from serious mental illness. Am J Orthopsychiatry 79:430–436. https://doi.org/10.1037/a0016812
24. Baxter E, Diehl S (1998) Emotional stages: consumers and family members recovering from the trauma of mental illness. Psychiatr Rehabil J 21:349–355. https://doi.org/10.1037/h0095289
25. Spaniol L (2010) The pain and the possibility: the family recovery process. Community Ment Health J 46:482–485. https://doi.org/10.1007/s10597-010-9315-3
26. Aldersey H, Whitley R (2014) Family influence in recovery from severe mental illness. Community Ment Health J 51:467–476. https://doi.org/10.1007/s10597-014-9783-y
27. Foster K, Goodyear M, Weimand B, Nicholson J (2018) Family-focused practice with ease: a practice framework for strengthening recovery when mental health consumers are parents. Int J Ment Health Nurs 28:351–360. https://doi.org/10.1111/inm.12535
28. Maybery D, Goodyear M, Sheen J, Cann W, Dalziel K, Tchernagovski P, Doussa H (2017) Developing an Australian-first recovery model for parents in Victorian mental health and family services: a study protocol for a randomised controlled trial. BMC Psychiatry 17:198. https://doi.org/10.1186/s12888-017-1357-4
29. Mayer L, Corrigan P, Eisheuer D, Oexle N, Rüsch N (2021) Attitudes towards disclosing a mental illness: impact on quality of life and recovery. Soc Psychiatry Psychiatr Epidemiol 57:363–374. https://doi.org/10.1007/s00127-021-02081-1
30. Andrews J, Brown L, Hawley M, Astell A (2019) Older adults' perspectives on using digital technology to maintain good mental health: interactive group study. J Med Internet Res 21:11694. https://doi.org/10.2196/11694
31. Naslund J, Aschbrenner K, Kim S, McHugo G, Unützer J, Bartels S, Marsch L (2017) Health behavior models for informing digital technology interventions for individuals with mental illness. Psychiatr Rehabil J 40:325–335. https://doi.org/10.1037/prj0000246
32. Tremain H, McEnery C, Fletcher K, Murray G (2020) The therapeutic alliance in digital mental health interventions for serious mental illnesses: narrative review. JMIR Ment Health 7:17204. https://doi.org/10.2196/17204
33. Torous J, Wisniewski H, Liu G, Keshavan M (2018) Mental health mobile phone app usage, concerns,

and benefits among psychiatric outpatients: comparative survey study. JMIR Ment Health 5:11715. https://doi.org/10.2196/11715
34. Lipschitz J, Miller C, Hogan T, Burdick K, Lippin-Foster R, Simon S, Burgess J (2019) Adoption of mobile apps for depression and anxiety: cross-sectional survey study on patient interest and barriers to engagement. JMIR Ment Health 6:11334. https://doi.org/10.2196/11334
35. Sheehan R, Hassiotis A (2017) Digital mental health and intellectual disabilities: state of the evidence and future directions. Evid Based Ment Health 20:107–111. https://doi.org/10.1136/eb-2017-102759
36. Terry N, Gunter T (2018) Regulating mobile mental health apps. Behav Sci Law 36:136–144. https://doi.org/10.1002/bsl.2339
37. Williams A, Farhall J, Fossey E, Thomas N (2019) Internet-based interventions to support recovery and self-management: a scoping review of their use by mental health service users and providers together. BMC Psychiatry 19(1):191. https://doi.org/10.1186/s12888-019-2153-0
38. Sherifali D, Ali MU, Ploeg J, Markle-Reid M, Valaitis R, Bartholomew A, Fitzpatrick-Lewis D (2018) Impact of internet-based interventions on caregiver mental health: systematic review and meta-analysis. J Med Internet 20:10668. https://doi.org/10.2196/10668
39. Gay K, Torous J, Joseph A, Pandya A, Duckworth K (2016) Digital technology use among individuals with schizophrenia: results of an online survey. JMIR Ment Health 3(2):e15. https://doi.org/10.2196/mental.5379
40. Villani M, Kovess-Masfety V (2017) How do people experiencing schizophrenia spectrum disorders or other psychotic disorders use the internet to get information on their mental health? Literature review and recommendations. JMIR Ment Health 4:e1. https://doi.org/10.2196/mental.5946
41. Noel V, Acquilano SC, Carpenter-Song E, Drake RE (2019) Use of mobile and computer devices to support recovery in people with serious mental illness: survey study. JMIR Men 6:12255. https://doi.org/10.2196/12255
42. Arjadi R, Nauta M, Bockting C (2018) Acceptability of internet-based interventions for depression in Indonesia. Internet Interv 13:8–15. https://doi.org/10.1016/j.invent.2018.04.004
43. Arjadi R, Nauta M, Chowdhary N, Bockting C (2015) A systematic review of online interventions for mental health in low and middle income countries: a neglected field. Global Ment Health 2:e12. https://doi.org/10.1017/gmh.2015.10
44. Størksen HT, Haga SM, Slinning K, Drozd F (2020) Health personnel's perceived usefulness of internet-based interventions for parents of children younger than 5 years: cross-sectional web-based survey study. JMIR Ment 7:15149. https://doi.org/10.2196/15149
45. Fineberg NA, Pellegrini L, Clarke A, Perera U, Drummond LM, Albert U, Laws KR (2022) Meta-analysis of cognitive behaviour therapy and selective serotonin reuptake inhibitors for the treatment of hypochondriasis: implications for trial design. Compr Psychiatry 118:152334. https://doi.org/10.1016/j.comppsych.2022.152334
46. Vismara M, Varinelli A, Pellegrini L, Enara A, Fineberg NA (2022) New challenges in facing Cyberchondria during the COVID-19 pandemic. Curr Opin Behav Sci 46:101156. https://doi.org/10.1016/j.cobeha.2022.101156
47. Egeland KM, Hauge M-I, Ruud T, Ogden T, Heiervang KS (2019) Significance of leaders for sustained use of evidence-based practices: a qualitative focus-group study with mental health practitioners. Community Ment Health J 55(8):1344–1353. https://doi.org/10.1007/s10597-019-00430-8
48. Xie H (2021) Mental health and its correlates: perspectives from two countries. Ment Health Rev J 26(1):100–112. https://doi.org/10.1108/mhrj-08-2020-0058
49. DeMartini L, Mizock L, Drob SL, Nelson A, Fisher WH (2022) The barriers and facilitators to serious mental illness: recovery postincarceration. Psychol Serv 19(2):261–270. https://doi.org/10.1037/ser0000431
50. Andersson G, Titov N (2014) Advantages and limitations of internet-based interventions for common mental disorders. World Psychiatry 13(1):4–11. https://doi.org/10.1002/wps.20083
51. Wiersma D, Fokko Nienhuis CJS, Giel R (1998) Natural course of schizophrenic disorders: a 15-year followup of a Dutch incidence cohort. Schizophr Bull 24(1):75–85. https://doi.org/10.1093/oxfordjournals.schbul.a033315
52. Lewis S, Ainsworth J, Sanders C, Stockton-Powdrell C, Machin M, Whelan P, Hopkins RS (2020) Smartphone-enhanced symptom management in psychosis: open, randomized controlled trial. J Med Internet 22:17019. https://doi.org/10.2196/17019
53. Bidargaddi N, Schrader G, Myles H, Schubert KO, Kasteren Y, Zhang T, Bastiampillai T (2021) Demonstration of automated non-adherence and service disengagement risk monitoring with active follow-up for severe mental illness. Aust N Z J Psychiatry 55(10):976–982. https://doi.org/10.1177/0004867421998800
54. Mudakavi I, Rentala S (2021) Relapse prevention in mental illnesses: concepts, issues and strategies with perspectives of psychiatric nursing—review article. Indian J Forensic Med Toxicol 15:134. https://doi.org/10.37506/ijfmt.v15i4.16674
55. Tlhowe TT, Plessis E, Koen MP (2017) Strengths of families to limit relapse in mentally ill family members. Health Sa Gesondheid 22:28–35. https://doi.org/10.4102/hsag.v22i0.1019
56. Muryani NMS, Putra IGY, Artawan IK (2022) Family experience dealing with relapse in people with men-

tal disorders. Babali Nurs Res 3(2):135–142. https://doi.org/10.37363/bnr.2022.32106
57. Mueser KT, Corrigan PW, Hilton DW, Tanzman B, Schaub A, Gingerich S, Essock SM, Tarrier N, Morey B, Vogel-Scibilia S, Herz MI (2002b) Illness management and recovery: a review of the research. Psychiatr Serv 53:1272
58. Mueser KT, Corrigan PW, Hilton D, Tanzman B, Schaub A, Gingerich S, Essock SM (2002a) Illness management and recovery: a review of the research. Psychiatric Serv 53(10):1272–1284
59. Agenagnew L, Kassaw C (2020) The lifetime prevalence and factors associated with relapse among mentally ill patients at Jimma University Medical Center, Ethiopia: cross sectional study. J Psychosoc Rehabil Ment Health 7(3):211–220. https://doi.org/10.1007/s40737-020-00176-7
60. Wang K, Link BG, Corrigan PW, Davidson L, Flanagan EH (2018) Perceived provider stigma as a predictor of mental health service users' internalized stigma and disempowerment. Psychiatry Res 259:526–531. https://doi.org/10.1016/j.psychres.2017.11.036
61. Daniel M, Kumar A (2018) Experiences of stigma among outpatients with psychotic illnesses in a tertiary hospital. Indian J Psychiatric Soc Work 9. https://doi.org/10.29120/ijpsw.2018.v9.i1.52
62. Agustina HS, Suryani S, Widianti E (2019) Nurses' life experiences as persons in charge of mental health programs in community health center. Jurnal Keperawatan Padjadjaran 2(7):200–210. https://doi.org/10.24198/jkp.v7i2.1113
63. Mak WWS, Chan RCH (2017) Perceived primal threat of mental illness and recovery: the mediating role of self-stigma and self-empowerment. Am J Orthopsychiatry 87(1):44–51. https://doi.org/10.1037/ort0000202
64. Resnick SG, Rosenheck RA, Lehman AF (2004) An exploratory analysis of correlates of recovery. Psychiatric Serv 55(5):540–547. https://doi.org/10.1176/appi.ps.55.5.540
65. Hamann J, Bühner M, Rüsch N (2017) Self-stigma and consumer participation in shared decision making in mental health services. Psychiatr Serv 68(8):783–788. https://doi.org/10.1176/appi.ps.201600282
66. Sullivan WP, Floyd DF (2013) Spirit lifting: hope and recovery in case management practice. Fam Soc 94(1):38–44. https://doi.org/10.1606/1044-3894.4262
67. Yang D, Tu C-C, Guo Z, Dai X, Tu CF (2023) Moderating mechanism in the relationship between social isolation and mental health among college students during high-risk period of covid-19 transmission in Hubei, China. Int J Ment Health Promot 25(2):193–206. https://doi.org/10.32604/ijmhp.2022.022130
68. Xiong R, Xia Y, Beihai T (2022) Social disconnectedness and mental health problems during the covid-19 pandemic in China: a moderated mediation model. Int J Public Health 67:1604742. https://doi.org/10.3389/ijph.2022.1604742
69. Cheng X, Cosco TD, Ariyo T (2021) Decreasing social isolation to enhance mental health among older adults in China: a mediation analysis of aging attitude. Front Psychol 12:735740. https://doi.org/10.3389/fpsyg.2021.735740
70. Pai NB (2022) The physical and mental health consequences of social isolation and loneliness in the context of COVID-19. Curr Opin Psychiatry 35:305. https://doi.org/10.1097/yco.0000000000000806
71. Stotland NL (2012) Recovery from depression. Psychiatr Clin North Am 35:37–49
72. Eaton WW, Shao H, Nestadt G, Lee HB, Bienvenu OJ, Zandi P (2008) Population-based study of first onset and chronicity in major depressive disorder. Arch Gen Psychiatry 65(5):513–520
73. Judd LL, Akiskal HS, Maser JD, Zeller PJ, Endicott J, Coryell W, Paulus MP, Kunovac JL, Leon AC, Mueller TI, Rice JA, Keller MB (1998a) A prospective 12-year study of subsyndromal and syndromal depressive symptoms in unipolar major depressive disorders. Arch Gen Psychiatry 55(8):694–700
74. Ten Have M, de Graaf R, van Dorsselaer S, Tuithof M, Kleinjan M, Penninx BWJH (2018) Recurrence and chronicity of major depressive disorder and their risk indicators in a population cohort. Acta Psychiatr Scand 137(6):503–515
75. Judd LL, Akiskal HS, Maser JD, Zeller PJ, Endicott J, Coryell W, Paulus MP, Kunovac JL, Leon AC, Mueller TI, Rice JA, Keller MB (1998b) Major depressive disorder: a prospective study of residual subthreshold depressive symptoms as predictor of rapid relapse. J Affect Disord 50(2–3):97–108
76. Nil R, Lütolf S, Seifritz E (2016) Residual symptoms and functionality in depressed outpatients: a one-year observational study in Switzerland with escitalopram. J Affect Disord 197:245
77. Verhoeven FEA, Wardenaar KJ, Ruhé HGE, Conradi HJ, Jonge P (2018) Seeing the signs: using the course of residual depressive symptomatology to predict patterns of relapse and recurrence of major depressive disorder. Depress Anxiety 35(2):148–159
78. Anthony WA (1993) Recovery from mental illness: the guiding vision of the mental health system in the 1990s. Innov Res 2:17–24
79. Frank E, Prien RF, Jarrett RB, Keller MB, Kupfer DJ, Lavori PW, Rush AJ, Weissman MM (1991) Conceptualization and rationale for consensus definitions of terms in major depressive disorder. Remission, recovery, relapse, and recurrence. Arch Gen Psychiatry 48(9):851–855
80. Habert J, Katzman MA, Oluboka OJ, McIntyre RS, McIntosh D, MacQueen GM, Khullar A, Milev RV, Kjernisted KD, Chokka PR, Kennedy SH (2016) Functional recovery in major depressive disorder: focus on early optimized treatment. Prim Care Companion CNS Disord 18(5)

81. Salzmann-Erikson M (2013) An integrative review of what contributes to personal recovery in psychiatric disabilities. Issues Ment Health Nurs 34:185–191
82. Solomon DA, Keller MB, Leon AC, Mueller TI, Lavori PW, Shea MT, Coryell W, Warshaw M, Turvey C, Maser JD, Endicott J (2000) Multiple recurrences of major depressive disorder. Am J Psychiatry 157(2):229–233
83. van Grieken RA, Kirkenier AC, Koeter MW, Nabitz UW, Schene AH (2015) Patients' perspective on self-management in the recovery from depression. Health Expect 18:1339–1348
84. Rush AJ, Trivedi MH, Wisniewski SR et al (2006) Acute and longer-term outcomes in depressed outpatients requiring one or several treatment steps: a STAR*D report. Am J Psychiatry 163(11):1905–1917
85. van Randenborgh A, Hüffmeier J, Victor D, Klocke K, Borlinghaus J, Pawelzik M (2012) Contrasting chronic with episodic depression: an analysis of distorted socio-emotional information processing in chronic depression. J Affect Disord 141:177–184
86. Keller MB (2004) Remission versus response: the new gold standard of antidepressant care. J Clin Psychiatry 4:53–59
87. Bakish D (2001) New standard of depression treatment: remission and full recovery. J Clin Psychiatry 26:5–9
88. Kelsey JE (2001) Clinician perspective on achieving and maintaining remission in depression. J Clin Psychiatry 26:16–21
89. Nierenberg AA, Wright EC (1999) Evolution of remission as the new standard in the treatment of depression. J Clin Psychiatry 22:7–11
90. Conradi HJ, Ormel J, Jonge P (2011) Presence of individual (residual) symptoms during depressive episodes and periods of remission: a 3-year prospective study. Psychol Med 41(6):1165–1174
91. Lee RS, Hermens DF, Porter MA, Redoblado-Hodge MA (2012) A meta-analysis of cognitive deficits in first-episode major depressive disorder. J Affect Disord 140:113
92. Saragoussi D, Touya M, Haro JM, Jönsson B, Knapp M, Botrel B, Florea I, Loft H, Rive B (2017) Factors associated with failure to achieve remission and with relapse after remission in patients with major depressive disorder in the PERFORM study. Neuropsychiatr Dis Treat 13:2151–2165
93. Bortolato B, Miskowiak KW, Köhler CA, Maes M, Fernandes BS, Berk M, Carvalho AF (2016) Cognitive remission: a novel objective for the treatment of major depression? BMC Med 14:9
94. McIntyre RS, Cha DS, Soczynska JK, Woldeyohannes HO, Gallaugher LA, Kudlow P (2013) Cognitive deficits and functional outcomes in major depressive disorder: determinants, substrates, and treatment interventions. Depress Anxiety 30:515–527
95. Trivedi MH, Greer TL (2014) Cognitive dysfunction in unipolar depression: implications for treatment. J Affect Disord 154:19–27. https://doi.org/10.1016/j.jad.2013.09.012
96. Fiorillo A, Carpiniello B, Giorgi S, Pia S, Maina G, Sampogna G, Spina E, Tortorella A, Vita A (2018) Assessment and management of cognitive and psychosocial dysfunctions in patients with major depressive disorder: a clinical review. Front Psychiatry 9:493
97. Lam RW, McIntosh D, Wang J, Enns MW, Kolivakis T, Michalak EE, Sareen J, Song WY, Kennedy SH, MacQueen GM, Milev RV, Parikh SV, Ravindran AV, Group, C.A.N.M.A.T.D.W (2016) Canadian Network for Mood and Anxiety Treatments (CANMAT) 2016 clinical guidelines for the management of adults with major depressive disorder: section 1. Disease burden and principles of care. Can J Psychiatry 61(9):510–523
98. Malhi GS, Bell E, Bassett D, Boyce P, Bryant R, Hazell P, Hopwood M, Lyndon B, Mulder R, Porter R, Singh AB, Murray G (2021) The 2020 Royal Australian and New Zealand College of Psychiatrists clinical practice guidelines for mood disorders. Aust N Z J Psychiatry 55(1):7–117
99. Cavelti M, Kvrgic S, Beck EM (2011) Assessing recovery from schizophrenia as an individual process. A review of self-report instruments. Eur Psychiatry 27:19–32
100. Andresen R, Oades L, Caputi P (2003) The experience of recovery from schizophrenia: towards an empirically-validated stage model. Aust N Z J Psychiatry 37:586–594
101. Leamy M, Bird V, Le Boutillier C, Williams J, Slade M (2011) Conceptual framework for personal recovery in mental health: systematic review and narrative synthesis. Br J Psychiatry 199:445–452
102. World Health Organization (2010) User empowerment in mental health—a statement by the WHO regional Office for Europe. World Health Organization, Washington, DC
103. System N.H. (2012) Liberating the NHS: no decision about me without me. Government response. Department of Health
104. Luciano M, Sampogna G, Del Vecchio V, Loos S, Slade M, Clarke E, Nagy M, Kovacs A, Munk-Jørgensen P, Krogsgaard Bording M, Kawohl W, Rössler W, Puschner B, Fiorillo A, C.E.D.A.R.S Group (2020) When does shared decision making is adopted in psychiatric clinical practice? Results from a European multicentric study. Eur Arch Psychiatry Clin Neurosci 270(6):645–653
105. Llewellyn-Beardsley J, Rennick-Egglestone S, Bradstreet S, Davidson L, Franklin D, Hui A, McGranahan R, Morgan K, Pollock K, Ramsay A, Smith R, Thornicroft G, Slade M (2020) Not the story you want? Assessing the fit of a conceptual framework characterising mental health recovery narratives. Soc Psychiatry Psychiatr Epidemiol 55:295–308. https://doi.org/10.1007/s00127-019-01791-x

106. Schrank B, Slade M (2007) Recovery in psychiatry. Psychiatr Bull 31:321–325
107. Morin L, Franck N (2017) Rehabilitation interventions to promote recovery from schizophrenia: a systematic review. Front Psychiatry 8:100
108. Happell B (2008) Who cares for whom? Re-examining the nurse-patient relationship. Int J Ment Health Nurs 17:381–382
109. Burgess P, Pirkis J, Coombs T, Rosen A (2011) Assessing the value of existing recovery measures for routine use in Australian mental health services. Aust N Z J Psychiatry 45:267–280
110. Leamy M, Clarke E, Le Boutillier C (2016) Recovery practice in community mental health teams: national survey. Br J Psychiatry 209:340–346
111. Dunn EC, Wewiorski NJ, Rogers ES (2008) The meaning and importance of employment to people in recovery from serious mental illness: results of a qualitative study. Psychiatr Rehabil J 32:59–62
112. Sells DJ, Stayner DA, Davidson L (2004) Recovering the self in schizophrenia: an integrative review of qualitative studies. Psychiatry Q 75:87–97
113. Whitley R, Drake RE (2010) Recovery: a dimensional approach. Psychiatr Serv 61(12):1248–1250
114. Richardson K, Barkham M (2017) Recovery from depression: a systematic review of perceptions and associated factors. J Ment Health 6:1–13
115. Van Eck RM, Burger TJ, Schenkelaars M, Vellinga A, de Koning MB, Schirmbeck F, Kikkert M, Dekker J, de Haan L (2018a) The impact of affective symptoms on personal recovery of patients with severe mental illness. Int J Soc Psychiatry 64:521–527
116. Van Eck RM, Burger TJ, Vellinga A, Schirmbeck F, de Haan L (2018b) The relationship between clinical and personal recovery in patients with schizophrenia spectrum disorders: a systematic review and meta-analysis. Schizophr Bull 44:631–642
117. Brugha TS, Bebbington PE, Sturt E et al (1990) The relation between life events and social support networks in a clinically depressed cohort. Soc Psychiatry Psychiatr Epidemiol 25:308–313
118. George LK, Blazer DG, Hughes DC, Fowler N (1989) Social support and the outcome of major depression. Br J Psychiatry 154:478–485
119. Gladstone GL, Parker GB, Malhi GS, Wilhelm KA (2007) Feeling unsupported? An investigation of depressed patients' perceptions. J Affect Disord 103:147–154
120. Bukh JD, Bock C, Vinberg M, Kessing LV (2013) The effect of prolonged duration of untreated depression on antidepressant treatment outcome. J Affect Disord 145(1):42–48
121. Okuda A, Suzuki T, Kishi T, Yamanouchi Y, Umeda K, Haitoh H, Hashimoto S, Ozaki N, Iwata N (2010) Duration of untreated illness and antidepressant fluvoxamine response in major depressive disorder. Psychiatry Clin Neurosci 64(3):268–273
122. Szegedi A, Jansen WT, Willigenburg AP, Meulen E, Stassen HH, Thase ME (2009) Early improvement in the first 2 weeks as a predictor of treatment outcome in patients with major depressive disorder: a meta-analysis including 6562 patients. J Clin Psychiatry 70(3):344–353
123. Villaggi B, Provencher H, Coulombe S, Meunier S, Radziszewski S, Hudon C, Roberge P, Provencher MD, Houle J (2015) Self-management strategies in recovery from mood and anxiety disorders. Glob Qual Nurs Res 2:2333393615606092
124. Battle CL, Uebelacker L, Friedman MA, Cardemil EV, Beevers CG, Miller IW (2010) Treatment goals of depressed outpatients: a qualitative investigation of goals identified by participants in a depression treatment trial. J Psychiatr Pract 16:425
125. Baune BT, Christensen MC (2019) Differences in perceptions of major depressive disorder symptoms and treatment priorities between patients and health care providers across the acute, post-acute, and remission phases of depression. Front Psychiatry 10:335
126. Zimmerman M (2012) Discordance between researchers and patients in defining remission from depression. J Clin Psychiatry 73(9):1262–1263
127. Demyttenaere K, Donneau AF, Albert A et al (2015) What is important in being cured from depression? Discordance between physicians and patients. J Affect Disord 174:390–396
128. Christensen MC, Wong CMJ, Baune BT (2020) Symptoms of major depressive disorder and their impact on psychosocial functioning in the different phases of the disease: do the perspectives of patients and healthcare providers differ? Front Psychiatry 11:280
129. Maj M, Stein DJ, Parker G, Zimmerman M, Fava GA, Hert M, Demyttenaere K, McIntyre RS, Widiger T, Wittchen HU (2020) The clinical characterization of the adult patient with depression aimed at personalization of management. World Psychiatry 19(3):269–293
130. Dell'Osso B, Albert U, Carrà G, Pompili M, Nanni MG, Pasquini M, Poloni N, Raballo A, Sambataro F, Serafini G, Viganò C, Demyttenaere K, McIntyre RS, Fiorillo A (2020) How to improve adherence to antidepressant treatments in patients with major depression: a psychoeducational consensus checklist. Ann General Psychiatry 19:61
131. Rush AJ (2015) Distinguishing functional from syndromal recovery: implications for clinical care and research. J Clin Psychiatry 76:e832–e834
132. Cuijpers P (2011) Prevention of depressive disorders: towards a further reduction of the disease burden of mental disorders. Early Interv Psychiatry 5:179–180
133. Salkovskis P, Rimes K, Stephenson D (2006) A randomized controlled trial of the use of self-help materials in addition to standard general practice treatment of depression compared to standard treatment alone. Psychol Med 36:325–333
134. Loos S, Clarke E, Jordan H et al (2017) Recovery and decision-making involvement in people with

severe mental illness from six countries: a prospective observational study. BMC Psychiatry 17:38
135. Slade M (2017) Implementing shared decision making in routine mental health care. World Psychiatry 16:146–153
136. Slade M, Amering M, Oades L (2008) Recovery: an international perspective. Epidemiol Psichiatr Soc 17:128–137
137. Whitley R, Shepherd G, Slade M (2019) Recovery colleges as a mental health innovation. World Psychiatry 18(2):141–142
138. Doughty C, Tse S, Duncan N, McIntyre L (2008) The wellness recovery action plan (WRAP): workshop evaluation. Australas Psychiatry 16(6):450–456
139. Slade M, Bird V, Le Boutillier C, Williams J, McCrone P, Leamy M (2011) REFOCUS trial: protocol for a cluster randomised controlled trial of a pro-recovery intervention within community based mental health teams. BMC Psychiatry 11:185

GPSR Compliance

The European Union's (EU) General Product Safety Regulation (GPSR) is a set of rules that requires consumer products to be safe and our obligations to ensure this.

If you have any concerns about our products, you can contact us on ProductSafety@springernature.com

In case Publisher is established outside the EU, the EU authorized representative is:

Springer Nature Customer Service Center GmbH
Europaplatz 3
69115 Heidelberg, Germany

Batch number: 10732801

Printed by Printforce, the Netherlands